Neuropsychiatry of Traumatic Brain Injury

Neuropsychiatry of Traumatic Brain Injury

Edited by
Jonathan M. Silver, M.D.,
Stuart C. Yudofsky, M.D., and
Robert E. Hales, M.D.

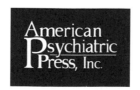

American Psychiatric Press, Inc.

Washington, DC
London, England

Copyright © 1994 American Psychiatric Press, Inc.
ALL RIGHTS RESERVED
Manufactured in the United States of America on acid-free paper
97 96 95 94   4 3 2 1
First Edition

American Psychiatric Press, Inc.
1400 K Street, N.W., Washington, DC   20005

Library of Congress Cataloging-in-Publication Data
Neuropsychiatry of traumatic brain injury / edited by Jonathan M.
   Silver, Stuart C. Yudofsky, and Robert E. Hales. — 1st ed.
      p. cm.
   Includes bibliographical references and index.
   ISBN 0-88048-538-8 (alk. paper)
   1. Brain damage. 2. Neuropsychiatry.   I. Silver, Jonathan M.
1953– . II. Yudofsky, Stuart C. III. Hales, Robert E.
   [DNLM: 1. Brain Injuries—diagnosis. 2. Brain Injuries—therapy.
WL 354 N494425 1994]
RC387.5.N477 1994
616.8—dc20
DNLM/DLC
for Library of Congress   93-11646
                                                                    CIP

British Library Cataloguing in Publication Data
A CIP record is available from the British Library.

Dedication

To our children,
Elliot, Benjamin, and Leah;
Elissa, Lynn, and Emily;
and Julia, with love.

To children with traumatic brain injury,
with love and hope.

To the parents of children with traumatic brain injury,
with love, hope, and admiration.

Contents

Section I
Assessment of Traumatic Brain Injury

Section II
Psychiatric Symptomatologies Associated
With Traumatic Brain Injury

Section III
Special Populations

Section IV
Treatment of Traumatic Brain Injury

Contributors

Gregory W. Albers, M.D.
Stanford University Medical Center
Palo Alto Veterans Affairs Medical Center
Palo Alto, California
Assistant Professor of Neurology and Neurological Sciences and
  Director Stanford Stroke Center
Stanford, California

Boris Birmaher, M.D.
Associate Professor of Psychiatry
Department of Psychiatry
University of Pittsburgh School of Medicine
Western Psychiatric Institute and Clinic
Pittsburgh, Pennsylvania

Maritza Cabrera, M.A., C.R.C.
Injury Prevention Liaison
Southwest Regional Brain Injury Rehabilitation and Prevention
  Center
Institute for Rehabilitation and Research
Houston, Texas

John W. Cassidy, M.D.
HCA Medical Center Hospital
Del Oro Institute for Rehabilitation
Clinical Assistant Professor of Restorative Neurology and Human
  Neurobiology
Baylor College of Medicine
Houston, Texas

Marie M. Cavallo, M.A.
Department of Rehabilitation Medicine
New York University Medical Center
New York, New York

Patrick W. Corrigan, Psy.D.
Director and Assistant Professor of Clinical Psychiatry
University of Chicago Center for Psychiatric Rehabilitation
Tinley Park, Illinois

James Duffy, M.D.
Associate Clinical Director
Allegheny Neuropsychiatric Institute
Oakdale, Pennsylvania

Richard S. Epstein, M.D.
Clinical Associate Professor
Department of Psychiatry
F. Edward Hebert School of Medicine
Uniformed Services University of the Health Sciences
Bethesda, Maryland

Barry S. Fogel, M.D.
Associate Director
Center for Gerontology and Health Care Research
Professor of Psychiatry and Human Behavior
Brown University
Providence, Rhode Island

Michael D. Franzen, Ph.D.
West Virginia University
Chestnut Ridge Hospital
Associate Professor of Behavioral Medicine and Psychiatry
West Virginia University
Morgantown, West Virginia

Robert E. Hales, M.D.
Chief, Department of Psychiatry
California Pacific Medical Center
Clinical Professor of Psychiatry
University of California, San Francisco
San Francisco, California

Lawrence S. Honig, M.D., Ph.D.
Clinical Assistant Professor of Neurology and
   Neurological Sciences
Stanford University Medical Center
Stanford, California

Marjory Jakus, B.A.
Research Associate
University of Chicago Center for Psychiatric Rehabilitation
Tinley Park, Illinois

Ricardo Jorge, M.D.
Fellow, University of Iowa College of Medicine
Iowa City, Iowa

Thomas Kay, Ph.D.
Assistant Professor of Clinical Rehabilitation Medicine
Department of Rehabilitation Medicine
New York University Medical Center
New York, New York

Jess F. Kraus, MPH, Ph.D.
Professor of Epidemiology, School of Public Health
University of California, Los Angeles
Los Angeles, California

Mark R. Lovell, Ph.D.
Medical College of Pennsylvania–Allegheny Campus
Allegheny General Hospital
Assistant Professor of Psychiatry (Psychology)
Medical College of Pennsylvania
Pittsburgh, Pennsylvania

Thomas W. McAllister, M.D.
Associate Professor of Psychiatry
Dartmouth Medical School
Director, Section of Neuropsychiatry
New Hampshire Hospital and Dartmouth-Hitchcock Medical
 Center
Hanover, New Hampshire

Norman S. Miller, M.D.
Associate Professor of Psychiatry and Neurology
Department of Psychiatry
University of Illinois at Chicago
Chicago, Illinois

Shannon C. Miller, M.D.
Wright-Patterson Medical Center/Wright State University
Psychiatry Residency Training Program
Dayton, Ohio

Henry A. Nasrallah, M.D.
Professor and Chairman
Department of Psychiatry
Ohio State University Medical Center
Columbus, Ohio

Vernon M. Neppe, M.D., Ph.D.
Director, Pacific Neuropsychiatric Institute
Seattle, Washington

Alison Moon O'Shanick, M.S., C.C.C.-S.L.P.
Center for Neurorehabilitation Services
Richmond, Virginia

Gregory J. O'Shanick, M.D.
Center for Neurorehabilitation Services
Richmond, Virginia

Irwin W. Pollack, M.D.
Professor of Psychiatry and Neurology
Robert Wood Johnson Medical Center
University Medicine and Dentistry of New Jersey
New Brunswick, New Jersey

Trevor R. P. Price, M.D.
Chairman, Department of Psychiatry
Professor and Chairman of Psychiatry
Allegheny Campus
Medical College of Pennsylvania
Pittsburgh, Pennsylvania

Jack Rattok, Ph.D.
Transitions of Long Island
Long Island Jewish Medical Center
Manhasset, New York

Robert G. Robinson, M.D.
Professor and Chairman
University of Iowa Hospital and Clinics
University of Iowa College of Medicine
Iowa City, Iowa

Barbara Ross, Ph.D.
Psychserve Co.
New York, New York

Jonathan M. Silver, M.D.
Associate Professor of Clinical Psychiatry
Columbia University–College of Physicians and Surgeons
Director of Neuropsychiatry
Columbia-Presbyterian Medical Center
New York, New York

Robert I. Simon, M.D.
Clinical Professor of Psychiatry
Director, Program in Psychiatry and Law
Georgetown University School of Medicine
Washington, D.C.

Donald J. Smeltzer, M.A.
Associate Professor of Psychiatry
Associate Director of Training and Education
Department of Psychiatry
Ohio State University
Columbus, Ohio

Susan B. Sorenson, Ph.D.
Assistant Research Epidemiologist, School of Public Health
University of California, Los Angeles
Los Angeles, California

Craig A. Taylor, M.D.
Assistant Professor of Psychiatry and Neurological Surgery
University of Pittsburgh School of Medicine
Medical Director, Brain Injury Program
Western Psychiatric Institute and Clinic
Pittsburgh, Pennsylvania

Paula T. Trzepacz, M.D.
Associate Professor of Psychiatry
University of Pittsburgh School of Medicine
Western Psychiatric Institute and Clinic
Pittsburgh, Pennsylvania

Gary J. Tucker, M.D.
Professor and Chairman
Department of Psychiatry and Behavioral Sciences
University of Washington
Seattle, Washington

Robert J. Ursano, M.D.
Professor and Chairman
Department of Psychiatry
F. Edward Hebert School of Medicine
Uniformed Services University of the Health Sciences
Bethesda, Maryland

Daniel T. Williams, M.D.
Associate Clinical Professor of Psychiatry
Columbia University–College of Physicians and Surgeons
Columbia Presbyterian Medical Center
New York, New York

Stuart A. Yablon, M.D.
Assistant Professor
Department of Physical Medicine and Rehabilitation
University of Texas Medical School at Houston
Baylor College of Medicine
Co-Director, Brain Injury Program
The Institute for Rehabilitation and Research
Houston, Texas

Stuart C. Yudofsky, M.D.
Professor and Chairman
Department of Psychiatry and Behavioral Sciences
Baylor College of Medicine
Houston, Texas

Nathan D. Zasler, M.D.
Executive Medical Director, National NeuroRehabilitation
    Consortium
Director, Concussion Care Center of Virginia
Co-Director, Richmond Rehabilitation Physicians
Richmond, Virginia

Foreword

For too long, the role and importance of neuropsychiatry in the treatment of persons with traumatic brain injury have been ignored. Little attention has been paid to the need for a neuropsychiatric assessment or for involvement of a psychiatrist in developing plans from the perspectives of professional assessment and treatment of people with brain injury. It has been as if the person who sustains a traumatic brain injury only requires physical and cognitive care for rehabilitation.

At the National Head Injury Foundation, the most frequent request for information and assistance from the "800 Helpline" involves problems of personality, mood, and behavior. People with traumatic brain injury and their families know only too well that the subsequent changes in personality, intelligence, mood, anxiety, and impulsivity that so frequently occur are by far the most disabling aspects of the illness.

No publication currently available will have the impact on the well-being of persons who have sustained a traumatic brain injury as will *Neuropsychiatry of Traumatic Brain Injury*. This book firmly establishes the importance of neuropsychiatry in the care, treatment, and rehabilitation of patients with traumatic brain injury. It is a rich resource and is must reading for family members, rehabilitation professionals, providers of rehabilitation services, case managers, educators, vocational rehabilitation counselors, and those concerned with public policy and service for persons with traumatic brain injury.

At the National Head Injury Foundation, *Neuropsychiatry of Traumatic Brain Injury* will help us recruit and utilize psychiatrists as a resource in the treatment of traumatic brain injury and will help us meet our mission: to enhance the quality of life for persons with traumatic brain injury and their families. This is a comprehensive resource that in one place addresses the whole person, including personality, emotions, moods, and behavior.

I want to thank the editors and contributing authors for assembling this most comprehensive book, which firmly establishes the importance of neuropsychiatry in the treatment of persons with traumatic brain injury. Thousands and thousands of persons with traumatic brain injury and their families will be the beneficiaries of this book.

George A. Zitnay, Ph.D.
President and Chief Executive Officer
National Head Injury Foundation
Washington, DC

Preface

Each year in the United States, more than three million people sustain a traumatic brain injury (TBI). In this population, the psychosocial and psychological deficits are the major source of disability to the patient and of stress to the family. Patients may have difficulties in many vital areas of functioning, including family, interpersonal, work, school, and recreational activities. Many have extreme personality changes. Unfortunately, the psychiatric impairments caused by TBI often are unrecognized because of the deficiency of appropriate education in this area for psychiatrists and other mental health professionals. Most clinicians lack experience in the treatment and evaluation of patients with TBI and are, therefore, unaware of the many subtle, but disabling, symptoms. Unfortunately, there has been no single source that provides assessment and treatment of psychiatric symptoms and syndromes associated with TBI and provides guidelines based on current scientific knowledge. Neuropsychiatry of Traumatic Brain Injury has been written to fill this void.

This book was conceived to be a comprehensive data-based text that serves as a clinically relevant and practical guide to the neuropsychiatric assessment and treatment of patients with TBI. We have endeavored to assemble authors who are authoritative and renowned in their areas. We hope that this book will be used by psychiatrists, neuropsychologists, clinical psychologists, physiatrists, neurologists, and other professionals, including residents and trainees, involved in brain injury rehabilitation.

The book is divided into four sections: Assessment, Psychiatric Symptomatologies, Special Populations, and Treatment. The first section, Assessment of Traumatic Brain Injury, is a review of the epidemiology, neuropathology, neuropsychiatric, and neuropsychological assessment of patients with TBI. The second section, Psychiatric Symptomatologies, reviews the specific neuropsychiatric problems that patients develop after TBI: personality and intellectual changes, delirium, mood disorders, psychotic disorders, anxiety disorders, and aggression. The third section, Special Populations, covers areas of minor brain injury, TBI in children and adolescents, TBI in elderly patients, sexual disorders, alcohol and drug disorders, seizures, family issues, and legal and ethical issues. The final section, Treatment of Traumatic Brain Injury, is designed to be practical in its clinical application and includes chapters on pharmacology, individual psychotherapy, cognitive rehabilitation, behavioral treatment, neuropharmacological treatment for acute brain injury, and prevention.

Section I begins with a review of the epidemiology of TBI by Kraus and Sorenson from the University of California, Los Angeles, School of Public Health. This is followed by comprehensive discussions of the neuroanatomic consequences of TBI by Cassidy. Taylor and Price's chapter on the neuropsychiatric assessment and Lovell and Franzen's chapter on neuropsychological testing have been written to provide clear clinical guidelines for a comprehensive evaluation of the patient who has sustained TBI.

Section II begins with a review by O'Shanick and O'Shanick of the personality and intellectual changes that occur after TBI. Trzepacz discusses the phenomenology and pathophysiology of posttraumatic delirium, which overlaps with the concept of posttraumatic amnesia. Robinson and Jorge, who have conducted careful research on affective disorders after brain injury, discuss the implications of their work on the treatment of mood disorders in this population. Smeltzer, Nasrallah, and Miller have written, to the best of our knowledge, the most current and comprehensive review assembled of the occurrence of psychosis after TBI. Similarly, Epstein and Ursano provide a unique overview of the presence of anxiety—including posttraumatic stress disorder—after TBI. Finally, Silver and Yudofsky discuss the phenomenology and treatment of aggression that frequently occurs with TBI.

McAllister's chapter on minor brain injury and the postconcussive syndrome initiates Section III. The problems of TBI are different when they occur in children and adolescents or in the elderly; Birmaher and Williams and Fogel and Duffy have written excellent chapters in these respective areas. Zasler, who has written extensively in the area of sexual dysfunction that occurs after TBI, has contributed a review of this area. Many victims of TBI have either a current or past history of alcohol or drug disorders; Miller discusses the implications of these disorders in TBI and how treatment must be tailored to meet the needs of these patients. Tucker and Neppe provide an excellent overview of the effect of posttraumatic seizures in TBI. TBI has significant impact in the family members of the injured person, and Kay and Cavallo discuss methods for family assessments and effective interventions. Finally, the section ends with Simon's unique and highly focussed contribution on ethical and legal issues related to patients with TBI.

Section IV presents specific treatment modalities and provides specific guidelines for the use of these interventions. Silver and Yudofsky write a detailed review of the scientific literature on the pharmacotherapy of psychiatric symptoms and provide specific guidelines for the use of psychoactive drugs. The application of individual psychotherapies is richly described in the chapter by Pollack. Cognitive rehabilitation is reviewed by Rattok and Ross, so that the reader gains an understanding of when this modality can and cannot be effectively applied. Behavioral treatments can be particularly useful in the treatment of inappropriate behaviors that may occur after TBI; Corrigan and Jakus have written a practical guide to the understanding and application of behavioral interventions. There have been exciting new research developments in the application of neuropharmacological interventions that can be used for acute brain injury to prevent secondary neuronal damage; Honig and Albers have written a scholarly overview of this area. Lastly, we recognize that the most effect intervention is in the prevention of TBI. Yablon, Cabrera, Yudofsky, and Silver conclude the volume with an overview of preventative measures that clinicians may and should utilize in their practices.

We have learned from readers' comments in our other books, such as *The American Psychiatric Press Textbook of Neuropsychiatry,* that very few people read a textbook from cover to cover. Most read only one or several chapters during any particular period. Consequently, we strived to ensure that each chapter would be complete in itself. As a result there is some unavoidable overlap among chapters, but we have judged that this was necessary from an information-retrieving standpoint and to prevent readers from having to "jump" from section to section, while reading about a particular subject. For example, the Glasgow Coma Scale is found in both Chapter 1 and Chapter 3. The table for treatment of psychosis developed by Smeltzer, Nasrallah, and Miller in Chapter 8 has been reprinted in the chapter on psychopharmacology by Silver and Yudofsky (Chapter 19). Further, although each chapter on symptomatology provides treatment guidelines, the chapters within the section on Treatment of Traumatic Brain Injury comprehensively discuss the application of treatment for these problems.

This book would not have been possible without the help and support of many people. First we thank the many chapter authors who labored diligently to produce contributions that we consider unique, scholarly, and enjoyable to read. We spent countless hours on the telephone with the authors reviewing their chapters and providing suggestions, usually agreed on, but occasionally disputed. Their continued willingness to answer our calls and letters was greatly appreciated.

We appreciate the efforts of Paul Berger-Gross, Eric Redlener, and Gerald Hurowitz, of the Neuropsychiatry Service at Allen Pavilion of Columbia-Presbyterian Medical Center, who provided thoughtful and practical comments on many chapters. Ron McMillen and his staff at the American Psychiatric Press, Inc., were extremely helpful and responsive, especially Pamela Harley, the Managing Editor; Edward Winkleman, the Project Editor; and Claire Reinburg, the Editorial Director for this book. Frances Rivera, at Allen Pavilion, patiently coordinated communications among editors and chapter authors. Lastly, and most importantly, we thank our patients with TBI and their families, who have been our greatest source of inspiration to further our knowledge on presentation, assessment, and effective treatment of the psychiatric symptoms and syndromes associated with TBI. We hope that the efforts of all of us who have participated in this book will result in reducing your suffering and enhancing your recovery.

Jonathan M. Silver, M.D.
Stuart C. Yudofsky, M.D.
Robert E. Hales, M.D.

Assessment of Traumatic Brain Injury

Chapter 1

Epidemiology

Jess F. Kraus, M.P.H., Ph.D.
Susan B. Sorenson, Ph.D.

In this chapter we synthesize the basic epidemiological literature of the last 10–15 years and examine four fundamental characteristics of brain injuries: 1) the occurrence or incidence of new cases of medically attended brain injury in the population, 2) the characteristics of high-risk groups and high-risk exposures, 3) the types and severity of brain injuries, and 4) the consequences or results of brain injury at hospital discharge or posthospital follow-up. The literature on brain injury expands annually but most of the published information is specific to hospitalized patients. Although the clinical literature has inherent value for the practitioner, the epidemiological literature provides a broader and more accurate assessment of the occurrence, characteristics, and consequences of brain injury in the population. Unfortunately, the epidemiological literature on brain injury is restricted to a handful of studies conducted primarily in the

We acknowledge the background work and data preparation by Craig Anderson, Linda Lange, David McArthur, Soumitra Sarkar, and Haikang Shen. New information in this chapter comes from the San Diego County cohort study of brain injury of the early 1980s. Special thanks to Hal Morgenstern for assisting in the estimation of brain injury disabilities in the United States. Work on this chapter was supported by the Southern California Injury Prevention Research Center (Centers for Disease Control, Grant R49/CCR903622).

late 1970s and early 1980s in the United States (Annegers et al. 1980; Cooper et al. 1983; Jagger et al. 1984; Kalsbeek et al. 1980; Klauber et al. 1981; Kraus et al. 1984; Whitman et al. 1984). Two other reports (Fife et al. 1986; MacKenzie et al. 1989), although population based, relied exclusively on computerized hospital discharge information. The findings of these two later studies have value, but the reader should be cautioned that the databases were generated for reasons other than to evaluate brain injury incidence and, therefore, have inherent limitations.

In assessing the literature, including studies cited in this chapter, the reader should be mindful that there are many differences among the research papers, making direct comparisons of their results problematic. Studies differ on a number of methodological parameters, such as how brain injury is defined, methods of case ascertainment, and how the medical information is collected and categorized. A major definition difficulty in many studies is that brain injuries often are subsumed under the term *head injury*. Although it is clear that many of the authors intended to study only neurological trauma, some case definitions (e.g., Annegers et al. 1980, Whitman et al. 1984) allow the inclusion of nonneurological head injuries such as fractures of the skull or face or damage to soft tissues of the head or face.

Case definitions and inclusion criteria vary from one study to another (see Table 1–1). In some studies (e.g., Auer et al. 1980; Bruce et al. 1979; Rimel 1981), the research populations are comprised of patients who were referred to neurosurgical intensive care units. In other studies (e.g., Gronwall and Wrightson 1974; Plaut and Gifford 1976), patients treated in emergency departments and released for outpatient observation have been included in the study base. And in still other studies (e.g., Jennett et al. 1979), patients with immediate death or death on arrival at the emergency department were excluded. Therefore, it is important to evaluate case definition and information collection across studies before comparing their results.

Various methods have been used over the past decade to measure the amount of brain damage (Table 1–1), including a newer proposal to classify severe brain injury using computed tomogra-

Table 1–1. Case identification and brain injury severity criteria and scoring: selected United States incidence studies

Study	Location and years	Case definition	Severity criteria/scoring
Annegers et al. 1980	Olmsted County, MN, 1965–1974	Head injury with evidence of presumed brain involvement (i.e., concussion with LOC, PTA, or neurological signs of brain injury or skull fracture)	1) Fatal (< 28 days) 2) Severe: intracranial hematoma, contusion, or LOC > 24 hours, or PTA > 24 hours 3) Moderate: LOC or PTA 30 minutes to 24 hours, skull fracture, or both 4) LOC or PTA < 30 minutes without skull fracture
Klauber et al. 1981	San Diego County, CA, 1978	ICD A-8 Codes 800, 801, 804, 806, and 850–854 with hospital admission diagnosis or cause of death with skull fracture, LOC, PTA, neurological deficit or seizure (no gunshot wounds)	GCS (3, 4–5, 6–7, 8–15)
Rimel 1981	Central Virginia 1977–1979	CNS referral patients with significant head injury admitted to neurosurgical service	GCS (3–5, 6–8, 9–11, 12–15) severe = ≤ 8; moderate = 9–11; mild = 12–15
Kraus et al. 1984	San Diego County, CA, 1981	Physician-diagnosed physical damage from acute mechanical energy exchange resulting in concussion, hemorrhage, contusion, or laceration of brain	Modified GCS (severe = ≤ 8; moderate = 9–15 plus hospital stay of 4–8 hours and brain surgery, or abnormal CT, or GCS 9–12; mild = all others, GCS 13–15)

Table 1–1. Case identification and brain injury severity criteria and scoring: selected United States incidence studies (*continued*)

Study	Location and years	Case definition	Severity criteria/scoring
Whitman et al. 1984	Chicago area 1979–1980	Any hospital discharge diagnosis of ICD-9-CN 800–804, 830, 850–854, 873, 920, 959.0. Injury within 7 days prior to hospital visit and blow to head/face with LOC, or laceration of scalp or forehead	1) Fatal 2) Severe = intracranial hematoma, LOC/PTA > 24 hours contusion, 3) Moderate = LOC or PTA 30 minutes to ≤ 24 hours 4) Mild = LOC to PTA < 30 minutes 5) Trivial = remainder
MacKenzie et al. 1989	Maryland 1986	ICD-9-CM codes 800, 801, 803, 804, 850–854	ICDMAP—converts ICD codes to Abbreviated Injury Severity Scores (Association for the Advancement of Automotive Medicine [1990]) of 1–6

Note. LOC = loss of consciousness; PTA = posttraumatic amnesia; GCS = Glasgow Coma Scale (Jennett and Teasdale 1981); ICD = International Classification of Diseases; ICD-9-CM = International Classification of Diseases, 9th Revision, Clinical Modification (Commission on Professional and Hospital Activities 1986); CNS = central nervous system; CT = computed tomography.

phy (Marshall et al. 1991). The Glasgow Coma Scale (GCS; Jennett and Teasdale 1981) is now commonly used for the initial assessment of severity. The GCS, a clinical prognostic indicator, is an important contribution to standardizing early assessment of the severity of brain injury (Table 1–2). Although its application was intended to be repeated, typical current practice generally consists of a single observation. Herein lies one of the major difficulties in the application of the GCS: not knowing in various studies when the GCS was administered during emergency treatment. In some studies, this was done at the scene of the injury or during emergency transport, whereas in others it was done on arrival at the emergency department or just before hospital admission; in still others, the time of assessment was not reported.

Obviously, GCS results during the hospital course will change according to patient improvement or deterioration. For proper comparison of research findings, the GCS should be measured at about the same time postinjury. Assessment on arrival at the emergency room is recommended.

Table 1–2.   Glasgow Coma Scale

Eye opening (E)	Spontaneous	4
	To speech	3
	To pain	2
	Nil	1
Best motor response (M)	Obeys	6
	Localizes	5
	Withdrawn	4
	Abnormal flexion	3
	Extensor response	2
	Nil	1
Verbal response (V)	Orientated	5
	Confused conversation	4
	Inappropriate words	3
	Incomprehensive sounds	2
	Nil	1
Coma score (E + M + V) = 3 to 15		

Source. Adapted from Jennett and Teasdale 1981.

An inherent weakness of the GCS is its limited relevance to some patients with brain injuries. The GCS is difficult or impossible to apply to very young children, patients with significant facial swelling from blunt trauma, patients under the influence of alcohol or other substances, and patients who are not able to respond to the verbal component because of language differences or an inability to comprehend. The current emergency department practice of immediate intubation or sedation may further invalidate (or restrict) GCS measurements. Regardless of these restrictions, the GCS remains one of the most consistently utilized measures of brain injury severity.

Epidemiological studies of patients with brain injuries are infrequently undertaken, and, as noted, research is difficult to assess because of differences in the types of patients included in follow-up. In addition, tests that can accurately assess cognitive, psychosocial, or physical outcomes have been inconsistently applied, making outcome assessments difficult to interpret.

In discussing the nature and severity of injury, we have drawn information from a large brain injury cohort study conducted in San Diego County, California, during the early 1980s (Kraus et al. 1984). For the purposes of this chapter, we focus on the specifics of diagnosis, considering skull fracture status as an important confounding factor. In addition, we provide basic information on the relationship between demographic characteristics such as age, sex, and socioeconomic status and the severity and type of brain injury. Finally, we develop a predictive model for outcome at hospital discharge.

All epidemiological studies on people hospitalized with brain injury indicate that a large majority of patients treated in emergency departments and admitted to hospitals (for observation or treatment) have sustained what has been termed *mild* brain injury, that is, one with a GCS score of 13–15. Because the magnitude of the occurrence of this injury is so extensive and the information on the injuries and outcomes is so incomplete, a special section addressing the nature of the available data and selected aggregate findings on outcome parameters has been included toward the end of this chapter.

Estimates of Occurrence of Brain Injury

Incidence

Data summarized in Figure 1–1 show that brain injury occurrence rates range from a low of 132 per 100,000 population in Maryland (MacKenzie et al. 1989) to a high of 367 per 100,000 population in the Chicago area (Whitman et al. 1984). Caution must be taken in interpreting these findings because brain injury definitions and criteria for diagnoses were not the same in all studies (see Table 1–1).

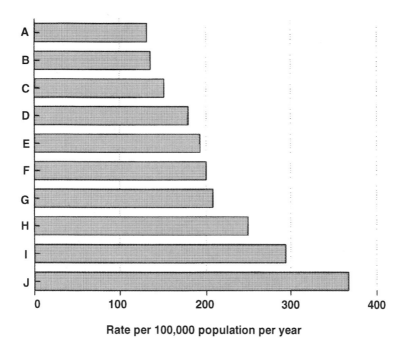

Rate per 100,000 population per year

Figure 1–1. Brain injury rates: selected United States studies. *A* = Maryland 1986 (MacKenzie et al. 1989); *B* = United States estimate 1981 (Fife 1987); *C* = Rhode Island 1979–1980 (Fife et al. 1986); *D* = San Diego County, CA, 1981 (Kraus et al. 1986); *E* = Olmsted County, MN, 1965–1974 (Annegers et al. 1980); *F* = United States estimate 1974 (Kalsbeek et al. 1980); *G* = Virgina 1978 (Jagger et al. 1984); *H* = Bronx, NY, 1980–1981 (Cooper et al. 1983); *I* = San Diego County, CA, 1978 (Klauber et al. 1981); *J* = Chicago area 1979–1980 (Whitman et al. 1984).

In addition, the precision of population-at-risk estimates varied considerably (i.e., some rates were based on "catchment area" population estimates in noncensus years).

Nevertheless, an average rate of fatal plus nonfatal hospitalized brain injury reported in all United States studies is about 237 per 100,000 population per year. If the highest and lowest estimates are excluded from consideration, the estimated rate is about 220 per 100,000 per year. A conservative estimate used in this chapter for purposes of disability estimation is 200 per 100,000 per year.

Brain Injury Death and Death Rates

In 1991, almost 148,500 people died from acute traumatic injury—about 8% of all deaths in the United States (Centers for Disease Control 1993). The exact percentage involving significant brain injury is unknown, but data from Olmsted County, Minnesota, (Annegers et al. 1980) and San Diego County, California, (Kraus et al. 1984) suggest that about 50% are caused by trauma to the brain. National Center for Health Statistics multiple-cause-of-death data indicate that about 28% of all injury deaths involve significant brain trauma (as cited in Sosin et al. 1989). This percentage is probably incorrect because, as the investigators pointed out, the case-finding process relied on a limited set of specific injury diagnoses. Furthermore, the actual death certificate was not examined—a crucial problem when "massive multiple trauma" is recorded on the death certificate but specific body locations and types of trauma are not recorded. Sosin et al. (1989) reported a possible underestimate in the actual proportion of fatal brain injury of 23% to 44%.

The reported brain injury fatality rate varies from 14 to 30 per 100,000 population per year. The range in rates probably reflects a lack of specificity of diagnosis on some death certificates (Figure 1–2).

Nonfatal Brain Injury

The only national estimate of nonfatal brain injury for the United States was derived from the National Health Interview Survey (NHIS) for 1985–1987 (Collins 1990) and is extrapolated to the 1990

U.S. Census estimated population of about 249,000,000 residents. The NHIS reported that about 1,975,000 head injuries occur per year (Collins 1990). Unfortunately, this estimate includes self-reported concussions and skull fractures, as well as a mixture of different types of intracranial injuries requiring professional medical care, some with and some without neurological trauma. The extent of emergency room and non-emergency-room diagnosis and treatment of brain injury is unknown.

On a reexamination of the NHIS data base, Fife (1987) concluded that only 16% of all head injuries resulted in an admission to a hospital. Hence, only one of six people with head (not necessarily

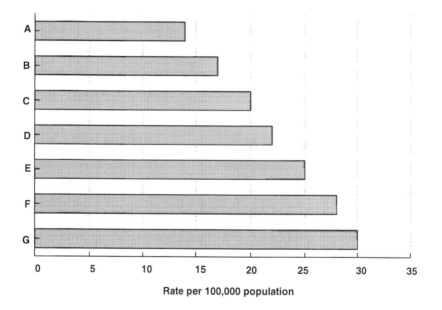

Figure 1–2. Brain injury fatality rates: selected United States studies. *A* = Virginia 1978 (Jagger et al. 1984); *B* = United States 1974 (Fife 1987); *C* = Olmsted County, MN, 1965–1974 (Annegers et al. 1980); *D* = San Diego County, CA, 1978 (Klauber et al. 1981); *E* = Chicago area 1979–1980 (Whitman et al. 1984); *F* = Bronx, NY, 1980–1981 (Cooper et al. 1983); *G* = San Diego County, CA, 1981 (Kraus et al. 1984).

brain) injury require hospitalization Because the number of individuals who seek medical care from non-emergency-room facilities is unknown, the figure of 1.95 million injuries from the NHIS remains an uncertain estimate of the true incidence in the population.

An estimate derived from published sources (summarized in Figure 1–3 and Table 1–3) suggests that about 373,000 people are discharged from a hospital each year in the United States with a brain injury diagnosis; using 1990 census data, that equals a hospital admission rate of about 150 per 100,000 population per year. The hospital discharge rate is useful for estimating the annual disability rate from injury (discussed below). The difference in estimates, using average incidence values in aggregate United States studies versus data from hospital discharges or visits, is due to definitional variation. The actual United States incidence rate is presumed, therefore, to range from 180 to 220 per 100,000 population per year.

The relative importance of brain injury discharge frequencies is illustrated in Table 1–3. As seen, the brain injury discharge rate is

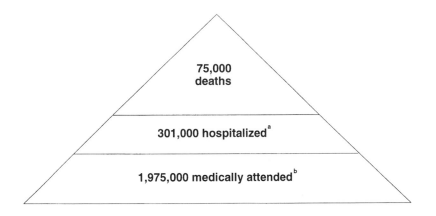

Figure 1–3. Estimated annual brain injury frequency (1990).
[a] *Source.* National Center for Health Statistics National Hospital Discharge Survey, 1990 (Graves 1992).
[b] *Source.* National Center for Health Statistics National Hospital Discharge Survey, 1988 (Collins 1990) extrapolated to 1990. This estimate includes both emergency department and other sources of emergency medical care.

higher than that for any other major central nervous system (CNS) diseases. The hospital discharge count (or rate) shown in Figure 1–3 and Table 1–3 is not the true figure because not all cases are found within the International Classification of Diseases (ICD) discharge diagnoses used to identify brain injury cases. The value of information on brain injury occurrence rates is threefold: to monitor changes in incidence in the population, to evaluate the effect of specific countermeasures, and to identify high- (or low-) risk groups or exposure circumstances.

Table 1–3. Frequency of selected first-listed diagnoses for inpatients discharged from short-stay, non-federal hospitals

ICD-9-CM code[a]	Diagnosis	Number discharges (× 1,000)	Discharge rate (per 100,000 population)
Multiple[b]	Brain injury	373	149.6
191	Malignant neoplasm of brain	30	12.1
295	Schizophrenic disorders	212	85.2
331	Cerebral degeneration (nonchildhood)	20	8.0
331.0	Alzheimer's disease	7	2.8
332	Parkinson's disease	14	5.6
340	Multiple sclerosis	32	12.9
345	Epilepsy	92	37.0
346	Migraine	50	20.1
430	Subarachnoid hemorrhage	20	8.0
431, 432	Intracerebral and intracranial hemorrhage	74	29.8
434	Occlusion of cerebral arteries	240	96.5
436, 437	Other cerebrovascular disease	208	83.6

Note. "Brain injuries" include *any* listed diagnoses.
[a]International Classification of Diseases, 9th Revision, Clinical Modification (ICD-9-CM; Commission on Professional and Hospital Activities 1986)
[b]Includes ICD-9-CM codes 800, 801, 803, 804, 850, 851, 852, 853, 854, 905, 907. These codes may not include all admissions with brain injuries but include diagnoses such as skull fracture with and without concussion, contusion, or hemorrhage and late effects of skull fracture or intracranial injury.
Source. National Hospital Discharge Survey, U.S. 1990 (Graves 1992).

Characteristics of High-Risk Groups

Age

All studies of brain injury occurrence in the United States show that people 15 to 24 years old are at the highest risk. Patterns in age-specific rates (Figure 1–4) illustrate this high-risk age period and demonstrate a decline in rates in the middle-age years and an increase in rates after about age 60. It is noteworthy that rates for people under age 10 (and particularly those under age 5) are high across all studies reporting age-specific data. Injury rates quickly increase, reaching a peak after age 15 and then declining after age 24. The age-related risk distribution reflects differences in exposure, particularly to motor vehicle crashes.

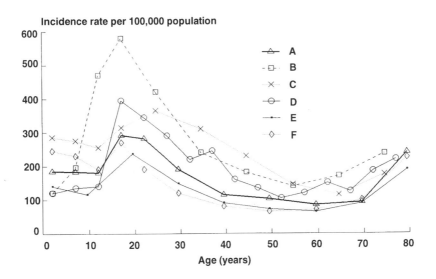

Figure 1–4. Age-specific brain injury incidence rates per 100,000 population: selected United States studies. *A* = San Diego County, CA, 1981 (Kraus et al. 1986); *B* = San Diego County, CA, 1978 (Klauber et al. 1981); *C* = Bronx, NY, 1980–1981 (Cooper et al. 1983); *D* = Virgina 1978 (Jagger et al. 1984); *E* = Maryland 1986 (MacKenzie et al. 1989); *F* = Rhode Island 1979–1980 (Fife et al. 1986).

Sex

All incidence reports published worldwide indicate that brain injuries are far more frequent among men than among women, with a rate ratio of approximately 2.0 to 2.8 (Figure 1–5). Although variation in rate ratios exist, it cannot be attributed solely to reporting differences. The differences in rate ratios may reflect different exposure levels. For example, there may be a higher proportion of injuries connected with motor vehicle crashes (which involve more males) as compared with injuries connected with falls in the home (which involve more females).

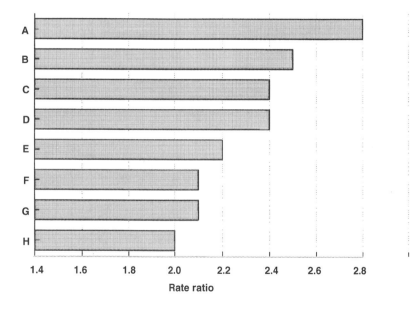

Figure 1–5. Male/female brain injury rate ratios: selected United States studies. *A* = Virginia 1978 (Jagger et al. 1984); *B* = Rhode Island 1979–1980 (Fife et al. 1986); *C* = San Diego County, CA, 1981 (Kraus et al. 1986); *D* = Maryland 1986 (MacKenzie et al. 1989); *E* = United States 1974 (Kalsbeek et al. 1980); *F* = Bronx, NY, 1980–1981 (Cooper et al. 1983) (age adjusted); *G* = Chicago area 1979–1980 (Whitman et al. 1984) (age adjusted); *H* = Olmsted County, MN, 1965–1974 (Annegers et al. 1980) (age adjusted).

Race or Ethnicity

Although some studies show excess brain injury incidence in non-whites compared with whites, there is justifiable concern over the quality of the data used to derive the rates. Because hospital reporting practices vary widely in recording ethnicity or race in medical records, racial or ethnic differences in brain injury rates have yet to be determined accurately.

Alcohol

The positive association between blood alcohol concentration (BAC) and risk of injury is well established for all external causes of injuries, including motor vehicle crashes, general aviation crashes, drownings, and violence (Smith and Kraus 1988). Less studied is the role of alcohol and the outcome of specific kinds or anatomic locations of injuries such as CNS trauma or burns. Although animal studies demonstrate a variety of physiological effects of alcohol on CNS injuries, human data are equivocal. In one study (Kraus et al. 1989), 56% of adults with a brain injury diagnosis had a positive BAC test result. It is noteworthy that 49% of those adults tested had a BAC that was at or above the legal level (0.10%). The prevalence of a positive BAC varied by severity of brain injury; highest prevalence of BAC was among those with mild brain injury compared with those with moderate or severe brain injury (71% versus 49%, respectively). However, selection bias may occur in emergency department BAC testing of injured people with different severities or types of injuries or different inherent sociodemographic or external cause features. For example, blood testing was less frequent for males, young adults, people with mild brain injuries, and those injured from falls. Despite this potential bias, Kraus et al. (1989) found that BAC level was positively associated with physician-diagnosed neurological impairment and length of hospitalization.

Socioeconomic Status

The NHIS for 1985–1987 (Collins 1990) showed that the estimated average annual number of injuries and the rates per 100 people per year are highest in families at the lowest income levels. This finding was also observed by Kraus et al. (1986) in San Diego County, California, and by Whitman et al. (1984) in two socioeconomically different communities in Chicago. In the Kraus et al. (1986) study, the surrogate for individual socioeconomic status was median family income per census tract. Findings did not change when race or ethnicity was considered. Multivariate analysis suggested that using race and/or ethnicity as a proxy for socioeconomic status may be inappropriate. Other aspects of exposure nested within the "socioeconomic environment" should be explored.

Characteristics of High-Risk Exposures

Published studies use different external cause of injury classifications, which restricts any meta-analysis of cause of brain injury. Broad groupings of external causes (Figure 1–6) can be used to make general statements about the nature of the exposures associated with brain injury.

Despite the limitations of the categorization of external cause, available data suggest that the most frequent exposure associated with fatal and nonfatal brain injury is transport. Transport includes automobiles, bicycles, motorcycles, aircraft, watercraft, and others (e.g., farm equipment). The most common transport-related external cause is motor vehicle crashes (Figure 1–7).

Falls are the second-leading cause of brain injury and are associated most frequently with older age (see Figure 1–6). Assault-related brain injury, most frequently involving the use of firearms, is an important factor in penetrating brain injuries (Cooper et al. 1983; Kraus et al. 1984; Whitman et al. 1984). It is not possible to identify brain injuries related to sports or recreation in some studies because they have been grouped into an "other" category. In at least three studies (Annegers et al. 1980; Kraus et al. 1984; Whitman et al. 1984), sports were identified as a significant exposure for brain injury. A major caveat here is that in some studies all bicycle-related exposures have been classified as transportation related. Kraus et al. (1987) found that approximately two-thirds of the brain injuries related to bicycles are not due to collisions with motor vehicles. The dominant form of exposure in motor vehicle crashes is as an occupant of a road vehicle. Classification difficulties across studies do not allow for characterization of occupant location (i.e., driver versus passenger side), but it is possible to categorize motor vehicle–related exposures into three general groups: vehicle occupants, riders on motorcycles, and pedestrians or bicyclists. Brain injuries are most frequent in the vehicle occupants group. Motorcyclists also frequently sustain brain injuries. Unfortunately there are no data on the actual number of people who are occupants or riders on motorcycles; hence, data on specific rates of occurrence are not possible to derive. Special note should be made of the report from Taiwan

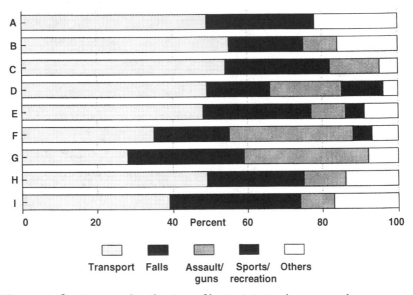

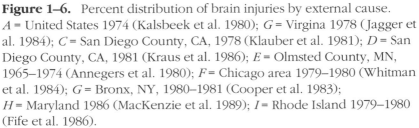

Figure 1–6.   Percent distribution of brain injuries by external cause. *A* = United States 1974 (Kalsbeek et al. 1980); *G* = Virgina 1978 (Jagger et al. 1984); *C* = San Diego County, CA, 1978 (Klauber et al. 1981); *D* = San Diego County, CA, 1981 (Kraus et al. 1986); *E* = Olmsted County, MN, 1965–1974 (Annegers et al. 1980); *F* = Chicago area 1979–1980 (Whitman et al. 1984); *G* = Bronx, NY, 1980–1981 (Cooper et al. 1983); *H* = Maryland 1986 (MacKenzie et al. 1989); *I* = Rhode Island 1979–1980 (Fife et al. 1986).

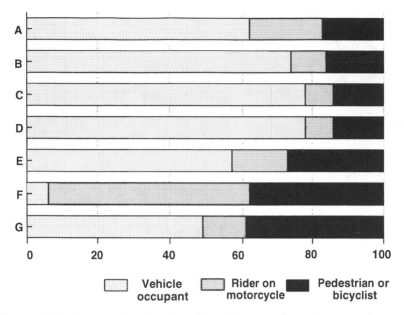

Figure 1–7. Percent distribution of brain injuries for subcauses of motor vehicle–related exposures. *A* = San Diego County, CA, 1981 (Kraus et al. 1986); *B* = San Diego County, CA, 1978 (Klauber et al. 1981); *C* = Olmsted County, MN, 1965–1974 (Annegers et al. 1980); *D* = Virginia 1978 (Jagger et al. 1984); *E* = Seattle 1981 (Gale et al. 1983); *F* = Taiwan 1977–1987 (Lee et al. 1990); *G* = Norway 1974 (Nestvold et al. 1988).

(Lee et al. 1990) where motorcyclists, including scooter riders, formed the largest portion of the motor vehicle–related brain injury problem in the population.

Severity and the Types of Brain Injury

Severity Distributions

All studies show that the greatest proportion of brain injuries are "mild" (i.e., generally a GCS score of 13–15). The distribution of the severity of brain injury, as assessed by the GCS, is shown in Figure

1–8. In terms of emergency department visits and hospital admissions, the majority of brain injuries are of mild severity. Among those people admitted to a hospital alive, the severity distribution is approximately 80% mild (GCS score of 13–15), 10% moderate (GCS score of 9–12), and 10% severe (GCS score of 8 or less). The lower proportion of mild brain injuries (and higher proportion of moderate and severe injuries) found in the Virginia study (Jagger et al. 1984) reflects the nature of the referral institution (i.e., serious injuries were more likely to be referred to the University of Virginia Hospital from the surrounding catchment area).

Hospital Discharges and Diagnoses

Information on people discharged from short-care non-federal hospitals in the United States in 1990 is available through the National

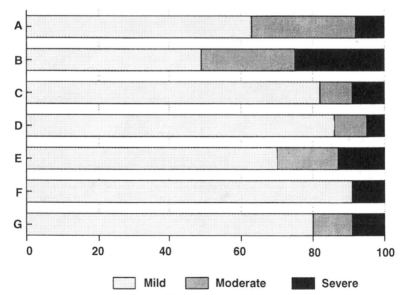

Figure 1–8. Percent severity distribution of brain injuries. *A* = Olmsted County, MN, 1965–1974 (Annegers et al. 1980); *B* = Virginia 1978 (Jagger et al. 1984); *C* = San Diego County, CA, 1981 (Kraus et al. 1986); *D* = Chicago area 1979–1980 (Whitman et al. 1984); *E* = Maryland 1986 (MacKenzie et al. 1989); *F* = San Diego County, CA, 1978 (Klauber et al. 1981); *G* = France 1986 (Tiret et al. 1990) (case series).

Hospital Discharge Survey (NHDS) (Graves 1992). This data source provides information on any listed diagnosis of brain injury coded according to the International Classification of Diseases, 9th Revision, Clinical Modification (ICD-9-CM; Commission on Professional and Hospital Activities 1986). Data on discharge rates with any listed brain injury diagnosis are summarized in Figures 1–9 and 1–10. The rate for those discharged with a brain injury from short-stay hospitals during 1990 was about 150 per 100,000 population. The rate for males was approximately twice as high as that for females. Figure 1–10 shows that most people discharged from a hospital with a brain injury were diagnosed as having a concussion without fracture of the skull. Approximately 30% of the discharges involved "other intracranial injury" without skull fracture; intracranial injury with fracture represented less than 13% of all hospital discharges.

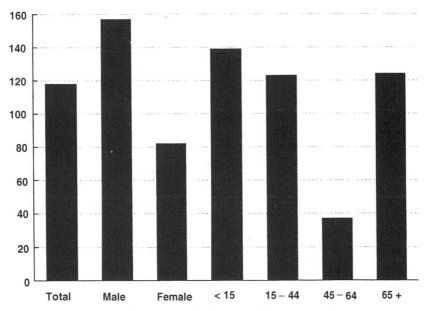

Figure 1–9. Sex- and age-specific (in years) brain injury hospital discharges per 100,000 population: United States 1990. All listed diagnoses. *Source.* Graves 1992.

Unfortunately, the only age-specific national data on hospital discharges are grouped into four generally heterogeneous age groups (see Figure 1–9). Those under age 15 (showing the highest discharge rates in Figure 1–9) include infants, toddlers, young children, and adolescents; each group has various types of exposures. The age 15–44 group combines people in their late 20s, 30s, and early 40s with those who are generally at highest risk of brain injury (i.e., those age 15–24), thus dramatically reducing the incidence shown in Figure 1–9 for this larger age range. It should be noted that the aggregate age-specific injury incidence rates reported above (Figure 1–4) are considerably higher than the age-specific discharge rates from the NHDS (Figure 1–9). One possible explanation for the high brain injury rate among hospital discharges for infants is "birth trauma," a diagnosis that is excluded from most brain injury data

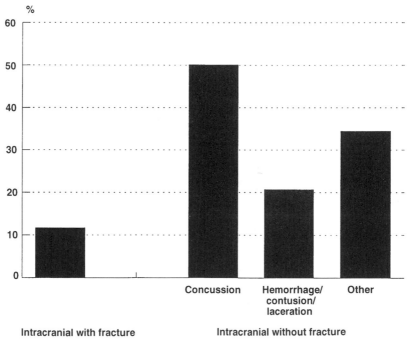

Figure 1–10. Percent brain injury hospital discharges by diagnoses (any listed diagnoses): United States 1990. All listed diagnoses. *Source.* Graves 1992.

bases. Those who died at the scene, during emergency transport, or in the emergency facility, are not included in the estimates.

In evaluating these data, it should be noted that NHDS data are based on *discharges* from short-stay hospitals, but some injured people may have been admitted to multiple hospitals or to the same hospital on multiple occasions for the same injury. Hence, the discharge does not represent a mutually exclusive occurrence, and a patient who had one or more admissions to one or more hospitals during the observation period is counted multiple times. Independent information from our studies suggests that multiple hospital admissions are relatively common, particularly in today's climate of payment requirements for public versus private institutions.

Types of Brain Lesions

Although the literature is replete with reports describing brain trauma, each report typically is based on a clinical series from a single institution. Few epidemiological studies have addressed the question of the nature and severity of the brain lesion, and, for this purpose, specific data were retrieved from the 1981 San Diego County cohort study (Kraus et al. 1984). In this study, clinical information was uniformly recorded from the physician's notes in the medical record. The reader should be aware that these data refer to a single time period from all hospitals in the region and, hence, are population based. Also, the data reported in Table 1–4 and Figure 1–11 represent only adults age 15 years and older. The information on pediatric brain injury can be found elsewhere (Kraus et al. 1990).

The matrix in Table 1–4 shows the distribution of brain injury lesions according to fracture status and type. Slightly less than half of all hospital-admitted brain injuries are concussions without a concurrent fracture to the head. Nearly 11% of those with a contusion or laceration of the brain do not have a concurrent fracture. Similarly, among those diagnosed with a brain hemorrhage, half do not have a concurrent skull fracture.

The distribution of types of fractures associated with focal and diffuse lesions of the brain is shown in Figure 1–11. In all four major brain lesion categories, at least half of the cases do not have a

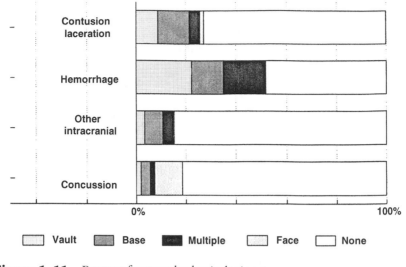

Figure 1–11. Percent fracture by brain lesion type.

concurrent fracture of the skull. Fracture is much less common among patients with concussion or other cranial injury than among those with contusion, laceration, or hemorrhage.

ICD-9-CM allows for a classification of "other intracranial injury." This nosological category is nonspecific and serves as a catchall for other and unspecified brain injuries. This coding needs to be refined to enhance the specificity of the nature of the brain lesion, a revision that will lead to better epidemiological studies. Our clinical colleagues may need to record more specific detail on the nature of the lesions to provide hospital medical record reviewers and coders with sufficient information to accurately code the injuries.

The Consequences of Brain Injury

Immediate Outcomes: Case Fatality Rates

One immediate outcome after brain injury is death. Whereas the fatality rate (Figure 1–2) provides an idea of the level or magnitude of severity in the general population, the case fatality rate after hospital admission measures the immediate gross consequences of the trauma.

Case fatality data are available from six United States population-based incidence studies (Figure 1–12). Case fatality rates range from approximately 3 per 100 hospitalized cases in Rhode Island (Fife et al. 1986) to about 8 per 100 hospitalized cases in the Bronx, New York (Cooper et al. 1983). However, these case fatality rates were not severity adjusted, which precludes adequate comparison across studies. Hospitals that admit a high proportion of patients with severe or moderate brain injury would be expected to have higher case fatality rates, compared with those admitting a large proportion of patients with mild brain injury, who sustain fewer

Table 1–4.   Number (and percent) of brain injuries by fracture status and anatomic location, San Diego County, CA, 1981

Brain injury (code)[a]	Vault (800)	Base (801)	Multiple/ unspecified (803, 804)	Face (802)	No fracture	Total n
			n **fractures**			
Contusion-laceration (851)	35	50	17	6	288	396
	1.3%	1.9%	0.6%	0.2%	10.9%	14.9%
Hemorrhage (852, 853)	72	41	54	0	156	323
	2.7%	1.5%	2.0%	—	5.9%	12.2%
Other intracranial (854)	12	27	17	1	311	368
	0.5%	1.0%	0.6%	—	11.7%	13.9%
Concussion (850)	28	58	30	174	1,274	1,564
	1.15	2.2%	1.1%	6.6%	48.1%	59.0%
Total *n*	147	176	118	181	2,029	2,651
	5.5%	6.6%	4.4%	6.8%	76.5%	100%

[a]International Classification of Diseases, 9th Revision, Clinical Modification (ICD-9-CM; Commission on Professional and Hospital Activities 1986) injury codes.
Source. Unpublished data from the San Diego County Brain Injury Cohort Study (see Kraus et al. 1984).

deaths. Figure 1–12 also shows a case fatality rate from a report from Taiwan (Lee et al. 1990). This high case fatality rate illustrates further the difficulties in comparing rates across study centers where severity mixes in patient populations have not been standardized. For this reason, it is not appropriate to suggest that differences in outcome after hospitalization relate to differences in quality of care.

Measurement of Long-Term Consequences

One widely used scale in assessing outcome of acute brain injury is the Glasgow Outcome Scale (GOS; Jennett and Teasdale 1981). The GOS is a crude indicator of medical (neurological) complications or

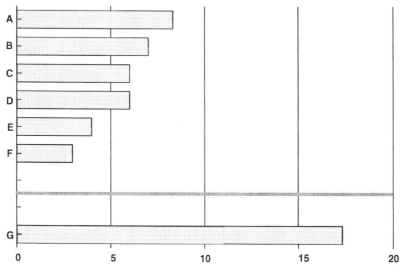

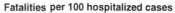

Fatalities per 100 hospitalized cases

Figure 1–12. Case fatality rate for brain injuries: selected studies. *A* = Bronx, NY, 1980–1981 (Cooper et al. 1983); *B* = Virginia 1978 (Jagger et al. 1984); *C* = San Diego County, CA, 1981 (Kraus et al. 1986); *D* = Maryland 1986 (MacKenzie et al. 1989); *E* = San Diego County, CA, 1978 (Klauber et al. 1981); *F* = Rhode Island 1979–1980 (Fife et al. 1986); *G* = Taiwan 1977–1987 (Lee et al. 1990) (case series).

residual effects at time of discharge from the primary treatment center. The major classifications of the GOS are 1) death, 2) persistent vegetative state (i.e., no cerebral cortical function as judged behaviorally), 3) severe disability (conscious but dependent on 24-hour care), 4) moderate disability (disabled but capable of independent care), and 5) good recovery (mild impairment with persistent sequelae but able to participate in normal social life).

The major difficulty with the GOS is the inability to properly classify patients because of the lack of specific objective criteria that separate severe from moderate or moderate from good recovery. Good recovery does not mean, nor was it intended to mean, complete recovery. Hence, it is important to assess GOS findings with some degree of caution.

Consequences of Mild Brain Injury

Understanding the sequelae of mild brain injury is complicated by the many differences among research investigations. Study differences include how the sample was identified and drawn, how *mild brain injury* was defined, the length of follow-up, and what outcome measures were employed. As shown in Figures 1–13 and 1–14, in research reports from 1984 to early 1991, definitions for *mild brain injury* in children, adolescents, and adults encompassed broad ranges of the length of loss of consciousness (from none to 60 minutes) and the GCS scores (from 15 only to a range of 8–15). Injury severity varied considerably across these studies, which all purported to study "mild" brain injury. The variation is regrettable, given that the severity of the injury appears to be a primary factor in long-term recovery.

Evidence on the frequency and nature of negative cognitive outcomes after mild brain injury is far from clear. As shown in Figure 1–15, most reports have assessed motor skills or a combination of learning and motor skills. A review of 13 recent outcome studies (Bassett and Slater 1990; Bawden et al. 1985; Costeff et al. 1988; Dennis and Barnes 1990; Ewing-Cobbs et al. 1985, 1987; Gulbrandson 1984; Hannay and Levin 1988; Jordan and Murdoch 1990; Jordan et al. 1988; Levin et al. 1987, 1988; Tompkins et al.

1990) indicated that children with mild brain injury scored worse than their noninjured counterparts on measures of general intelligence, language, and a combination of learning and motor skills. In contrast, most studies indicated that adults with mild brain injury did not differ from noninjured individuals on measures of motor and spatial skills. Thus results were not consistent for mental functioning among skills as diverse as language, learning and memory, motor skills, and spatial skills. Furthermore, these studies are plagued by a common threat to validity—all assessments were made postinjury so the groups may have differed on the variables of interest before the brain injury occurred.

The current scientific literature contains studies with small numbers of subjects, retrospective study designs, and inadequate control or comparison groups. Small numbers of study subjects and many different outcome measures compromise the researcher's ability to detect differences. Almost no studies were designed to

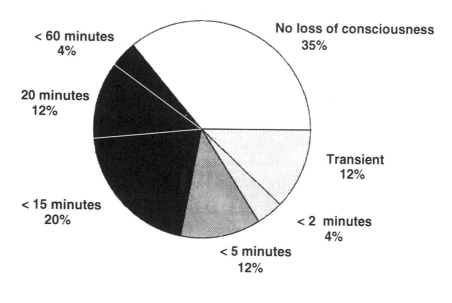

Proportion of studies

Figure 1–13. Mild head injury: loss of consiousness criterion.

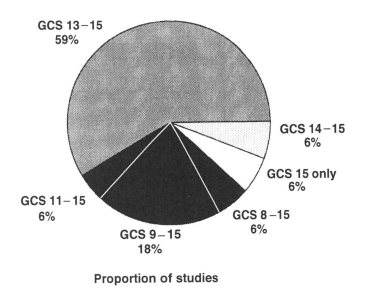

Figure 1–14. Mild head injury: Glasgow Coma Scale (GCS; Jennett and Teasdale 1981) criterion.

---

adequately identify differences between people who had sustained a mild brain injury and those who had not. Given that there is not a sufficient body of literature to draw conclusions with confidence about the negative consequences of mild brain injury, the task of future research is to use sufficiently sophisticated research methods to detect these consequences if they exist.

Predicting Initial Consequences of Brain Injury

It would be very useful to know which factors predict unfavorable consequences after acute brain injury. Not all of the potential predictive factors from the moment of injury through emergency transport, emergency department treatment, and definitive care have been adequately measured or evaluated. A few factors, however, are available to help predict severe outcome after trauma. For this

discussion, we divided outcomes into three general categories:
1) death; 2) an unfavorable GOS score of moderate disability,
severe disability, or persistent vegetative state; and 3) presence of
any neurological deficit or limitation on discharge. As mentioned
above, it is difficult to evaluate all variables in cross-institutional
comparisons because they have not been assessed in a similar way.
Hence, for this illustration, we use the information from the 1981
San Diego County brain injury cohort study (Klauber et al. 1981).
Variables for which verification was complete include age, sex, GCS
score, Maximum Abbreviated Injury Severity (MAIS; Association for
the Advancement of Automotive Medicine 1990) for non-head injury, fracture status, and type of brain lesion (i.e., concussion, hemorrhage, contusion, laceration, or other intracranial injury).

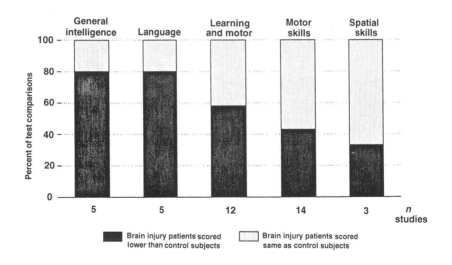

Figure 1–15. Consequences of mild brain injury: summary of findings
from 13 studies.
Source. Bassett and Slater 1990; Bawden et al. 1985; Costeff et al. 1988;
Dennis and Barnes 1990; Ewing-Cobbs et al. 1985, 1987; Gulbrandson
1984; Hannay and Levin 1988; Jordan and Murdoch 1990; Jordan et al.
1988; Levin et al. 1987, 1988; Tompkins et al. 1990.

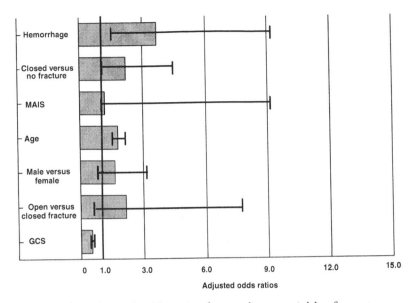

Figure 1–16. Adjusted odds ratios for predictor variables for outcome: death following brain injury. MAIS = Maximum Abbreviated Injury Severity (Association for the Advancement of Automotive Medicine 1990); GCS = Glasgow Coma Scale (Jennett and Teasdale 1981). *Source.* Unpublished data from the San Diego County Brain Injury Cohort Study (see Kraus et al. 1984).

Figures 1–16, 1–17, and 1–18 and Table 1–5 provide adjusted odds ratios[1] for an unfavorable outcome (see above). The adjusted odds ratios show that hemorrhage and fracture are important predictive factors for all unfavorable outcome measures. Age (in 10-year increasing increments), the GCS score, and the MAIS are other factors that independently predict an unfavorable outcome. Although these data are not likely to apply to all brain injury populations, they illustrate the potential for using patient-descriptive and diagnostic measures to assist in identifying factors that need in-

---

[1] The ratio of unfavorable outcome (e.g., death) to a favorable outcome when injury severity, age, sex, and so on, are controlled.

creased clinical attention in the effort to improve current outcomes for brain injury.

Table 1–5 presents significant findings for three measures of outcome (i.e., death, a poor GOS score, and neurological limitation) for the matrix of brain injury types and fracture status. Patients with a concussion without a fracture are the reference group. The reader should recall that all of the adjusted odds ratios take into consideration the MAIS (in another body segment), age, sex, and open versus closed fracture status. Contusion and/or laceration or hemorrhage of the brain have poor outcomes independent of other factors measured.

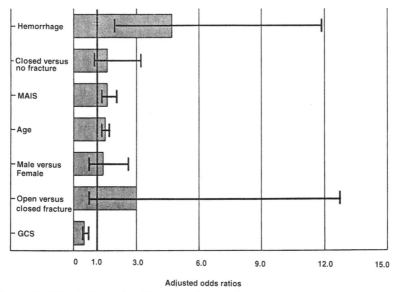

Figure 1–17. Adjusted odds ratios for predictor variables for outcome: Glasgow Outcome Scale (Jennett and Teasdale 1981) less than good recovery. MAIS = Maximum Abbreviated Injury Severity (Association for the Advancement of Automotive Medicine 1990); GSC = Glasgow Coma Scale (Jennett and Teasdale 1981).
Source. Unpublished data from the San Diego County Brain Injury Cohort Study (see Kraus et al. 1984).

Estimating Brain Injury Disability in the Population

▮ **Estimation of the number of new disabilities.** Several assumptions are necessary to devise an estimate of the number of new disabilities (i.e., neurological deficits or limitations) each year after head injury (the incidence rate being based on a pooled estimate from all incidence studies reported earlier in this chapter):

1. Brain injury incidence = 200/100,000
2. United States population size, 1990 = 250 million
3. Total new cases in 1990 = (200 × 2,500) = 500,000
4. Prehospital brain injury deaths = (.0002 × 250,000,000) = 50,000
5. Total cases admitted to hospital alive = 450,000
6. United States hospital admissions by severity:
   Mild: 80% × 450,000 = 360,000
   Moderate: 10% × 450,000 = 45,000
   Severe: 10% × 450,000 = 45,000
7. Discharge rate (alive) (Kraus et al 1984; Levin et al. 1987; MacKenzie et al. 1989) by severity of brain injury:
   Mild = 100%
   Moderate = 93%
   Severe = 42%

Table 1–5.   Adjusted odd ratios for three outcomes after brain injury

Brain injury	Vault	Base	Multiple/ unspecified	Face	No fracture
Contusion and/ or laceration	N	GN	GN	—	GDN
Hemorrhage	N	GDN	GDN	—	GDN
Other intracranial	—	N	—	—	—
Concussion	—	N	—	—	ref

Note. Odds ratios adjusted for Maximum Abbreviated Injury Severity (MAIS; Association for the Advancement of Automotive Medicine 1990), age, sex, and open versus closed fracture. G = a poor Glasgow Outcome Scale (Jennett and Teasdale 1981) score; D = death; N = neurological limits; ref = reference group.
Source. Unpublished data from the San Diego County Brain Injury Cohort Study (see Kraus et al. 1984).

If 80% of all new hospital-admitted patients have mild injuries, 360,000 (100% × 360,000) are discharged alive. If 10% of all new hospital cases have moderate injuries, 45,000 (10% × 450,000) are admitted to a hospital and 41,850 (93% × 45,000) are discharged alive. If 10% of all brain injuries are severe, 45,000 (10% × 450,000) are admitted to a hospital annually, but only 18,900 (42% × 45,000) are discharged alive. Hence, the total pool of people discharged alive from a hospital by severity of admission is 420,750 (360,000 [mild] + 41,850 [moderate] + 18,900 [severe]).

The disability rate varies by severity of brain injury. If we assume that 10% of those with mild brain injury will have some neurological limitation, then 36,000 people are afflicted. Also, if two-thirds of those with moderate brain injury are disabled, 27,901

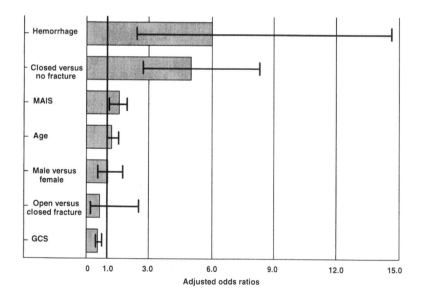

Figure 1–18. Adjusted odds ratios for predictor variables for outcome: neurological limits. MAIS = Maximum Abbreviated Injury Severity (Association for the Advancement of Automotive Medicine 1990); GSC = Glasgow Coma Scale (Jennett and Teasdale 1981).
Source. Unpublished data from the San Diego County Brain Injury Cohort Study (see Kraus et al. 1984).

have some disability. Finally, if 100% of severely injured patients have residual effects, 18,900 can be expected to have some form of disability. The total number of new disabilities from brain injuries for 1990 is about 82,800, a rate of about 33 per 100,000 population.

This estimating procedure can be summarized as follows (see Figure 1–19):

Let BID equal the number of brain injured patients who are discharged alive from hospitals each year with disability

n = size of population (i.e., United States 1990, 250,000,000)

H = *hospitalization admission rate* of brain injury patients in the population (i.e., 0.0018/year)

p_i = proportion of brain injury patients in the i-th severity group (i = 1...k, where k = 3), where p_1 = .80, p_2 = .10, p_3 = .10

F_i = cumulative hospital fatality for the i-th group where F_1 = 0, F_2 = .07, F_3 = .58)

P_i = posthospital prevalence of disability in the i-th group where P_1 = 0.1, P_2 = 0.667, P_3 = 1.0

If

  BID = n brain injury patients with disability

  n = population

  H = hospital admission rate

  p_i = proportion in severity groups
  (mild, moderate, severe)

  F_i = hospital case fatality rate for severity groups in pi

  P_i = posthospital prevalence of disability in each
  severity group

Then

$$BID = Hn \sum_{i=1}^{k} p_i (1-F_i) P_i$$

Figure 1–19. Estimating model.

Hence

$$BID = Hn \sum_{i=1}^{k} p_i(1 - F_i)P_i$$

that is,

$$BID = .0018\ (250{,}000{,}000)\ [.8\ (1 - 0)(.1) + .1\ (1 - .07)(.6667)$$
$$+\ .1\ (1 - .42)(1)] = 82{,}800$$

■ **Cost of head injury.** Almost no information was available on the economic impact of head injuries until Max et al. (1991) provided the first clear insight into the financial impact of head injuries in the population. The data show that the average lifetime cost for head injury was approximately $85,000 per person during 1985. Max et al. pointed out that the lifetime costs for minor, moderate, and severe head injury are surprisingly close, ranging from about $77,000 to $93,000 (Figure 1–20). This finding illustrates the problem associated with mild head injury, namely, that specific treatment costs are nearly as high as those for moderate and severe brain injury because the mild injury incurs other associated treatment costs and affects full-time employment. The lifetime cost for a brain injury fatality is approximately $357,000, a figure not much higher

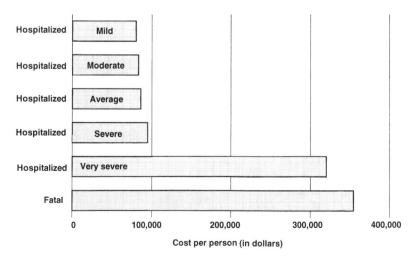

Figure 1–20. Lifetime costs of head injury, 1985 (by severity of injury). *Source.* Max et al. 1991.

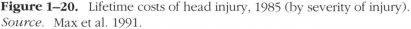

than the $325,000 for a very severe nonfatal brain injury.

The lifetime costs of head injury by age (Figure 1–21) are much higher for people between the ages of 15 and 44 than for those in younger or older age groups. Although the data have not been severity adjusted, they reflect costs associated with loss of productivity (and physical, as well as psychosocial, limitations) during the middle, most productive years.

Total costs for all 328,000 head injuries occurring in 1985 are estimated to be $37.8 billion (Max et al. 1991). About 65% of the total costs are accrued among those who survive a head injury, the remainder is associated with head injury deaths.

Summary and Conclusions

The current brain injury research literature should be read cautiously because of the wide differences in the research methods and interpretation of clinically based, as opposed to epidemiologically based, data. This is especially important in the consideration of the

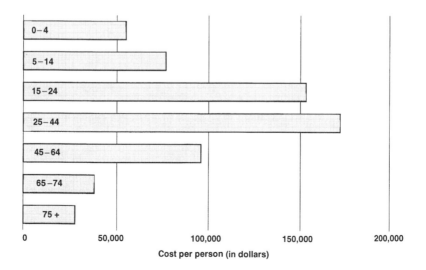

Figure 1–21. Lifetime cost of head injury, 1985 (by age, in years). *Source.* Max et al. 1991.

definition of brain trauma and the ways in which injury severity is measured. The results of these methodological inconsistencies (points of interpretation) make cross-study comparisons extremely difficult, if not impossible. The epidemiological literature is far less prevalent than the clinical literature. Since the mid-1970s, there has been only a handful of studies that incorporated sound epidemiological methods in case definition, case ascertainment, severity definition, incidence measurement, and risk marker or risk factor evaluation. There are even fewer studies that address the long-term sequelae of brain injury that are population based and have standardized and rigorous forms of cohort follow-up.

Despite these limitations, there are some findings that can be summarized from the available literature. Aggregate average incidence values are approximately 200 per 100,000 population per year, which includes fatal and nonfatal hospitalized cases. The estimates based solely on hospital discharge data are an undercount of the true incidence because of difficulties in definition and ascertainment of nonrepetitive admitted patients to a single institution. The epidemiological data suggest that the age of highest occurrence is in the late teens and early twenties with a second period of high frequency after age 65. Males have two to three times the frequency of brain injury as do females. Most studies show that transport-related causes are a dominant form of exposure. Almost all population-based incidence studies show that approximately 80% of brain injuries (average of all hospital admitted cases) are mild, 10% are moderate, and approximately 10% are severe.

The most frequent diagnosis on hospitalized cases is concussion. Less than 30% of all cases have concurrent fracture of the vault or base of the skull. Case fatality rates vary considerably across different studies with a range of 3–8 per 100 patients admitted to a hospital. The literature is inconclusive with regard to the long-term effects in patients with short-time loss of consciousness and a GCS of 13 to 15. Methodological difficulties hamper a scientific assessment of this question. Available data suggest that hemorrhage, closed versus absence of fracture, MAIS, and age are independent predictors of unfavorable outcome after brain injury. Hemorrhage is the single most important of all outcome predictive factors.

An algorithm to estimate brain injury disability suggests that approximately 80,000 to 85,000 individuals each year who sustain a brain injury will have neurological deficit or disability. This cumulative prevalence is noteworthy because of the current pressures for effective delivery of long-term health care. The designation of the decade of the 1990s for head injury research by the National Institutes of Health is a timely if not crucial commitment of the federal government to control this tragic form of human affliction.

References

Annegers JF, Grabow JD, Kurland LT, et al: The incidence, causes, and secular trends in head injury in Olmsted County, Minnesota, 1965–1974. Neurology 30:912–919, 1980

Association for the Advancement of Automotive Medicine: The Abbreviated Injury Scale, 1990 Revision. Des Plaines, IL, 1990

Auer LM, Gell G, Richling B, et al: Predicting lethal outcome after severe head injury: a computer-assisted analysis of neurological symptoms and laboratory values. Acta Neurochir 52:225–238, 1980

Bassett SS, Slater J: Neuropsychologic function in adolescents sustaining mild closed head injury. J Pediatr Psychol 15:225–236, 1990

Bawden HN, Knights RM, Winogron HW: Speeded performance following head injury in children. J Clin Exp Neuropsychol 7:39–54, 1985

Bruce DA, Raphaely RC, Goldberg AI, et al: Pathophysiology, treatment and outcome following severe head injury in children. Childs Brain 5:74–191, 1979

Centers for Disease Control: Monthly Vital Statistics Report 42 (suppl 2), 1993

Collins JG: Types of Injuries by Selected Characteristics: United States, 1985–1987 (Vital and Health Statistics, Series 10: Data From the National Health Survey, No 175) (DHHS Publication No [PHS]91-1503). Hyattsville, MD, US Department of Health and Human Services, 1990

Commission on Professional and Hospital Activities: International Classification of Diseases, 9th Revision, Clinical Modification (ICD-9-CM). Ann Arbor, MI, 1986

Cooper JD, Tabaddor K, Hauser WA: The epidemiology of head injury in the Bronx. Neuroepidemiology 2:70–88, 1983

Costeff H, Abraham E, Brenner T, et al: Late neuropsychologic status after childhood head trauma. Brain Dev 10:381–384, 1988

Dennis M, Barnes MA: Knowing the meaning, getting the point, bridging the gap, and carrying the message: aspects of discourse following closed head injury in childhood and adolescence. Brain Lang 39:428–446, 1990

Ewing-Cobbs L, Fletcher JM, Landry SH, et al: Language disorders after pediatric head injury, in Speech and Language Evaluation in Neurology. Edited by Darby JK. New York, Grune & Stratton, 1985, pp 71–89

Ewing-Cobbs L, Levin HS, Eisenberg HM, et al:: Language functions following closed-head injury in children and adolescents. J Clin Exp Neuropsychol 9:575–592, 1987

Fife D: Head injury with and without hospital admission: comparisons of incidence and short-term disability. Am J Public Health 77:810–812, 1987

Fife D, Faich G, Hollenshead W, et al: Incidence and outcome of hospital-treated head injury in Rhode Island. Am J Public Health 76:773–778, 1986

Gale JL, Dikmen S, Wyler A, et al: Head injury in the Pacific Northwest. Neurosurgery 12:487–491, 1983

Graves E: Detailed Diagnoses and Procedures (Vital and Health Statistics, Series 13: Data From the National Health Survey, No 113). Hyattsville, MD, US Department of Health and Human Services, 1992

Gronwall SL, Wrightson P: Delayed recovery of intellectual function after minor head injury. Lancet 2:605–609, 1974

Gulbrandson GB: Neuropsychological sequelae of light head injuries in older children 6 months after trauma. J Clin Exp Neuropsychol 6:257–268, 1984

Hannay HJ, Levin HS: Visual continuous recognition memory in normal and closed-head-injured adolescents. J Clin Exp Neuropsychol 11:444–460, 1988

Jagger J, Levine J, Jane J, et al: Epidemiologic features of head injury in a predominantly rural population. J Trauma 24:40–44, 1984

Jennett B, Murry A, Carlin J, et al: Head injuries in three Scottish neurosurgical units. BMJ 2:955–958, 1979

Jennett B, Teasdale G: Management of Head Injuries. Philadelphia, PA, FA Davis, 1981

Jordan FM, Murdoch BE: Linguistic status following closed head injury in children: a follow-up study. Brain Inj 4:47–54, 1990

Jordan FM, Ozanne AE, Murdoch BE: Long-term speech and language disorders subsequent to closed head injury in children. Brain Inj 2:179–185, 1988

Kalsbeek WD, McLauren RL, Harris BSH, et al: The national head and spinal cord injury survey: major findings. J Neurosurg 53 (suppl):19–31, 1980

Klauber MR, Barrett-Connor E, Marshall LF, et al: The epidemiology of head injury: a prospective study of an entire community: San Diego County, California, 1978. Am J Epidemiol 113:500–509, 1981

Kraus JF, Black MA, Hessol N, et al: The incidence of acute brain injury and serious impairment in a defined population. Am J Epidemiol 119:186–201, 1984

Kraus JF, Fife D, Ramstein K, et al: The relationship of family income to the incidence, external causes and outcome of serious brain injury, San Diego County, California. Am J Public Health 76:1345–1347, 1986

Kraus JF, Fife D, Conroy C: Incidence, severity and outcomes of brain injuries involving bicycles. Am J Public Health 77:76–78, 1987

Kraus JF, Morgenstern H, Fife D, et al: Blood alcohol tests, prevalence of involvement, and outcomes following brain injury. Am J Public Health 79:294–299, 1989

Kraus JF, Rock A, Hemyari P: Brain injuries among infants, children, adolescents, and young adults. Am J Dis Child 144:684–691, 1990

Lee S, Lui T, Chang C, et al: Features of head injury in a developing country: Taiwan (1977–1987). J Trauma 30:194–199, 1990

Levin HS, Mattis S, Ruff RM, et al: Neurobehavioral outcome following minor head injury: a three-center study. J Neurosurg 66:234–243, 1987

Levin HS, High WM, Ewing-Cobbs L, et al: Memory functioning during the first year after closed head injury in children and adolescents. Neurosurgery 22:1043–1052, 1988

MacKenzie EJ, Edelstein SL, Flynn JP: Hospitalized head-injured patients in Maryland: incidence and severity of injuries. Maryland Medical Journal 38:725–732, 1989

Marshall L, Marshall S, Klauber M, et al: A new classification of head injury based on computerized tomography. J Neurosurg (suppl) 75:s1–s66, 1991

Max W, MacKenzie E, Rice D: Head injuries: costs and consequences. Journal of Head Trauma Rehabilitation 6:76–91, 1991

Nestvold K, Lunder T, Blikra G, et al: Head injuries during one year in a central hospital in Norway: A prospective study: epidemiologic features. Neuroepidemiology 7:134–144, 1988

Plaut MR, Gifford RRM: Trivial head trauma and its consequences in a perspective of regional health care. Milit Med 141:244–247, 1976

Rimel RW: A prospective study of patients with central nervous system trauma. Journal of Neurosurgical Nursing 13:132–141, 1981

Smith GS, Kraus JF: Alcohol and residential, recreational and occupational injuries: a review of the epidemiologic evidence. Am J Public Health 79:99–121, 1988

Sosin D, Sacks J, Smith S: Head injury-associated deaths in the United States from 1979 to 1986. JAMA 262:2251–2255, 1989

Tiret L, Hausherr E, Thioipe M, et al: The epidemiology of head trauma in Aquitaine (France) 1986: a community-based study of hospital admissions and deaths. Int J Epidemiol 19:133–140, 1990

Tompkins CA, Holland AL, Ratcliff G, et al: Predicting cognitive recovery from closed head injury in children and adolescents. Brain Cogn 13:86–97, 1990

Whitman S, Coonley-Hoganson R, Desai BT: Comparative head trauma experiences in two socioeconomically different Chicago-area communities: a population study. Am J Epidemiol 119:570–580, 1984

Chapter 2

Neuropathology

John W. Cassidy, M.D.

Neuroanatomic and Functional Bases of Behavior

The human central nervous system (CNS) consists of a vast array of hierarchically controlled structures that subserve behavioral regulation. Classical anatomists consider the whole modern human brain to consist of five subdivisions based on their distinct embryologic origins (Horstadius 1950). Three of these subdivisions are contained in the brain stem, which subserves vegetative functions such as the regulation of respiration, heart rate, and blood pressure. The brain stem consists of the myelencephalon (medulla), the metencephalon (pons and cerebellum), and the mesencephalon (midbrain), and includes the reticular formation, which extends the length of the three regions. The more rostral diencephalon consists of the thalamus and hypothalamus, as well as the hypophysis (pituitary gland) and the epiphysis (pineal gland). Structures in this subdivision are considered to be intermediary links between higher brain regions and lower brain regions. Finally, the telencephalon, the most advanced brain region (both phylogenetically and ontologically), consists of the entire cerebrum, including the neocortex, subcortical nuclear complexes, and the internal capsule. This subdivision therefore includes the brain sites that mediate both cognitive processing and emotional behavior. This classical scheme of structural organization has proven to be useful for describing and topographically categorizing the hard wiring of neuroanatomy. However, the clinician trying to design a rehabilitation program for a patient with brain injury will often have difficulty associating structural impairment with functional deficit. To understand the anatomic bases of complex behavior, it is more useful to consider a conceptual model of the human brain that is based on a functional paradigm.

To associate form with function, neurobiologist Paul MacLean proposed a triunal model of brain and behavior (MacLean 1973). The human brain evolved, increasing in both size and complexity, by *adding on* to more primitive structures. Hence beneath a mantle of distinctly human neocortex, the modern human brain still retains the highly conserved archetypical patterns of structural organization that are reflections of reptilian and primitive mammalian ancestry.

Based on the triunal model, the brain may be divided, both anatomically and functionally, into three basic levels: reptilian, paleomammalian, and neomammalian (see Figure 2–1). The reptilian component corresponds to the brain stem and consists of not only medulla, pons, and midbrain, but basal ganglia as well. Therefore, not only vegetative functions, but also many volitional behaviors such as feeding, drinking, and sexual aggression may be considered to be phylogenetic legacies of our cold-blooded ancestors.

Correspondingly, the paleomammalian brain is characterized by the primitive cortex of the limbic lobe (described by Broca in 1878), the prominent convolution that surrounds the rostral brain stem of all mammalian brains (*limbic* means "forming a border around"). Structures of the limbic cortex subserve primitive but distinctly mammalian behaviors such as hoarding and parental care of offspring.

Finally, the outermost neomammalian brain, the neocortex, subserves the uniquely human behaviors such as cognition and speech. The modern human brain, then, may be conceptually divided into three functional divisions: the brain stem, the limbic system, and the neocortex.

The Brain Stem

Both anatomically and physiologically, the brain stem marks a transitional zone between brain and spinal cord. In fact, much of the substance of the brain stem is devoted to ascending and descending tracts connecting the upper and lower divisions of the CNS. Because of its vulnerability to rotational accelerative forces and the density of critical life-sustaining fiber tracts in the region, traumatic injuries to the brain stem carry a high probability for morbidity and mortality.

The brain stem as a unit is densely packed with many vital structures. In addition to the long ascending and descending pathways, several specific nuclear groups, including the nuclei of the cranial nerves, are found there. The central core of the brain stem is occupied by the reticular formation, diffuse aggregations of cells surrounded by myriad interlacing fibers. Centers within the brain

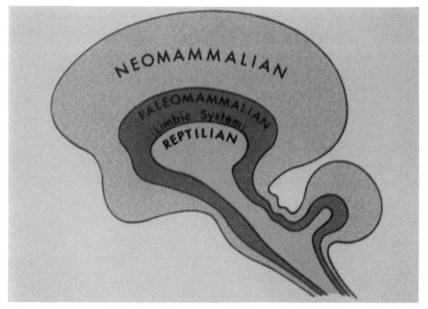

Figure 2–1. Symbolic representation of the triune brain.
Source. Reprinted from MacLean PD: *Triune Concept of Brain and Behavior.* Toronto, Canada, University of Toronto Press, 1973, p. 9. Used with permission.

stem subserve not only the primary vegetative functions but motor activities and mechanisms related to sleep and consciousness as well (Table 2–1).

Although the monoamine neurotransmitters (dopamine, epinephrine, and serotonin) are widely distributed in the CNS, the cell groups from which the monoaminergic pathways arise are almost without exception located within the brain stem (Carpenter 1976). The monoaminergic systems participate in the regulation of sleep-wake cycles, feeding behaviors, motor and neuroendocrine regulation, reward mechanisms, and probably many other functions.

The caudal portion of the brain stem is the *medulla oblongata*. At the level of the medulla, both the descending motor pyramidal tracts and the ascending sensory dorsal columns decussate. In the dorsal medulla, the motor nuclei of the vagus, spinal accessory, and hypoglossal cranial nerves lie medially, whereas portions of nuclei of sensory cranial nerves (trigeminal and the vestibular complex) lie laterally. The ventral surface of the medulla lies against the basilar portion of the occipital bone, whereas the dorsal surface and the fourth ventricle are lodged in a groove on the anterior surface of the cerebellum (Figure 2–2).

The *pons* ("bridge") of the brain stem is named for the massive

Table 2–1.   Localization of brain stem functions

Region	Nuclear groups	Prominent fiber tracts
Medulla oblongata	Vagus, spinal accessory, and hypoglossal motor nuclei; Trigeminal and vestibular sensory nuclei	Descending motor pyramidal and ascending sensory dorsal columns
Pons	Trigeminal, abducens, and facial motor nuclei; Superior vestibular sensory nuclei	Pontocerebellar tracts; corticopontine, corticobulbar, and corticospinal tracts
Midbrain	Oculomotor and trochlear motor nuclei; reflex centers for vision and audition; Substantia nigra	Medial longitudinal fasciculus; cerebral peduncles

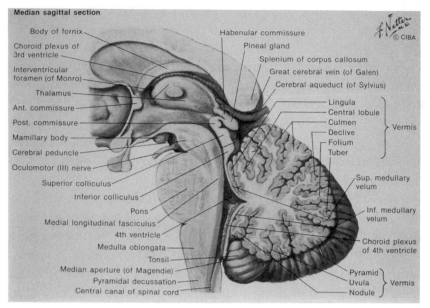

Median sagittal section

Body of fornix

Choroid plexus of 3rd ventricle

Interventricular foramen (of Monro)

Thalamus

Ant. commissure

Post. commissure

Mamillary body

Cerebral peduncle

Oculomotor (III) nerve

Superior colliculus

Inferior colliculus

Pons

Medial longitudinal fasciculus

4th ventricle

Medulla oblongata

Tonsil

Median aperture (of Magendie)

Pyramidal decussation

Central canal of spinal cord

Habenular commissure

Pineal gland

Splenium of corpus callosum

Great cerebral vein (of Galen)

Cerebral aqueduct (of Sylvius)

Lingula

Central lobule

Culmen

Declive

Folium

Tuber

Vermis

Sup. medullary velum

Inf. medullary velum

Choroid plexus of 4th ventricle

Pyramid

Uvula

Nodule

Vermis

Figure 2–2.　Median sagittal section of the caudal brain.
Source.　Reprinted from Netter FH: *CIBA Collection of Medical Illustrations,* Volume I: *Nervous System;* Part I: *Anatomy and Physiology.* Summit, NJ, CIBA, 1983, p. 32. Used with permission.

bundles of transversely oriented fibers that originate in the pontine nuclei and enter the cerebellum via the middle cerebellar peduncles. These pontocerebellar fibers form the second link in a pathway between the cerebral cortex and the cerebellum. Longitudinally oriented pontine fiber bundles include the corticopontine, corticobulbar, and corticospinal tracts. Cranial nerve nuclei located in the pons include the trigeminal, abducens, facial, and superior vestibular. The pons occupies the central part of the ventral brain stem, resting against the clivus of the occipital bone (Figure 2–2).

The dorsal *midbrain* contains the reflex centers for visual and auditory impulses in the superior and inferior colliculi respectively. Beneath the colliculi are the nuclei of the oculomotor and trochlear cranial nerves. Running longitudinally through the area is the medial longitudinal fasciculus. This complex bundle of fibers, connecting the oculomotor apparatus with the vestibular nuclei and motor centers in the cervical cord, is essential for the coordination of eye and head movement. The ventral portion of the midbrain is dominated by the cerebral peduncles, parallel massive bundles carrying several ascending and descending tracts. The substantia nigra and red nucleus are deep to the peduncles.

The *reticular formation* is located in the central region of the brain stem, extending from the medulla to the rostral midbrain. It is characterized by diffuse aggregations of cells intermeshed among multidirectional fibers. Discrete populations of cells are grouped as either small, localized cells (the lateral parvocellular zone) or large arborizing cells that connect to long ascending and descending pathways (the medial magnocellular zone) characterized by elaborate perpendicular interconnections. The extensive overlapping of these fibers facilitates the widespread convergence of afferent impulses.

The concept of the *ascending reticular activating system* (ARAS) is based on evidence of an arousal zone in the brain stem (Moruzzi and Magoun 1949). It is a physiological concept with anatomic correlates represented by discrete areas of the brain stem reticular formation, as well as specific ascending pathways to the thalamus and cortex. The ARAS is critical for maintaining a state of wakefulness. The regulation of the conscious state, however, is an extremely complex function, in which many parts of the CNS are involved. In addition, areas of special importance for sleep have been identified in the ARAS, as well as in the thalamus and the hypothalamus. The anatomic components of the ARAS lie in a narrow isthmus between the cerebellum in the infratentorial compartment and the cerebrum in the supratentorial compartment. This location renders the ARAS vulnerable to trauma resulting from rotational and accelerating forces.

A number of neuron groups located primarily in the brain stem have been characterized according to the three monoaminergic neurotransmitters: serotonin (5-hydroxytryptamine, 5-HT), norepinephrine, and dopamine (Table 2–2). There are some notable anatomic differences among the three neurotransmitter systems. In the serotonin and norepinephrine systems, the cells of origin are located within or near the reticular formation whereas their projections are widespread throughout the CNS. On the other hand, the dopamine-specific cells are located in the substantia nigra and nearby ventral areas of the midbrain, as well as in some hypothalamic nuclei. Axons of these cells project to specific areas of the CNS in a highly ordered topographic fashion.

The cells of origin of the serotonin system are located primarily in the raphe nuclei, an extensive, continuous collection of cell groups close to the midline throughout the brain stem (Azmitia 1987). Their axons project both caudally and rostrally, extending to the forebrain, the cerebellum, and the spinal cord. These pathways have been implicated in pain mechanisms, changes in mood and behavior (via projections to limbic structures), and sleep induction.

Norepinephrine fibers arise from special cells in the pontine and medullary reticular formation, the nucleus locus ceruleus, located beneath the floor of the fourth ventricle (Janowsky and Sulser 1987). Projections from the locus ceruleus are characterized by widespread distribution of norepinephrine fibers via profuse branching of a limited number of neurons. This system participates in the regulation of cerebral blood flow, alertness, spinal cord locomotion, mood, memory, and hormonal modulation.

Table 2–2.   Neurotransmitters of the brain stem

Neurotransmitter	Location of cells of origin	Functions
Serotonin	Raphe nuclei of the reticular formation	Pain mechanisms, changes in mood and behavior, sleep
Norepinephrine	Locus ceruleus of the reticular formation	Regulation of cerebral blood flow, alertness, mood, memory, and hormonal modulation
Dopamine	Substantia nigra, ventral tegmental area of the midbrain, and hypothalamus	Motor control, mentation, and hormonal regulation

Most dopaminergic cells are located in the substantia nigra or the ventral tegmental area of the midbrain. Traditionally, two dopaminergic systems are described (Creese 1987). The nigrostriatal dopaminergic system originates primarily in the pars compacta of the substantia nigra and ends in the dorsal striatum. Loss of neurons in this system results in Parkinson's disease. The mesolimbic dopaminergic system originates in the ventral tegmental area of the midbrain and projects to the striatum, septum, amygdala, and the frontal lobe. Some evidence suggests that excessive activity in the mesolimbic system is involved in the genesis of psychosis. A dopaminergic pathway from the posterior hypothalamus to dorsal and intermediate cell columns of the spinal cord has also been identified.

The Limbic System

The term *limbic system* was coined by MacLean in 1952 to describe the limbic lobe and those anatomic structures with which it has primary connections. More often, however, this "system" is defined functionally rather than anatomically to include those regions associated with affective and motivational behaviors.

The *limbic lobe* includes a large part of the basomedial telencephalon (Figure 2–3). Hence its primary components, visible on the medial hemispheric surface, include the cingulate and the parahippocampal gyri (which together loop around the medial diencephalic components) and the septal region (which includes the midline septum pellucidum and the septal nuclei).

In a behavioral sense, the primary components of the limbic system include, in addition to the various regions of the limbic lobe, the amygdala and the hippocampal formation (Table 2–3). These structures are located within the cerebral temporal lobe and are continuous with adjacent cerebral cortex. They also have extensive interconnections with other cortical and subcortical structures via numerous reciprocal pathways. In addition, these structures (as well as limbic lobe regions) are extensively connected to the hypothalamus, the primary brain structure involved in the integration of autonomic effects that accompany emotional expression (Figure 2–4).

The *amygdala* is actually a large heterogeneous nuclear complex, which occupies the dorsomedial portion of the temporal lobe immediately deep to the uncus. It contains several different cellular subgroups, which exhibit distinctly different cytoarchitectural and

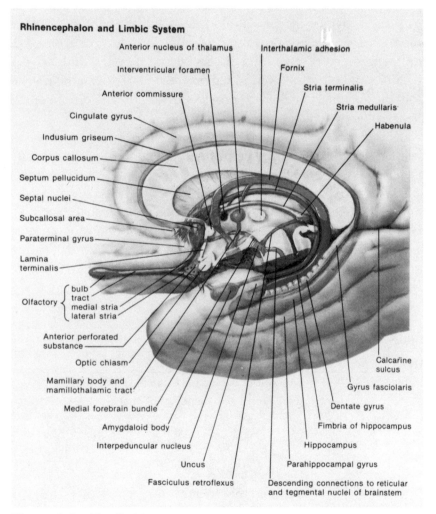

Figure 2–3. The limbic system.
Source. Reprinted from Netter FH: *CIBA Collection of Medical Illustrations,* Volume I: *Nervous System;* Part I: *Anatomy and Physiology.* Summit, NJ, CIBA, 1983, p. 27. Used with permission.

histochemical characteristics and connections. Bilateral ablation studies have implicated the amygdala in sensory-affective associations: the relation of sensory information to past experience. Thus aggressive, sexual, and eating behaviors are specifically related to amygdaloid activities. In addition, a widespread system of amygdalocortical fibers allows the amygdala to modulate and influence the activities in cortical association areas, known to be of importance for higher-order sensory functions such as storage of long-term memory. By virtue of close associations with the hypothalamus and other subcortical regions related to drive and motivation, the amygdala is likely to provide an emotional component to the learning experience.

The *hippocampal formation* is laid down embryonically when, on the medial wall of the hemisphere, the choroid plexus invaginates into the ventricle. The resultant fissure (the hippocampal sulcus) is carried downward and forward, forming an arch as the temporal lobe develops. The name *hippocampus* ("seahorse") derives from the convoluted appearance of the structure in coronal sections. The hippocampus appears immediately caudal to the amygdaloid complex in the temporal lobe. The primary components of the hippocampal formation include the hippocampus, the

Table 2–3.	Localization of limbic functions
Area	**Functions**
Limbic lobe[a]	Elevation or depression of arterial blood pressure
	Inhibition or acceleration of respiration
Amygdala	Aggression
	Sexual behavior
	Eating behavior
	Long-term memory
	Emotional component
Hippocampal formation	Learning
	Memory
	Spatial orientation

[a]Cingulate gyrus, parahippocampal gyrus, and septal region (septum pellucidum and septal nuclei).

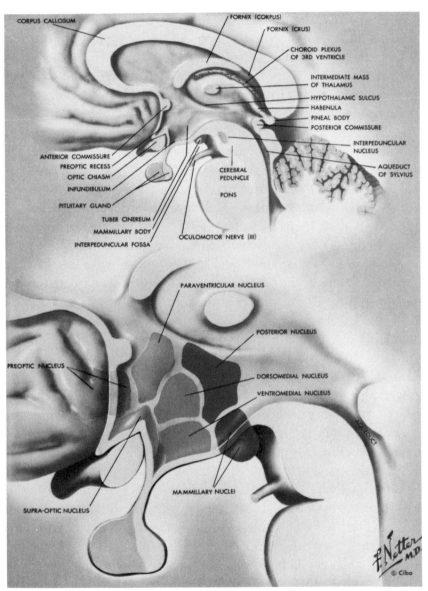

Figure 2–4. The hypothalamus.
Source. Reprinted from Netter FH: *CIBA Collection of Medical Illustrations,* Volume I: *Nervous System;* Part I: *Anatomy and Physiology.* Summit, NJ, CIBA, 1953, p. 76. Used with permission.

parahippocampal gyrus, the dentate gyrus, and the fornix.

The hippocampus proper is traditionally divided into three fields (CA$_1$, CA$_2$, and CA$_3$), based on cytoarchitonic differences (Carpenter 1976). The dentate gyrus, which interlocks with the concave surface of the hippocampus proper, is characterized primarily by cells that project into the hippocampus. The fornix is the massive fiber bundle that connects the hippocampal formation with a variety of subcortical structures, including the septum, the hypothalamus, and the anterior thalamic nucleus.

In addition to their extrinsic connections, the components of the hippocampal formation possess a complex intrinsic neuronal circuit. The dentate gyrus is richly innervated by projections from the parahippocampal gyrus, which has numerous connections with sensory cortical areas. The fibers of the dentate gyrus project, via interconnections with the hippocampus proper and the alveus, to the subiculum. The fornix, the subiculum, and the hippocampus itself send feedback projections to the sensory cortex. Behaviorally, the hippocampus is traditionally implicated in learning and memory functions. In addition, physiological studies of single hippocampal neurons indicate a critical involvement in spatial orientation mechanisms that permit recognition and prediction of environmental relationships and events.

Several other regions of the forebrain and brain stem are frequently described as components of the limbic system, based on functional associations, as well as extensive anatomic interconnections. These limbic system affiliates include neocortical areas in the basal frontotemporal region, the olfactory cortex, ventral parts of the striatum, the anterior and medial thalamic nuclei, the habenula, and parts of the medial midbrain. However, inclusion of these structures under the aegis of "limbic system" is variable (Mesulam 1985).

The Cerebral Cortex

The human cerebral cortex, a convoluted mantle six cell layers (2–4 mm) thick, is densely and richly connected to most of the lower structures of the CNS: the numerous complex cortical projections reflect the degree of cortical influence, either directly or indirectly, on practically every functional system of the entire CNS (Figure 2–5). In addition, the intrinsic circuitry of the cerebral cortex, with its myriad interneurons, collateral pathways, and synaptic relationships, provides an almost infinite number of possibilities for impulse transmission.

The cortex may be conceptually divided into motor, sensory, and association areas. Whereas primary motor function and sensory function are generally localized to specific regions of the frontal or parietal cortex according to Brodmann's cytoarchitectural mapping scheme, association areas are represented by more general territories in the frontal lobe (the prefrontal cortex) and by extensive parietotemporal regions. Association cortex, then, is involved in associative functions such as the analysis and elaboration of sensory information.

Information about the localization of cortical functions in humans has depended historically on lesion or cortical stimulation studies. More recently, radiographic technologies have permitted the dynamic mapping of brain function based on measurements of cerebral blood flow or metabolic rate. General concepts correlating cortical regions with specific behavioral characteristics have been established, although the macroscopic boundaries by which hemispheric lobes and gyri are defined do not necessarily indicate strict functional boundaries (Table 2–4).

That portion of the *frontal lobe* located immediately anterior to the central sulci is related to control of movement; this is true of all mammalian brains. However, the prefrontal cortex, occupying approximately a quarter of the total cerebral cortex, has increased dramatically in size and complexity in humans. Prefrontal cortical function is subtle and therefore difficult to describe with a high degree of specificity. Some insights have been gained, however, from studying patients who have experienced frontal lobe damage or psychosurgical procedures. Based on these analyses, the frontal lobe seems to be crucially involved in the organization and control of both intellectual and emotional factors of behavior. Many aspects of personality seem to be mediated by prefrontal cortex, including the perceptions of self-awareness and of the consequences of one's behavior. In fact, via numerous connections with the major cortical

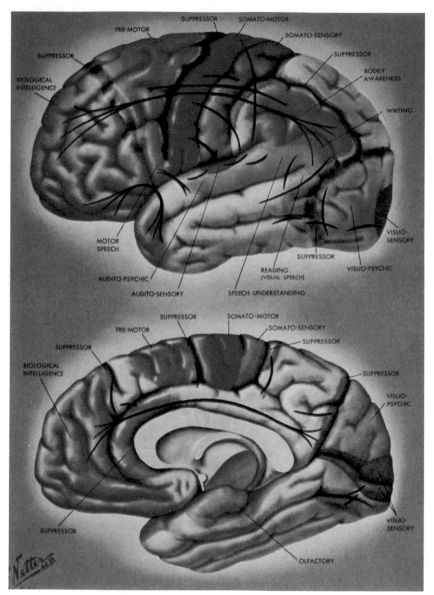

Figure 2–5. The cerebral cortex.
Source. Reprinted from Netter FH: *CIBA Collection of Medical Illustrations,* Volume I: *Nervous System,* Part I: *Anatomy and Physiology.* Summit, NJ, CIBA, 1953, p. 74. Used with permission.

and subcortical regions of the brain, the frontal cortex can continuously monitor internal and external stimuli; the close topographic association with motor control areas facilitates the behavioral response to such input.

In the *parietal lobe*, the postcentral gyrus has been well characterized as the terminal target tissue of ascending tactile and proprioceptive impulses. Most of the remainder of the lobe, the extensive posterior parietal association cortex, is generally considered to be a sensory association area for higher-order processing such as the integration of visual, auditory, and somatosensory stimuli.

The *temporal lobe* contains receiving areas for the olfactory (in the region of the uncus) and auditory (deep to the lateral fissure) systems. In addition, the posterior temporal lobe is involved in language functions, as are the nearby occipital and parietal areas. Interestingly, extensive areas on the underside of the temporal and occipital lobes are of special importance for facial recognition.

Due to the subcortical temporal loci of the amygdala and the hippocampal formation, the temporal lobe is considered to be intricately involved in memory functions. Not surprisingly, some of the cortical areas in the temporal lobe have been identified as neocorticolimbic associative areas.

Table 2–4.   Localization of cortical functions

Area	Functions
Frontal lobe	
Precentral gyrus	Motor control
Prefrontal cortex	Organization and control of intellectual and emotional factors of behavior
Parietal lobe	
Postcentral gyrus	Tactile sensation and perception
Sensory associative area	Integration of visual, somatosensory, and auditory stimuli
Temporal lobe	Olfaction
	Audition
	Language
	Memory
	Facial recognition

The Pathophysiology of Brain Injury

Two distinct components contribute to the pathophysiology of brain injury: 1) the immediate trauma resulting from the biomechanical forces applied to the cranial contents and 2) the secondary complications that develop from the subsequent metabolic perturbations. The first component is a function of an accidental event and cannot yet be affected by treatment. On the other hand, prompt and appropriate medical or surgical intervention often plays a key role in alleviating secondary complications and improving the potential for recovery of a patient with brain injury.

The Primary Effects of Brain Injury

The initial assessment of any head injury begins with the determination of the type and degree of structural damage sustained by the protective skull. Hence an "open" head injury results from the penetration of the cranium and durae, as in the case of missile wounds such as gun shots. Generally, these injuries tend to be more focal, damaging discrete regions of tissue; critical care calls for immediate attention to the likely presence of foreign bodies, hemorrhage, and tissue contamination. On the other hand, "closed" head injuries are likely to be much more subtle, with the foci of lesions difficult, perhaps impossible, to pinpoint either by clinical examination or with current neuroimaging techniques. Nonetheless, closed head injuries are far more common in most clinical settings, and will therefore be the focus of the following discussion. The principal hallmarks of closed head injuries are contusional damage and diffuse axonal injury.

∎ **Contusions.** The physical forces that are applied to the head during trauma are both translational and angular. Hence when they occur as a result of acceleration, as in the case of motor vehicle accidents, the resultant brain damage is likely to be greater than that produced by crushing injuries to the stationary head. Two factors must be considered in analyzing the association between physical forces and brain injury: the energetics of brain tissue displacement and the spatial environment of the cranial cavity. Although translational acceleration is produced by a force vector applied through the center of gravity of a rigid body, rotational acceleration occurs when the force vector does not pass through the object's center of gravity. Under this circumstance, the object will rotate around its own center of gravity. In most clinical circumstances, forces applied to the head produce both translational and angular acceleration.

The pathology produced by translational acceleration is due to the differences between the densities of the skull and the brain. In response to a blow to the head, the skull itself and the soft tissue contents are propelled forward at different rates. Hence the displacement of bone with respect to the brain causes abrasive frictional forces that damage the brain surface. In addition, when the forward momentum of the skull is abruptly stopped by contact with an immovable object, the brain continues forward until it collides with the internal surface of the skull opposite the point of initial impact. Due to the relative elasticity of the cranial contents, the abrasive and collisional forces will be repeated through several oscillations during deceleration. Hence during the dynamic interval of asynchronous skull and brain acceleration and deceleration, the friable cortical surface is exposed to repeated impacts. Therefore, contusional lesions are commonly seen in brain tissues that interface with unyielding edges, ridges, and protuberances within the cranial cavity: the irregular orbital plate of the frontal bone, the sphenoidal ridge, the petrous portion of the temporal bone, and the sharp edges of the falces (see Figure 2–6). Therefore, the basal and polar portions of the frontal and temporal lobes, because of their topographic proximity to these unyielding structures, are particularly vulnerable to contusional injury (see Figure 2–7) (Courville 1937).

However, not all contusional lesions are confined to cortical areas that interface with rigid structures. The cavitation theory explains the common presence of surface injuries removed from any abrasive bony surfaces (Pang 1989). Based on a theoretical model of an aqueous solution contained within an inextensible shell, it may be predicted that, upon external impact, the fluid molecules will translocate toward the impact pole and away from the opposite pole, creating a pressure gradient. Hence as brain tissue displaces toward the site of impact, negative pressure causes a spontaneous but transient liquid-to-gas phase shift among aqueous molecules in

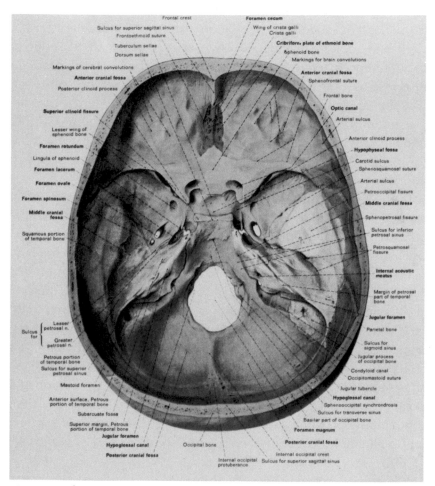

Figure 2–6. The base of the skull: internal aspect (*superior view*).
Source. Reprinted from Clemente CD: *Anatomy: A Regional Atlas of the Human Body.* Philadelphia, PA, Lea & Febiger/Munich, Germany, Urban & Schwarzenberg, 1975 (Figure 480). Used with permission.

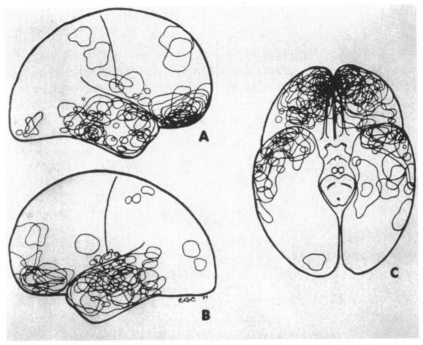

Figure 2–7. Composite views demonstrating contusional localization.

the region of the opposite pole. The explosive nature of the phase shift and the concomitant abrupt pressure changes result in the "contrecoup" lesions in the brain regions opposite impact sites (Figure 2–8). Because brain tissue has been shown to withstand positive pressure much better than negative pressure, brain regions near the site of impact (coup lesions) are generally spared the serious injury caused by translational trauma.

The radius of curvature of the brain surface and the configuration of area gyri are also factors contributing to the regional severity of brain injury. The net effect of cavitation is accentuated in large flat regions with shallow sulci, where superficial surface area is maximal. This factor contributes to the extensive damage frequently seen on the basal surface of the frontal lobes. Pressure gradients also affect the microvasculature of the brain. Cavitation injures the capillary endothelium, often resulting in small focal hemorrhages.

■ **Diffuse axonal injury.** Diffuse axonal injury can be produced either biomechanically or neurochemically. Biomechanically, the shearing forces between brain tissues of different densities may physically damage cellular structure. Neurochemically, cytotoxic factors released into the cellular milieu at the time of impact may

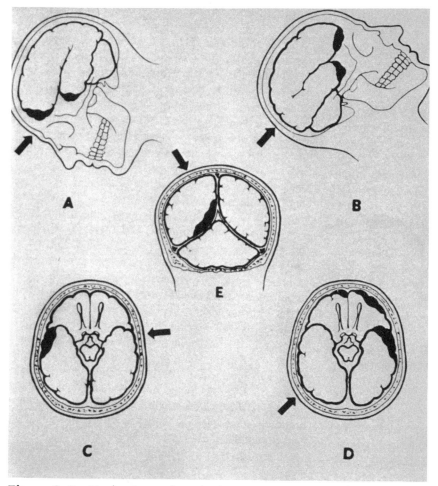

Figure 2–8. Mechanisms of cerebral contusion. *Arrows* indicate force vector. *Darkened areas* indicate contusional location.
Source. Reprinted from Adams R, Victor M: *Principles of Neurology.* New York, McGraw-Hill, 1985, p. 646. Used with permission.

initiate a cascade of metabolic events that eventually lead to neuronal death. Paradoxically, these devastating injuries are rarely detectable despite the use of modern diagnostic imaging techniques.

Deep brain lesions are thought to result from rotational forces that produce shearing between structures of varying densities and differential mobility (Alexander 1982). These effects are most prominent at junctures between gray matter and white fiber tracts. Tissues found in each of the three functional divisions of the brain are particularly vulnerable to this type of injury, including the reticular formation and the superior cerebellar peduncles (of the brain stem), regions of the basal ganglia, hypothalamus, and fornices (of the limbic system), and the corpus callosum (of the cerebral hemispheres). Widespread tissue disruption may occur at these sites, accompanied by microhemorrhages and eventual axonal degeneration (Figure 2–9). The composite effect of these lesions includes acute and chronic disturbances of consciousness, vestibular dysfunction, and a variety of motor impairments. The most devastating long-term consequences, however, arise from the resultant disconnection syndromes that dissociate higher, modulatory cortical structures from their lower, drive-producing counterparts. It is this disconnection that accounts for much of the psychiatric morbidity seen in patients with brain injury.

Another phenomenon producing diffuse axonal injury is delayed cell degeneration. This construct first attracted interest when it became clear that not all diffuse axonal injuries could be attributed to acute shearing forces (Pilz 1983). The apparent lag time between the acute injury and the development of delayed sequelae suggested the potential for medical intervention to improve outcomes (Povlishock 1991). It has been hypothesized that traumatic brain injury focally alters the axonal cytoskeleton resulting in impaired axoplasmic transport (Povlishock 1992). This leads to axonal swelling, which eventuates in axonal detachment approximately 6 to 12 hours after the injury. The proximal axonal segment attached to the neuronal soma collapses and undergoes Wallerian degeneration.

In addition to these biomechanical perturbations, the effect of massive neuroexcitation has been studied in an attempt to under-

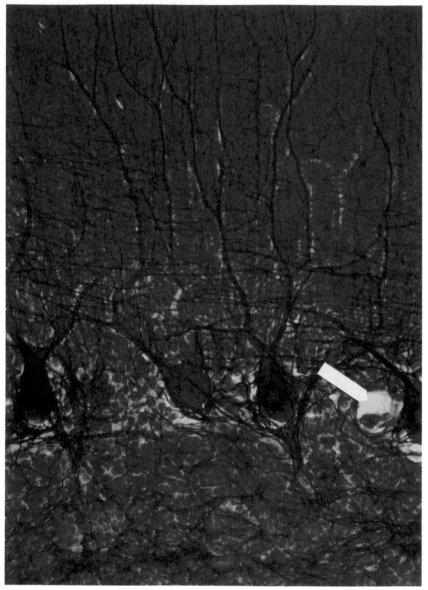

Figure 2–9. Retraction ball indicating axonal degeneration.
Source. Photo copyright by Manfred Kage, Peter Arnold Inc., 1984.
Used with permission.

stand the changes associated with diffuse injury. Calcium, magnesium, free radicals, and excitatory neurotransmitters such as acetylcholine, *N*-methyl-D-aspartate (NMDA), and glutamate have all been implicated in this process. Because much of the total energy expenditure of neurons is devoted to the tight control of intracellular concentrations of ions, the loss of ion gradients across the plasma membrane is indicative of energy failure and incipient necrosis. In terms of the response to brain injury, perturbations in intracellular concentrations of calcium and magnesium have received the most attention.

Normally, calcium plays a major role in neuronal synaptic activity by serving as a second messenger that can trigger the activity of phosphatases, kinases, lipases, and proteases. Cellular function and viability are highly dependent, therefore, on tightly controlling the intracellular concentrations of the ion against a very steep (23,000 to 1) calcium gradient between the extracellular and intracellular compartments (Siegel et al. 1981). During normal neuronal transmission, a stimulus triggers a modulated influx of ion through calcium-specific channels. Following its function as a second messenger, calcium is actively extruded (principally via a Ca^{2+}/Na^+ antiport system) or sequestered intracellularly. The disruption of these regulatory mechanisms leads to a rapid increase in the intracellular concentration of calcium, activating a variety of lipases and proteases. The effects of uncontrolled calcium influx are exacerbated by the presence of free radicals, highly reactive charged molecules, which tend to bind to and degrade cell membranes. The synergy of calcium with free radicals produces arachidonic acid, which in turn is converted to the vasoactive metabolites, prostaglandins and leukotrienes. These products further compromise blood flow to already ischemic neural tissue (Faden et al. 1989).

In normal brain tissue, magnesium plays a role in a number of ATP-mediated cellular processes. Electrochemical gradients across the plasma membrane maintain intracellular concentrations approximately 50 times greater than those in extracellular stores. Vink et al. (1988) have demonstrated that following brain injury, intracellular levels of magnesium decline sharply with the decay of the membrane potential, in close correlation with the severity of injury.

Thus the unavailability of magnesium is probably a key factor in the failure of a number of intracellular mechanisms, including membrane integrity, ATPase functioning, cofactor synthesis, and mitochondrial respiration (McIntosh et al. 1989, 1990).

Whereas calcium and magnesium may be the final common pathways to neuronal destruction, excitatory neurotransmitters certainly play a role in setting the cascade in motion. Acetylcholine was the first neurotransmitter to be systematically evaluated in this regard (Hayes et al. 1984). In a series of elaborate studies, Lyeth et al. (1988) demonstrated that acetylcholine is responsible for transient behavioral suppression following mild to moderate brain injury. It appears that this effect is mediated by an inhibitory cholinergic system located in the rostral pons and exacerbated by the disruption of the blood-brain barrier, which permits an influx of peripherally produced acetylcholine into the CNS. In addition, muscarinic receptors, binding sites for free acetylcholine, may mediate the permeability characteristics of cell membranes throughout the CNS. Therefore, damage to the acetylcholine system contributes to the overall disruption of ion homeostasis.

Excitatory amino acids have little effect on consciousness, but perturbations in their concentrations seem to produce long-term behavioral effects. Although the exact mechanisms have not been established, glutamate and aspartate analogs have been shown to cause postsynaptic dendritic swelling and cell death in proportion to their potential for excitation (Olney 1983). Other putative excitatory amino acids appear to function as endogenous cytotoxins: kainic acid, NMDA, and homocysteic acid, as well as glutamate (Faden et al. 1989).

Intracranial Secondary Effects of Brain Injury

Although some new acute management protocols are being evaluated at several neurotrauma centers throughout the United States, the primary damage resulting from head injury begins instantaneously and, therefore, at this time, cannot be directly addressed therapeutically. Thus initial trauma care is directed toward preventing or limiting the secondary damage that occurs over time subsequent to the initial injury. Secondary processes of significance within the CNS include traumatic hematomas, cerebral edema, hydrocephalus, and increased intracranial pressure, which can lead not only to ischemia, but also to a number of herniation syndromes (Table 2–5). Intracranial infection and a number of systemic factors may also affect the potential for CNS recovery.

❚ **Traumatic hematomas.** Traumatic hematomas result from lacerations or shear stress to the vasculature supplying the brain. About 90% of *epidural hematomas* (characterized by bleeding between the skull and the dura) are associated with skull fractures (Ford and Mclaurin 1963). Generally, bleeding may originate from lacerated dural vessels or from ruptured venous sinuses. Arterial bleeding results in rapidly expanding extravasation, which creates a mass lesion that requires immediate evacuation. Whereas epidural hematomas along the cranial convexity tend to diffuse spatially, clots located in either the temporal region or the posterior fossa of the cranial cavity tend to form bulky boluses, which may cause brain stem herniation. In a few instances, epidural hematomas may occur without concomitant skull fracture, as a result of oozing from damaged epidural veins; such lesions are generally asymptomatic and resolve spontaneously without surgical intervention.

 Subdural hematomas result from lacerated cortical vessels that bleed into the subdural space, exposing the cortex itself to blood and blood products. These lesions are more common than epidural hematomas and produce greater morbidity and higher mortality. The vascular damage is usually associated with underlying cortical contusion and parenchymal edema. Surgical intervention therefore involves both the evacuation of the clot and the resection of necrotic brain tissue. Patient outcome therefore depends not only on expeditious neurosurgical intervention, but also on the location and extent of the lesion and the degree of edema (Miller et al. 1990). In addition, because the dura must be surgically penetrated, infection is another potential complication.

 Intracerebral hematomas are vascular extravasations within the substance of the brain itself. Depressed skull fractures and missile wounds produce the largest of these lesions. However, deep shear-

Table 2–5. Secondary effects of brain injury

Secondary injury	Site	Anatomic involvement	Clinical effects
Hematomas			
Epidural	Between skull and dura	Lacerated veins or dural sinuses	Expanding mass lesions, herniation
Subdural	Arachnoid space	Lacerated cortical arteries	Cortical contusions, parenchymal edema
Intracerebral	Within brain parenchyma	Vascular occlusion at arterial border zones	Bleeding and herniation
Cerebral edemas			
Vasogenic	Extracellular space	Disruption of blood-brain barrier	Increased intracranial pressure
Cytotoxic	Intracellular space	Disruption of cell membrane gradients	Edema, ischemia
Hydrocephalus	Arachnoid villi or ventricular system	Blockage of cerebrospinal fluid circulation	Increased intracranial pressure
Increased intracranial pressure	Global	Ischemia	Ischemic encephalopathy, herniations
Herniations			
Subfalcine	Midsagittal hemispheric surface	Displacement of cingulate gyrus	Contralateral motor impairment
Transtentorial	Midbrain Pons Ascending reticular activating system Hippocampus	Shearing of ascending and descending pathways, entrapment of oculomotor nerve	Decerebrate rigidity coma, memory loss, oculomotor compression syndrome
Tonsillar	Brain stem Upper spinal cord	Trauma to medulla and cerebellar tonsils	Loss of vasomotor and respiratory control centers

ing injuries are the most common and dangerous cause of smaller intracerebral hematomas. These infarctions often occur at the border zone between regions supplied by the anterior cerebral and middle cerebral arteries. Within several days of the initial trauma, these small lesions may coalesce into a large hematoma that can lead to rapid herniation. This emergency is often precipitated by renewed bleeding as vessels previously tamponaded by edema and vasospasm continue to deteriorate over time (Teasdale and Mendelow 1984).

∎ **Cerebral edema.** Cerebral edema is another secondary process that can produce significant complications following traumatic brain injury. It is best understood as an increase in the total volume of water in the brain. Two types of brain edema, vasogenic and cytotoxic edema, are relevant to the clinical outcome following head trauma (Miller 1979).

Vasogenic edema is characterized by the accumulation of excess water in the extracellular space. Whereas systemic capillaries are fenestrated to allow both lipid- and water-soluble molecules to diffuse freely between the plasma and the tissue compartments, the blood-brain barrier of the CNS has tight junctions that block the passive transport of most water-soluble molecules. Following any significant degree of brain trauma, however, the blood-brain barrier is disrupted, permitting the passive diffusion of solutes and water across the endothelial lining according to their concentration gradients. The clinical manifestations of vasogenic edema gradually evolve during the first several hours following the primary injury. These processes generally peak within a few days, assuming that no further insults occur to the CNS and herniation syndromes do not develop. If autoregulatory mechanisms survive, homeostasis may be reestablished as excess fluids and solutes enter the ventricular system and are reabsorbed back into the intravascular space. If the blood-brain barrier is reestablished, clinical management may involve the use of intravenous hyperosmolar agents such as mannitol to enhance the intravascular osmotic gradients, permitting free water to be preferentially absorbed from the extravascular space back into the plasma. However, if the blood-brain barrier is severely damaged, hyperosmolar agents may filter into the extravascular space, increasing the water content of that compartment and leading to unintended and unwanted increases in intracranial pressure (Klatzo and Seitelberger 1967).

In *cytotoxic edema,* the membranes of individual cells (neurons, astroglia, and endothelia) are impaired so that water diffuses from the extracellular to the intracellular space. Normally, energy-dependent ion pumps in the cell membrane maintain an electrochemical gradient between the external and internal cellular milieus. If the ion gradients are disrupted, normally excluded ions flood into the cell; osmotic gradients are perturbed, cellular energy stores are depleted, and water passively enters the cell. As endothelial cells swell, capillary lumina are blocked, setting up a lethal cycle of edema and ischemia. This condition cannot be treated by hyperosmotic agents, which function by setting up concentration gradients between the vascular and extracellular compartments.

∎ **Hydrocephalus.**   Hydrocephalus is characterized by an excessive amount of cerebrospinal fluid in the ventricular system. The condition may occur following head injury when the arachnoid villi become blocked by blood or other foreign substances that interfere with the normal absorption of cerebrospinal fluid. In addition, any swelling or distortion of the cranial contents may result in the blockage of the narrow passageways of the ventricular system, notably the interventricular foramina and the cerebral aqueduct.

∎ **Increased intracranial pressure.**   Hematomas, edema, and hydrocephalus (each of them alone or in combination) may potentially increase intracranial pressure. Because the skull is essentially inextensible, an increase in the volume of any of the intracranial contents, including glia, neurons, blood, cerebrospinal fluid, and extracellular fluid, may lead to elevated intracranial pressure. Increases in intracranial pressure are not directly linear with respect to intracranial volume, however. Normally, the CNS is inherently capable of compensating for increases in one compartment by concomitantly decreasing the pressure in others. However, once these compensatory mechanisms begin to fail, as they frequently do in severe brain injury, intracranial pressure begins to rise dramatically (Miller and Adams 1984). As the brain becomes increasingly inelastic, damage to the brain mounts exponentially.

Increases in intracranial pressure will ultimately diminish cerebral blood flow, leading to ischemia. The CNS has substantial autoregulatory capabilities over a wide range of systemic mean arterial pressures, as it does over a range of intracranial pressures. However, following brain trauma, autoregulation is generally impaired so that even relatively small elevations in intracranial pressure will result in significant reductions in cerebral blood flow. When increases in intracranial pressure are accompanied by decreases in systemic blood pressure, cerebral blood flow is critically reduced and ischemic encephalopathy is likely to result.

In addition to causing ischemia, increases in intracranial pressure can cause physical shifts of brain tissue from one intracranial compartment to another, leading to a number of herniation syndromes. These shifts may be unilateral or bilateral. There are three common sites of tissue displacement, based on the vector of herniation generated by the foci of increased pressure, as well as the conformation of the partitions of the cranial cavity (Pang 1989). The most common of these shifts is a *subfalcine herniation*: an asymmetric mass lesion forces the tissue of the cingulate gyrus under the edge of the falx cerebri into the contralateral hemispheric space. This type of herniation is often asymptomatic, although visible in neuroimaging studies. At times, however, the anterior cerebral artery may be entrapped, compromising blood flow to the motor cortical areas and producing symptoms in the contralateral lower extremity.

Transtentorial herniation is likely to result in much more grave consequences. In this case, basal portions of the temporal lobe are displaced medially and caudally, insinuating between the midbrain and the tentorial margin. The clinical effects of this syndrome include ptosis, pupillary dilation, and ocular paralysis as a result of oculomotor nerve compression. Brain stem distortion and the concomitant vascular occlusion frequently lead to decerebrate rigidity as a result of disruption of inhibitory influences from higher centers. Irreversible damage to pontine blood vessels and subsequent ischemia in the region of the reticular activating system account for the progressively deeper coma that may ensue. Because the hippocampal formation may be damaged by this process, memory difficulties are frequent among those who survive this complication.

Tonsillar herniation results from the extrusion of the medulla and the cerebellar tonsils through the foramen magnum. The lower brain stem and the upper spinal cord may be crushed against the bony ring of the occipital bone. Damage to the vagal motor nuclei in the medulla can lead to death as a result of loss of vasomotor and respiratory control centers.

∎ **Infection.** Intracranial infections, in the form of brain abscess or meningitis, may develop a few days after severe head injury (Miller 1976). Infectious organisms are most often introduced into the cranial cavity by compound depressed fractures of the calvarium or by fractures of the skull base and nasal sinuses. General impairment of the systemic immune responses resulting from severe trauma of any kind may also contribute to the development of intracranial infections. The mass effect of brain abscesses may lead to increased intracranial pressure, herniation syndromes, or both. Meningitis is a more diffuse process, commonly resulting in increased intracranial pressure and hydrocephalus. Antibiotic therapies must take into consideration the likely impairment of the blood-brain barrier, which generally accompanies severe head trauma and its sequelae.

Systemic Secondary Effects

Accidents that result in brain trauma often involve injuries to other parts of the body as well. These systemic effects may exacerbate the neurobehavioral sequelae of brain injury and complicate rehabilitation efforts. Some of the primary extracranial factors that may play a significant role in brain injury (described by Miller et al. 1990) are

- Hypoxemia
- Hypotension
- Hypercapnia

- Anemia
- Hyponatremia
- Hypoglycemia
- Infection

Sixty percent of severe and 40% of moderate brain injuries are accompanied by one or more systemic complications (Pang 1989). In particular, the presence of systemic hypoxemia and/or hypotension may significantly complicate traumatic brain injuries.

▌ **Hypoxemia.** Hypoxemia occurs in more than 30% of severe traumatic brain injuries. Oxygen deficiency can occur as a result of obstruction or injury to any component of the respiratory system. Foreign bodies, blood, or vomitus, as well as the tongue, may obstruct airways. In the acute critical care of accident victims, the recognition and remediation of respiratory distress is a top priority in minimizing CNS damage, with or without direct head trauma. Aspiration of liquids can severely compromise pulmonary functioning, as can chest trauma that causes pneumo- or hemothoraxes. Pulmonary edema and adult respiratory distress syndrome may be seen in patients with brain injury despite the absence of chest trauma (Miller et al. 1990).

Even if the lungs themselves are undamaged, head injury may impair the central mechanisms that control the depth and rhythm of respiration, leading to imbalances between ventilation and perfusion. The net effect of this type of injury is a general systemic reduction in partial pressure of oxygen (PO_2). Normally, autoregulatory mechanisms in the CNS compensate for a wide range of PO_2 levels; if PO_2 falls below 55 torr, vasodilation (which increases the volume of blood delivered to the brain) and desaturation (which causes the erythrocytes to release more oxygen to the tissues) permit adequate ventilation of brain tissues (Teasdale and Mendelow 1984). However, the impairment of the autoregulatory mechanisms caused by brain stem injury leads to ischemia, especially in those regions with the highest metabolic requirements. Because areas of the temporal lobes have the highest metabolic rate of all brain regions, the temporolimbic structures that are involved in learning and memory are particularly vulnerable to hypoxemic damage, which often produces a profound amnestic syndrome.

■ **Hypotension.** Significant hypotension can be associated with a number of systemic complications: intra-abdominal or thoracic visceral injuries, pelvic fractures, and major long bone fractures. In fact, these complications are seen in 15%–20% of patients presenting to neurotrauma centers following brain injury. A mean arterial blood pressure of less than 80 torr will lead to a reduction in cerebral blood flow; therefore, if systolic blood pressure falls below 100 torr in adults, a careful search must be undertaken to rule out occult sources of systemic hemorrhage.

General medical management of patients in neurotrauma centers requires close monitoring of all the primary extracranial factors listed above. In particular, fluid and electrolyte imbalances often occur as a result of pituitary dysfunction associated with traumatic brain injury. Infection, especially of pulmonary etiology, can significantly compound the metabolic demands and compromise ventilation efforts.

Electrophysiological Abnormalities Following Brain Injury

One of the most enduring problems arising from CNS trauma is the occurrence of electrophysiological abnormalities that may eventuate in seizures. The presence of seizures within the first week following traumatic injury is not by itself predictive of the development of posttraumatic epilepsy (Young et al. 1983). However, the occurrence of early seizures is one risk factor for its development, following closed head injury in particular (Jennett 1975). Other risk factors and their relative weightings in the production of posttraumatic epilepsy are listed in Table 2–6 (Feeney and Walker 1979).

The onset of frank posttraumatic epilepsy often occurs during the first year following traumatic brain injury, but it may be discovered much later. This is especially true of complex partial epilepsy emanating from a temporolimbic focus. The prevalence of epilepsy following all closed head injuries ranges from 2% to 5% (Annegers et al. 1980; Jennett 1987). However, with severe injuries the risk may rise to 7% during the first year and to nearly 12% by the fifth year (Annegers et al. 1980).

Epilepsy following brain injury can take several forms. Many patients may exhibit more than one type of seizure. Some focal features are noted, especially at the onset of seizure, in approximately half of those individuals who develop posttraumatic epilepsy. However, in most cases, seizures will tend to spread and become more generalized. Classic major motor epilepsy without focal onset occurs in another 40%–50% of patients and is the most physically disabling form of traumatic epilepsy (Jennett 1990). However, complex partial epilepsy, which develops in 30%–50% of cases, is the most psychiatrically devastating type of seizure disorder.

Over 30% of patients with epilepsy are at risk of developing severe psychiatric sequelae (Ferguson and Rayport 1984), including psychosis. Even in the absence of frank epilepsy, temporolimbic

Table 2–6. Risk factors and their relative weightings in the production of posttraumatic epilepsy

Risk factors	Relative weightings
Centroparietal lesion	.25
Dural penetration	.20
Hemiparesis or aphasia	.20
Hemorrhage	.20
Early seizures	.15
Temporal lesion	.15
Depressed skull fracture	.10
Persistent EEG abnormality	.10
Prefrontal lesion	.10
Occipital lesion	.10
Central nervous system infection	.10
Loss of consciousness, PTA > 1 hour	.05
Linear skull fracture	.05

Note. EEG = electroencephalogram; PTA = posttraumatic amnesia.

dysrhythmias have been associated with neurologically mediated forms of aggression. In fact, if a patient's neuropsychiatric status deteriorates during the postacute phase of rehabilitation, one should always suspect the evolution of an underlying seizure diathesis. Anticonvulsant prophylaxis for this patient population remains an area of continuing controversy. See Chapter 16 for further elaboration of these issues.

In conclusion, Sir Charles Symonds put it well in 1937 when he wrote,

> The later effects of head injury can only be properly understood in the light of a full psychiatric study of the individual patient, and in particular, his constitution. In other words, it is not only the kind of injury that matters, but also the kind of head.

In this chapter I have focused on the injury characteristics that lead to the functional and behavioral constraints imposed by traumatic head injury on its survivors. The care and neuropsychiatric management of patients with brain injury must, therefore, take into consideration not only the cognitive, behavioral, and emotional sequelae of the primary and secondary injuries, but also the structural, metabolic, and biochemical perturbations that underlie the condition. Subsequent chapters will integrate these concepts into therapeutic paradigms, which should ultimately mediate the neurobehavioral rehabilitation of these individuals.

References

Adams R, Victor M: Principles of Neurology. New York, McGraw-Hill, 1985

Alexander MP: Traumatic brain injury, in Psychiatric Aspects of Neurologic Disease, Vol II. Edited by Benson DF, Blumer E. New York, Grune & Stratton, 1982, pp 219–248

Annegers JF, Grabow JD, Groover RV, et al: Seizures after head injury in a population study. Neurology 30:683–689, 1980

Azmitia ED: The CNS serotonergic system: progression toward a collaborative organization, in Psychopharmacology, The Third Generation of Progress. Edited by Meltzer HY. New York, Raven Press, 1987, pp 61–73

Broca P: Anatomic comparee circonvolutions cerebrales. Le grad lobe limbique et la scissure limbique dans la serie des mammiferes. Revue d'Anthropologie 1 (ser 2):384–498, 1878

Carpenter MB: Human Neuroanatomy. Baltimore, MD, Williams & Wilkins, 1976

Clemente CD: Anatomy: A Regional Atlas of the Human Body. Philadelphia, PA, Lea & Febiger/Munich, Germany, Urban & Schwarzenberg, 1975

Courville CG: Pathology of the Central Nervous System, Part IV. Mountain View, CA, Pacific, 1937

Creese I: Biochemical properties of CNS dopamine receptors, in Psychopharmacology, The Third Generation of Progress. Edited by Meltzer HY. New York, Raven Press, 1987, pp 257–264

Faden A, Demediuk P, Panter S, et al: The role of excitatory amino acids and NMDA receptors in traumatic brain injury. Science 244:798–800, 1989

Feeney DM, Walker AE: The prediction of posttraumatic epilepsy: a mathematical approach. Arch Neurol 36:8–12, 1979

Ferguson SM, Rayport M: Psychosis in epilepsy, in Psychiatric Aspects of Epilepsy. Edited by Blumer D. Washington, DC, American Psychiatric Press, 1984, pp 229–270

Ford LE, Mclaurin RL: Mechanisms of extradural hematomas. J Neurosurg 20:760–769, 1963

Hayes RL, Pechura CM, Katayama Y, et al: Activation of pontine cholinergic sites implicated in unconsciousness following cerebral concussion in the cat. Science 233:301–303, 1984

Horstadius S: The Neural Crest. London, Oxford University Press, 1950

Janowsky A, Sulser F: Alpha and beta adrenoreceptors in brain, in Psychopharmacology, The Third Generation of Progress. Edited by Meltzer HY. New York, Raven Press, 1987, pp 249–256

Jennett B: Epilepsy after Non-Missile Head Injuries, 2nd Edition. London, Heinemann, 1975

Jennett B: Epilepsy after head injury and intracranial surgery, in Epilepsy. Edited by Hopkins AP. London, Chapman Hall, 1987, pp 401–411

Jennett B: Post-traumatic epilepsy, in Rehabilitation of the Adult and Child with Traumatic Brain Injury. Edited by Rosenthal M, Griffith ER, Bond MR, et al. Philadelphia, PA, F.A. Davis Company, 1990, pp 89–93

Klatzo I, Seitelberger F: Brain Edema. New York, Springer-Verlag, 1967

Lyeth BG, Dixon CE, Hamm RJ, et al: Effects of anticholinergic treatment on transient behavioral suppression and physiological responses following concussive brain injury to the rat. Brain Res 448:88–97, 1988

MacLean PD: Some psychiatric implications of physiological studies on frontotemporal portions of limbic system (visceral brain). Electroencephalogr Clin Neurophysiol 4:407–418, 1952

MacLean PD: A Triune Concept of the Brain and Behavior. Toronto, Canada, University of Toronto Press, 1973

McIntosh T, Vink R, Soares H, et al: Effects of *N*-Methyl-D-Aspartate receptor blocker MK-801 on neurologic function after experimental brain injury. J Neurotrauma 6:247–259, 1989

McIntosh T, Vink R, Soares H, et al: Effects of noncompetitive blockade of *N*-Methyl-D-Aspartate receptors in neurochemical sequelae of experimental brain injury. J Neurochem 55:1170–1179, 1990

Mesulam MM: Patterns in behavioral neuroanatomy: association areas, the limbic system, and hemispheric specialization, in Principles of Behavioral Neurology. Edited by Mesulam MM. Philadelphia, PA, F.A. Davis Company, 1985, pp 1–70

Miller JD: Infection in head injury, in Handbook of Neurology, Vol 24. Injuries of the Brain and Skull, Part II. Edited by R. Braakman. Amsterdam, North Holland, 1976, pp 215–230

Miller JD: Clinical management of cerebral oedema. Br J Hosp Med 21:152–166, 1979

Miller JD, Adams JH: The pathophysiology of raised intracranial pressure, in Greenfield's Neuropathology, 4th Edition. Edited by Adams JH, Corsellis JAN, Duchen LW. London, Edward Arnold, 1984, pp 53–84

Miller JD, Pentland B, Berol S: Early evaluation and management, in Rehabilitation of the Adult and Child with Traumatic Brain Injury, 2nd Edition. Edited by Rosenthal M, Griffith ER, Bond MR, et al. Philadelphia, PA, F.A. Davis Company, 1990, pp 21–51

Moruzzi G, Magoun HW: Brainstem reticular formation and activation of the EEG. Electroencephalogr Clin Neurophysiol 1:455–473, 1949

Netter FH: CIBA Collection of Medical Illustrations, Volume I: Nervous System; Part I: Anatomy and Physiology. Summit, NJ, CIBA, 1983

Olney JW: Excitotoxins: an overview, in Excitotoxins. Edited by Fuxe K, Roberts P, Schwarcz R. New York, MacMillan, 1983, pp 82–96

Pang D: Physics and pathophysiology of closed head injury, in Assessment of the Behavioral Consequences of Head Trauma. Edited by Lezak MD. New York, Alan R. Liss, Inc., 1989, 1–17

Pilz P: Axonal injury in head injury. Acta Neurochir Suppl 32:119–124, 1983

Povlishock J: Current concepts on axonal damage due to head injury. Proceedings of the XIth International Congress of Neuropathy 4 (suppl):749–753, 1991

Povlishock J: Traumatically induced axonal injury: pathogenesis and pathobiological implications. Brain Pathology 2:1–12, 1992

Siegel GJ, Stahl WL, Swanson PD: Ion transport, in Basic Neurochemistry. Edited by Siegal GJ, Albers RW, Agranoff BW, et al. Boston, MA, Little, Brown & Co., 1981, pp 107–143

Symonds C: Mental disorder following head injury (1937), in Studies in Neurology. London, Oxford University Press, 1970, pp 128–142

Teasdale G, Mendelow D: Pathophysiology of head injuries, in Closed Head Injury: Psychological, Social, and Family Consequences. Edited by Brooks N. Oxford, Oxford University Press, 1984, pp 4–36

Vink R, McIntosh TK, Demediuk P, et al: Decline in intracellular free Mg^{++} is associated with irreversible tissue injury following brain trauma. J Biol Chem 263:757–761, 1988

Young B, Rapp RP, Norton JA, et al: Failure of prophylactically administered phenytoin to prevent late post-traumatic seizures. J Neurosurg 58:236–241, 1983

Chapter 3

Neuropsychiatric Assessment

Craig A. Taylor, M.D.
Trevor R. P. Price, M.D.

A traumatic brain injury (TBI) is a significant event that may result in dramatic alterations in the individual's cognition, behavior, and emotion. The neuropsychiatric manifestations of such an injury depend on several factors: 1) preexisting variables such as the patient's personality before the injury, family psychiatric history, and previous psychiatric, medical, and neurological history; 2) the patient's psychosocial, economic, and vocational status at the time of injury; 3) the type, location, and severity of the brain injury; 4) the emotional and psychological responses of the individual to the TBI-mediated disturbances in cognition and behavior; and 5) the impact of such changes on personal and professional roles, relationships, and family. The multiple variables that result in these neurobehavioral disturbances subsequent to TBI require a comprehensive and integrated approach to data collection, diagnostic formulation, and treatment.

Clinical Assessment:
The Biopsychosocial Approach

A useful conceptual framework for the neuropsychiatric assessment is the biopsychosocial model. The biopsychosocial model integrates clinical data from three interrelated domains: 1) biological disturbances in brain function; 2) the patient's emotional and psychological reaction to impairments in cognition and behavior, including his or her awareness and acceptance of these deficits; and 3) the disruptions of interpersonal relationships, family interactions, and work capacities. A comprehensive, integrated clinical assessment based on such a framework will lead to the identification of specific problem areas, a multidimensional formulation of etiology, and development of treatment approaches that focus narrowly and specifically on the patient's problems.

In this chapter we describe the neuropsychiatric evaluation of the patient with TBI. Fundamental to a comprehensive neuropsychiatric evaluation of the patient with TBI is a thorough understanding of the neurobehavioral phenomena that are associated with the type and location of the traumatic lesion, the severity of the brain injury, and the phase of recovery. The patient's symptomatology occurs in the context of alterations in brain function that lead to acquired biologically-mediated disturbances in cognition, emotion, and behavior. This biopsychosocial model forms a framework for recognizing and understanding the neuropsychological and neurocognitive factors that affect a patient's adjustment and function.

History Related to the Brain
Injury and Recovery Period

There are a number of questions and concerns that are particularly relevant to the neuropsychiatric assessment of the patient with TBI. Traditionally the clinical database begins with the elicitation of the patient's chief complaint, which may or may not include a spontaneous report of a history of TBI. Therefore, the clinician must specifically inquire as to whether there is any history of TBI. The clinician should ask about automobile, bicycle, and motorcycle accidents, as well as falls, assaults, and sports or recreational accidents. If there is a history of TBI, the clinician should attempt to delineate the type, severity, and location of the injury.

A temporal relationship should be established between the onset of current signs and symptoms and the occurrence of the traumatic injury. This information helps to differentiate the personality and psychiatric variables before the accident from those arising after the brain injury. Careful consideration of temporal relationships also must address the phase of recovery and associated behavioral changes. The clinician should focus attention on the patient's psychological reactions and adjustment to and acceptance of the injury-induced cognitive and emotional changes, as well as their impact on interpersonal relationships, family dynamics, and employment status.

It is helpful to categorize observed signs and symptoms into the broad domains of cognition, memory, behavior, impulse control, emotion, and affect and thought processes. This categorization permits more precise formulation and diagnosis of the patient's problems and assists in the determination of appropriate treatment.

Because awareness of and insight into disturbances of cognition, behavior, and emotional state are often compromised in patients with brain injury, it is incumbent on the clinician to verify from collateral sources the accuracy of the patient's history and complaints. Prigatano demonstrated that the greater the severity of the brain injury, particularly when the frontal lobes are involved, the less aware the patient is of his or her neurobehavioral deficits (Prigatano 1988; Prigatano et al. 1991).

The clinician must recognize that the patient's current neurobehavioral status represents a vector of change resulting from the interaction of premorbid factors, including temperament, personality, intelligence, and character structure with the acquired consequences of the brain injury (Bond 1984; Lishman 1988). Any number of emotional and behavioral difficulties that existed in milder form before the brain injury can be accentuated after it. Thus, virtually any psychiatric or behavioral disturbance can occur in the context of a brain injury. This recognition is particularly important in predicting functional outcome (Lishman 1988; Rutter 1981).

▮ **Importance of collateral history.** As noted above, patients with TBI often experience disturbances in cognition, particularly involving memory, conceptual flexibility, concentration, and speed of information processing (Levin 1989; Levin et al. 1990). In cases of severe TBI, there is rarely recall of the incidents surrounding the injury. This disturbance in recall of the incident, in conjunction with the patient's decreased awareness of and appreciation for his or her deficits (especially with more severe injuries) makes collateral history important. Collateral history includes information obtained from family members and friends who have had frequent enough contact with the patient over a sufficiently long period of time to be able to offer accurate descriptions of changes in behavior, cognition, memory, personality characteristics, and general level of functioning that have resulted subsequent to the brain injury.

For example, Oddy et al. (1985) found that 40% of relatives of patients with TBI reported that their relative acted childishly, whereas no patients reported this behavior symptom. Twenty-eight percent of patients reported vision problems after the injury, but none of their relatives reported this difficulty. Patients generally view cognitive problems as being more serious than emotional changes (Hendryx 1989); yet families consider mood problems and decreased frustration tolerance as more serious than cognitive problems (Rappaport et al. 1989). The observations of allied health care professionals, such as speech therapists, physical therapists, occupational therapists, and other similar individuals can provide valuable descriptions of current behavior and important details about the course of recovery.

Hospital records related to the acute treatment of a TBI provide invaluable information about the traumatic event. This information includes the nature of the trauma (e.g., motor vehicle accident, fall, or blunt trauma), severity (Glasgow Coma Score, period of unconsciousness, presence of traumatically related seizures, duration of retrograde and posttraumatic amnesia, medical complications, and course of recovery), time of onset and types of neurobehavioral changes that occurred during the acute and postacute phases of recovery, results of neurodiagnostic studies delineating the location and extent of injury, and type and extent of cognitive and memory impairment as revealed by delineating the location and extent of injury, and previous neuropsychological testing.

Medical and psychiatric records for the period before the trauma are also helpful, in relating current signs and symptoms to past psychiatric disturbances and premorbid personality, and can assist in ascertaining the relative contributions of antecedent variables, the brain injury itself, and current psychosocial parameters to the observed neurobehavioral changes.

If available, posttrauma psychiatric records help delineate the course of the patient's recovery, including the acute versus chronic nature of presenting psychiatric complaints, and provide a source of additional behavioral observations. Relevant posttrauma records also should be reviewed for the emergence of subsequent medical problems, results of neurodiagnostic studies, and indications of the efficacy and adverse effects of various treatments the patient may have received.

▌ **Current psychiatric symptoms.** By applying the above principles, the clinician can better understand the patient's current psychiatric symptoms in the context of the past history, the location and severity of the injury, and the phase of recovery, and can then attempt to group signs and symptoms into the domains of cognition, memory, behavior, impulse control, emotion, and affect and thought disturbances. Each symptom or symptom cluster is further delineated with regard to duration, mode of expression, degree of change over time, and relationship to other clinical factors.

The kinds of psychiatric symptoms seen during the acute phase of recovery from a TBI are a function of the severity of the injury. The severity of brain injuries has been assessed in different ways over the years, using criteria that have varied from one study to the next. Since its introduction by Teasdale and Jennett (1974), the Glasgow Coma Scale (GCS) (see Table 1–2 in Chapter 1) has become a commonly used measure of the severity of an injury, and is now the standard used by most clinicians. Based on the GCS, mild brain injury is associated with a score of 13–15 (and in association with loss of consciousness not exceeding 20 minutes and hospitalization less than 48 hours (Barth et al. 1983). Moderate brain injury is associated with a score of 9–12 (Rimel et al. 1982). Williams et al. (1990) suggest that the designation of moderate closed head injury also should include patients with mild impairment of consciousness (GCS Score of 13–15) and a concomitant intracranial lesion. Severe closed head injury is defined as posttraumatic amnesia or loss of consciousness for one week or longer, and a GCS score of less than 10.

Within days of a mild to moderate TBI, a significant number of patients will experience headaches, fatigue, dizziness, decreased attention, memory disturbance, slowed speed of information processing, and distractibility (Levin et al. 1987a; McLean et al. 1983). Other symptoms that frequently occur within the first few days after such an injury include hypersensitivity to noise and light, irritability, easy loss of temper, sleep disturbances, and anxiety (Binder 1986). These symptoms, which are often referred to as "postconcussive" symptoms, and their relative frequencies are shown in Table 3–1.

Although there are some discrepancies in the results of available follow-up outcome studies, it is apparent that most patients experience substantial resolution of cognitive, somatic, and emotional symptoms within 1 to 6 months after a mild brain injury (Barth et al. 1983; Rimel et al. 1981). However, there is a subgroup of patients who will experience persistent difficulties with reasoning, information processing, memory, vigilance, and attention, as well as symptoms of depression and anxiety for up to 2 years after the injury (Hall and Bornstein 1991; Leininger et al. 1990; Yarnell and Rossie 1988). The symptom profile with moderate TBI is generally similar to that seen with minor TBI, but the frequency of symptoms is greater, and they tend to be more severe (Rimel et al. 1982).

Severe TBI is associated with a large number of chronic neurobehavioral changes, acute as well as delayed in onset. These symptoms and their relative frequencies are shown in Table 3–2. Recovery from severe TBI is typically marked by a number of stages that can be documented using the Rancho Los Amigos Cognitive Scale (Table 3–3).

After a brief loss of consciousness, recovery can be rapid, and the specific stages of recovery not easily discernible. On the other hand, recovery after prolonged periods of unconsciousness is slow and gradual, and the stages are more clearly identifiable (Alexander 1982).

Coma is the first stage of recovery and is characterized by a loss of consciousness and responsiveness to the environment. The duration and depth of loss of consciousness can be quite variable (Alexander 1982). A simple but useful measure of the depth of coma is the GCS, which assesses eye opening, gross motor activity, and verbalization (Teasdale and Jennett 1974). As noted above, the GCS correlates with the severity of TBI and can be useful in predicting

Table 3–1.   Neurobehavioral symptoms associated with mild brain injury

Symptoms	Relative frequencies
Cognitive	
Trouble concentrating	33%–52%
Forgetfulness	42%–45%
Trouble handling information	32%–41%
Behavioral	
More easily angered	37%–44%
Yelling or striking out	10%–32%
Impulsivity	14%–31%
Change in behavior	29%–43%
Emotional	
Depressed	33%–51%
Anxiety	36%–43%
Mood fluctuations	27%–48%
Somatic	
Headaches	20%–39%
Fatigue	50%–55%
Dizziness	7%–39%
Blurred vision	17%–35%
Noise sensitivity	10%–19%
Light sensitivity	13%–24%
Trouble sleeping	33%–53%
Irritability	33%–42%

Source.   C. A. Taylor, R. B. Fields, unpublished data, March 1993.

outcome in severe cases of TBI (Jennett 1979).

Upon emerging from deep coma, the patient enters the second stage of recovery, a state of unresponsive vigilance, marked by apparent gross wakefulness with eye tracking, but without purposeful responsiveness to the environment. The third stage of recovery is characterized by mute responsiveness, in which there are no vocalizations but the patient responds to commands. Identification of this stage depends on demonstrating the patient's capacity to carry out simple commands that will not be confused with reflex activity and do not depend upon intact language function, because the patient may have an aphasia or apraxia. Requesting the patient to carry out various eye movements is often the best task to use and can range from simple to complex (Alexander 1982).

Table 3–2.   Neurobehavioral symptoms associated with severe brain injury

Symptoms	Relative frequencies during postinjury period		
	6 months	12 months	2 years
Forgetfulness			54%
Slowness	69%	69%	33%–65%
Tiredness	69%	69%	28%–30%
Irritability	69%	53%–71%	38%–39%
Memory problems	59%	69%–87%	68%–80%
Decreased initiative		53%	
Impatience	64%	57%–71%	
Anxiety	66%	58%	16%–46%
Temper outbursts	56%	50%–67%	28%
Personality change	58%	60%	
Depressed mood	52%	57%	19%–48%
Headaches	46%	53%	23%
Childishness			60%
Emotional lability			21%–40%
Restlessness			25%
Poor concentration			33%–73%
Lack of interest			16%–20%
Dizziness			26%–41%
Light sensitivity			25%
Noise sensitivity			23%

Source.   Adapted from Jacobs 1987; Mauss–Clum and Ryan 1981; McKinlay et al. 1981; Thomsen 1984; Van Zomeren and Van Den Berg 1985.

Table 3–3.	Rancho Los Amigos Cognitive Scale

   I. **No response:** Unresponsive to any stimulus

  II. **Generalized response:** Limited, inconsistent, and nonpurposeful responses—often to pain only

 III. **Localized response:** Purposeful responses; may follow simple commands; may focus on presented object

 IV. **Confused, agitated:** Heightened state of activity; confusion and disorientation; aggressive behavior; unable to do self-care; unaware of present events; agitation appears related to internal confusion

  V. **Confused, inappropriate:** Nonagitated; appears alert; responds to commands; distractible; does not concentrate on task; agitated responses to external stimuli; verbally inappropriate; does not learn new information

 VI. **Confused, appropriate:** Good directed behavior, needs cuing; can relearn old skills as activities of daily living; serious memory problems, some awareness of self and others

VII. **Automatic, appropriate:** Appears appropriately oriented; frequently robotlike in daily routine; minimal or absent confusion; shallow recall; increased awareness of self and interaction in environment; lacks insight into condition; decreased judgment and problem solving; lacks realistic planning for future

VIII. **Purposeful, appropriate:** Alert and oriented; recalls and integrates past events; learns new activities and can continue without supervision; independent in home and living skills; capable of driving; defects in stress tolerance, judgment, and abstract reasoning persist; may function at reduced levels in society

Source. Reprinted with permission from the Adult Brain Injury Service of the Rancho Los Amigos Medical Center, Downey, California.

The next phase of recovery is characterized by the return of speech and language function. During this stage, the patient begins to demonstrate a confusional state as indicated by impairments in attention and orientation and an incoherent stream of thought. The confused or delirious patient usually displays distractibility, perseveration, and a disturbance in the usual sleep/wake cycle. Such patients may become agitated and demonstrate increased psychomotor activity. This stage is also frequently associated with sensory misperceptions, hallucinations, confabulation, and denial of illness (Alexander 1982).

During the stage of confusion, the patient is not able to form new memories in a normal fashion and is disoriented. This stage is the period when posttraumatic anterograde amnesia is prominent. Posttraumatic amnesia is considered to be present until the patient is consistently oriented and can recall particulars of his or her environment in a consistent manner. The duration of posttraumatic amnesia can be assessed with the Galveston Orientation and Amnesia Test (Levin et al. 1979a, 1979b) (see Table 4–1 in Chapter 4), which monitors both the degree of orientation and recall of newly learned material. The length of posttraumatic amnesia is one of the best indicators of the severity of injury and is a clinically useful predictor of outcome. Further, the length of posttraumatic amnesia may correlate with the occurrence of psychiatric and behavioral sequelae.

When the stage characterized by posttraumatic amnesia resolves, attention and concentration improve, the sleep/wake cycle normalizes, and there is a decrease in confabulation. These changes mark a major transition from the acute to the subacute and chronic phases of recovery. This transition phase is characterized by persistent, though less severe, disturbances in attention and concentration, memory impairments, and limited awareness by the patient of the presence of other disturbances of cognitive function. Some patients also experience retrograde amnesia, which rapidly shrinks and is usually relatively short in duration. Patients may also complain of headache and dizziness during this phase (Alexander 1982; Long and Webb 1983).

As the chronic phase of recovery unfolds, changes in personality, behavior, and emotions may emerge and be superimposed on the cognitive disturbances. Patients with severe TBI experience more emotional withdrawal, motor retardation, and impairment in self-appraisal, poorer planning skills, and greater disinhibition than patients with mild to moderate TBI (Levin and Grossman 1978; Levin et al. 1987a). Many patients with severe TBI complain of forgetfulness, irritability, slowness, poor concentration, fatigue, and dizziness, in addition to headache, mood lability, apathy, depressed mood, and anxiety (Hinkeldey and Corrigan 1990; Thomsen 1984; Van Zomeren and Van Den Burg 1985).

The types of signs and symptoms that may occur are, in part, related to the type of injury and its anatomical location. Symptoms that are thought to be associated with diffuse axonal injury include mental slowness, decreased concentration, and decreased arousal (Alexander 1982; Gualtieri 1991).

Focal lesions involving the convexities of the frontal lobes are typically associated with decreased initiation, decreased interpersonal interaction, passivity, mental inflexibility, and perseveration. Focal lesions involving the orbitofrontal surfaces are associated with disinhibition of behavior, dysregulation of mood and anger, impulsivity, and sexually and socially inappropriate behavior (Cummings 1985; Gualtieri 1991; Mattson and Levin 1990). More specifically, right orbitofrontal lesions tend to be associated with increased edginess (anxiety) and depression, whereas left dorsolateral lesions tend to be associated with increased anger and hostility (Grafman et al. 1986).

Temporal lobe lesions are often associated with memory disturbances (left-sided lesions interfering with verbal memory and right-sided lesions with nonverbal memory), increased emotional expressiveness, uncontrolled rages, sudden changes in mood, unprovoked crying and laughing, manic symptoms, and delusions (Gualtieri 1991). Bilateral temporal lobe injuries may cause a Klüver-Bucy-like syndrome, characterized by placidity, hyperorality, increased exploratory behavior, memory disturbance, and hypersexuality (Cummings 1985; Gualtieri 1991).

Clearly, there are numerous changes in cognition, behavior, and emotion that can result from TBI. The severity and chronicity of symptoms appear to be related to both the severity and the location of the brain injury. However, some of the signs and symptoms result from the patient's emotional and psychological responses to having suffered a TBI and having to deal with its negative interpersonal and social consequences.

Patients with TBI may experience frustration, anxiety, anger, depression, irritability, isolation, withdrawal, and denial in response to the losses they have experienced. These losses may include former functional capacities, former relationships, the ability to accomplish tasks that were formerly easy to do, the ability to meet their own and others' expectations, both former and current, and the ability to cope with new demands and stressful life circumstances (Fordyce et al. 1983; Prigatano 1985).

Studies assessing neurobehavioral changes subsequent to TBI have not thus far used standardized psychiatric diagnostic interviews to assess psychiatric syndromes. In fact, the array of psychiatric and behavioral symptoms demonstrated by patients with TBI do not always cluster in a definitive syndromic fashion (with the possible exception of the postconcussive syndrome in mild head injury), nor do they always allow for a specific diagnosis based on DSM-IV criteria (American Psychiatric Association 1994), other than that of the category known as "secondary organic personality change due to a general medical condition." This category has several specific subtypes: labile, disinhibited, aggressive, apathetic, and paranoid. However, TBI may often be associated with the delayed onset of a number of psychiatric disorders, including depression and dysthymia (Silver et al. 1991), mania (Shukla et al. 1987; Starkstein et al. 1988) and psychosis (Levine and Finklestein 1982; Nasrallah et al. 1981). In the future it will be important to use structured clinical interviews, such as the Structured Clinical Interview for DSM-III-R Diagnoses (SCID; Spitzer et al. 1986) to establish the presence of psychiatric syndromes.

■ **Current neurological symptoms.** Brain injuries cause a number of subtle and gross neurological disturbances, including visual and sensory disturbances, motor dysfunction, ataxias, tremor, aphasias, apraxias, and seizures. Inquiring about neurological symptoms and a neurological examination may shed light on the nature and extent of brain injury and focal neurological dysfunction. The neurological examination should assess various aspects of motor function, that is, strength, tone, gait, cerebellar function (ataxia), fine motor movements (speed and coordination), motor imitation, and reflexes. Vision should be tested to identify any field cuts or diminished acuity. Sensory function, including the sense of smell, should also be examined. Anosmia (the impairment of the sense of smell) may be correlated with poor recovery and may indicate damage to the orbitofrontal cortex where the olfactory nerves are located (Varney 1988). Frontal lobe damage or dysfunction may also be indicated by the presence of frontal-release signs, including the grasp reflex, Hoffmann's sign, palmomental reflex, and suck, snout, and rooting reflexes.

Patients with severe TBI may experience impairment in expressive speech and receptive language function (posttraumatic aphasias), which may be indicated by deficits in naming, repetition, and word fluency (Sarno 1980; Levin et al. 1976). Patients with frontal lobe lesions may produce speech that is simple in structure and poorly organized. Patients with orbitofrontal damage may demonstrate confabulation and digressive speech, whereas patients with left dorsolateral lesions may have linguistic deficits, marked perseveration, and difficulty initiating speech (Kaczmarek 1984).

The prevalence of posttraumatic seizure disorders is greater with penetrating than with closed head injuries. The prevalence of posttraumatic seizures subsequent to penetrating injuries is 53%, and is related to the depth of penetration, size of the lesion, and presence of focal neurological signs (Gualtieri 1991). The prevalence of posttraumatic seizures subsequent to closed head injuries is estimated to be 2%–5% in general, and for severe injuries 7.1% in the first year and up to 11.5% after five years (Gualtieri 1991). Predictive factors indicating that posttraumatic seizures may occur subsequent to a closed head injury include duration of coma, posttraumatic amnesia, focal cortical damage with a mass lesion or depressed skull fracture, focal neurological signs, and seizures during the first week after the injury (Gualtieri 1991). Complex partial seizures are the most commonly seen seizure type subsequent to a TBI (Alexander 1982). Seizures are associated with a variety of neuropsychiatric disorders, and may be etiologically important in the occurrence of some late onset post-TBI psychiatric syndromes.

History Before the Injury

▌ **Psychiatric disorders.** Although many neurobehavioral disturbances appear to result directly from damage to the brain, the contributions of premorbid personality features and antecedent psychiatric disturbances are also important in determining the nature of post-TBI psychiatric and behavioral syndromes, particularly in patients with mild to moderate brain injuries. Premorbid factors that may influence the presentation of TBI-associated neurobehavioral disturbances include a history of a psychiatric disturbance (neuroticism, anxiety, or depression), a history of alcohol abuse, and/or premorbid sociopathic personality traits (Bond 1984; Dunlop et al. 1991; Lishman 1988). Rutter (1981) has also reported that premorbid behavioral problems in children with severe TBI significantly influence the later development of psychiatric disturbances.

Neurobehavioral changes following recovery from TBI result from the interplay of underlying personality traits, premorbid coping mechanisms, direct alterations in brain function, and injury-related psychosocial stressors. Because all of these factors contribute to outcome, they must all be assessed in the gathering of a clinical database. Significantly, many recent studies of patients with TBI do not include those patients with previous psychiatric disorders or substance abuse. However, clinical experience indicates that premorbid personality traits are exacerbated after TBI, possibly due to damage to inhibitory frontal lobe function.

∎ **Drug and alcohol abuse.** Alcohol use is estimated to be a contributing factor in at least 50% of all traumatic brain injuries (Sparadeo et al. 1990). Among TBI patients with positive blood alcohol levels at the time of evaluation in the emergency room, 29%–56% were legally intoxicated (Sparadeo et al. 1990). Alcohol use at the time of injury is associated with a more complicated recovery, as indicated by longer hospitalization, longer periods of agitation, and more impaired cognitive function on discharge (Sparadeo et al. 1990). Brooks et al. (1989) observed that TBI patients with higher blood alcohol levels at the time of injury had poorer verbal learning and memory compared to those with lower blood alcohol levels. A history of excessive alcohol use before the brain injury is associated with an increase in mortality at the time of injury, greater risk of space-occupying, intracranial lesions acutely, and poorer overall outcome (Ruff et al. 1990). Continued excessive use of alcohol in TBI patients may further compromise their functional capacities and place them at greater risk for subsequent head injuries (Strauss and Sparadeo, 1988). Therefore, attention to pre- and postinjury substance use and abuse is important in assessing both current levels of functioning and prognosis for recovery. The abbreviated Michigan Alcohol Screening Test (Zung 1979) (see Table 15–3, this volume) and the CAGE (Ewing 1984) (see Table 15–4, this volume) are useful screening instruments in assessing patients for the presence of alcohol abuse.

Medical History

A thorough medical history and a careful review of systems are important parts of the neuropsychiatric evaluation. Detailed knowledge of prior, as well as current, medical problems, both related and unrelated to the brain injury, allows the clinician to assess their impact on the patient's overall neurobehavioral status and on recommendations with respect to safe and appropriate treatments.

History of early childhood illness, particularly seizure disorders and previous head injuries, should be assessed. The clinician must inquire specifically about situations that are associated with TBI (e.g., falls, bicycle accidents, and sports accidents). A history of prior head injuries has been associated with a subsequent increased incidence of moderate TBI (Rimel et al. 1982), a longer duration of postconcussive symptoms (Carlsson et al. 1987), and a poorer overall outcome (Levin 1989). TBI patients who eventually develop dementia are more likely to have had multiple previous brain injuries, alcoholism, and atherosclerosis (Gualtieri 1991). Assessment of developmental milestones and previous levels of cognitive and intellectual functioning also will provide the clinician with valuable baseline information against which to compare postinjury cognitive capabilities and coping strategies.

A detailed history of preinjury, idiopathic, or posttraumatic seizure disorders, and associated treatment, is important in understanding the impact of seizures and anticonvulsants on current cognitive and behavioral functioning. Detailed knowledge of seizure disorders and their current treatment is particularly important to the clinician in choosing safe and efficacious psychotropic medications.

Endocrine disturbances may be seen subsequent to TBI. These tend to appear during the acute phase of recovery, presumably secondary to diffuse axonal injury and shear-strain damage to the hypothalamus and pituitary stalk (Crompton 1971). Abnormalities in thyroid function, growth hormone release, and adrenal cortical function, as well as cases of hypopituitarism, hypothalamic hypogonadism, and precocious puberty, all have been described (Clark et al. 1988; Edwards and Clark 1986; Gottardis et al. 1990; Klingbeil and Cline 1985; Maxwell et al. 1990; Shaul et al. 1985; Sockalosky et al. 1987; Woolf et al. 1990). Patients also may experience CNS-mediated hyperphagia and temperature dysregulation (Glenn 1988). Further, TBI patients in the acute phase of recovery can develop the syndrome of inappropriate antidiuretic hormone, as well as diabetes insipidus (Bontke and Cobble 1991). In addition, women may experience menstrual irregularities subsequent to severe TBI, making inquiry about the menstrual cycle and reproductive function an important part of the history (Bontke and Cobble 1991).

∎ **Medications.** Obtaining a thorough history of past treatment trials with psychotropic drugs, as well as the current types and doses of such medications and their efficacy, is important in establishing the value of previous drug trials, the responsiveness of current neurobehavioral symptoms to medications, and the potential efficacy of pharmacotherapy in maintaining or enhancing current levels of functioning. Psychotropic agents, anticonvulsants, and many other kinds of medication can have important effects on cognition and behavior, and their contributions to the patient's current neurobehavioral status must be ascertained. Benzodiazepines can impair memory and interfere with coordination. Anticholinergic drugs can increase confusion. If a patient is being treated with anticonvulsants, the clinician needs to determine whether this is for prophylaxis (and the patient never had a seizure or had seizures only immediately after the TBI) or for a continuing seizure disorder. The clinician also should ascertain whether the

anticonvulsant is associated with cognitive and emotional disturbances. A careful review of the patient's medication history should
also reveal any drug allergies or drug intolerances.

❚ **Family psychiatric and medical history.** Knowledge of the
family psychiatric and medical history can help in differentiating the
increased risk of psychiatric disturbance due to genetic predisposition from that due to current psychosocial stressors or the TBI itself.
Familiarity with the family history of psychiatric disturbances, medical illness, deaths, and their causes, can provide a better understanding of the possible role these factors may be playing in current
abnormalities of emotional and psychological functioning.

Social History

Social history encompasses information on 1) family structure and
other support systems; 2) social, school, occupational, and recreational functioning; and 3) data on legal problems and personal
habits. The social history provides extremely important data on the
patient's level of current functioning, the nature and severity of
psychosocial stressors, the adequacy of coping mechanisms, and
characteristic patterns of adaptation. Psychopathological reactions
may result from the severe stresses associated with the disruption of
an individual's life caused by a TBI. TBI can have an enormous
impact on the patient's family (Mauss-Clum and Ryan 1981), as
illustrated by the symptoms reported by family members of patients
with TBI (see Table 3–4). The clinician must sensitively assess the
level of distress experienced by the family and should attempt to
understand the quality of the relationships between the TBI patient
and his or her spouse, children, parents, and siblings. Families are
generally more troubled by behavioral and personality changes that
occur in TBI patients than they are by their physical disabilities
(Brooks 1991). Understanding the nature of the stresses on the
family, and the family's concerns about the TBI patient will enable
the clinician to make appropriate referrals for family and/or couples
therapy. It will also allow for family members at risk and in need of
psychiatric treatment themselves to be identified. In addition to the

clinical interview, a number of self-report instruments, rater-administered scales, and structured interviews are available to assist in quantifying and monitoring family functions and adaptation over time (Bishop and Miller 1988).

■ **School functioning.**   Children and adolescents with TBI may experience disturbances in cognition and behavior that interfere with school functioning. Thus, careful inquiries about academic performance, social and interpersonal interactions with peers, and difficulties with school authorities or the law are important in understanding the role that the brain injury may be playing in neurobehavioral disturbances that are contributing to school difficulties. This information will guide recommendations for neuropsychological and educational testing, counseling, behavioral and pharmacologic treatments, and possible alternative special educational programming.

Assessment of cognitive function after TBI should be carried out only when a period of stability has been achieved—not during the phase of rapid recovery (Telzrow 1991). Periodic reassessments thereafter will be helpful in adjusting continuing intervention programs to achieve optimal levels. Formal assessment of cognition

Table 3–4.   Symptoms reported by family members of patients with severe brain injury

Reported symptom	Family member	
	Mother	Wife
Frustration	100%	84%
Irritability	55%	74%
Annoyance	55%	68%
Depression	45%	79%
Decreased social contact	27%	77%
Anger	45%	63%
Financial insecurity	18%	58%
Guilt	18%	47%
Feeling trapped	45%	42%

Source. Adapted from Mauss-Clum and Ryan 1981.

and behavior should be carried out as close to the start of an educational intervention as possible, to establish a baseline against which progress over time can be measured (Telzrow 1991).

Any child or adolescent presenting for evaluation of behavioral problems should be queried about previous head trauma, particularly when disturbances in attention or memory function, impulsive or aggressive behavior, mood lability, or impaired social skills are evident (Obrzut and Hynd 1987; Parmelee 1989).

▋ **Occupational functioning.** TBI often has a significant impact on the ability of the patient to maintain gainful employment. A number of studies have investigated the percentage of TBI patients returning to work, and the reported rates vary from 12% to 96% (Ben Yishay et al. 1987). These authors suggest that the reasons for this wide degree of variability include the broad range of severity of the TBI patients sampled, the absence of uniform criteria for defining return to work, the lack of verification of work performance and occupational status, and the lack of sufficiently long follow-up periods to establish reliable data.

Ben Yishay et al. (1987) cited a study of four comparable groups of 30 to 50 TBI patients with moderate to severe brain injury who had received extensive rehabilitation and were considered ready for vocational assessment and placement. When followed over time, less than 3% of the patients were able to achieve and maintain competitive employment for as long as one year. The high failure rate was attributed to cognitive impairments (deficits in attention, memory, and executive functioning complicated by distractibility and behavioral impersistence), problems with apathy and disinhibition, impaired interpersonal skills, lack of awareness and appreciation of the impact of the injury on functioning, and unrealistic expectations concerning the suitability of various types of employment.

Clearly then, occupational functioning is often severely compromised by TBI. Not surprisingly, TBI patients with greater memory, learning, and personality deficits show poorer work adjustment (Ben Yishay et al. 1987; Kay and Silver 1988). In fact, memory impairment, personality changes, slowed mental processes, social isolation, aspontaneity, and fatigue are the most significant hurdles that must be overcome by the TBI patient in returning to premorbid levels of occupational functioning (Ben Yishay et al. 1987; Kay and Silver 1988).

A TBI patient often has an intense desire to return to work despite obvious limitations in work capacities. The clinician faced with this situation must ascertain the patient's expectations, explore any associated behavioral and emotional disturbances, and obtain a comprehensive neuropsychological and functional assessment. Only with this data in hand can the clinician accurately assess the impact of the patient's deficits on current or future employability and make appropriate recommendations for 1) behavioral and/or pharmacologic therapy for psychiatric and behavioral disturbances, 2) supportive psychotherapy to address unrealistic expectations, 3) cognitive rehabilitation targeted at the patient's specific areas of dysfunction, and 4) vocational rehabilitation programming aimed at occupational assessment, retraining, and eventual reentry into the work place.

Behavioral Assessment

There are numerous rating scales with which to quantify various aspects of thought, emotion, and behavior (see other sections for specific scales for depression, mania, aggression, delirium, agitation, and others). Several rating scales have particular utility in evaluating behavior and cognition during the various phases of recovery from TBI.

In the assessment of coma, the GCS (Jennett 1979) is one of the most useful instruments for monitoring changes in levels of consciousness and the patient's emergence from coma. The GCS assesses eye movements, motor coordination, and verbal responses. The GCS severity index scores range from 3 to 15, with scores of 3–8 indicating severe, 9–12 moderate, and 13–15 mild injury.

After emergence from coma, the Galveston Orientation and Amnesia Test (GOAT) (see Table 4–1, this volume) can be used to follow the course of improvement in posttraumatic amnesia, and can be used to establish the end of this period (Levin et al. 1979b).

The GOAT is a 10-item, rater-administered questionnaire, which assesses orientation to person, place, and time, and recall of events before and after the injury. The score is calculated by subtracting error points from 100. A score of 65 or less is considered abnormal whereas borderline abnormal scores range from 65 to 75 (Levin et al. 1979a, 1979b). GOAT scores correlate with the severity of injury and because this test provides an assessment of the duration of posttraumatic amnesia, it is helpful in predicting long-term outcome.

As the period of posttraumatic amnesia ends, the patient enters the chronic phase of recovery, where assessment of TBI-related neurobehavioral and neurocognitive changes becomes especially important. The Rancho Los Amigos Scale is a useful tool in tracking cognitive and behavioral recovery. Levin et al. (1987b) developed the Neurobehavioral Rating Scale (see Table 3–5) to measure disturbances in behavior, cognition, emotion, thought content, and language function during the long-term recovery from brain injury. The Neurobehavioral Rating Scale is a rater-administered 7-point Likert scale on which ratings for each item range from not present to extremely severe. In a study of 101 TBI patients without previous psychiatric disorders, Levin et al. (1987b) found that scale items assessing conceptual disorganization, inaccurate self-appraisal, decreased initiative/motivation, and poor planning correlated best with the severity of injury. They also found that patients with mild TBI demonstrated greater somatic concern and anxiety. The Neurobehavioral Rating Scale is a useful tool in assessing neurobehavioral functioning in TBI patients and offers a way of quantifying change over time.

A thorough clinical neuropsychiatric evaluation requires careful assessment of cognitive functioning. The Neurobehavioral Cognitive Status Examination (NCSE), which can be completed in 5 to 20 minutes, is an extremely useful tool for rapid cognitive screening. The NCSE was developed by Kiernan and colleagues (Kiernan et al. 1987; Schwamm et al. 1987) to assess levels of consciousness, attention and orientation, language and visuoconstructional skills, memory, calculations, and abstract reasoning. Most of the NCSE's assessment categories begin with a screening item that is a relatively demanding test of the skill involved. If the screening item is suc-

Table 3–5. Neurobehavioral Rating Scale

DIRECTIONS: **Place an X in the appropriate box to represent level of severity of each symptom.**

	Not present	Very mild	Mild	Moderate	Moderately severe	Severe	Extremely severe
1. **Inattention/reduced alertness:** Fails to sustain attention, easily distracted, fails to notice aspects of environment, difficulty directing attention, and decreased alertness	☐	☐	☐	☐	☐		☐
2. **Somatic concern:** Volunteers complaints or elaborates about somatic symptoms (e.g., headache, dizziness, and blurred vision) and about physical health in general	☐	☐	☐	☐	☐	☐	☐
3. **Disorientation:** Confusion or lack of proper association for person, place, or time.	☐	☐	☐	☐	☐	☐	☐
4. **Anxiety:** Worry, fear, and overconcern for present or future	☐☐	☐☐	☐☐	☐☐	☐☐		☐☐
5. **Expressive deficit:** Word-finding disturbance, anomia, pauses in speech, effortful and agrammatic speech, and circumlocution							
6. **Emotional withdrawal:** Lack of spontaneous interaction, isolation, and deficiency in relating to others	☐	☐	☐	☐	☐	☐	☐
7. **Conceptual disorganization:** Thought processes confused, disconnected, disorganized, disrupted; tangential social communication; and perseverative	☐	☐	☐	☐	☐	☐	☐
8. **Disinhibition:** Socially inappropriate comments and/or actions, including aggressive/sexual content, or inappropriate to the situation, and outbursts of temper	☐	☐	☐	☐	☐	☐	☐
9. **Guilt feelings:** Self-blame, shame, and remorse for past behavior	☐	☐	☐	☐	☐	☐	☐
10. **Memory deficit:** Difficulty learning new information, rapidly forgets recent events, although immediate recall (forward digit span) may be intact	☐	☐	☐	☐	☐	☐	☐
11. **Agitation:** Motor manifestations of overactivation (e.g., kicking, arm flailing, picking, roaming, restlessness, and talkativeness)	☐	☐	☐	☐	☐	☐	☐
12. **Inaccurate insight and self-appraisal:** Poor insight, exaggerated self-opinion, and overrates level of ability and underrates personality change in comparison with evaluation by clinicians and family	☐	☐	☐	☐	☐	☐	☐

13. **Depressive mood:** Sorrow, sadness, despondency, and pessimism

14. **Hostility/uncooperativeness:** Animosity, irritability, belligerence, disdain for others, and defiance of authority

15. **Decreased initiative/motivation:** Lacks normal initiative in work or leisure, fails to persist in tasks, and is reluctant to accept new challenges

16. **Suspiciousness:** Mistrust, belief that others harbor malicious or discriminatory intent

17. **Fatigability:** Rapidly fatigues on challenging cognitive tasks or complex activities, lethargic

18. **Hallucinatory behavior:** Perceptions without normal external stimulus correspondence

19. **Motor retardation:** Slowed movements or speech (excluding primary weakness)

20. **Unusual thought content:** Unusual, odd, strange, and bizarre thought content

21. **Blunted affect:** Reduced emotional tone, reduction in normal intensity of feelings, and flatness

22. **Excitement:** Heightened emotional tone, increased reactivity

23. **Poor planning:** Unrealistic goals, poorly formulated plans for the future, disregards prerequisites (e.g., training), and fails to take disability into account

24. **Lability of mood:** Sudden change in mood which is disproportionate to the situation

25. **Tension:** Postural and facial expression of heightened tension, without the necessity of excessive activity involving the limbs or trunk

26. **Comprehension deficit:** Difficulty in undestanding oral instructions on single or multistage commands

27. **Speech articulation defect:** Misarticulation, slurring, or substitution

Source. Reprinted from Levin HS, High WM, Goethe KE, et al: "The Neurobehavioral Rating Scale: Assessment of the Behavioral Sequelae of Head Injury by the Clinician." *Journal of Neurology, Neurosurgery, and Psychiatry* 50:183–193, 1987. Used with permission.

cessfully completed, no further testing in that domain is required. This allows for rapid completion when there is little cognitive impairment. The NCSE generates a performance profile that reflects differentiated functioning and can be compared to group norms for various neuropsychiatric disorders. The NCSE is particularly useful as a screening tool in identifying patients for whom formal neuropsychological testing is indicated and is a valuable adjunct to other clinical neurodiagnostic studies when neuropsychological testing is not readily available. Scales for specific assessment of other psychiatric or behavioral problems are discussed elsewhere in this text (e.g., Overt Aggression Scale and the Hamilton Rating Scale for Depression).

Brain Imaging and Electrophysiological Studies in the Neuropsychiatric Diagnostic Assessment of TBI Patients

Powerful brain-imaging and electrophysiological neurodiagnostic techniques, currently available to the clinician, have become increasingly important in the neuropsychiatric diagnostic assessment of TBI patients and their concomitant psychiatric and behavioral symptoms. These diagnostic studies complement the basic clinical neuropsychiatric evaluation that we discussed in the first part of this chapter. The information made available by them provides the clinician with a better understanding of the neuroanatomic and neurophysiological substrates of the often confusing array of cognitive, emotional, and behavioral problems that occur in TBI patients.

The latest generation of largely noninvasive neurodiagnostic studies is more sensitive and specific than the older ones, which included plain skull films, routine electroencephalography (EEG), radioisotope brain scans, echoencephalography, and pneumoencephalography. These newer technologies are indispensable to clinicians who care for TBI patients with neuropsychiatric syndromes; the information provided by them is often critical in making difficult diagnoses, deciding on specific psychotherapeutic and/or pharmacotherapeutic approaches, and integrating these into ongoing comprehensive rehabilitative programs.

In the remainder of this chapter, we focus on these structural and functional brain imaging and electrophysiological neurodiagnostic techniques. We consider the indications for their use, including time and diagnostic considerations, information they may yield and its clinical utility, relative sensitivity and specificity, limitations to their use, and possible future applications. In the first section we discuss structural brain imaging techniques, including skull films, radioisotope brain scans, pneumoencephalography, cerebral arteriography, computed tomography, and magnetic resonance imaging. Next we discuss functional brain imaging techniques, including regional cerebral blood flow, single photon emission computed tomography, positron-emission tomography, and nuclear magnetic resonance spectroscopy. In the final section we focus on electrophysiological neurodiagnostic studies, including routine EEGs, with standard as well as special lead placements, split-screen video EEG monitoring, 24-hour ambulatory EEG studies, sleep studies, evoked potential studies, and quantitative computerized EEG.

Formal neuropsychological testing is an essential part of the neuropsychiatric evaluation of the TBI patient. In fact, it is often the single most sensitive indicator of subtle brain disturbances that may be contributing to the cognitive, emotional, and behavioral dysfunctions that bring TBI patients to the psychiatrist, especially those who have a history of only mild to moderate brain injury. Frequently both the nature and anatomical localization of neuropsychological abnormalities are consistent with the patient's clinical and behavioral symptomatology (Levin et al. 1982, 1985a, 1985b, 1987c; Schaffer et al. 1985; Shores et al. 1990; Strub and Black 1988).

Neuropsychological testing may reveal significant abnormalities in some cases when standard structural brain imaging techniques such as computed tomography and magnetic resonance imaging do not (Jenkins et al. 1986; Kwentus et al. 1985; Levin et al. 1987c; Riether and Stoudemire 1987; Schaffer et al. 1985; Shores et al. 1990;

Strub and Black 1988; Wilson et al. 1988). Some recent studies suggest that functional brain imaging studies, such as regional cerebral blood flow, single photon emission computed tomography, and positron-emission tomography correlate better with demonstrated neuropsychological deficits and clinical symptomatology than do the structural brain imaging techniques (Barclay et al. 1985; Clothier et al. 1990; Gray et al. 1990; Reid and Krelina 1990; Ruff et al. 1989; Shores et al. 1990). (Neuropsychological assessment of the TBI patient is discussed in detail in Chapter 4 of this text.)

Structural Brain Imaging

∎ **Skull films.** Skull films, with posterior-anterior, lateral, and Towne's views, are of their greatest value in the initial evaluation of acute mild to moderate head injuries. Their major value is in the diagnosis of skull fractures, especially depressed skull fractures that require immediate surgical intervention. Early diagnosis of skull fractures is also important because they are associated with a substantially increased risk of developing hematomas (either subdural or extradural) (Miller et al. 1990; Strub and Black 1988) and therefore indicate the need for prompt computed tomography scanning and neurosurgical consultation.

Acute subdural hematomas can be associated with abrupt, otherwise unexplained neurological deterioration and chronic subdural hematomas with fluctuating neurocognitive disturbances. Acute extradural hematomas can be life threatening, especially when the causal fracture involves the temporal or parietal bones, where laceration of the middle meningeal artery may result, or the occipital bone, where massive bleeding from the numerous diploic channels and venous sinuses located there may result in increased morbidity and mortality (Schaffer et al. 1985). Computed tomography scanning with bone windows can be helpful in diagnosing skull fractures, especially depressed fractures that are sometimes difficult to see on plain skull films (Miller 1990; Schaffer et al. 1985). In general, skull films have little to contribute to the evaluation of subacute and chronic behavioral disorders associated with TBI.

❚ **Radioisotope (^{99m}Tc) brain scans.** Before the introduction of computed tomography and magnetic resonance imaging, technetium-99m (^{99m}Tc) brain scans were widely employed in the diagnostic evaluation of a variety of different types of intracranial pathology, including that related to TBI. These scans were used in the diagnosis of trauma-related subdural hematomas, intracerebral hematomas, and brain contusions (Gilson and Gargano 1965). Now, however, radioisotope brain scans have been largely replaced by the newer techniques. Only in instances where computed tomography scanning is unavailable or unrevealing (due to the presence of an isodense subdural hematoma for example) and magnetic resonance imaging is not available, do brain scans still play a role in the diagnosis of subdural hematoma (Jennett 1987). The expected finding would be a marked increase in activity in the region of the lesion (Blankfein 1979). Otherwise, technetium brain scans play no role in the diagnosis of postacute and chronic neuropsychiatric syndromes in TBI patients.

❚ **Pneumoencephalography.** Pneumoencephalography (PEG) is an old and now virtually obsolete air contrast study of the brain. It involved introducing air into the lumbar sac and allowing it to rise to the head and fill the ventricular system and subarachnoid spaces. Films taken after the introduction of air showed brain tissue in clear contrast to the air in the spaces usually occupied by cerebrospinal fluid. PEGs allowed the identification of structural abnormalities of the ventricular system, cisterns, and subarachnoid spaces, as well as distortions or displacements of the structures surrounding them. Formerly helpful in the diagnosis of deep midline intracranial pathology or hydrocephalus, PEGs were technically difficult, invasive, and uncomfortable for the patient because they required a lumbar puncture for the introduction of air. More often than not, they were poorly tolerated because of severe headaches, nausea, and vomiting that often accompanied the procedure, and they also had a certain incidence of infectious complications following the procedure. With the introduction of computed tomography scanning, PEG has been largely abandoned as a neurodiagnostic technique (Gawler et al. 1976) and currently plays no role in the diagnosis of acute or postacute behavioral syndromes related to head trauma.

▋ **Cerebral arteriography.** Cerebral arteriography is used in the diagnosis of acute head trauma only in special circumstances and under the supervision of a consulting neurosurgeon. Arteriography may be helpful when computed tomography and magnetic resonance imaging are not available, radioisotope brain scanning is nondiagnostic, computed tomography findings are inconsistent with the patient's clinical status, or traumatic arterial injury, aneurysm, or vasospasm is suspected (Schaffer et al. 1985). Given the risks inherent with arteriography and the noninvasive nature and greater diagnostic accuracy of computed tomography and magnetic resonance imaging, the latter are the studies of choice in identifying structural brain changes in postacute TBI patients.

▋ **Computed tomography.** When magnetic resonance imaging is unavailable or contraindicated, computed tomography (CT) is the diagnostic study of choice in the initial evaluation of minor head injuries with significant neurological signs and symptoms or with radiological or clinical evidence of a skull fracture, especially when it involves the cranial bones over the middle meningeal artery distribution. Epidural and subdural hematomas may occasionally develop in a delayed fashion (Blankfein 1979; Schaffer et al. 1985), and in such cases, the initial CT may be normal, but after an asymptomatic interval of a few minutes to a few hours, the patient experiences rapid clinical deterioration. This sequence of events suggests the delayed development of an epidural or subdural hematoma, which may now be visible by CT. The presence of an epidural or significant subdural hematoma requires prompt surgical intervention.

Vague fluctuating neurological, cognitive, and behavioral symptoms may gradually appear, especially in elderly or alcoholic patients, days to weeks after a blow to the head and an initially negative CT scan (Deitch and Kirshner 1989). In such cases a repeat CT at the time the new symptoms appear may reveal the presence of a delayed-onset, subacute or chronic subdural hematoma

(Deitch and Kirshner 1989), which, if large enough, should be evacuated (see Figure 3–1). Surgical drainage may result in significant symptomatic improvement.

Subacute and chronic unilateral subdural hematomas may be isodense and thus undetectable by CT scanning unless there is an associated shift or distortion of the ventricular system or other intracranial structures. Similarly, bilateral isodense subdural hematomas may be difficult to diagnose with CT. In such cases, magnetic resonance imaging, radioisotope brain scanning, or arteriography

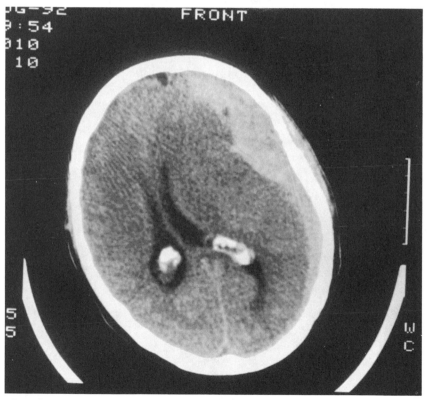

Figure 3–1. Computed tomography scan showing a large left-hemispheric subdural hematoma with midline shift, resulting from traumatic brain injury.
Source. Photograph courtesy of A. Goldberg, Allegheny General Hospital, Pittsburgh, Pennsylvania.

(if magnetic resonance imaging is unavailable) will help establish the diagnosis (see Figure 3–2).

CT is superior to magnetic resonance imaging in the diagnosis of skull fractures (especially when bone windows are employed), acute subarachnoid or parenchymal hemorrhages, acute intracerebral hematomas, and associated acute injuries to other organ systems (see Figures 3–3 and 3–4) (Garber et al. 1988; Yoshino and Seeger 1989).

∎ **Magnetic resonance imaging.** Magnetic resonance imaging (MRI) has been shown to be at least twice as sensitive as CT in the diagnosis of intracranial soft tissue abnormalities in TBI patients (Alavi 1989; Levin et al. 1992), except when they are calcified (Garber et al. 1988; Oot et al. 1986), in which case CT is preferred. Specifically, MRI is superior to CT in the diagnosis of the following

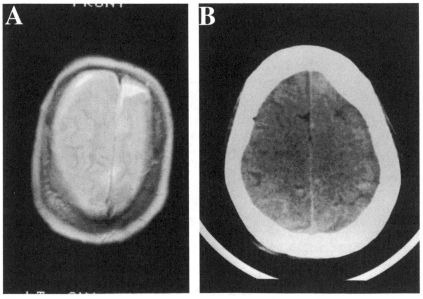

Figure 3–2. Magnetic resonance imaging scan (*panel A*) demonstrating a left frontal subdural hematoma that appears isodense on a computed tomography scan (*panel B*).
Source. Photograph courtesy of A. Goldberg, Allegheny General Hospital, Pittsburgh, Pennsylvania.

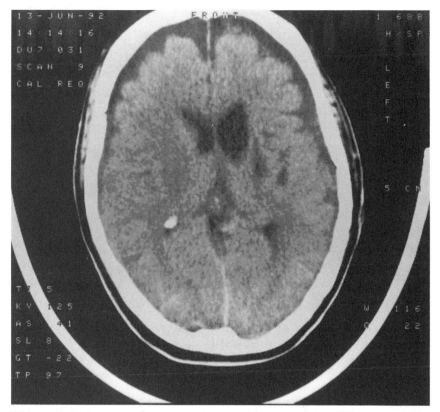

Figure 3–3. Computed tomography scan demonstrating diffuse axonal injury resulting from traumatic brain injury.
Source. Photograph courtesy of A. Goldberg, Allegheny General Hospital, Pittsburgh, Pennsylvania.

conditions: vertical, skull base, posterior fossa, and brain stem soft tissue abnormalities, because bone artifact does not interfere with soft tissue imaging with MRI; brain contusions; diffuse axonal injury involving the deep white matter, corpus callosum, or brain stem due to shearing injuries; and cerebral and other intracranial hemorrhages, especially small or isodense subdural hematomas (see Figures 3–2 and 3–5) (Alavi 1989; Baker et al. 1985; Consensus Development Panel 1987; DeMyer et al. 1985; Gandy et al. 1984; Levin et al. 1985a, 1987c; Ram et al. 1989; Schaffer et al. 1985; Shores et al. 1990; Thatcher et al. 1989; Wilberger et al. 1987; Yoshino and Seeger 1989). In one study MRI was ten times more sensitive than CT in identifying diffuse axonal injury involving the deep white matter, a type of injury that appears to be highly correlated with the depth and duration of unconsciousness after an acute TBI in primates (Gennarelli et al. 1982).

In a recent comparative study of patients with mild to moderate brain injuries (GCS of 9–15), MRI revealed lesions in 80% of the cases, whereas CT scanning was abnormal in only 20% (Levin et al.

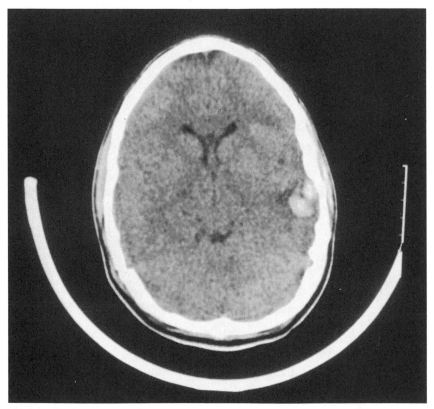

Figure 3–4. Computed tomography scan showing an intracerebral contusion resulting from a traumatic brain injury.
Source. Photograph courtesy of A. Goldberg, Allegheny General Hospital, Pittsburgh, Pennsylvania.

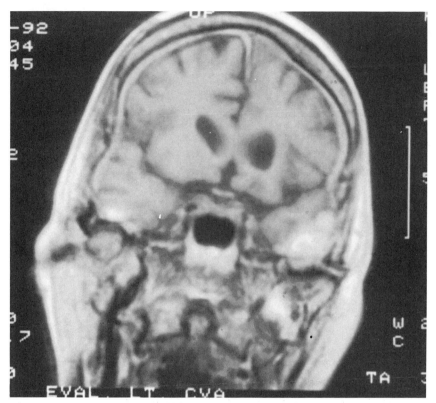

Figure 3–5. Magnetic resonance imaging coronal section demonstrating bilateral contusions of the anterior temporal lobes resulting from traumatic brain injury.
Source. Photograph courtesy of A. Goldberg, Allegheny General Hospital, Pittsburgh, Pennsylvania.

1992). Neuropsychological tests administered at the same time revealed pervasive abnormalities with respect to cognition and memory, but no consistent relationship between observed neuropsychological abnormalities and expected lesion location. Follow-up MRI studies 1 to 3 months later revealed substantial improvement in the previously demonstrated structural lesions with concomitant improvement in neuropsychological abnormalities, although the absence of the expected relationship between them and lesion location persisted.

Although MRI is generally superior to CT in the diagnostic assessment of the TBI patient, this is not the case during the first 1 to 3 days after the injury, during which time CT is more sensitive than MRI (Chakares and Bryan 1986; Consensus Development Panel 1987; Garber et al. 1988; Gawler et al. 1976). MRI is more helpful than CT in determining the age of intracranial collections of blood (Alavi 1989) and is more accurate than CT in delineating the extent of brain damage during the postacute healing period after a head injury (Baker et al. 1985; Levin et al. 1985a, 1987c; Ram et al. 1989; Shores et al. 1990; Wilberger et al. 1987).

MRI has also been shown (Wilson et al. 1988) to reveal deep white matter lesions and ventricular enlargement on follow-up examination between 5 and 18 months (median time of 11 months) after mild to moderate brain injuries (GCS of 8–15) that were not present on the initial MRI. These late MRI findings were correlated with poorer clinical outcome and more impaired neuropsychological test performance than were indicated by early CT or MRI abnormalities, which did not correlate with outcome or performance. Thus it appears that some functionally important MRI abnormalities may be revealed only on late follow-up scanning.

Overall, except during the first 1 to 3 days after the injury or where calcified lesions are expected to be present, MRI is the preferred structural imaging technique in the evaluation of acute and chemical brain injuries. Although clearly the study of choice for diffuse axonal injury, it is important to bear in mind that MRI may not demonstrate pathology in some cases of very severe head injury (Alavi 1989). The main disadvantages of MRI include its higher cost and more limited availability, slower acquisition time, the technical limitations related to the diagnosis of acutely head-injured patients who are being maintained on complex life support equipment, and lack of diagnostic sensitivity with bony injuries (Yoshino and Seeger 1989).

Functional Brain Imaging

▌ **Cerebral blood flow.** Global cerebral blood flow (CBF) is diminished immediately after acute head injury but tends to return toward normal during the recovery period as the patient's level of consciousness improves (Fieschi et al. 1974; Obrist et al. 1979a, 1979b; Overgaard and Tweed 1974). Regional CBF is often acutely decreased in the anatomic region where the brain injury is located, although this is not a consistent finding (Bruce et al. 1973; Obrist et al. 1979a, 1979b).

Decreased blood flow has also been reported in chronic brain injury patients as late as 12 months after regaining consciousness and 13 months after sustaining the injury (Barclay et al. 1985). In this study both global and regional CBF, which reflect global and regional cerebral metabolism respectively, were decreased in the patients compared to age-matched controls, and the CBF findings correlated with neuropsychological abnormalities. In a subsample of patients with neuropsychological abnormalities who were re-studied after intervals of 5 to 14 weeks, there had been improvement in neuropsychological test results, which was associated with a concomitant increase in CBF.

The above studies suggest a potentially useful role for CBF studies in combination with neuropsychological testing (Alavi 1989) in the diagnostic assessment of subacute and chronic neurocognitive and neurobehavioral syndromes associated with brain injuries, and in tracking their improvement over time.

■ **Single photon emission computed tomography.** Single photon emission computed tomography (SPECT) scanning, a nuclear medicine technique that can be used to assess both structural and functional changes in the CNS, is carried out with easily obtainable isotopes and equipment that is routinely available in most departments of nuclear medicine. Thus, unlike positron-emission tomography scanning, which requires sophisticated, expensive equipment and highly trained specialized personnel, thus severely limiting its clinical availability, SPECT imaging is or should be available in most hospitals.

Although it provides a lesser degree of spatial resolution than positron-emission tomography, SPECT provides images, especially with the newest generation of scanners, that are precise enough to allow for diagnostically useful visualization and localization of abnormalities of cerebral blood flow (see Figure 3–6), brain metabolic activity, and potentially even CNS neurotransmitter receptor function. Its role in the diagnostic evaluation of brain injuries has not yet been fully explored, but it appears that SPECT may be quite helpful in the assessment of subacute and chronic neurocognitive and neurobehavioral abnormalities associated with brain metabolic abnormalities (Clothier et al. 1990; Gray et al. 1990, 1992; Reid and Krelina 1990; Van Heertum and Tikofsky 1989; Wiedmann et al. 1989).

These studies suggest that in patients with subacute and chronic brain injuries, the anatomic localization of SPECT abnormalities often correlates better with specific behavioral abnormalities and neuropsychological deficits than do those revealed by CT and MRI, and that some of these SPECT abnormalities may reflect local metabolic derangements (created via the mechanism of diaschisis), resulting from distant structural lesions that can be identified by CT or MRI.

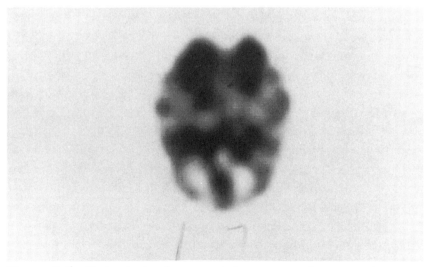

Figure 3–6. Brain single photon emission computed tomography demonstrating bifrontal hypoperfusion as a result of an anoxic brain injury.
Source. Photograph courtesy of Andy Goldberg, Allegheny General Hospital, Pittsburgh, Pennsylvania.

In two related studies of 36 patients 3 to 14 months after severe brain injury (mean GCS = 6.6), both lowered frontal and thalamic blood flow by SPECT correlated with neuropsychological evidence of executive dysfunction, whereas only decreased thalamic blood flow correlated with greater degrees of neurological and cognitive impairment (Goldenberg et al. 1992). In a related study decreased frontal blood flow was correlated with disinhibited behavior and decreased left-hemisphere blood flow was associated with social isolation, whereas decreased right-hemisphere blood flow was associated with aggressive behavior (Oder et al. 1992). Interestingly, there was no correlation between the degree of memory impairment and observed changes in blood flow in the temporal lobes.

Information about the localization of brain metabolic abnormalities provided by SPECT may thus complement data on the localization of structural abnormalities revealed by CT and MRI. Such complementary information may be helpful in the diagnosis and clinical management of subacutely or chronically brain-injured patients with psychiatric and behavioral symptoms or neuropsychological and neurocognitive dysfunctions.

▌ **Positron-emission tomography.** Like SPECT, positron-emission tomography (PET) scanning yields simultaneous information about the anatomic structure, as well as metabolic function, of superficial cortical and deep subcortical brain regions. Depending on the technique and type of positron-emitting ligand used, PET can be used to measure CBF, oxygen utilization, glucose metabolism, or specific neurotransmitter receptor functions (Rosse and Morihisa 1988). It can do these things more rapidly, with a higher degree of spatial resolution, and a broader array of currently available ligands, than can SPECT. It is the most sensitive tool we have at present for determining the nature and extent of persistent metabolic abnormalities in patients with brain injuries.

PET has been shown to provide potentially clinically valuable information in the diagnosis and management of patients with either acute or chronic brain injury. In studies using the [^{18}F]fluoro-2-deoxy-D-glucose (FDG) technique, PET has revealed regional (focal) and global (diffuse) decreases in brain glucose metabolism in patients with acute brain injury, with the degree of decreased metabolic activity closely corresponding to the severity of the brain injury as reflected by the GCS score (Alavi 1989). These studies have shown that areas of decreased brain metabolic activity demonstrated by PET tend to improve over time in conjunction with clinical improvement of the patient, but that some focal or diffuse regions of hypometabolism may persist, indicating the location of areas of probable permanent focal or diffuse brain damage (Alavi 1989).

It has been reported that areas of focally decreased metabolism in the occipital cortex, for reasons that are not yet fully understood, may distinguish patients with diffuse axonal injury from those with other types of acute brain injuries with a high degree of consistency (Alavi 1989).

Available data suggest that PET may be considerably more sensitive than CT or MRI in identifying brain abnormalities in TBI patients (Alavi 1989; Langfitt et al. 1986; Ruff et al. 1989). In two studies of patients with acute brain injury with known structural lesions on CT or MRI, PET revealed additional, unsuspected metabolic abnormalities in one-third of the cases. PET abnormalities without corresponding structural lesions by CT or MRI were also found in 42% of these patients (Alavi et al. 1986, 1988). Not surprisingly, PET abnormalities bear a high degree of correspondence to functional abnormalities revealed by neuropsychological testing (Ruff et al. 1989).

In the future, PET may have important applications in the clinical diagnosis and treatment of specific psychiatric, behavioral, and neurocognitive syndromes in postacute brain injury patients. For example, a patient who had suffered an acute, traumatic, subcortical contusion of the right frontal lobe was recently reported to have developed secondary mania (Starkstein et al. 1990). A PET scan revealed an area of hypometabolism in a right basotemporal region, anatomically distant from the injury-related subcortical contusion demonstrated by CT and MRI, and localized to the anatomic region presumed to be causally involved in a number of other similar cases of secondary mania described in the same article (Starkstein et al. 1990). In the patient with brain injury, as well as in the two other cases where there was focal right basotemporal hypometabolism by PET without evidence of concomitant structural lesions by CT or MRI, diaschisis was suggested to be the underlying mechanism.

The extent to which PET will play a role in such cases in the future depends on clearly establishing its clinical usefulness through further research, and whether or not its clinical availability can be increased.

▮ **Nuclear magnetic resonance spectroscopy.** Nuclear magnetic resonance spectroscopy (NMRS) is a promising though at the present time largely experimental, noninvasive metabolic imaging technique (Guze 1991; Keshavan et al. 1991), which may eventually be helpful in the diagnostic assessment and management of preventable sequelae of acute brain injury caused by oxygen free radicals (Ikeda and Long 1990). NMRS holds the promise of providing information that may be helpful in limiting the extent of acute brain damage that develops after an injury, thereby decreasing the subsequent chronic neurobehavioral and neurocognitive symptoms and disabilities that TBI patients might otherwise develop. Its future clinical role is unknown at present.

Electrophysiological Diagnosis in Brain Injury

▮ **EEG.** The clinical value of routine EEG in the evaluation of minor head injuries is generally limited (Strub and Black 1988). However, it may be quite helpful in monitoring postoperative patients with severe brain injuries who are comatose, in making the diagnosis of status epilepticus, in recognizing posttraumatic seizure foci that require anticonvulsant treatment, or in revealing focal slow wave activity at the site of the brain injury. Seizures occurring during the first week after an acute brain injury tend to be focal. Such early posttraumatic focal seizures are a risk factor for the subsequent occurrence of generalized persistent posttraumatic epilepsy (Schaffer et al. 1985). Late posttraumatic epilepsy is characterized by generalized centrencephalic seizures with loss of consciousness. Up to 7% of patients who have head injuries develop posttraumatic epilepsy (Schaffer et al. 1985).

Routine EEGs may be helpful in the diagnosis of severe or persistent postconcussive syndromes, especially when they are accompanied by paroxysmal symptoms such as memory lapses or dizzy spells, which may be indicative of a seizure disorder (Riether and Stoudemire 1987). The likelihood of finding an abnormality on a routine EEG can be increased by using nasopharyngeal, anterior temporal, or sphenoidal leads (Goodin et al. 1990), or by recording the EEG when the patient is hyperventilating or has been sleep deprived.

In some cases of diagnostically unclear paroxysmal behavioral disturbances, split-screen video-EEG monitoring (Therapeutics and Technology Assessment Subcommittee of the American Academy of Neurology 1989), 24-hour ambulatory EEG recordings, and pre- and postepisode blood prolactin levels may be helpful in establishing the presence of a seizure disorder. Although such studies may be of value in the diagnostic evaluation of paroxysmal disturbances in patients with postacute or chronic brain injury, it must be borne in mind, especially with 24-hour ambulatory EEG studies, that their value is highly dependent on the skill and experience of the person interpreting them.

∎ **Polysomnography.** Preliminary data suggest that polysomnography or diagnostic sleep studies may be helpful in the evaluation of the atypical sleep disturbances that commonly occur in patients with brain injury. Night terrors have been described in adult patients who have sustained brain injury (Marshall 1975). A more recent study reported that more than half (9 of 17) of the patients in the sample studied had heterogeneous sleep disorders when studied with polysomnography (Herman et al. 1990). These included nocturnal myoclonus, sleep apnea, idiopathic daytime hypersomnolence, and restless legs syndrome, all of which were responsive to specific treatment.

∎ **Evoked potentials.** Evoked potentials can be elicited in comatose patients, and they have been shown to reliably localize injuries to various afferent neural pathways and cerebral cortical regions, especially when multimodality evoked potentials (visual, somato-sensory, and brain stem auditory evoked responses) are employed (Schaffer et al. 1985). Brain stem auditory evoked responses are particularly helpful in the diagnosis of brain stem pathology. Some preliminary data suggest that passive P300 evoked responses may be clinically useful in the evaluation of severely brain-injured patients in vegetative states (Rappaport et al. 1991). Long-latency evoked potentials, on the other hand, are generally considered to be investigational at this point (Therapeutics and Technology Assessment Subcommittee of the American Academy of Neurology 1989).

▌ **Computerized quantitative EEG.** Computerized quantitative EEG (qEEG) is a potentially powerful technology currently in search of clearly defined clinical application. Its noninvasive nature and ability to rapidly analyze enormous amounts of electrophysiological data derived from complex brain electrical activity hold great promise for the future. Nonetheless, established indications for its clinical use are quite limited at the present time (Therapeutics and Technology Assessment Subcommittee of the American Academy of Neurology 1989). It has been shown that qEEG studies in patients with brain injury often reveal abnormalities indicative of organic impairment but that such findings are nonspecific and require careful clinical correlation (Therapeutics and Technology Assessment Subcommittee of the American Academy of Neurology 1989). qEEGs should always be done in conjunction with routine EEG testing and should be interpreted by a qualified electro-encephalographer fully trained and experienced in the reading of qEEGs.

qEEG may be useful as an adjunctive diagnostic technique in the evaluation of slow-wave abnormalities associated with brain injuries (American Psychiatric Association Task Force on Quantitative Electrophysiological Assessment 1991) and may be helpful in the diagnosis of some cases of posttraumatic temporal lobe epilepsy that cannot be diagnosed by routine EEG testing (Garber et al. 1989). Computer-generated discriminant functions based on power spectral analyses have been developed that appear to be of prognostic value in patients with mild brain injuries (Thatcher et al. 1989).

qEEG is not currently a standard part of the neuropsychiatric evaluation of postacute and chronic neurobehavioral and neurocognitive syndromes in patients with brain injury. However, when carefully applied and thoughtfully interpreted in relation to the results of the other currently available structural and functional imaging studies and neuropsychological test results, it may yield additional information that can be beneficial in diagnosis and management.

∎ **Magnetoencephalography.**   Magnetoencephalography is technically complicated, time-consuming, and very expensive, and thus currently available only as a research tool. It has the potential to localize, noninvasively and in three dimensions, small regions of brain dysfunction, including those in deep subcortical and superficial cortical locations (Reeve et al. 1989). This suggests that it may have an important future role in the evaluation of both acute traumatic brain injuries and their postacute and chronic psychiatric and behavioral sequelae.

Summary

Comprehensive neuropsychiatric assessments of patients experiencing neurocognitive and neurobehavioral symptomatology and/or functional disability subsequent to traumatic brain injuries are essential.

Such assessments should elicit and integrate clinical data from each of the three major biopsychosocial domains as they apply to patients with traumatic brain injures: 1) the biologically based brain dysfunction; 2) the patient's awareness and acceptance of and psychological reactions to injury-related cognitive, behavioral, and functional impairments; and 3) the disruptions of interpersonal, family, and work-related interactions resulting from the brain injury and its consequences.

Favorable outcomes from neuropsychiatric treatment depend on careful clinical evaluations that are based on in-depth medical, neurological, psychiatric, and substance abuse histories, with special emphasis on premorbid functioning, detailed inquiry into the acute traumatic event, delineation of the time-course of development of posttraumatic neurocognitive and neurobehavioral problems, and precise elicitation of the patient's current psychiatric and behavioral symptomatology. Careful physical, neurological, and mental status examinations, formal neuropsychological testing, additional history form collateral sources including friends, family members, and co-workers, detailed reviews of all available old medical records, and appropriate structural and functional brain imaging and electrophysiological diagnostic studies are all essential components of a comprehensive neuropsychiatric assessment.

Correlation of the patient's symptoms with the type and location of abnormalities revealed by neuropsychological testing and brain-imaging studies should enable the clinician to characterize more precisely the nature and duration of the patient's neurocognitive and neurobehavioral impairments and psychiatric and behavioral symptoms, thereby determining whether they are a result of the brain injury, were present premorbidly and therefore largely unrelated to it, or, as is often the case, an admixture of both.

A comprehensive yet individualized neuropsychiatric assessment should assist the clinician in choosing therapeutically optimal combinations of pharmacotherapy and individual, group, and family psychotherapy. Such combinations of treatments may substantially ameliorate psychiatric and behavioral symptoms, improve the patient's interactions with spouses, family members, co-workers, and others, and sometimes even decrease the patient's neurocognitive and neurobehavioral impairments (and related functional disabilities) when these have been exacerbated as a result of a reversible organically based psychiatric disturbance. Psychotropic drugs can often be administered with a minimum of side effects if the clinician 1) is aware that the patient may be suffering from residual trauma-related organic brain symptoms, 2) understands that patients with coarse brain disease tend to experience side effects and may have favorable therapeutic responses with lower-than-usual doses of psychotropic medications, and 3) makes adjustments in dose levels and/or dosing intervals accordingly.

Comprehensive individualized neuropsychiatric evaluations are the cornerstone of accurate diagnosis and the basis for the safe and effective treatment of many of the neuropsychiatric, neurocognitive, and functional disturbances and disabilities that occur in the aftermath of a TBI.

References

Alavi A: Functional and anatomic studies of head injury. J Neuropsychiatr Clin Neurosci 1 (Suppl 1):S45–S50, 1989

Alavi A, Langfitt T, Fazekas F, et al: Correlation studies of head trauma with PET, MRI, and XCT. J Nucl Med 27:919–920, 1986

Alavi A, Alves W, Fazekas F, Langfitt T, et al: Comparison of CT, MRI, and PET brain imaging in acute head injury (abstract). J Nucl Med 29:910, 1988

Alexander MP: Traumatic brain injury, in Psychiatric Aspects of Neurologic Disease, Volume II. Edited by Benson DF, Blumer D. New York, Grune & Stratton, 1982, pp 219–249

American Psychiatric Association: Diagnostic and Statistical Manual of Mental Disorders, 4th Edition. Washington, DC, American Psychiatric Association, 1994

APA Task Force on Quantitative Electrophysiological Assessment: Quantitative electroencephalography: a report on the present state of computerized EEG techniques. Am J Psychiatry 148:961–964, 1991

Baker HL, Berquist TH, Kispert DB, et al: Magnetic resonance imaging in a routine clinical setting. Mayo Clinic Proceedings 60:75–90, 1985

Barclay L, Zemcov A, Reichert W, et al: Cerebral blood flow decrements in chronic head injury syndrome. Biol Psychiatry 20:146–157, 1985

Barth JT, Macciocchi SN, Giordani B, et al: Neuropsychological sequelae of minor head injury. Neurosurgery 13:529–533, 1983

Ben Yishay Y, Silver SM, Piasetsky E, et al: Relationship between employability and vocational outcome after intensive holistic cognitive rehabilitation. Journal of Head Trauma Rehabilitation 2(1):35–48, 1987

Binder LM: Persisting symptoms after mild head injury: a review of the postconcussive syndrome. J Clin Exp Neuropsychol 8:323–346, 1986

Bishop DS, Miller IW: Traumatic brain injury: empirical family assessment techniques. Journal of Head Trauma Rehabilitation 3(4):16–30, 1988

Blankfein RJ: Head trauma, II: classification of injuries to the brain. Hospital Physician 15:65–73, 1979

Bond M: The psychiatry of closed head injury, in Closed Head Injury: Psychological, Social, and Family Consequences. Edited by Brooks N. London, Oxford University Press, 1984, pp 148–178

Bontke CF, Cobble ND: Rehabilitation in brain disorders, II: clinical manifestations and medical issues. Arch Phys Med Rehabil 72 (suppl):S320–S323, 1991

Brooks DN: The head-injured family. J Clin Exp Neuropsychol 3:155–188, 1991

Brooks N, Symington C, Beattie A, et al: Alcohol and other predictors of cognitive recovery after severe head injury. Brain Inj 3:235–246, 1989

Bruce DA, Langfitt TW, Miller JD, et al: Regional cerebral blood flow, intracranial pressure, and brain metabolism in comatose patients. J Neurosurg 38:131–144, 1973

Carlsson GS, Svardsudd K, Welin L: Long term effects of head injures sustained during life in the male populations. J Neurosurg 67:197–205, 1987

Chakares DW, Bryan RN: Acute subarachnoid hemorrhage: in vitro comparison of MR and CT. A J Neurorad 7:223–228, 1986

Clark JDA, Raggatt PR, Edwards OM: Hypothalamic hypogonadism following major head injury. Clin Endocrinol 29:153–165, 1988

Clothier JL, Freeman TW, Cassidy J, et al: Clinical neuroimaging in traumatic brain injury (abstract). APA 143rd Annual Meeting New Research Program and Abstracts. Washinton, DC, American Psychiatric Association, 1990, p 299

Consensus Development Panel (Abrams HD [Chairperson]): Magnetic Resonance Imaging: NIH Consensus Development Conference Statement. 6:14:1–31, 1987

Crompton M: Hypothalamic lesions following closed head injury. Brain 94:165–172, 1971

Cummings JL: Clinical Neuropsychiatry. New York, Grune & Stratton, 1985

Deitch D, Kirshner HS: Subdural hematoma after normal CT. Neurology 39:985–987, 1989

DeMyer MK, Hendrie HC, Gilmor RL, et al: Magnetic resonance imaging in psychiatry. Psychiatric Annals 15:262–267, 1985

Dunlop TW, Udvarhelyi GB, Stedem AFA, et al: Comparison of patients with and without emotional/behavioral deterioration during the first year after traumatic brain injury. Journal of Neuropsychiatry and Clinical Neuroscience 3:150–156, 1991

Edwards OM, Clark JDA: Post-traumatic hypopituitarism: six cases and a review of the literature. Medicine 65:281–290, 1986

Ewing J: Detecting alcoholism: The CAGE Questionnaire. JAMA 252:1905–1907, 1984

Fieschi C, Battistini N, Beduschi A, et al: Regional cerebral blood flow and intraventricular pressure in acute head injuries. J Neurol Neurosurg Psychiatry 37:1378–1388, 1974

Fordyce DJ, Roueche JR, Prigatano GP: Enhanced emotional reactions in chronic head trauma patients. J Neurol Neurosurg Psychiatry 46:620–624, 1983

Gandy SE, Snow RB, Zimmerman RD, et al: Cranial nuclear magnetic resonance imaging in head trauma. Ann Neurol 16:254–257, 1984

Garber HJ, Weilburg JB, Buonanno, FS, et al: Use of magnetic resonance imaging in psychiatry. Am J Psychiatry 145.164–171, 1988

Garber HJ, Weilburg JB, Duffy FH, et al: Clinical use of topographic brain electrical activity mapping in psychiatry. J Clin Psychiatry 50:205–211, 1989

Gawler J, Du Boulay GH, Bull JWD, et al: Computerized tomography (the EMI scanner): a comparison with pneumoencephalography and ventriculography. J Neurol Neurosurg Psychiatry 39:203–211, 1976

Gennarelli TA, Thibault LE, Adams JH, et al: Diffuse axonal injury and traumatic coma in primates. Ann Neurol 12:564–574, 1982

Gilson AJ, Gargano FP: Correlation of brain scans and angiography in intracranial trauma. Am J Roentg 94:819–827, 1965

Glenn MB: Pharmacologic interventions in neuroendocrine disorders following traumatic brain injury, part I. Journal of Head Trauma Rehabilitation 3(2):87–90, 1988

Goldenberg G, Oder W, Spatt J, et al: Cerebral correlates of disturbed executive function and memory in survivors of severe closed head injury: a SPECT study. J Neurol Neurosurg Psychiatry 55:362–368, 1992

Goodin DS, Aminoff MJ, Laxer KD: Detection of epileptiform activity by different noninvasive EEG methods in complex partial epilepsy. Ann Neurol 27:330–334, 1990

Gottardis M, Nigitsch C, Schmutzhard, et al: The secretion of human growth hormone stimulated by human growth hormone releasing factor following severe cranio-cerebral trauma. Intensive Care Med 16:163–166, 1990

Grafman J, Vance SC, Weingartner H, et al: The effects of lateralized frontal lesions on mood regulation. Brain 109:1127–1148, 1986

Gray B, Ichise M, Chung D, et al: TC-99m HM-PAO SPECT in the evaluation of patients with a remote history of traumatic head injury: a comparison with computed tomography (abstract). Eur J Nucl Med 16 (suppl):S22, 1990

Gray BG, Ichise M, Chung D, et al: Technetium-99m-HMPAO SPECT in the evaluation of patients with a remote history of traumatic brain injury: a comparison with X-ray computed tomography. J Nucl Med 33:52–58, 1992

Gualtieri CT: Neuropsychiatry and Behavioral Pharmacology. New York, Springer Verlag, 1991

Guze BH: Magnetic resonance spectroscopy. Arch Gen Psychiatry 48:572–574, 1991

Hall S, Bornstein RA: The relationship between intelligence and memory following minor or mild closed head injury: greater impairment in memory than intelligence. J Neurosurg 75:378–381, 1991

Hendryx PM: Psychosocial changes perceived by closed-head-injured adults and their families. Arch Phys Med Rehabil 70:526–530, 1989

Herman R, McAllister TW, James S: Sleep EEG findings in behaviorally disturbed, brain-injured patients with sleep complaints (abstract). Biol Psychiatry 27 (suppl A):55A, 1990

Hinkeldey NS, Corrigan JD: The structure of head-injured patients' neurobehavioral complaints: a preliminary study. Brain Inj 4:115–133, 1990

Ikeda Y, Long DM: The molecular basis of brain injury and brain edema: the role of oxygen free radicals. Neurosurgery 27:1–11, 1990

Jacobs HE: The Los Angeles Head Injury Survey: project rationale and design implications. Journal of Head Trauma Rehabilitation 2(3):37–50, 1987

Jenkins A, Teasdale G, Hadley DM, et al: Brain lesions detected by magnetic resonance imaging in mild and severe head injuries. Lancet 2:445–446, 1986

Jennett B: Predictors of recovery in evaluation of patients in coma. Adv Neurol 22:129–135, 1979

Jennett B: Head injuries in the older patient. Geriatric Medicine Today 6:41–52, 1987

Kaczmarek BL: Neurolinguistic analysis of verbal utterances in patients with focal lesions of the frontal lobes. Brain Lang 21:52–58, 1984

Kay T, Silver SM: The contribution of the neuropsychological evaluation to the vocational rehabilitation of the head-injured adult. Journal of Head Trauma Rehabilitation 3(1):65–76, 1988

Keshavan MS, Kapur S, Pettegrew JW: Magnetic resonance spectroscopy in psychiatry: potentials, pitfalls, and promise. Am J Psychiatry 148:976–985, 1991

Kiernan RJ, Mueller J, Langston JW, et al: The neurobehavioral cognitive status examination: a brief but differentiated approach to cognitive assessment. Ann Intern Med 107:481–485, 1987

Klingbeil GEG, Cline P: Anterior hypopituitarism: a consequence of head injury. Arch Phys Med Rehabil 66:44–46, 1985

Kwentus JA, Hart RP, Peck ET, et al: Psychiatric complications of closed head trauma. Psychosomatics 26:8–17, 1985

Langfitt TW, Obrist WD, Alavi A, et al: Computerized tomography, magnetic resonance imaging and positron emission tomography in the study of brain trauma. J Neurosurg 64:760–767, 1986

Leininger BE, Gramling SE, Farrell AD, et al: Neuropsychological deficits in symptomatic minor head injury patients after concussion and mild concussion. J Neurol Neurosurg Psychiatry 53:293–296, 1990

Levin HS: Neurobehavioral outcome of mild to moderate head injury, in Mild to Moderate Head Injury. Edited by Hoff JT, Anderson TE, Cole TM. London, Blackwell Scientific Publications, 1989, pp 153–185

Levin HS, Grossman RG: Behavioral sequelae of closed head injury: a quantitative study. Arch Neurol 35:720–727, 1978

Levin HS, Grossman RG, Kelly PJ: Aphasic disorder in patients with closed head injury. J Neurol Neurosurg Psychiatry 39:1062–1070, 1976

Levin HS, Grossman RG, Rose JE, et al: Long-term neuropsychological outcome of closed head injury. J Neurosurg 50:412–422, 1979a

Levin HS, O'Donnell VM, Grossman RG: The Galveston Orientation and Amnesia Test: a practical scale to assess cognition after head injury. J Nerv Ment Dis 167:675–684, 1979b

Levin HS, Benton Al, Grossman RG: Neurobehavioral Consequences of Closed Head Injury. New York, Oxford University Press, 1982

Levin HS, Handel SF, Goodman AM, et al: Magnetic resonance imaging after 'diffuse' nonmissile head injury: a neurobehavioral study. Arch Neurol 42:963–968, 1985a

Levin HS, High HM, Meyers CA, et al: Impairment of remote memory after closed head injury. J Neurol Neurosurg Psychiatry 48:556–563, 1985b

Levin HS, Mattis S, Ruff RM, et al: Neurobehavioral outcome following minor head injury: a three-center study. J Neurosurg 66:234–243, 1987a

Levin HS, High WM, Goethe KE, et al: The neurobehavioral rating scale: assessment of the behavioral sequelae of head injury by the clinician. J Neurol Neurosurg Psychiatry 50:183–193, 1987b

Levin HS, Amparo E, Eisenberg HM, et al: Magnetic resonance imaging and computerized tomography in relation to the neurobehavioral sequelae of mild and moderate head injuries. J Neurosurg 66:706–713, 1987c

Levin HS, Gary HE, Eisenberg HM, et al: Neurobehavioral outcome 1 year after severe head injury: experience of the traumatic coma data bank. J Neurosurg 73:699–709, 1990

Levin HS, Williams DH, Eisenberg HM, et al: Serial MRI and neurobehavioral findings after mild to moderate closed head injury. J Neurol Neurosurg Psychiatry 55:255–262, 1992

Levine DN, Finklestein S: Delayed psychosis after right temporoparietal stroke or trauma: relation to epilepsy. Neurology 32:267–73, 1982

Lishman WA: Physiogenesis and psychogenesis in the 'post-concussional syndrome'. Br J Psychiatry 133:460–469, 1988

Long CJ, Webb WL Jr: Psychological sequelae of head trauma. Psychiatr Med 1:35–77, 1983

Marshall JR: The treatment of night terrors associated with the posttraumatic syndrome. Am J Psychiatry 132:293–295, 1975

Mattson AJ, Levin HS: Frontal lobe dysfunction following closed head injury. J Nerv Ment Dis 178:282–291, 1990

Mauss-Clum N, Ryan M: Brain injury and the family. Journal of Neurosurgical Nursing 13:165–169, 1981

Maxwell M, Karacostas D, Ellenbogen RG, et al: Precocious puberty following head injury. J Neurosurg 73:123–129, 1990

McKinlay W, Brooks D, Bowd M, et al: The short-term outcome of severe blunt head injury as reported by relatives of the injured persons. J Neurol Neurosurg Psychiatry 44:527–533, 1981

McLean A Jr, Temkin NR, Dikmen S, et al: The behavioral sequelae of head injury. Journal of Clinical Neuropsychology 5:361–376, 1983

Miller JD: Assessing patients with head injury. Br J Surg 77:241–242, 1990

Miller JD, Murray LS, Teasdale GM: Development of a traumatic intracranial hematoma after a 'minor' head injury. Neurosurgery 27:669–673, 1990

Nasrallah HA, Fowler RC, Judd LL: Schizophrenia-like illness following head injury. Psychosomatics 22:359–361, 1981

Obrist WD, Dolinskas CA, Gennarelli TA, et al: Relation of cerebral blood flow to CT scan in acute head injury, in Neural Trauma. Edited by Popp AJ. New York, Raven Press, 1979a, pp 41–50

Obrist WD, Gennarelli TA, Segawa H, et al: Relation of cerebral blood flow to neurological status and outcome in head-injury patients. J Neurosurg 51:292–300, 1979b

Obrzut JE, Hynd GW: Cognitive dysfunction and psychoeducational assessment in individuals with acquired brain injury. Journal of Learning Disabilities 20:596–602, 1987

Oddy M, Coughlan T, Tyerman A, et al: Social adjustment after closed head injury: a further follow-up seven years after injury. J Neurol Neurosurg Psychiatry 48:564–568, 1985

Oder W, Goldenberg G, Spatt J, et al: Behavioral and psychosocial sequelae of severe closed head injury and regional cerebral blood flow: a SPECT study. J Neurol Neurosurg Psychiatry 55:475–480, 1992

Oot RF, New PFJ, Pile-Spellman J, et al: The detection of intracranial calcifications by magnetic resonance imaging. AJNR 20:571–576, 1987

Overgaard J, Tweed WA: Cerebral circulation after head injury: cerebral blood flow and its regulation after closed head injury with emphasis on clinical correlations. J Neurosurg 41:531–541, 1974

Parmelee DX: Neuropsychiatric sequelae of traumatic brain injury in children and adolescents. Psychiatr Med 7:11–16, 1989

Prigatano GP: Neuropsychological Rehabilitation After Brain Injury. Baltimore, MD, Johns Hopkins University Press, 1985

Prigatano GP: Anosognosia, delusions, and altered self-awareness after brain injury: a historical perspective. BNI Quarterly 4:40–48, 1988

Prigatano GP, Altman IM, O'Brien KP: Behavioral limitations traumatic brain-injured patients tend to underestimate. BNI Quarterly 7:27–33, 1991

Ram Z, Hadani M, Spiegelman R, et al: Delayed nonhemorrhagic encephalopathy following mild head trauma. Ann Neurol 71:608–610, 1989

Rappaport M, Herrero-Backe C, Rappaport ML, et al: Head injury outcome up to ten years later. Arch Phys Med Rehabil 70:885–892, 1989

Rappaport M, McCandless KL, Pond W, et al: Passive P300 response in traumatic brain injury patients. J Neuropsychiatry Clin Neurosci 3:180–185, 1991

Reeve A, Rose DF, Weinberger DR: Magnetoencephalography. Arch Gen Psychiatry 48:573–576, 1989

Reid RH, Krelina ME: Tc-99m HMPAO brain imaging post head trauma evaluation of the chronic psychiatric sequelae (abstract). Eur J Nucl Med 16 (suppl):S111, 1990

Riether A, Stoudemire A: Surgery and trauma, in Principles of Medical Psychiatry. Edited by Stoudemire A, Fogel B. New York, Grune and Stratton, 1987, pp 423–450

Rimel RW, Giordani B, Barth JT, et al: Disability caused by minor head injury. Neurosurgery 9:221–228, 1981

Rimel RW, Giordani B, Barth JT, et al: Moderate head injury: completing the clinical spectrum of brain trauma. Neurosurgery 11:344–351, 1982

Rosse RB, Morihisa JM: Laboratory and other diagnostic tests in psychiatry, in The American Psychiatric Press Textbook of Psychiatry. Edited by Talbott JA, Hales RE, Yudofsky SC. Washington, DC, American Psychiatric Press, 1988, pp 247–277

Ruff RM, Buchsbaum MS, Troster AI, et al: Computerized tomography, neuropsychology, and positron emission tomography in the evaluation of head injury. Neuropsychiatry, Neuropsychology, and Behavioral Neurology 2:103–123, 1989

Ruff RM, Marshall LF, Klauber MR, et al: Alcohol abuse and neurological outcome of the severely head injured. Journal of Head Trauma Rehabilitation 5(3):21–31, 1990

Rutter M: Psychological sequelae of brain damage in children. Am J Psychiatry 138:1533–1544, 1981

Sarno MT: The nature of verbal impairment after closed head injury. J Nerv Ment Dis 168:685–692, 1980

Schaffer L, Kranzler LI, Siqueira EB: Aspects of evaluation and treatment of head injury. Neurol Clin 9:259–273, 1985

Schwamm LH, Van Dyke C, Kiernan RJ, et al: The neurobehavioral cognitive status examination: comparison with the cognitive capacity screening examination and the mini-mental state. Ann Intern Med 107:486–491, 1987

Shaul PW, Towbin RB, Chernausek SD: Precocious puberty following severe head trauma. Am J Dis Child 139:467–469, 1985

Shores A, Krajuhin C, Zurynski Y, et al: Neuropsychological assessment and brain imaging technologies in evaluation of the sequelae of blunt head injury. Aust N Z J Psychiatry 24:133–138, 1990

Shukla S, Cook BL, Mukherjee S, et al: Mania following head trauma. Am J Psychiatry 144:93–96, 1987

Silver JM, Yudofsky SC, Hales RE: Depression in traumatic brain injury. Neuropsychiatry, Neuropsychology, and Behavioral Neurology 4:12–23, 1991

Sockalosky JJ, Kriel RL, Krach LE, et al: Precocious puberty after traumatic brain injury. J Pediatr 110:373–377, 1987

Sparadeo FR, Strauss D, Barth JT: The incidence, impact, and treatment of substance abuse in head trauma rehabilitation. Journal of Head Trauma Rehabilitation 5(3):1–8, 1990

Spitzer R, Williams JB, Gibbon M: Structured Clinical Interview for DSM-III-R. New York, Biometric Research Department, New York State Psychiatric Institute, 1986

Starkstein SE, Boston JD, Robinson RG: Mechanisms of mania after brain injury: 12 case reports and review of the literature. J Nerv Ment Dis 176:87–100, 1988

Starkstein SE, Mayberg HS, Berthier ML, et al: Mania after brain injury: neuroradiological and metabolic findings. Ann Neurol 27:652–659, 1990

Strauss D, Sparadeo FR: The incidence, impact and treatment of substance abuse in head trauma rehabilitation: proceedings from the NHIF Task Force on Substance Abuse, White Paper, Southborough, MA 1988

Strub RL, Black FW: Neurobehavioral Disorders: A Clinical Approach. Philadelphia, PA, FA Davis, 1988

Teasdale G, Jennett B: Assessment of coma and impaired consciousness: a practical scale. Lancet 2:81–84, 1974

Telzrow CF: The school psychologist's perspective on testing students with traumatic brain injury. Journal of Head Trauma Rehabilitation 6:23–34, 1991

Thatcher RW, Walker RA, Gerson I, et al: EEG discriminant analyses of mild head trauma. Electroencephalogr Clin Neurophysiol 73:94–106, 1989

Therapeutics and Technology Assessment Subcommittee of the American Academy of Neurology: Assessment: EEG brain mapping. Neurology 39:1100–1101, 1989

Therapeutics and Technology Subcommittee of the American Academy of Neurology: Assessment: intensive EEG/video monitoring for epilepsy. Neurology 39:1101–1102, 1989

Thomsen IV: Late outcome of very severe blunt head trauma: a 10–15 year second follow-up. J Neurol Neurosurg Psychiatry 47:260–268, 1984

Van Heertum RL, Tikofsky RS (eds): Advances in Cerebral SPECT Imaging: An Atlas and Guideline for Practitioner. New York, Trivirum Publishing Company, 1989, pp 98–101

Van Zomeren AH, Van Den Burg W: Residual complaints of patients two years after severe head injury. J Neurol Neurosurg Psychiatry 48:21–28, 1985

Varney NR: Prognostic significance of anosmia in patients with closed-head trauma. J Clin Exp Neuropsychol 10:250–254, 1988

Wiedmann KD, Wilson JTL, Wyper D, et al: SPECT cerebral blood flow, MR imaging, and neuropsychological findings in traumatic head injury. Neuropsychology 3:267–281, 1989

Wilberger JE, Deeb Z, Rothfus W: Magnetic resonance imaging in cases of severe head injury. Neurosurgery 20:571–576, 1987

Williams DH, Levin HS, Eisenberg HM: Mild head injury classification. Neurosurgery 27:422–428, 1990

Wilson JTL, Wiedman KD, Hadley DM, et al: Early and late magnetic resonance imaging and neuropsychological outcome after head injury. J Neurol Neurosurg Psychiatry 51:391–396, 1988

Woolf PD, Cox C, Kelly M, et al: The adrenocortical response to brain injury: correlation with the severity of neurologic dysfunction, effects of intoxication, and patient outcome. Alcoholism: Clinical and Experimental Research 14:917–921, 1990

Yarnell PR, Rossie GV: Minor whiplash head injury with major debilitation. Brain Inj 2:255–258, 1988

Yoshino MT, Seeger JF: CT still exam of choice in closed head trauma. Diagnostic Imaging 11:88–92, 1989

Zung B: Psychometric properties of the MAST and two briefer versions. J Stud Alcohol 40:845–850, 1979

Chapter 4

Neuropsychological Assessment

Mark R. Lovell, Ph.D.
Michael D. Franzen, Ph.D.

Traumatic brain injury (TBI) can cause deficits in many different domains of cognitive functioning. The extent of impairment is affected by a number of factors including the type (e.g., penetrating or closed head, focal or diffuse), the severity, and the site of the injury. In this chapter we review the cognitive sequelae of TBI, focusing specifically on the clinical neuropsychological assessment of the patient with brain injury and the regional effects of TBI. We also discuss the implications of neuropsychological assessment for the legal process.

Neuropsychological Assessment of Specific Areas of Function

Premorbid Level of Functioning

One of the most fundamental aspects of the clinical neuro-psychological evaluation of the patient with brain injury is the establishment of the patient's likely level of functioning prior to the injury. Although neuropsychological tests are designed to provide precise information about the level of cognitive functioning in the individual at a given point in time, test results must be contrasted with the estimated level of functioning before the injury. This is a difficult task because often little data exist that provide the basis for direct comparison. In fact, very few patients with brain injury have undergone neuropsychological evaluation prior to injury, which makes a direct comparison with postinjury testing impossible. However, as intellectual and achievement testing has become more popular in the schools, this information has become more readily available to the neuropsychologist and is often helpful in establishing a preinjury level of functioning. In the context of the clinical evaluation of a patient with brain injury, the neuropsychologist is often required to make a series of judgments or educated guesses about the likely loss of function through careful consideration of a number of factors.

One traditional method of estimating level of preinjury functioning is a pattern analysis of psychometric test scores. This approach is based on the premise that TBI often has differential effects on neuropsychological skills. For instance, some processes such as basic reading skills and vocabulary tend to be less affected by TBI than are skills in other areas (except in certain instances of specific posterior left-hemisphere damage). This has led to the recommendation of the use of reading tests to estimate premorbid functioning (Wilshire et al. 1991). Lezak (1983) suggested using the highest current score on intelligence battery subtests or the highest level of functioning. However, this may lead to an overestimate of premorbid functioning because of naturally occurring variability among intelligence subtest scores, even in healthy subjects (Mortensen et al. 1991).

Additional methods of establishing the level of premorbid functioning are based on other correlates of intelligence such as demographic variables, attitudes, and interests (Wilson et al. 1979). Gouvier et al. (1983) developed a regression model using demographic variables of TBI patients, but found that the accuracy of this model was not sufficient to recommend it for clinical use. Barona et al. (1984) also developed a demographic model for estimating pre-morbid intellectual function that was later cross-validated by Eppinger et al. (1987). However, this model overestimated the level of preinjury functioning. Schlottmann and Johnsen (1991) suggested the use of an interest and attitude scale to estimate premorbid IQ. Although their method appears to be more accurate than the demographic methods as applied to subjects without brain injury, it appears to be less accurate as applied to patients who have sustained brain damage.

Because proven clinical advantage has not been demonstrated for any single method of estimating preinjury level, the clinician should use information from multiple areas in making this assessment. A synthesis of information about the patient's level of education, performance in school, occupational attainment, and specific neuropsychological test performance is the most prudent approach to resolving this difficult but extremely important issue.

Posttraumatic Amnesia

Traumatic injury to the brain often results in acute or time-limited cognitive difficulties, as well as more long-term, chronic impairments in functioning. It is extremely important to separate the acute from the chronic sequelae of TBI when attempting to determine the prognosis for recovery, or when designing an effective rehabilitation program. Posttraumatic amnesia is an acute and usually time-limited period during which the patient's memory for ongoing events is disrupted. During posttraumatic amnesia, the patient is disoriented and confused, and his or her ability to learn and remember new information is disrupted. The duration of posttraumatic amnesia can be an important prognostic indicator of recovery from brain injury; episodes that are longer than 1 to 2 weeks are predictive of poor recovery (Brooks 1989). Undertaking a more extensive neuropsychological evaluation while a patient is experiencing posttraumatic amnesia leads to a misunderstanding and an exaggeration of deficits. This can lead to an inaccurate understanding of long-term consequences of the brain injury and the impact upon the patient's resumption of preinjury lifestyle and occupational pursuits. The measurement of posttraumatic amnesia can also assist in the accurate documentation of mental status changes that occur as a result of a previously undiagnosed hematoma or increase in intracranial pressure. For example, if a patient appears to be improving daily following a TBI and suddenly becomes more disoriented, this may signal an acute neurological disorder.

Posttraumatic amnesia is effectively measured using a standardized questionnaire such as the Galveston Orientation and Amnesia Test or GOAT (Levin et al. 1979) (see Table 4–1). The GOAT assesses the patient's current level of orientation and recall of events that occurred before and after the accident. The GOAT is most useful if the patient is evaluated daily to index recovery from the acute consequences of the brain injury and to indicate the value of undertaking more specific neuropsychological testing.

Attentional Processes

As the patient with brain injury emerges from posttraumatic amnesia, a more detailed neuropsychological evaluation can be initiated. This should include the careful assessment of attentional processes, which are often disrupted after TBI. This assessment is imperative for two reasons. First, evaluation of other domains of cognitive functioning is, to a significant extent, dependent on the patient's ability to focus his or her attention and to participate actively in the testing. Second, impairment of attentional processes may mimic impairment in other areas of cognitive functioning. This is particularly true for memory. Apparent difficulties in learning and remembering new information may be due to an inability to attend to the information rather than to disruption of memory processes per se.

Despite the prevalence of disorders of attention following TBI, this domain of cognitive functioning remains poorly understood by many clinicians. Attention is not a unitary function, but rather consists of multiple processes that appear to reflect separate but related neural systems (Nissen 1986). In fact, attentional processes do not appear to be localizable to one area of the brain, but instead appear to be subserved by multiple areas (Auerbach 1986). Therefore, lesions in many areas of the brain will result in impaired attention.

Table 4–1.	Galveston Orientation and Amnesia Test (GOAT)

Name: _____ Date of test: _____

Age: _____ Sex: M   F   Day of the week: S M T W Th F S

Date of birth:_____ /_____ /_____   Time: _____ A.M. _____ P.M.

Diagnosis: _____ Date of injury: _____ /_____ /_____

Instructions: Error Points (shown in parentheses after each question) are scored for *incorrect* answers and are entered in the two columns on the extreme right side of the test form. Enter the total error points accrued for the 10 items in the lower right hand corner of the test form. The GOAT score equals 100 minus the total error points. Recovery of orientation is depicted by plotting serial GOAT scores on at least a daily basis.

	Error	Points
1. What is your name? (2) When were you born? (4) Where do you live? (4)		
2. Where are you now? (5) city (5) hospital (unnecessary to state name of hospital)		
3. On what date were you admitted to this hospital? (5) How did you get here? (5)		
4. What is the first event you can remember *after* the injury? (5) Can you describe in detail (e.g., date, time, companions) the first event you can recall *after* the injury? (5)		
5. Can you describe the last event you recall *before* the accident? (5) Can you describe in detail (e.g., date, time, companions) the first event you can recall *before* the injury? (5)		
6. What time is it now? (1) for each 1/2 hour *removed* from correct time to maximum of 5		
7. What day of the week is it? (1) for each day *removed* from correct one to a maximum of 5		
8. What day of the month is it? (1) for each day *removed* from correct date to a maximum of 5		
9. What is the month? (5) for each month *removed* from correct one to a maximum of 15		
10. What is the year? (10) for each year *removed* from correct one to a maximum of 30		
Total		

Source. Reprinted from Levin HS, O'Donnell VM, Grossman RG: "The Galveston Orientation and Amnesia Test: A Practical Scale to Assess Cognition After Head Injury." *Journal of Nervous and Mental Disease* 167:675–684, 1979. Used with permission.

It is important clinically to evaluate multiple components of attentional processes and different tests are used to evaluate different aspects of attention (Table 4–2). First, it is necessary to establish the patient's general level of arousal, or readiness of the individual to process incoming information (Nissen 1986). Second, it is important to test the individual's attention span, which can be accomplished using various digit span or visual span tests. These procedures help evaluate the density of attention, or how many "bits" of information can be held in attention at one time. It is also very important to establish the patient's ability to maintain attention under conditions of distraction or divided attention, such as occur when the individual is presented with multiple pieces of information and is required to discriminate or shift back and forth between them. This is particularly important because patients with brain injury often complain that they can attend to one piece of information (e.g., a conversation with one person) but not to multiple stimuli (e.g., a group conversation).

An information processing deficit is indicated by impairment of the ability to attend to incoming information, particularly when this information is presented at a rapid rate and a distracting stimulus is introduced (Gronwall and Wrightson 1980). Impairment of information processing may lead to poor performance in other cognitive

---

Table 4–2.   Evaluation of attentional processes: selected procedures

Span procedures	Visual Memory Span (Wechsler Memory Scale–Revised [WMS-R; Wechsler 1987])
	Digit Span (WMS-R)
	Knox Cube Test (Arthur 1947)
Sustained attention and/or vigilance	Digit Symbol (Wechsler Adult Intelligence Scale–Revised [WAIS-R; Wechsler 1981])
	Continuous Performance Test (Rosvold et al. 1956)
	Cancellation tests
Divided attention	Consonant Trigrams (Peterson and Peterson 1959)
	Paced Auditory Serial Addition Test (PASAT; Gronwall 1977)
	Stroop Color and Word Test (Golden 1978)

domains due to a decrease in the rate of processing new information. For example, a patient who is unable to perform arithmetic problems may appear to have difficulty with numerical processes, when this problem is due to an information processing deficit. Similarly, a patient with TBI who appears to have a receptive aphasia may actually have difficulty understanding what is said due to impairment in information processing, rather than language-related problems. To assess information processing deficits in patients with brain injury, Gronwall and colleagues developed the Paced Auditory Serial Addition Test (PASAT) (Gronwall 1977). The PASAT consists of a series of single-digit numbers that are presented at increasing rates of speed to the patient via a tape recorder. The patient is required to add each digit to the preceding digit, instead of to the total. Although this task can be challenging even to individuals who are not brain injured, it is often extremely difficult for patients with TBI and has been successfully employed as a measure of recovery from mild brain injury. The PASAT also has been demonstrated to be sensitive to the subtle but meaningful deficits that may occur following multiple head injuries (Gronwall 1977).

Another aspect of attentional processes that may be impaired following TBI is vigilance or sustained attention. Vigilance is often affected in cases of closed head injury, and deficits in this area are easily missed in the course of a traditional neuropsychological evaluation. The Continuous Performance Test (Rosvold et al. 1956) is one commonly used measure of vigilance. One recent computerized version of this test (Loong 1988) requires the patient to respond only under certain conditions (e.g., when he or she sees an "A" after the letter "X"). Choice reaction time apparatus is also used to measure vigilance as are more simple paper and pencil tasks such as the letter and number cancellation tests. The comparison of the performance of TBI patients on these tests to established norms allows an evaluation of the extent of vigilance deficits.

Memory Processes

Impairment of memory is probably the most frequent complaint subsequent to TBI. Memory processes are susceptible to temporary disruption (as in the case of posttraumatic amnesia), as well as more permanent impairment. In fact, at least 25% of patients with severe TBI may have disabling memory disorders subsequent to their injury (Levin 1989). Although there are many different forms of memory impairment, they are usually classified as either retrograde or anterograde amnesia.

∎ **Retrograde amnesia.**　Retrograde amnesia refers to the partial or complete loss of memory for a period of time before the traumatic event. Retrograde amnesia usually shrinks or diminishes within the first several days after the injury with chronologically more distant memories returning first and with orientation returning usually in the sequence of person, place, and time (Levin 1989). Often a residual period of retrograde amnesia remains for the period that immediately preceded the injury. Administration of the GOAT can assist in documenting the resolution of retrograde amnesia.

∎ **Anterograde amnesia.**　Anterograde amnesia refers to the loss of memory for events occurring after a TBI. As mentioned previously, anterograde amnesia can occur only within the context of posttraumatic amnesia or can be more permanent. The clinical distinction between temporary and more chronic memory impairment following TBI is an extremely important one, with implications for the rehabilitation process, and significance related to legal compensation issues following brain injury.

As is the case with attention, memory is not a unitary process but instead involves multiple cognitive processes and underlying brain structures. Furthermore, our existing base of knowledge concerning the nature of memory impairment following TBI is still evolving. Our continued understanding of how TBI affects memory reflects advances in cognitive psychology (Levin 1989). This approach attempts to understand how information is processed in healthy individuals and how these processes are affected by TBI.

Memory processes should be assessed across several dimensions. First, TBI may lead to impairment in the acquisition, retention, and retrieval of newly learned information (Table 4–3). All of these dimensions should be evaluated clinically. Although the acquisition of new information may be preserved, delayed recall of this information is likely to be impaired in individuals with brain injury (Brooks 1975). Second, TBI may lead to material-specific deficits in learning and remembering, where the individual's ability to recall certain information (e.g., verbal material) is impaired but his or her capacity to process and remember other information (e.g., spatial material) is preserved. This type of specific memory difficulty is particularly common after focal brain injury, when verbal memory deficits are associated with dominant hemisphere dysfunction and spatial memory deficits are associated with non-dominant hemisphere dysfunction (Milner 1971). Global amnestic states are more common after more generalized brain injury, especially when this injury is bilateral and affects subcortical structures (Scoville and Milner 1957).

In addition to the assessment of material specific memory processes, the clinician should assess the patient's ability to organize by category or to semantically cluster verbal information, because recent research suggests that TBI patients show deficits in these organizational skills compared to individuals who have not sustained brain injury. These findings have been cited as evidence of

Table 4–3.   Evaluation of memory processes: selected procedures

General memory	Memory Assessment Scales (Williams 1991)
	Wechsler Memory Scale–Revised (WMS-R; Wechsler 1987)
Verbal memory	Hopkins Verbal Learning Test (Brandt 1991)
	Rey Auditory-Verbal Learning Test (Rey 1964)
	California Verbal Learning Test (Delis et al. 1987)
	Selective Reminding Test (Bushke and Fuld 1974)
Nonverbal memory	Continuous Visual Memory Test (Trahan and Larrabee 1978)
	Rey-Osterrieth Complex Figure (recall condition) (Osterrieth 1944)
	Corsi blocks (Milner 1971
	Benton Visual Retention Test (recall conditions) (Benton et al. 1983)

the involvement of the frontal lobes in memory processes (Levin 1989).

There are a large number of procedures that assess various dimensions of memory processes. Included among these procedures are two batteries of tests, as well as individual tests of more circumscribed memory function. The Wechsler Memory Scale–Revised (WMS-R; Wechsler 1987) and the Memory Assessment Scales (Williams 1991) both assess multiple aspects of learning and recall (both immediate and delayed) for verbal and visual modalities. The Rey Auditory-Verbal Learning Test (Rey 1964) is a very popular memory test, which indexes the patient's ability to memorize a list of 15 words, over 5 presentations. The California Verbal Learning Test (Delis et al. 1987) is a particularly useful measure of verbal memory, because it provides information on the acquisition and retention dimensions of memory and on the patient's ability to cluster verbal material semantically. Semantic clustering refers to the strategy of grouping information by category. For example, on the California Verbal Learning Test, a list of 16 words is read to the patient over 5 consecutive trials. The words belong to one of four semantic categories ("tools," "clothing," "herbs and spices," or "fruits"). A semantic clustering strategy groups each of the words by one of these categories rather than attempting to remember each word individually. The ability to semantically cluster new information can have important implications for the development of rehabilitation strategies for individual patients, because patients can be taught to facilitate the learning of verbal material by employing clustering strategies (Levin 1989). The Selective Reminding Test (Bushke and Fuld 1974) also provides valuable information on verbal learning ability and is commonly employed in the assessment of TBI. This test differs from the California Verbal Learning Test in that the patient is asked to recall only words that were not recalled on the previous trial instead of the entire list of words after each trial. Although widely used in the assessment of head injury, the California Verbal Learning Test and the Selective Reminding Test may be too challenging for some TBI patients, particularly if the patient is evaluated only days or weeks after his or her brain injury. In this case a shorter procedure such as the Hopkins Verbal

Learning Test (Brandt 1991) can be useful. This recently developed test employs a list of 12 words, instead of 15 or 16, and also has six equivalent forms, which minimizes practice effects if the patient is evaluated more than once.

The clinical assessment of visual memory processes typically includes several procedures, but most frequently either construction (e.g., drawing) or recognition memory tasks are used. The Rey-Osterrieth Complex Figure (Osterrieth 1944) tests the patient's ability to reproduce line drawings at different time intervals after presentation (Figure 4–1). The Visual Reproduction items from the Wechsler Memory Scale (Wechsler 1945) and the Revised version of this test (Wechsler 1987) also are used frequently, although these scales have been criticized because they can be verbally encoded and hence may not be pure measures of visual memory (Brooks

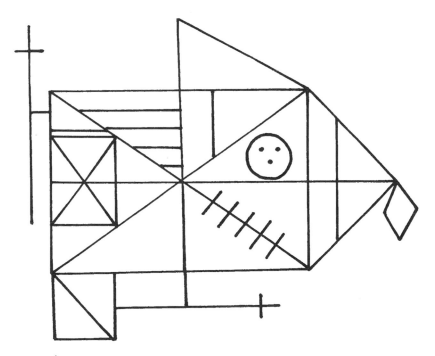

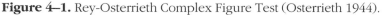

Figure 4–1. Rey-Osterrieth Complex Figure Test (Osterrieth 1944).

1989). Other tests for visual memory assess continuous visual memory (Hannay et al. 1979; Trahan and Larrabee 1988). In this procedure recurring pictures and designs are presented to the patient and his or her recognition memory is tested both immediately after presentation and 20 to 30 minutes later. The designs are highly abstract and therefore less likely to be encoded verbally. Also the procedure uses a recognition format that does not require the patient to draw the remembered material, thus allowing the separation of cognitive deficits that are due to visuoconstructional impairment from true visual memory deficits.

Executive Functioning, Concept Formation, and Planning

Deficits in executive functioning, concept formation, and planning are common after TBI. Executive functions can be divided into four components: 1) goal formulation, 2) planning, 3) carrying out goal-directed plans, and 4) effective performance (Lezak 1983).

Understanding the nature of executive functioning deficits is critical to understanding the individual patient within the broader context of the neuropsychiatric evaluation. Deficits in any of these areas have important implications for the patient's behavior, and for his or her potential for vocational rehabilitation (Cicerone and Wood 1987). Executive functioning deficits can occur in disparate behavioral systems, involving motor, verbal, or conceptual processes (Goldberg and Tucker 1979). Because many traditional neuropsychological measures may be insensitive to impairment of executive functions, the tasks specifically designed to assess these processes should be utilized. Table 4–4 lists commonly used tests of executive functioning.

One of the most pervasive executive functioning deficits following TBI is perseveration, or the inability to terminate a sequence of behavior. This problem is particularly common after injury to the prefrontal cortex (Goldberg and Costa 1981). The Wisconsin Card Sorting Test (Berg 1948) is a useful measure of perseveration and in addition provides information across multiple behavioral domains including the patient's 1) ability to form concepts, 2) problem-solving ability, 3) ability to learn from experience, and 4) capacity to shift conceptual sets. In this test 128 cards differing in color (green, red, blue, or yellow), form (crosses, squares, circles, or triangles), or number of forms (one, two, three, or four) are sorted and matched to one of four stimulus cards. The patient is not told how to accomplish the task but is told after each match whether the response was correct. The criterion for correct performance is changed by the examiner without informing the patient so the patient must adapt to this "set shift." The Wisconsin Card Sorting Test is unstructured and therefore provides valuable information on how the patient solves problems when placed in a novel situation. The Category Test (Halstead 1947) is another widely used test of problem solving that requires the patient to learn by trial and error and think abstractly. The Goldberg Executive Control Battery (E. Goldberg, R. Bilder, J. Jaeger, unpublished battery, 1981) is an extensive group of tests that tap motoric, as well as other, dimensions of executive functioning. The Trail Making Test—Part B (Reitan 1958) is one commonly used executive functioning task that can be administered in a brief period of time. This test requires the patient to connect a sequence of numbers and letters in alternating order while being timed, and thus provides information on the patient's ability to work with several types of information simultaneously under time pressure.

The inability to formulate goals, plan effectively, and carry out these plans commonly follows TBI. Planning can be evaluated

---

Table 4–4.   Evaluation of executive functions, concept formation, and planning: selected procedures

Wisconsin Card Sorting Test (Berg 1948)
Goldberg Executive Control Battery (Goldberg et al. 1981)
Design fluency (Jones-Gotman and Milner 1977)
Controlled Oral Word Association Test (Benton and Hamsher 1978)
Trail Making Test–Part B (Reitan 1958)
Tinkertoy Test (Lezak 1983)
Tower of London Test (Shallice 1982)
Porteus Maze Test (Porteus 1965)
The Category Test (Halstead 1947)

clinically using maze learning tasks such as the Porteus Maze Test (Porteus 1965). The Tower of London Test (Shallice 1982) and the Tinker Toy Test (Lezak 1983) can provide valuable qualitative information about the patient's use of strategies and ability to carry out effective plans of action.

Language Disorders

Language processes are often disrupted following TBI, particularly if the injury is of a focal or penetrating nature and involves the language-dominant (usually left) hemisphere. A complete discussion of syndromes of aphasia is beyond the scope of this chapter. For a more extensive discussion of language disturbance following brain injury, see Benson (1979).

Language disorders following TBI vary greatly depending on the nature, localization, and severity of the brain injury. Probably the two most common variants of language disturbance are expressive aphasia and receptive aphasia. Expressive (Broca's) aphasia is characterized by nonfluent speech with intact comprehension of spoken information, whereas receptive (Wernicke's) aphasia disrupts language comprehension but leaves fluency intact. Conduction aphasia is characterized by fluent but paraphasic verbal output, normal comprehension, and impaired repetition. The paraphasia often seen in conduction aphasia is referred to as "literal" and is characterized by phonemic (sound) distortion of the word (e.g., "spikologist" for "psychologist"). This type of response can be contrasted with "verbal" paraphasia, which is indicated by the incorrect substitution of a lexical item (e.g., referring to a "screwdriver" as a "hammer") (Goodglass 1986). Other relatively common forms of aphasia are anomic aphasia, transcortical aphasia, and global aphasia. Although the above nomenclature can be useful in diagnosing the language disorder, the categories are not mutually exclusive, and "pure" cases of aphasia are more the exception than the rule. This is especially true for language deficits following TBI, where the structural damage is likely to be diffuse rather than localized and the manifest language disruption may be in part secondary to confusion and impairment in other cognitive systems.

The evaluation of language processes assesses spontaneous speech, repetition of spoken information, comprehension, naming, reading, and writing. A number of aphasia test batteries have been developed that measure language processes in addition to a number of individual tests that can be useful in specific situations (see Table 4–5). The Reitan-Indiana Aphasia Screening Test (Reitan 1984) is a useful screening instrument, which can often uncover language deficits deserving of further evaluation. More in-depth assessment of the individual's language disturbance can be tested using The Boston Diagnostic Aphasia Examination (Goodglass and Kaplan 1972), Western Aphasia Battery (Kertesz 1979), and the Multilingual Aphasia Examination (Benton and Hamsher 1978), each of which can be administered in less than an hour.

Visuospatial and Visuoconstructional Disorders

TBI can result in impairment of visual perception and processing. Disorders of visuospatial and visuoconstructional processes can occur as a result of disruption of any number of cognitive systems involved in visual perception. Hence these processes should be evaluated in the TBI patient across multiple dimensions. In the assessment of visuoperceptive processes, visual acuity should be tested to assure that the patient can see the test stimuli. In addition, visual recognition, often including angulation and facial recognition (Benton et al. 1983), visual organization (i.e., the ability of the patient to organize fragmented or otherwise degraded visual stimuli), and visual scanning (Lezak 1983) should be tested. Commonly used procedures are listed in Table 4–6.

Table 4–5.   Evaluation of language: selected procedures

Boston Diagnostic Aphasia Examination (Goodglass and Kaplan 1972)
Multilingual Aphasia Evaluation (Benton and Hamsher 1978)
Reitan-Indiana Aphasia Screening Test (Reitan 1984)
Western Aphasia Battery (Kertesz 1979)

Constructional disorders indicate impairment of the ability to draw or assemble visual material into a meaningful form. This group of disorders is quite diverse and is not necessarily secondary to impairment of visuospatial processes. The evaluation of constructional disorders usually includes engaging the patient in at least two types of activities, drawing and building or assembling (Lezak 1983). Drawing can be assessed using tasks in which the patient reproduces line drawings, such as the Benton Visual Retention Test (Benton et al. 1983) or the Rey-Osterrieth Complex Figure (Osterrieth 1944). Building or assembling can be assessed using the Block Design and Object Assembly subtests of the Wechsler Adult Intelligence Scale–Revised (WAIS-R; Wechsler 1981), as well as three-dimensional block design or individualized block or stick building tests.

Evaluation of Regional Brain Dysfunction Following TBI

Another way to conceptualize the effects of TBI on neuropsychological functioning is to consider the effects of localized

Table 4–6.	Evaluation of visuospatial and visuoconstructional processes: selected procedures
Visuospatial	Visual Form Discrimination Test (Benton et al. 1983)
	Judgment of Line Orientation Test (Benton et al. 1983)
	Facial Recognition Test (Benton et al. 1983)
	Hooper Visual Organization Test (Hooper 1958)
Visuoconstructive	Rey-Osterrieth Complex Figure (Osterrieth 1944) (copy condition)
	Visual Retention Test (Benton et al. 1983) (copy condition)
	Block Design (Wechsler Adult Intelligence Scale–Revised [WAIS-R; Wechsler 1981])
	Object Assembly (WAIS-R)
	Three-Dimensional Block Construction (Lezak 1983)

lesions on test performance. TBI frequently results in widespread damage from diffuse axonal injury as commonly occurs in acceleration/deceleration injuries. However, there also may be focal contusions or other lesions that are responsible for additional cognitive deficits. Hence the neuropsychological consequences of TBI often may reflect multiple and additive areas of brain dysfunction/pathology. A careful neuropsychological evaluation in combination with other neurodiagnostic procedures can be integral to identifying and localizing areas of brain dysfunction. Although an in-depth discussion of the behavioral geography of the brain is beyond the scope of this chapter, a brief review is presented below. Table 4–7 highlights some of the common neuropsychological sequelae of TBI.

Table 4–7.   Common sequelae of traumatic brain injury

Brain region	Neuropsychological deficit
Diffuse damage	Information processing deficit, impairment of attention, impairment of memory, decreased motor speed, decreased reaction time
Frontal lobes	Executive functioning deficits (inability to formulate goals, to plan, and to effectively carry out these plans), decreased oral fluency (dominant hemisphere), decreased design fluency (nondominant hemisphere), motor perseveration, impersistence, inability to "hold conceptual set," Broca's aphasia, contralateral hemiparesis, decreased motor strength and speed
Temporal lobes	Wernicke's aphasia, decreased verbal memory (dominant hemisphere), decreased spatial/configural memory (nondominant hemisphere), auditory agnosia, amusia (nondominant hemisphere)
Parietal lobes	Constructional dyspraxia, visuospatial impairment, agraphesthesia, astereognosis, denial of illness (anosognosia), finger agnosia, apraxia, writing impairment (agraphia), reading impairment (alexia), prosopagnosia, right-left confusion, impaired calculation abilities (acalculia)
Occipital lobes	Alexia, agraphia, prosopagnosia, construction apraxia, Anton's syndrome, cortical blindness, homonymous hemianopsia

For a more complete review of the neuropsychological correlates of brain injury, see Tranel (1992).

Frontal Lobe Functions

The frontal and especially the prefrontal areas of the cerebral cortex are particularly susceptible to traumatic injury; the orbitofrontal cortex is especially vulnerable to damage due to contusion, hematoma, and hemorrhage (Levin et al. 1987). In addition to direct traumatic injury to the prefrontal cortex, the disruption of connections between the frontal lobes and subcortical structures is also a potential source of neuropsychological dysfunction (Ommaya and Gennarelli 1974; Auerbach 1986).

The neuropsychiatric sequelae associated with frontal lobe damage will be discussed in Chapter 5 of this textbook. Cognitive deficits associated with frontal dysfunction are no less distinct and most often involve impairment of attentional processes and executive functioning. The patient with orbitofrontal damage may have a deficit in selective attention that affects his or her performance on all other neuropsychological measures. Problem solving and reasoning tasks are likely to be approached in a disorganized and impulsive manner. On the other hand, damage to the dorsolateral frontal cortex is likely to result in impaired ability to shift conceptual sets, excessive behavioral rigidity, and perseveration (Benson et al. 1981). Decreased fluency is also a common consequence of injury to the prefrontal cortex. Verbal fluency is particularly impaired following injury to the dominant (usually left) prefrontal cortex (Milner 1964; Perret 1974), whereas design fluency is impaired following nondominant (usually right) prefrontal injury (Jones-Gotman and Milner 1977). In addition to impairment of speech fluency, patients with frontal lobe damage may show aprosodia, a disruption of the rate, rhythm, or intonation pattern of speech, leading to speech that is monotonous or mechanical sounding (Goodglass 1986).

Impairment of attentional processes and executive functioning is commonly observed following prefrontal brain injury, and disruption of motor functioning, particularly the motor processes necessary for speech, is known to follow injury to the posterior frontal cortex. Broca's aphasia is a common consequence of injury to the posterior frontal cortex and often follows infarction of the middle cerebral artery or a penetrating injury to this area.

Temporal Lobe Functions

Lesions in the temporal lobes are also a common consequence of TBI, due to the vulnerability of this area to contusion and the susceptibility of mesial temporal brain structures to hypoxic injury (Auerbach 1986). Because the temporal lobes are involved in language and memory processes, traumatic injury often leads to deficits in these areas. Receptive or Wernicke's aphasia is common following traumatic injury to the language-dominant temporal cortex, whereas nondominant temporal lobe brain injury may lead to impairment of the patient's ability to process nonspeech sounds. Verbal or nonverbal memory may be differentially affected, depending on the site of injury. Dominant temporal lobe dysfunction is likely to be associated with disruption of verbal learning processes, whereas nondominant temporal lobe injury may lead to deficits in acquiring and retaining nonverbal material (Butters 1979).

Parietal Lobe Functions

Parietal lobe injury may result in a variety of neuropsychological impairments. Inability of the individual to perceive objects placed in the hand (astereognosis) may be seen with injury to the contralateral parietal lobe cortex. Difficulty in the recognition of shapes, letters, and numbers (or agraphesthesia) may also be seen with parietal lobe injury. Apraxias, which are disorders of willful movement, may also occur. Traumatic injury to the parietal lobe may affect the patient's ability to perform visuospatial and visuoconstructive operations, especially when the lesion is localized to the nondominant hemisphere (Warrington and Rabin 1970). Impairment of facial recognition may also occur with damage to the parietal lobe.

One consequence of parietal lobe injury that is of particular importance to the neuropsychiatrist is the denial of illness or anosognosia. Although a lesion in virtually any area of the brain may be followed by a denial, minimization, or lack of awareness of a cognitive deficit, the dramatic syndrome of neglect that is characterized by inattention to the side of the body contralateral to the injured hemisphere (anosognosia) is often associated with parietal lobe injury.

Occipital Lobe Functions

Traumatic injury to the occipital cortex results in difficulties in cognitive and perceptual processes secondary to impairment of visuoperceptive processes. A typical finding in patients who have occipital damage is the loss of one half of the visual field in each eye (homonymous hemianopsia). Patients may also be unable to recognize items visually (visual agnosia) (Lezak 1983). Patients who have incurred injury to the primary visual cortex in the occipital lobe may show cortical blindness. The patient may lose the ability to distinguish form but may retain some sensitivity to light and dark. In Anton's syndrome, which also occurs following injury to the occipital lobe, the patient may deny blindness and behave as if sighted.

Neuropsychological Functioning and Pathophysiology of TBI

Traumatic injury to the brain can have disparate effects on cognitive functioning depending on the type of injury (e.g., closed head vs. penetrating injury), severity of the brain lesion, location of the lesions, and factors such as the patient's age and premorbid level of functioning. Although brain injuries are often described as diffuse or focal in nature, in reality many traumatic brain injuries have both focal and diffuse components.

Contusion

Cerebral contusions are often associated with TBI and result from "bruising" of the surface of the brain. Contusions often produce focal neuropsychological deficits, with the type of deficit determined by the location of the contusion. According to Auerbach (1986), several generalizations can be made about the distribution of cerebral contusions: contusions can occur from impact to the head if the trauma is significant enough to produce a deformity of the skull; 2) contusions are usually found in the frontal and temporal areas, which may be independent of the site of impact; and 3) contusions are often bilateral but not symmetrical. The point of impact of the blow is referred to as coup whereas the contusion in the brain area opposite the initial point of impact is referred to as contrecoup. Coup-contrecoup injuries are commonly observed in the temporal lobes and in the frontal-occipital plane, and often occur in motor vehicle accidents that result in rapid deceleration of the brain within the skull cavity. There may be little or no loss of consciousness following cerebral contusion and no posttraumatic amnesia. This is thought to result from the absence of damage to the mesencephalic reticular activating system (Auerbach 1986). Focal cognitive deficits associated with contusion of the brain are dependent on the location and severity of the lesion. As is the case with other types of "focal" brain injury such as stroke or brain laceration, contusion of a particular area of the brain is likely to produce corresponding neuropsychological deficits. Executive functioning deficits are common following frontal injury and memory difficulties often occur following temporal lobe contusion.

Hematoma

Cerebral hematoma occurs as a result of hemorrhage following TBI (Rosenblum 1989). As the hematoma grows in size, brain tissue is compressed. This can lead to cognitive deficits secondary to focal brain injury and diffuse deficits due to increased intracranial pressure and brain herniation. As is the case with contusions of the brain, hematomas are most commonly seen following trauma to the frontal and temporal lobes and result in the characteristic neuropsychological sequelae described earlier. Increases in intracranial pressure as a result of hematoma may also lead to cognitive impairment if not treated promptly.

Diffuse Axonal Injury

Whereas contusions and hematomas often occur as a result of direct trauma to the skull, more diffuse injury to the brain occurs as a result of damage to axons throughout the brain. This type of brain injury is associated with high-speed acceleration-deceleration injuries that occur in motor vehicle and sports-related accidents (Auerbach 1986). The neuropsychological sequelae of diffuse axonal injury are well documented and often begin with posttraumatic amnesia. As the posttraumatic amnesia resolves, other cognitive changes may be present, with particular difficulty evident in attentional processes (Van Zomeren et al. 1984) and information processing (Gronwall 1977). Patients with diffuse axonal injury may perform adequately on standard tests of intellectual functioning, language, and memory, and their deficits will be apparent only on specific neuropsychological indices such as PASAT (Stuss et al. 1985).

Hypoxia

Dramatic decreases in blood pressure and excessive blood loss during TBI may result in hypoxic brain damage. The hippocampal areas of the cortex are particularly sensitive to injury due to oxygen deprivation (Brierley 1976). A variety of cognitive impairments occur, including concentration difficulties, deficits in new learning, and problems with executive functioning and planning (Lezak 1983).

Forensic Issues in the Neuropsychological Assessment of TBI

TBI can occur as a result of an error in judgment or excessive risk taking. The injuries may occur as a result of a motor vehicle accident, an industrial work-site accident, or may be sports-related. In these cases, there may be legal attempts to assign blame and therefore financial responsibility for the resulting disability. This situation may result in attempts by the patient to feign or exaggerate a brain injury. The possibility of the dissimulation or malingering of cognitive deficits should always be considered in cases of alleged brain injury. Alternately, the TBI patient may not be capable of returning to his or her employment and prior lifestyle, and issues of disability and financial compensation naturally arise. For all of these reasons, the neuropsychological evaluation of patients with TBI is frequently utilized in the forensic arena.

The most fundamental analysis of the patient's reported versus actual level of cognitive impairment is the comparison of the patient's functioning "in the real world" with performance on formal neuropsychological testing. This requires a careful investigation in which the clinician should interview the patient's friends and family and evaluate other supporting documentation (e.g., school transcripts, work records). For example, an individual who is suing for damages due to an alleged brain injury may perform in the severely brain impaired range on neuropsychological testing but may be performing successfully in college. The lack of agreement between results of neuropsychological testing and performance in college level classes suggests an attempt to malinger.

One of the most frequently employed neuropsychological techniques to measure dissimulation is the "memorization of 15 items" paradigm described by Lezak (1983). This technique is based on the principle that patients who are attempting to feign a brain injury perform more poorly than most patients with severe brain injury. In this procedure, the patient is presented with a card that has five rows of three stimuli that are actually sequentially organized (e.g., A,B,C; 1,2,3; or a,b,c). To perform this task, the patient must remember only several concepts and even patients with severe brain impairment can recall most of the information. Failure to do so should alert the examiner to the possibility of malingering.

More recently, Franzen et al. (1990) reviewed the current methods available to detect malingering and suggested some directions for future research. Among the most promising methods is the forced-choice recognition memory test (Iverson et al. 1991), in which a word list is read to the subject, and then the subject is tested for free recall of the list; then the list is presented with a matched distracter list in a forced-choice recognition format (i.e., the patient must choose one of the words). A chance level of performance on this task is 50%; scores that fall significantly below this may suggest malingering. Iverson et al. were able to correctly classify 100% of both control subjects and subjects with memory impairment, and 65% of healthy subjects who had been instructed to malinger.

Regarding the forensic evaluation of the TBI patient, it must be stressed that the methods of investigating malingering that are currently available are far from perfect and often require the use of existing empirical, objective methods of detecting malingering and careful documentation of the cognitive and emotional sequelae of the trauma via serial neuropsychological evaluation. Given the high probability of litigation following TBI, the neuropsychologist should perform every evaluation as if he or she will eventually be asked to testify in court.

Conclusions

Traumatic brain injury can have multiple neuropsychological sequelae. These sequelae are related to the synergistic effects of both diffuse and focal injury that often result in variable cognitive deficits. In addition to the effects of direct injury to the brain, the range and extent of cognitive sequelae after TBI depend on premorbid level of functioning and type of injury. A thorough neuropsychological evaluation should take all these factors into account.

References

Arthur G: A Point Scale of Performance Tests, Revised Form II. New York, Psychological Corporation, 1947

Auerbach SH: Neuroanatomical correlates of attention and memory disorders in traumatic brain injury: an application of neurobehavioral subtypes. Journal of Head Trauma Rehabilitation 1(3):1–12, 1986

Barona A, Reynolds CR, Chastain R: A demographically based index of premorbid intelligence for the WAIS-R. J Consult Clin Psychol 52:885–887, 1984

Benson DF: Aphasia, in Clinical Neuropsychology. Edited by Heilman K, Valenstein E. New York, Oxford University Press, 1979, pp 29–38

Benson DF, Stuss DT, Naeser MA, et al: The long-term effects of prefrontal leukotomy. Arch Neurol 38:165–169, 1981

Benton AL, Hamsher K: Multilingual Aphasia Examination. Iowa City, IA, The University of Iowa Press, 1978

Benton AL, Hamsher K, Varney NR, et al: Contributions to Neuropsychological Assessment: A Clinical Manual. New York, Oxford University Press, 1983

Berg GE: A simple objective test for measuring flexibility in thinking. J Gen Psychol 39:15–22, 1948

Brandt J: The Hopkins verbal learning test: development of a new memory test with six equivalent forms. The Clinical Neuropsychologist 5:125–142, 1991

Brierley JB: Cerebral hypoxia, in Greenfield's Neuropathology. Edited by Blackwood W, Cersellis A. Edinburgh, Edward Arnold Publishers, 1976, pp 43–85

Brooks N: Long- and short-term memory in head injured patients. Cortex 11:329–340, 1975

Brooks N: Closed head trauma: assessing the common cognitive problems, in Assessment of the Behavioral Consequences of Head Trauma. Edited by Lezak MD. New York, Alan R Liss, 1989, pp 137–152

Bushke H, Fuld PA: Evaluating storage, retention, and retrieval in disordered memory and learning. Neurology 14:1019–1025, 1974

Butters N: Amnestic disorders, in Clinical Neuropsychology. Edited by Heilman K, Valenstein E. New York, Oxford University Press, 1979, pp 439–474

Cicerone KD, Wood JC: Planning disorder after closed head injury: a case study. Arch Phys Med Rehabil 68:111–115, 1987

Delis DC, Kramer JH, Kaplan E, et al: The California Verbal Learning Test—Adult Version. San Antonio, TX, The Psychological Corporation/Harcourt Brace Jovanovich, 1987

Eppinger MG, Russell PL, Adams RL, et al: The WAIS-R index for estimating premorbid intelligence: cross-validation and clinical utility. J Consult Clin Psychol 55:86–90, 1987

Franzen MD, Iverson GL, McCracken LM: The detection of malingering in neuropsychological assessment. Neuropsychology Review, 1:247–279, 1990

Goldberg E, Costa LD: Hemispheric differences in the acquisition and use of descriptive systems. Brain Lang 14:144–173, 1981

Goldberg E, Tucker D: Motor perseveration and long-term memory for visual forms. Journal of Clinical Neuropsychology, 4:273–288, 1979

Golden CJ: The Stroop Color and Word Test: A Manual for Clinical and Experimental Use. Chicago, IL, Stoelting, 1978

Goodglass H: The assessment of language after brain damage, in Handbook of Clinical Neuropsychology, Vol 2. Edited by Filskov SB, Boll TJ. New York, Wiley, 1986, pp 172–197

Goodglass H, Kaplan E: Assessment of Aphasia and Related Disorders. Philadelphia, PA, Lea and Febiger, 1972

Gouvier WD, Bolter JF, Veneklasen JA, et al: Predicting verbal and performance IQ from demographic data: further findings with head trauma patients. Journal of Clinical Neuropsychology, 5:119–121, 1983

Gronwall D: Paced Auditory Serial Addition Test: A measure of recovery from concussion. Percept Mot Skills 44:367–373, 1977

Gronwall D, Wrightson P: Duration of post-traumatic amnesia after mild head injury. Journal of Clinical Neuropsychology, 2:51–60, 1980

Halstead WC: Brain and Intelligence. Chicago, IL, University of Chicago Press, 1947

Hannay HJ, Levin HS, Grossman RG: Impaired recognition memory after head injury. Cortex 15:269–283, 1979

Hooper HE: The Hooper Visual Organization Test Manual. Los Angeles, CA, Western Psychological Services, 1958

Iverson GL, Franzen MD, McCracken LM: Evaluation of an objective assessment technique for the detection of malingered memory deficits. Law and Human Behavior 15:667–676, 1991

Jones-Gotman M, Milner B: Design fluency: the invention of nonsense drawings after focal cortical lesions. Neuropsychologia 15:653–674, 1977

Kertesz A: Aphasia and Associated Disorders. New York, Grune and Stratton, 1979

Levin HS: Memory deficit after closed head injury. J Clin Exp Neuropsychol 12:129–153, 1989

Levin HS, O'Donnell VM, Grossman RG: The Galveston Orientation and Amnesia Test: a practical scale to assess cognition after head injury. J Nerv Ment Dis 167:675–684, 1979

Levin HS, Amparo E, Eisenberg HM, et al: Magnetic resonance imaging and computerized tomography in relation to the neurobehavioral sequelae of mild and moderate head injuries. J Neurosurg 66:706–713, 1987

Lezak MD: Neuropsychological Assessment, 2nd Edition. New York, Oxford University Press, 1983

Loong JWK: The Continuous Performance Test. San Luis Obispo, CA, Wang Neuropsychological Laboratory, 1988

Milner B: Some effects of frontal lobectomy in man, in The Frontal Granular Cortex and Behavior. Edited by Warren JM, Akert K. New York, McGraw-Hill, 1964, pp 126–142

Milner B: Interhemispheric differences in the localization of psychological processes in man. Br Med Bull 27:272–277, 1971

Mortensen EL, Gade A, Reinisch JM: A critical note on Lezak's Best Performance Method in clinical neuropsychology. J Clin Exp Neuropsychol 13:361–371, 1991

Nissen MJ: Neuropsychology of attention and memory. Journal of Head Trauma Rehabilitation, 1(3):13–21, 1986

Ommaya AK, Gennarelli TA: Cerebral concussion and traumatic unconsciousness. Brain 97:633–654, 1974

Osterrieth PA: Le test de copie d'une figure complexe. Archives de Psychologie 30:206–356, 1944

Perret E: The left frontal lobe of man and the suppression of habitual responses in verbal categorical behavior. Neuropsychologia 12:323–330, 1974

Porteus SD: The Maze Test: Fifty Years Application. New York, Psychological Corp, 1965

Reitan RM: Validity of the Trail Making Test as an indicator of organic brain damage. Percept Mot Skills 8:271–276, 1958

Rey A: L'Examen Clinique En Psychologie. Paris, Presses Universitaires de France, 1964

Rosenblum WI: Pathology of human head injury, in Textbook of Head Injury. Edited by Becker DP, Gudeman SK. Philadelphia, PA, WB Saunders, 1989, pp 507–524

Rosvold HE, Mirsky AF, Sarason EF, et al: A continuous performance test of brain damage. J Consult Clin Psychol 20:343–350, 1956

Schlottmann RS, Johnsen DE: The Intellectual Correlates Scale and the prediction of premorbid intelligence in brain-damaged adults. Archives of Clinical Neuropsychology 6:363–374, 1991

Scoville WB, Milner B: Loss of recent memory after bilateral hippocampal lesions. J Neurol Neurosurg Psychiatry 20:11–24, 1957

Shallice T: Specific impairment in planning. Philos Trans R Soc Lond (Biol) 298:199–209, 1982

Stuss D, Ely BA, Hugenholtz H, et al: Subtle neuropsychological deficits in patients with good recovery after closed head injury. Neurosurgery 17:41–47, 1985

Trahan DE, Larrabee GJ: The Continuous Visual Memory Test. Odessa, TX, Psychological Assessment Resources, 1978

Tranel D: Functional neuroanatomy: neuropsychological correlates of cortical and subcortical damage, in The American Psychiatric Press Textbook of Neuropsychiatry, 2nd Edition. Edited by Yudofsky SC, Hales RE. Washington, DC, American Psychiatric Press, 1992, pp 57–88

Van Zomeren AH, Brouwer WH, Deelman BG: Attentional deficits: the riddles of selectivity, speed, and alertness, in Closed Head Injury: Psychological, Social and Family Consequences. Edited by Brooks N. New York, Oxford University Press, 1984, pp 74–107

Warrington EK, Rabin P: Perceptual matching in patients with cerebral lesions. Neuropsychologia 8:475–487, 1970

Wechsler D: A standardized memory scale for clinical use. J Clin Psychol 19:87–95, 1945

Wechsler D: WAIS-R Manual. New York, Psychological Corporation, 1981

Wechsler D: Wechsler Memory Scale—Revised Manual. San Antonio, TX, Psychological Corporation, 1987

Williams JM: Memory Assessment Scales—Professional Manual. Odessa, FL, Psychological Assessment Resources, Inc., 1991

Wilshire D, Kinsella G, Prior M: Estimating WAIS-R IQ from the National Reading Test: a cross-validation. J Clin Exp Neuropsychol 13:204–216, 1991

Wilson RS, Rosenbaum G, Brown G, et al: The problem of premorbid intelligence in neuropsychological assessment. J Clin Neuropsychol 1:49–54, 1979

Psychiatric Symptomatologies Associated With Traumatic Brain Injury

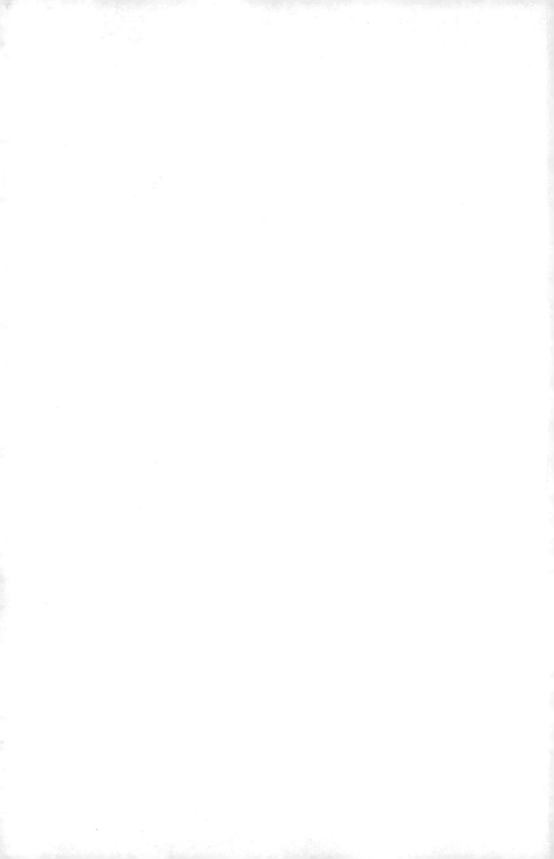

Chapter 5

Personality and Intellectual Changes

Gregory J. O'Shanick, M.D.
Alison Moon O'Shanick, M.S., C.C.C.-S.L.P.

Studies of individuals with traumatic brain injury (TBI) have found that personality changes are the most significant problems at 1, 5, and 15 years postinjury (Livingston et al. 1985; Tomsen 1984; Weddell et al. 1980). At one extreme, there may be subtle awareness on the part of the person and his or her most intimate friends of an attitudinal shift or interpersonal "clumsiness," whereas at the other extreme, there may be dramatic departures from socially acceptable norms of behavior. Such idiosyncratic changes in personality create substantial problems in quantifying these changes after TBI.

On the whole, these changes represent an exaggeration of premorbid traits. Focal cerebral contusions may elicit a pattern of behaviors that initially suggest a personality change. In the course of longitudinal contact with the individual, the therapist will often observe that these discrete areas existed in the context of the person's overall premorbid personality style. The manifestations of these personality changes vary as a function of fatigue, anxiety, styles of the other individuals involved, and environmental cues. Development of chameleon-like or "as if" attributes can create diagnostic confusion with patients who have disorders due to early disturbances of separation-individuation (Gunderson and Singer 1975; Mahler et al. 1975; Munro 1969). Patients may be diagnosed as having borderline personality disorder when they display the impulsivity, lack of empathy, lack of sense of self, and inability to self-monitor that are typical of frontal lobe dysfunction.

Developmental milestones during the life cycle mediate certain elements of personality change subsequent to TBI. An Eriksonian model provides a functional yardstick against which to measure such traits (Erikson 1950). The maturational arrests that are observed following TBI may, in part, be a function of a critical insult that stalls further developmental sequences. Actions that are acceptable from a 15-year-old adolescent are not congruent with those of a 35-year-old. Yet those who sustained their TBI in adolescence are caught in precisely this "time warp" that adversely affects their relationships.

Dissection of these issues requires a relationship between the physician and the individual that allows coping strategies to be observed and assessed in multiple settings and under varying conditions. By their very nature, personality changes show modest response to a crisis intervention approach of treatment. In this chapter we review the complexities of these personality alterations.

Personality Changes After TBI

In the motion picture entitled *Desperately Seeking Susan,* the protagonist, subsequent to a mild TBI, is dramatically transformed into a risk-taking, pleasure-seeking individual in contrast to her conforming preinjury style. Harlow (1868) describes a 19th century railroad worker, Phinaeous Gage, who suffered a penetrating brain injury with a tamping rod, and had personality alterations described as apathy, disinhibition, lability, and loss of appropriate social behavior. Such alterations are illustrative of the effects of both focal and diffuse changes that accompany TBI. Focal trauma to the tips of the temporal lobes, inferior orbital frontal regions, or frontal convexities may occur without neuroradiographic evidence of injury and yet may have devastating clinical ramifications for the patient and the family (Jenkins et al. 1986; Langfitt et al. 1986; Wilson and Wyper 1992). Diffuse axonal injury is the underlying pathophysiological change that accompanies TBI regardless of its severity (Strich 1956, 1961). Diffuse axonal injury results in the "unplugging" of neural networks from one another with a decrease or loss of the associational matrix within the central nervous system (CNS). These changes create "networking" lapses for the individual during functional activities. Lapses may vary from transient problems with initiation that affect one's ability to appropriately begin a pattern, such as a conversation or a problem-solving sequence, to more overt problems with stopping ongoing behaviors.

Judgment

Judgment may be impaired due to difficulty in accurately assessing a current situation based on previously acquired information from past situations. This requires the correct and efficient retrieval of information from long-term databanks and an active comparative process to assess similar and dissimilar elements of the setting. Difficulties in accurate scanning of the situation, assessing the relevant components of the situation, and impulsivity also may be manifested as impairments in judgment. These difficulties constitute neurolinguistic deficits associated with the pragmatics of language (see Table 5–1, adapted from Ehrlich and Sipesk 1985; see also Prutting and Kirchner 1983). A patient may accurately appraise a situation, effectively review past strategies for interaction, and still execute an inappropriate response due to a failure to coordinate propositional language with the intended prosodic component. This can occur when the patient misreads a sarcastic remark as one that is sincere.

Sense of Self

The "innate sense of self" or the individuality of the person rests with his or her idiosyncratic analytic capacities that are developed throughout life and represent an amalgamation of experience, genetic endowment, defensive structure, and social reinforcers at any point in time. Environmental cues play a major role in the regression observed in hospitalized patients without TBI (see Table 5–2, adapted from Strain and Grossman 1975). These same factors may influence individuals with a chronic medical disability such as TBI. Pressures to conform to an external set of behaviors in addition to the "chameleon-like" effect of TBI on personality further serve to confound the individual's sense of self. This "chameleon" quality relates to the patient's assuming the behavioral characteristics of individuals in the immediate environment. When in the presence of severely impaired psychotics, the patient's behavior is similarly impaired. When in the presence of more functional individuals, the patient shows a higher level of competence. Subtle deficits in executive functions that accompany frontal lobe injuries in mild TBI or concussive injuries may impact those individuals who rely primarily on these skills for vocational or interpersonal success, such as lawyers, health care professionals, and entrepreneurs. Integrative deficits in sensory areas may undermine the confidence and skills of craftsmen whose jobs rely on these functions, such as welders, electricians, and artists. The chronic and enduring nature of these deficits requires a reworking of the internal representation of oneself, which may be hindered by the impairment in self-appraisal.

Childish Behavior

Childish behavior results from a combination of changes after TBI that include language deficits, cognitive deficits, and egocentricity. Pragmatic language deficits (Table 5–1) are implicated most frequently in the childish behavior observed following TBI (Szekeres et al. 1987). From a developmental perspective, the same conversational or behavioral response is not expected from a 6-year-old as from a 30-year-old. Developmentally acquired skills such as taking turns, sharing, not interrupting, and inviting expansion on a conversational topic all require awareness of others and ongoing appraisal of the environment during social discourse. A childish style emerges when these elements are absent or diminished. Developmental arrests that result from hospitalization, as observed in infatuations with therapy staff or nurses, also may be perceived as childish.

One component of this type of childish behavior relates to the Eriksonian stage (Table 5–3) that is present at the highest risk period for the occurrence of TBI (15 to 24 years old). At that age, the stage of Identity versus Diffusion precedes the stage of Intimacy versus Isolation. A task of adolescence is to define oneself independent of one's parents, and then to share that self with another in an intimate relationship. In the setting of a rehabilitation hospital, the need for a strong therapeutic alliance between patient and therapist is critical, and similar to that required for successful psychotherapy. The patient needs to relinquish control to the therapist for a period of time and to suspend defensive barriers to permit the reeducation of a dysfunctional process. Similarly, both activities require delaying gratification and assuming a more vulnerable position relative to the therapist. The therapist, in both settings, must carefully avoid the creation of potentially damaging scenarios and misperceptions of the motivation behind the therapist's actions. Infatuations may arise out of a misguided enthusiasm for helping the patient, which is misinterpreted by the patient as a process that is more intimate than

---

Table 5–1.   Pragmatic language dysfunction after traumatic brain injury

---

Decreased intelligibility
Choppy rhythm
Impaired prosody
Limited gesturing with avoidant posturing
Limited affect and eye gaze
Constricted operational vocabulary
Use of ungrammatical syntax
Random, diffuse, and disjointed verbal style
Limited use of language with reliance on stereotypic uses
Abrupt shift of topic
Perseveration
Unable to alter message when communication failure occurs
Frequent interruptions of others
Limited initiation and/or listening

Source.   Adapted from Ehrlich and Sipesk 1985. Used with permission.

professional. Further complicating this set of interactions is the fact that the majority of traumatic brain injuries occur in young males whereas the staff caring for these patients are typically younger female professionals. The avoidance of such childish responses rests in large measure on the concurrent supervision of therapeutic

---

Table 5–2.   Manifestations of stress in hospitalized patients with traumatic brain injury

---

Threat to one's sense of self
  Change in self-identity
  Short-term memory impairment
  Disorientation
Stranger anxiety
  Short-term memory impairment
  Loss of anticipatory capacity
  Impaired visual memory or recognition
  Visual field cuts
  Inattention syndromes (anosognosia)
Separation anxiety
  Disorientation
  Loss of anticipatory capacity
  Short-term memory impairment
Fear of losing love or approval
  Social role disruption
  Interpersonal intrusiveness
  Loss of intimacy and approval
  Impaired self observational skills
Fear of losing control of developmentally mastered milestones
  Loss of impulse control
  Bowel or bladder incontinence
  Motor dysfunction (apraxia)
  Functional independence changes in activities of daily living
  Language disturbances (aphasia, aprosodia, and alexia)
Fear of loss of or injury to body parts
  Craniotomy scars
  PEG tube sites
  Tracheostomy scars
  Urinary catheters
Fears of retribution, guilt, or shame
  Retribution or expiation themes
  Survivor guilt

Source. Adapted from Strain and Grossman 1975. Used with permission.

staff by seasoned senior supervisors and the establishment of thera-peutic limits early in the treatment process. Mental health profes-sionals who have received psychotherapy supervision at some point in their training are often more aware of these elements in the therapeutic process. Utilization of this unique expertise by the reha-bilitation team can minimize staff and patient conflicts.

Frontal Lobe Syndromes

In 1978 Lezak described alterations in personality following TBI: 1) impaired social perceptiveness, 2) impaired self-control and regulation, 3) stimulus-bound behavior, 4) emotional change, and 5) inability to learn from social experience. These deficits, either singly or collectively, impair the ability of the individual to engage in an acceptable social interaction and create a high poten-tial for alienation from others. Frequently, the loss of self-monitor-ing is overtly manifest as the externalization of responsibility for failed social interactions. As a result, this behavior can appear similar to a narcissistic disorder. Whether this lack of interpersonal awareness or insight represents an organically based agnosia (fail-ure to recognize one's behavior) or is a result of a defensive use of denial is unclear (Sandifer 1946). The term "organic denial" has been proposed to describe this phenomenon.

The search for correlates between brain lesions and behavior following TBI resulted in a reworking and refinement of Lezak's work. Describing a population of individuals with frontal lobe inju-ries, Lezak (1982) defined the following attributes: 1) problems with

Table 5–3.   Eriksonian stages

Trust vs. Mistrust
Autonomy vs. Shame and doubt
Industry vs. Inferiority
Identity vs. Diffusion
Intimacy vs. Isolation
Generativity vs. Stagnation
Integrity vs. Despair

initiation, 2) inability to shift responses, 3) difficulty stopping ongoing behavior, 4) inability to monitor oneself, and 5) profound concreteness. These attributes mirror a behavioral equivalent of
parkinsonism (Table 5–4). The clinician often observes the apathetic, abulic patient who lacks sufficient "motivation" to get going
(similar to bradykinesia). Once involved in an activity, the patient
has difficulty changing focus. This may be seen in the spiraling
despair that may engulf the patient in the "catastrophic reaction"
defined by Goldstein (Goldstein 1942). The inability to stop the
behavioral descent resembles the festinating gait disturbance of the
patient with parkinsonism.

The definition of frontal lobe syndromes has been the subject of
multiple articles and a comprehensive work by Stuss and Benson
(1986). Functional correlates of regional changes in these lobes are
important with focal lesions such as arteriovenous malformations,
neoplastic disease, and focal hemorrhagic events. However, caution is advised when ascribing definitive importance of frontal lesions in TBI when the critical neuropathological change is diffuse
axonal injury. Nonetheless, some elements of frontal lobe localization may be evident following TBI. Orbital frontal lesions resulting
from contusions of neural tissue against the floor of the anterior
cranial vault can occur when an individual falls backwards striking
the occiput against a firm surface. A subtle dysfunction in olfaction
(CN I) may be detected as a result of either complete avulsion from
the cribiform plate or stretching of fibers on the inferior surface of
the frontal lobes (Costanzo and Zasler 1992). Such a finding is often
accompanied by neurobehavioral alterations including impulsivity,

---

Table 5–4.   Clinical symptoms of parkinsonism

Impaired initiation
Bradykinesia
Festination
"En bloc" turning
Masklike facies
Tremor
Rigidity

---

euphoria, and manic symptoms. These individuals also have been described as "pseudosociopathic" because they have diminished capacity for introspection and self-awareness. Damage to the medial surfaces or the frontal convexities define a syndrome of apathy, abulia, and indifference as described above. These individuals present in the "lobotomized" image much as Jack Nicholson portrayed in the closing scenes of *One Flew Over The Cuckoo's Nest*. The term *pseudodepressed* has been applied to this population.

Assessment of Personality

Personality changes following TBI have been assessed in many ways over the past 75 years. Projective tests such as the Rorschach were believed to have predictive validity regarding post-TBI personality disturbance (Perline 1979). A more neurologically-based approach was offered by Bender in the development of the test of visual motor gestalt (1938). Although this instrument tapped integrative deficits, it lacked an objective scoring strategy with a high degree of interrater reliability. Attempts to use large population-based measures such as the Minnesota Multiphasic Personality Inventory (MMPI) in individuals with TBI have created potential for misdiagnosis of response profiles for a variety of reasons (Levin et al. 1976). Foremost among these is the length of this instrument even in the shortened 168-item version published in 1974 (Vincent et al. 1984). In clinical use, the slowed rate of information processing that occurs in TBI results in an inordinate time for proper administration. Impulsivity results in invalid scores or inaccurate data. Language-mediated problems, which affect up to 85% of individuals post-TBI, may preclude adequate reading, comprehension, or analytic skills to honestly answer the items (Groher 1977).

At least one study (Kaimann 1983) has correlated elevations in MMPI scores with neuropathological findings on computed tomography. In this study, a high degree of correlation was noted between elevations of the depression scale and nondominant temporal lobe lesions, elevations of the psychoticism scale and periventricular lesions, and elevations of the psychopathic deviance scale and lesions of the frontal lobes. The exclusive use of the MMPI in lieu of a comprehensive clinical interview conducted by a skilled professional is to be absolutely avoided in the evaluation of individuals with TBI. Face-to-face interaction between the examiner and the patient is always indicated to allow the assessment of nonverbal elements. Due to the multiple problems with written and symbolic language that are found after TBI, a pencil-and-paper analysis alone will neglect intact communication pathways that may enable the patient to better communicate his or her strengths and weaknesses.

More recent efforts to objectively quantify personality changes following TBI have relied on factor analysis of multicenter studies such as the National Traumatic Coma Databank (Levin et al. 1990). One such instrument is the Neurobehavioral Rating Scale (Levin et al. 1987). This 27-item, observer-rated scale incorporates elements of the Brief Psychiatric Rating Scale (Overall and Gorham 1962) and provides a profile of personality and behavioral change that can demonstrate recovery over time. An assessment has been developed for the pediatric population that incorporates a more age-appropriate profile of memory changes (Ewing-Cobbs et al. 1990).

The clinical use of an Eriksonian model to identify the psychosocial stage of the patient in the rehabilitation setting provides a method of understanding the emotional recovery from the traumatic event. Development of basic trust in the form of a therapeutic alliance with the treatment team is the core necessity for successful outcome. Becoming increasingly independent in activities of daily living prepares the patient for the increasing complexity of group-based therapeutic activities. Competitive issues arise at this stage, which require caution on the therapist's part to avoid unduly frustrating the success. The individual gradually regains a sense of new identity, which incorporates elements of the preaccident style with the residua of the neurological damage. Attempts to seek intimacy with peers from the preinjury period may result in rejection due to antipathy for TBI changes or normal developmental maturation of those peers beyond the patient's current level. Creation of a productive enriching environment allows for continued growth and productivity with the resulting personal satisfaction.

Diagnostic categories for these changes in DSM-IV (American Psychiatric Association 1994) are included in the section "personality change due to a general medical condition." The elements are that a persistent disturbance in previous personality characteristics exists that is due to a nonpsychiatric medical condition. Marked impairment in social or occupational functioning or marked distress occurs. Subtypes are also proposed (Table 5–5).

Pathophysiology of Personality Changes

Localization of personality to any one structure or set of structures in the CNS is a difficult task. The set of characteristic reactions and psychological defenses to an anxiety-inducing stimulus results from a complex interaction among limbic-mediated drive states, paralimbic cortical inhibition of certain of those states, contextual elements relating to pattern recognition of similar past events, and selection of a response pattern predicated on a cost/benefit analysis for the event in question. All these cognitive events must occur subsequent to the sensory recognition of the provocative event. Diffuse injury that occurs in TBI can impact any of these events. Pathway reduplication and parallel systems in the CNS may contribute to the behavioral variability over time. This creates the potential for an irregularly irregular syndrome. Nondominant parietal structures and frontal executive structures may define awareness of body in space and integration of sensory signals. Indeed, damage to these regions can result in a syndrome of guarded hypervigilance similar to a paranoid style. Damage to temporal regions of the amygdala may effect the "coloration" or affective intensity of an event. Rage

Table 5–5. Secondary personality subtypes (DSM-IV)

Labile
Disinhibited
Aggressive
Apathetic
Paranoid
Other (e.g., associated with a seizure disorder)
Combined
Unspecified

Source. American Psychiatric Association 1994.

and fear responses associated with these lesions are discussed in Chapter 10.

The neurochemical basis of personality attributes is an emerging area of interest. Whereas models of dopamine receptor activity relating to vigilance, expectation, and reward have been proffered (Gershanik et al. 1983; McEntee et al. 1987), serotonin has recently been implicated in large scale studies of hostility in Type A personality (Tyrer and Seivewright 1988; Williams 1991). Of great clinical interest is the correlation between high circulating levels of catecholamines and their metabolites and a good outcome post-TBI (Clifton et al. 1981; Woolf et al. 1987). This laboratory finding supports the long held clinical wisdom that the patient who was agitated and "hit the ground running" had a much better prognosis than his lethargic apathetic counterpart.

Effect of Premorbid Personality

Controversy exists regarding the importance of premorbid personality in predicting the occurrence of TBI. Earlier studies suggested that TBI was not strictly a random event and tended to affect those with a proclivity for "living on the edge." More recent studies, however, find that there is no overrepresentation of risk takers or substance abusers in adolescents with TBI (Lehr 1990). More data is needed in this regard.

Premorbid personality factors mitigate the defense mechanisms used to cope with the stresses of TBI. The schema developed by Strain and Grossman (1975) for stresses of hospitalization, as shown in Table 5–2, can be adapted to focus on the stresses specific to the experience of TBI. The loss of self is a primary focus of individual psychotherapy as discussed in Chapter 20. The loss of narcissistic integrity pervades every aspect of life for those with TBI, resulting in significant anxiety. In an attempt to contain this anxiety, the patient uses the defenses that have the greatest past success in stress reduction. This exaggeration of premorbid style is identical to that described in a study of personality types in acutely ill medical patients (Kahana and Bibring 1964). These authors observed that these styles became exaggerated under stress. Because stress is reduced by the correction of Axis I or Axis III disturbances, the individual gradually returns to the pre-illness level of homeostasis. In the case of TBI, the level of stress becomes chronic because there is a seemingly permanent exaggeration of personality style.

Intellectual Changes After TBI

Changes of intellect have received vast interest as the development of more rigorously standardized assessment instruments have been introduced. As shown in Chapter 4, comprehensive neuropsychological evaluation has been the mainstay of TBI intellectual assessment for the past two decades. The ability to perform these evaluations over many points in time with minimal test-retest effect has aided in quantification of recovery curves. However, the efforts of multiple researchers have excluded to large degree the contributions of "non-neuropsychologists" in the evaluation of intellectual changes post-TBI (Levin et al. 1982, 1991; Prigatano 1986). Although neurolinguistic experts and those with neurosensory integration backgrounds have been consulted in the area of treatment of TBI in children, the developmental approach has, unfortunately, been neglected in the current evaluation and treatment in adults. In individuals who have sustained either classic concussive or mild TBI injuries, the sensitivity of standardized neuropsychological testing batteries may miss the "higher" cognitive problems that require more facile manipulation of symbolic language. A comprehensive evaluation includes the assessments of the psychiatrist, neuropsychologist, occupational therapist, physical therapist, and speech-language pathologist.

Arousal

Arousal or vigilance may range from heightened to impaired. Low-vigilance states are associated with a poorer prognosis for functional independence (Clifton et al. 1981; Woolf et al. 1987). These problems most frequently are correlated with reduction in dopaminergic activity (Feeney and Sutton 1988; Lal et al. 1988; Neppe 1988) or increases in cholinergic activity in the CNS (Nissen et al. 1987; Rusted and Warburton 1989). Hypervigilant states may portend a better clinical prognosis; however, the heightened arousal may predispose the patient to aggressive behavior (Eichelman 1987). Serotonergic and noradrenergic mechanisms have been implicated in aggressive states.

Attention

Disorders of attention are a common consequence and may be overlooked by the casual observer (Stuss et al. 1985, 1989; Van Zomeren 1981). The inability to attend to one distinct stimulus may be manifest in any sensory domain, including visual, auditory, and tactile. Whereas the neural substrate for the perception of the event may be intact, the capacity to "lock on" to the target is reduced. This reduction has been termed a *loss of phasic attention* by Van Zomeren (1981). This is in contrast to the phenomenon of an increased scanning attention whereby the person is seeking meaningful stimuli from the environment. The loss of filtering capacity is presumably mediated by descending pathways that suppress simultaneous reception of competing sensory stimuli. Clinically, this is displayed in the reduced capacity to converse in noisy settings (parties, malls), impaired ability to read maps and blueprints, and problems interpreting simultaneous sensory events.

Concentration is the capacity to maintain attention on a fixed stimulus for a given period of time. Although in certain frontal lobe syndromes concentration appears to be present, this actually represents the loss of capacity to stop ongoing behavior such as watching television. The deficits are believed to be due to damage to pathways that inhibit transmission of afferent impulses (Gualtieri and Evans 1988; Gualtieri et al. 1989).

Memory

The classically described memory change subsequent to TBI is a loss of short-term memory for events that transpire in the individual's immediate life, such as misplacing objects and the inability to recall lists of items. These occasions of memory loss arise from an impairment in the capacity for encoding incoming data, which presumably resides in the region of the hippocampus. The high frequency of this occurrence in TBI may be explained by the vulnerable location of the hippocampus. The hippocampus resides in the anterior temporal lobe where force vectors may propel neuronal tissue into the sphenoidal ridge. In fact, the presence of anterograde and retrograde amnesia has been a diagnostic requirement for TBI in multiple studies (Levin et al. 1979, 1982). This strict definition excludes countless numbers who have "near-concussive" injuries. The translation of information from storage to active memory also requires manipulation by hippocampal structures. Again, after TBI retrieval of data also may be faulty.

These changes in memory may be reflected in verbal and/or nonverbal functions. Attempts to define variations in memory capacity may lead to more efficient retraining strategies; however, from a clinical perspective such differences have not proven useful. Memory dysfunction also might be dichotomized as effortful versus incidental in nature. Effortful memory would involve those processes needed to respond accurately to a "fill in the blank" question. In this situation, the patient's recall process must conform to the external structure imposed by the examiner. Incidental memory, conversely, is demonstrated in the capacity to answer essay questions by using one's own idiosyncratic neural association pathways to arrive at the correct response. Following TBI, incidental memory is more intact than effortful memory. Therefore, the examiner may obtain more information using an open-ended design than a structured interview format, such as is required by the MMPI, Structured Clinical Interview for DSM-III-R (SCID; Spitzer et al. 1986), and Beck Depression Inventory, which may therefore produce inaccurate results. However, the open-ended design involves more investment in time for the examiner.

Cognition may be defined as the sum total of all processes involved in the analysis and management of data-based activity. This includes data acquisition through sensory inputs, discernment of a hierarchy of choice/nonchoice options based on a predefined set of comparisons, and execution of the option chosen. A further element of follow-up analysis also occurs that expands the pre-defined set of comparisons. These steps have been labeled "executive functions" (see Table 5–6). Disturbances in these functions occur after TBI in a frequency that approaches 100% (Szekeres et al. 1987).

Abstraction

The capacity for abstract thought may be reduced following TBI with injury to structures in the frontal lobes. This ability requires a multistep sequencing process that analyzes both face content and metaphoric elements. Because abstract reasoning represents the highest level of cognitive development on the Piagetian scale, this process is keenly vulnerable to attack. Loss of abstract reasoning also involves an impaired capacity to move from a linear analysis to one based on a systems analytic approach. For example, an individual may appreciate that an employer expects punctuality when he or she is present, but may not demonstrate the same time skills when the boss is on vacation. A recent text by Levin et al. (1991) provides the most appropriate treatment of this subject.

Problems in understanding abstract concepts, or concreteness, that occur in frontal lobe dysfunction result from the inability to maintain one set of information and to perform a simultaneous comparison with another set of data. The inability to perform divergent rather than linear analyses results in a "loss of the abstract attitude" and a decrease in sense of humor. Those individuals who

Table 5–6.	Executive functions

Setting goals
Assessing strengths and weaknesses
Planning and/or directing activity
Initiating and/or inhibiting behavior
Monitoring current activity
Evaluating results

Source. Adapted from Szekeres et al. 1987. Used with permission.

have maintained their humor following TBI may, in fact, have a better clinical prognosis. Premorbid capacity for humor and the social modeling of those with whom the individual resides are other important factors.

Language

Language disturbance is observed in 8%–85% of individuals following TBI (Groher 1977). Observed changes may include problems with verbal memory, auditory processing, integration and synthesis of linguistic information, word retrieval, and spelling. These problems most commonly arise from the combined effects of diffuse injury and focal cortical contusions. Loss of spontaneity of speech may occur in even the most trivial of injuries. Disturbances in the intonation of language (prosodic dysfunction) can influence both the ability to convey affect in speech (motor aprosodia) and to perceive affect in speech (sensory aprosodia). Cortical regions in analogous position to Broca's and Wernicke's areas in the nondominant hemisphere are believed to subserve expressive and receptive prosodic speech respectively. With motor aprosodia the patient may be misdiagnosed as depressed with blunted affect or thought disordered with flattened affect. The inability to impart tonal color to one's language often requires the use of either physical mannerisms (shaking fists or pounding the table) or invective to punctuate one's intended message clearly.

Pure sensory prosodic dysfunction is rarely observed. Substantial regions of the nondominant hemisphere and the inferior surfaces of both temporal lobes are involved in this process, possibly due to the adaptive evolutionary advantage that exists in the capacity to visually recognize affect in others. More commonly following TBI, dysfunction of auditory sensory prosody is seen and is manifest as the inability to correctly interpret affect in situations where visual cuing is absent. This typically would be encountered in telephone conversations and crowd settings where the capacity to lock on to one individual's face may be compromised. In such situations, the individual may respond out of context to another's conversation predicated on his or her own mood state.

Evaluation of post-TBI neurolinguistic problems mandates a comprehensive speech language assessment performed by a speech language pathologist with experience in TBI. Attention to developmental language issues is required to adequately define the context in which the TBI changes occur. Audiometric evaluation may also be needed to diagnose occult peripheral deficits that may further worsen language capability.

Perception

Perceptual problems arise post-TBI due to diffuse damage to subcortical pathways responsible for interpretation of visual, auditory, kinesthetic, olfactory, and gustatory stimuli. Although end organ damage may coexist to further compromise perception, deficient central processing occurs in most levels of TBI. Visual processing problems may be manifest by defects in visual organization, visual figure ground awareness, three-dimensional perception, and visual tracking. These changes are often so subtle that the individual fails to recognize the existence of any problem. Rather, the presenting complaint is often one of anxiety that is situation specific. For example, an interior designer decreased the complexity of wallpaper hung following the disastrous event of hanging an entire room upside down. In another situation, a seamstress pieced a pattern in such a manner that the sleeves were inside out.

Auditory perceptual problems include auditory figure ground, vigilance, and attention disturbances. Although the individual may possess intact afferent pathways for hearing, central integrative deficits may render the person functionally deaf (i.e., auditory agnosia or pure word deafness). Figure ground deficits render the individual unable to accurately perceive one voice amidst a crowd of many, as may occur at a party or mall. The inability to lock on to one stimulus source again is the underlying problem.

Olfactory disturbances may involve not only disruption of the olfactory nerve, but also perceptual changes due to injury to the rhinencephalic cortex. These deficits have significant survival ramifications as seen in the inability to smell smoke, food spoilage, or leaking natural gas. Adaptations to these might include the use of smoke detectors, visually inspecting the contents of a container prior to ingestion, and gas alarms to warn of leakage.

Treatment

All therapeutic interventions in traumatic brain injury combine the use of pharmacological manipulation with a series of structured exercises of graded difficulty designed to stimulate restitution of the CNS. The use of splints and adaptive equipment supports the maximal independence of the individual when total return to premorbid functional levels would otherwise be impossible. Just as TBI rarely results in an improved physical state, the patient's behavior is seldom improved after TBI. The goal of treatment is to return the person to his or her premorbid level of function. For the adult, this is to rehabilitate rather than habilitate.

Pharmacotherapy

Pharmacotherapy serves as a mechanism to provide a "splint" or "adaptive device" on the neurochemical milieu while the intrinsic healing of the CNS occurs. Selection of the agent is predicated on a cost-benefit analysis of desired therapeutic effects countered against the known side effects. This includes an awareness of the idiosyncratic responses observed in individuals after TBI (O'Shanick 1991).

Indications and contraindications relate to those agents that can adversely impact the recovery of the CNS. This might include dopamine antagonists, which may inhibit recovery curves in the acute phase postinjury (Feeney et al. 1982). Anticholinergic agents may in high concentrations induce delirium or worsen cognitive performance (Nissen et al. 1987; O'Shanick 1991; Rusted and Warburton 1989). Agents that lower seizure threshold require careful monitoring to prevent seizure induction (O'Shanick and Zasler 1990). Any medication that shares metabolic degradation pathways with an anticonvulsant in use requires scrutiny of levels early in the course of therapy and regularly thereafter (O'Shanick 1987).

Several agents are useful in increasing arousal, decreasing fatigue, and improving affective continence (Gualtieri et al. 1989; Lal et al. 1988; Neppe 1988; O'Shanick 1991) (see Tables 5–7 and 5–8). Stimulants exert their therapeutic effect primarily through augmenting the release of catecholamines into the synapse (Gualtieri and Evans 1988). Serotonergic actions have been described at higher concentrations. Dextroamphetamine is the prototype, although methylphenidate is a more potent releaser of dopamine from storage vesicles. Although pemoline has a longer half-life, it is seldom used because of the need to rapidly clear medication effects in the event of an adverse action. An alternative intervention for arousal and abulia is the use of agents that directly impact the synthesis of dopamine (Table 5–9). By increasing the precursor (as with Sinemet), reducing degradation through inhibition of monoamine oxidase (as with Eldepryl), or disrupting feedback inhibition of dopamine production (as with amantadine), a net gain can be attained. These strategies require an intact neuron for successful treatment. If substantial cell death has occurred, a limited response will be observed. The use of direct agents with a predominant agonist action will provide benefit. These include bromocriptine and pergolide (Berg et al. 1987; Crismon et al. 1988).

Table 5–7.   Target symptoms for stimulant therapy

Depression
Excessive daytime drowsiness
Fatigue
Impaired concentration
Decreased arousal
Decreased initiation

Table 5–8.   Doses of stimulants in traumatic brain injury

Drug	Dosage
Methylphenidate	5–15 mg per day to qid
Dextroamphetamine	15–20 mg per day to bid
Pemoline	18.75–75 mg per day

Opiate antagonists have been shown to be of benefit in situations involving hypothalamic dysregulation. Disorders of satiety that have been described as "organic bulimia" have shown response to naltrexone (Childs 1987). Self-injurious behaviors also respond to naltrexone much as has been described in the developmental disability literature (Herman et al. 1986) (Table 5–10).

Psychotherapy Treatment

Verbal therapies with individuals with TBI require careful monitoring to assure that auditory processing problems do not interfere with the therapeutic process.

Short-term memory problems also may be mistaken for resistance in the setting of a traditional psychotherapeutic relationship. The use of a notebook or audiotape for the patient's benefit remedies this problem. A flexible treatment schedule that also includes a period with an involved outside observer is advantageous in providing corroborating data unavailable to the patient due to frontal lobe injuries. Care with issues of a confidential nature that could

Table 5–9.   Dopamine agonist doses in traumatic brain injury

Drug	Dosage
Symmetrel (amantadine)	100 mg per day to tid
Eldepryl (L-deprenyl)	5–10 mg per day
Sinemet (L-dopa/carbidopa)	Up to a total daily dose of 100 mg L-dopa
Parlodel (bromocriptine)	2.5–30 mg per day to tid
Permax (pergolide)	0.05–1.5 mg per day to tid

Table 5–10.   Opiate antagonists

Indications:	Organic bulimia
	Self-injurious behavior
	Prader-Willi Syndrome
	? Other hypothalamic dysregulation
Dosage:	25–50 mg bid to qid

compromise the trust in the therapist is essential. A close alliance with healthy family members can provide the therapist with a base of understanding of the system needs and tolerances. Additional information concerning individual, behavioral, cognitive, and family therapies are addressed in Chapters 20, 21, and 22.

Conclusions

Personality and cognitive changes after TBI result from a complex array of forces that impact biological, psychological, and social spheres of the individual's life. Comprehensive evaluation based on an understanding of the myriad subtle changes in information processing is a mandatory prerequisite for therapeutic success. The astute clinician will consider these parameters not only in clearly identified situations of TBI, but also in those cases previously labelled as "functionally" disordered who have become "treatment refractory." In these cases, either misdiagnosis or insufficient diagnosis may subject an individual to inadequate if not harmful interventions.

References

American Psychiatric Association: Diagnostic and Statistical Manual of Mental Disorders, 4th Edition. Washington, DC, American Psychiatric Association, 1994

Bender L: A visual motor gestalt test and its clinical use. American Orthopsychiatric Association Research Monographs No 3, 1938

Berg MJ, Ebert B, Willis DK, et al: Parkinsonism-drug treatment, I: drug Intelligence and Clinical Pharmacy 21:10–21, 1987

Childs A: Naltrexone in organic bulimia: a preliminary report. Brain Inj 1:49–55, 1987

Clifton GL, Ziegler MG, Grossman RG: Circulating catecholamines and sympathetic activity after head injury. Neurosurgery 8:10–14, 1981

Costanzo RM, Zasler ND: Epidemiology and pathophysiology of olfactory and gustatory dysfunction in head trauma. Journal of Head Trauma Rehabilitation 7:15–24, 1992

Crismon ML, Childs A, Wilcox RE, et al: The effect of bromocriptine on speech dysfunction in patients with diffuse brain injury (akinetic mutism). Clin Neuropharmacol 11:462–466, 1988

Ehrlich J, Sipesk A: Group treatment of communication skills for head trauma patients. Cognitive Rehabilitation 13:32–37, 1985

Eichelman B: Neurochemical and psychopharmacologic aspects of aggressive behavior, in The Third Generation of Progress. Edited by Meltzer HY. New York, Raven Press, 1987, pp 697–704

Erikson E: Childhood and Society. New York, WW Norton, 1950

Ewing-Cobbs L, Levin HS, Fletcher JM, et al: The children's orientation and amnesia test: relationship to severity of acute head injury and to recovery of memory. Neurosurgery 27:683–691, 1990

Feeney DM, Sutton RL: Catecholamines and recovery of function after brain damage, in Pharmacological Approaches to the Treatment of Brain and Spinal Cord Injury. Edited by Stein DG, Sabel BA. New York, Plenum, 1988, pp 121–142

Feeney DM, Gonzalez A, Law WA: Amphetamine, haloperidol and experience interact to affect rate of recovery after motor cortex injury. Science 217:855–857, 1982

Gershanik O, Heikkila RE, Duvoisin RC: Behavioral correlates of dopamine receptor activation. Neurology 33:1489–1492, 1983

Goldstein K: Aftereffects of Brain Injuries in War. New York, Grune and Stratton, 1942

Groher M: Language and memory disorders following closed head trauma. J Speech Hearing Res 20:212–223, 1977

Gualtieri CT, Evans RW: Stimulant treatment for the neurobehavioural sequelae of traumatic brain injury. Brain Inj 2:273–290, 1988

Gualtieri CT, Chandler M, Coons TB, et al: Amantadine: a new clinical profile for traumatic brain injury. Clin Neuropharmacol 12:258–270, 1989

Gunderson JG, Singer MT: Defining borderline patients: an overview. Am J Psychiatry 132:1–10, 1975

Harlow JM: Recovery from the passage of an iron bar through the head. Publications of the Massachusetts Medical Society 2:327–346, 1868

Herman BH, Hammock MK, Arthur-Smith A, et al: A biochemical role for opioid peptides in self-injurious behavior. Paper presented at the annual meeting of the American Academy of Child and Adolescent Psychiatry, Los Angeles, CA, October 1986

Jenkins A, Teasdale G, Hadley MDM, et al: Brain lesions detected by magnetic resonance imaging in mild and severe head injuries. Lancet 2:445–446, 1986

Kahana R, Bibring G: Personality types in medical management, in Psychiatry and Medical Practice in a General Hospital. Edited by Zimberg NE. New York, International Universities Press, 1964, pp 108–123

Kaimann CR: A Neuropsychological Investigation of Multiple Sclerosis. Ph.D. Dissertation, Department of Psychology, University of Nebraska, Lincoln, Nebraska, December 1983

Lal S, Merbitz CP, Grip JC: Modification of function in head-injured patients with Sinemet. Brain Inj 2:225–233, 1988

Langfitt TW, Obrist WD, Alavi A, et al: Computerized tomography, magnetic resonance imaging, and positron emission tomography in the study of brain trauma. J Neurosurg 64:760–767, 1986

Lehr E: Incidence and etiology, in Psychological Management of Traumatic Brain Injuries in Children and Adolescents. Edited by Lehr E. Rockville, MD, Aspen Publishers, 1990, pp 1–13

Levin HS, Grossman RG, Kelley PJ: Aphasic disorders in patients with closed head injury. J Neurol Neurosurg Psychiatry 39:1062–1070, 1976

Levin HS, O'Donnell VM, Grossman RG: The Galveston Orientation and Amnesia Test: a practical scale to assess cognition after head injury. J Nerv Ment Dis 167:675–686, 1979

Levin HS, Benton AL, Grossman RG: Neurobehavioral Consequences of Closed Head Injury. New York, Oxford University Press, 1982

Levin HS, High WM, Goethe KE, et al: The Neurobehavioral Rating Scale: assessment of the behavioral sequelae of head injury by the clinician. J Neurol Neurosurg Psychiatry 50:183–193, 1987

Levin HS, Gary HE, Eisenberg HM: Neurobehavioral outcome one year after severe head injury: experience of the traumatic coma databank. J Neurosurg 73:699–709, 1990

Levin HS, Eisenberg HM, Benton AL: Frontal Lobe Function and Dysfunction. New York, Oxford University Press, 1991

Lezak MD: Living with the characterologically altered brain injured patient. J Clin Psychiatry 39:592–598, 1978

Lezak MD: The problem of assessing executive functions. International Journal of Psychology 17:281–297, 1982

Livingston M, Brooks N, Bond M: Patient outcome in the year following severe head injury and relatives' psychiatric and social functioning. J Neurol Neurosurg Psychiatry 48:876–881, 1985

Mahler MS, Pine F, Bergman A: The Psychological Birth of the Human Infant. New York, Basic Books, 1975

McEntee WJ, Mair RG, Langlais PJ: Neurochemical specificity of learning: dopamine and motor learning. Yale J Biol Med 60:187–193, 1987

Munro A: Parent-child separation—is it really the cause of psychiatric illness in adult life? Arch Gen Psychiatry 20:598–604, 1969

Neppe VM: Management of catatonic stupor with L-DOPA. Clin Neuropharmacol 11:90–91, 1988

Nissen MJ, Knopman DS, Schacter DL: Neurochemical dissociation of memory systems. Neurology 37:789–794, 1987

O'Shanick GJ: Clinical aspects of psychopharmacologic treatment in head-injured patients. Journal of Head Trauma Rehabilitation 2:59–67, 1987

O'Shanick GJ: Cognitive function after brain injury: pharmacologic interference and facilitation. Neurorehabilitation 1:44–49, 1991

O'Shanick GJ, Zasler ND: Neuropsychopharmacological approaches to traumatic brain injury, in Community Integration Following Traumatic Brain Injury. Edited by Kreutzer JS, Wehman P. Baltimore, MD, Brooks Publishing, 1990, pp 15–27

Overall JE, Gorham DR: The brief psychiatric rating scale. Psycholog Rep 10:799–812, 1962

Perline IH: Computer Interpreted Rorschach. Tempe, AZ, Century Diagnostics, 1979

Prigatano GP (ed): Neuropsychological Rehabilitation After Brain Injury. Baltimore, MD, Johns Hopkins University Press, 1986

Prutting C, Kirchner D: Applied pragmatics, in Pragmatic Assessment and Intervention Issues in Language. Edited by Gallagher T, Prutting L. San Diego, CA, College-Hill Press, 1983, pp 32–41

Rusted JM, Warburton DM: Cognitive models and cholinergic drugs. Neuropsychobiology 21:31–36, 1989

Sandifer P: Anosognosia and disorders of body scheme. Brain 69:122–137, 1946

Spitzer R, William JB, Gibbon M: Structured Clinical Interview for DSM-III-R. New York, Biometrics Research Department, New York State Psychiatric Institute, 1986

Strain J, Grossman S: Psychological reactions to medical illness and hospitalization, in Psychological Care of the Medically Ill: A Primer in Liaison Psychiatry. Edited by Strain J, Grossman S. New York, Appleton Century Crofts, 1975, pp 23–36

Strich S: Diffuse degeneration of the cerebral white matter in severe dementia following head injury. J Neurol Neurosurg Psychiatry 19:163–185, 1956

Strich SJ: Shearing of nerve fibers as a cause of brain damage due to head injury, a pathological study of twenty cases. Lancet 2:443–448, 1961

Stuss DT, Benson DF: The Frontal Lobes. New York, Raven Press, 1986

Stuss DT, Ely P, Hugenholtz H, et al: Subtle neuropsychological deficits in patients with good recovery after closed head injury. Neurosurgery 17:41–47, 1985

Stuss DT, Stethem LL, Hugenholtz H, et al: Reaction time after head injury: fatigue, divided and focused attention, and consistency of performance. J Neurol Neurosurg Psychiatry 52:742–748, 1989

Szekeres SF, Ylvisaker M, Cohen SB: A framework for cognitive rehabilitation therapy, in Community Reentry for Head Injured Adults. Edited by Ylvisaker M, Gobble EMR. Boston, MA, College-Hill Press, 1987, pp 87–136

Tomsen I: Late outcome of very severe blunt head trauma: a 10–15 year second follow-up. J Neurol Neurosurg Psychiatry 47:260–268, 1984

Tyrer P, Seivewright N: Pharmacological treatment of personality disorders. Clin Neuropharmacol 11:493–499, 1988

Van Zomeren AH: Reaction Time and Attention After Closed Head Injury. Lisse, Swets and Zeitlinger, 1981

Vincent KR, Castillo IM, Hauser RI, et al: MMPI-168: Codebook. Norwood, NJ, Ablex Publishing, 1984

Weddell R, Oddy M, Jenkins D: Social adjustment after rehabilitation: a two year follow-up of patients with severe head injury. Psychol Med 10:257–263, 1980

Williams R: A relook at personality type and coronary heart disease. Progress in Cardiology 4:91–97, 1991

Wilson JTL, Wyper D: Neuroimaging and neuropsychological functioning following closed head injury: CT, MRI, and SPECT. Journal of Head Trauma Rehabilitation 7:29–39, 1992

Woolf PD, Hamill RW, Lee LA, et al: The predictive value of catecholamines in assessing outcome in traumatic brain injury. J Neurosurg 66:875–882, 1987

Chapter 6

Delirium

Paula T. Trzepacz, M.D.

What Is Delirium?

Defining Delirium in Traumatic Brain Injury

Delirium is a psychiatric disorder that is common in medically ill patients. Approximately 18% of general hospital patients are delirious (Trzepacz et al. 1989a). Some surgical populations have an even higher incidence of delirium—approximately 30% in postcardiotomy patients (Smith and Dimsdale 1989) and 50% in elderly hip surgery patients (Williams et al. 1985). The incidence of delirium after traumatic brain injury (TBI) is uncertain because of classification issues in the TBI literature, but appears to be frequent, especially with severe injuries and loss of consciousness. Brief confusional periods can result from even seemingly minor concussions (Lipowski 1990; Teasdale and Jennett 1974). Russell stated that "disturbed consciousness is a feature found in most cases of head injury" (Russell and Smith 1961).

The term *delirium* is rarely used in TBI literature. Terms such as *states of impaired consciousness, posttraumatic amnesia, altered consciousness,* and *loss of consciousness* (coma) are used, often without clear definitions of signs and symptoms or, when defined, without a clear consensus as to usage or practical assessment

(Artiola et al. 1980; Gronwall and Wrightson 1980). The varying definitions and criteria make a review of delirium after TBI difficult and interpretation of research on posttraumatic amnesia (PTA) confusing.

The closest term to *delirium* in the TBI literature is *posttraumatic amnesia;* however, this is loosely used and may encompass coma at one extreme or only focal memory deficits at the other. In fact, *posttraumatic amnesia* is defined as the "time elapsed from injury until recovery of full consciousness and the return of ongoing memory" (Grant and Alves 1987). *Posttraumatic amnesia* also has been defined as "a period of clouded consciousness which precedes the attainment of full orientation and continuous awareness in persons recovering from head injuries" and as "characterized primarily by a failure of mnestic processes" (Mandleberg 1975). Thus PTA overlaps with coma, stupor, delirium, and amnestic syndrome, although its name would indicate synonymity only with an amnestic syndrome. However, that delirium ("confusion") is a separate state from either coma or amnesia in TBI patients was nicely diagrammed by Ommaya and Gennarelli (1974), along with the expected temporal relationship between them (Figure 6–1). This paradigm has not been well integrated into the literature, however.

Delirium is an abnormal state of consciousness that exists on a continuum between stupor or coma and normal consciousness (Figure 6–2). However, patients often progress directly from coma into delirium without a clearly defined stupor stage. The placement of a particular delirious episode along this continuum depends on the severity of that delirium. "Subclinical delirium" describes a phase before or during the resolution of an episode of diagnosable delirium that is less severe and detectable only by more subtle examination of the patient. This is an important concept in TBI because of the need to distinguish lingering amnestic deficits from a preceding possible delirium, in which the cognitive deficits were more generalized and were accompanied by other behavioral symptoms.

Signs and Symptoms of Delirium

Diffuse cognitive deficits are a hallmark of delirium that differentiates it from other psychiatric disorders (Table 6–1), except for the

more advanced dementias. (The temporal history usually distinguishes it from dementias, where the onset of delirium is acute or
even abrupt.) These cognitive deficits include disorientation to
time, place, and person (usually in that order), deficits in attention
and concentration, deficits in short-term memory with an inability
to learn and retain new information, deficits in long-term memory,
reduced ability to abstract, conceptualize, and sequence using
higher order thought, reduced mental flexibility for switching mental sets, and reduced visuoconstructional ability. Some or all of
these cognitive deficits may be present in delirium. It is unlikely that
delirium is a disorder only of attention.

In addition to these cognitive deficits, delirium involves many
other neuropsychiatric symptoms (Table 6–2). These include an
alteration in mood (anxious, depressed, irritable, hostile), affective
lability (sometimes to the proportions of pseudobulbar palsy), and
mood incongruency. Thinking is disorganized, and may be rambling, tangential, or even loosely associated; in the most severe

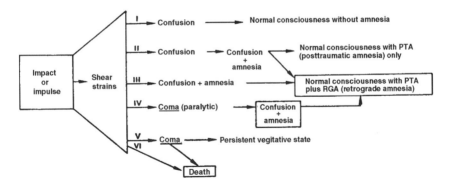

Figure 6–1. Coma and levels of confusion (delirium) following
traumatic brain injury, with posttraumatic amnesia (PTA) occurring after
resolution of delirium and in the context of normal consciousness,
according to Ommaya and Gennarelli (1974). This differentiates PTA
from delirium states.
Source. Reprinted from Ommaya AK, Gennarelli TA: "Cerebral
Concussion and Traumatic Unconsciousness." *Brain* 97:633–654, 1974.
Used with permission of Oxford University Press.

cases, speech resembles a fluent or a global aphasia. Language abnormalities are variable, but can include word-finding difficulty, paraphasias, dysnomia, dysgraphia, impaired repetition, impaired articulation, impaired comprehension, and perseveration of words or phrases; or language may be relatively intact. Psychomotor behavior may evidence retardation or agitation, often mixed together (related concepts are the variants of delirium, called hypoactive or hyperactive); patients may appear depressed and withdrawn, or may be agitated and remove intravenous lines, or wander or pace around. Perceptual disturbances are common and may take the form of either illusions or hallucinations; visual and tactile hallucinations strongly suggest delirium, although auditory hallucinations or illusions also occur in delirium. Suspiciousness and persecutory delusions are common, but the latter usually are poorly formed and not well systematized, often incorporating many of the caregivers

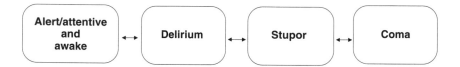

Figure 6–2. Delirium and continuum of levels of consciousness. Delirium occurs on a continuum between normal consciousness and stupor and/or coma. Delirium often has a prodrome of milder symptoms, called *subclinical delirium,* as an intermediate state between full-blown delirium and normal consciousness; subclinical delirium also occurs during the resolution of an episode of delirium.

Table 6–1.   Cognitive deficits in delirium

Disorientation
Attentional deficits
Memory defects
Deficits in higher-order thinking
Visuoconstructional dysfunction

Note. Some or all deficits may occur.

into the delusional ideation. Patients may refuse tests because of suspiciousness, thus interfering with their own medical care. The sleep-wake cycle is disrupted and fragmented throughout the 24-hour period, with napping and nocturnal arousals that are often accompanied by nocturnal confusion and an inability to distinguish nightmares or dreams from reality.

These symptoms of delirium classically wax and wane during a 24-hour period, with phases of increased lucidity alternating with increased impairment. This waxing and waning makes it more difficult to assess the severity of delirium and complicates determining when the episode has ended.

DSM-IV criteria (American Psychiatric Association 1994) for diagnosing delirium require the presence of disturbance of consciousness and attentional deficits, disorganized thinking, a fairly abrupt onset with a fluctuating course, and physical factors that can be implicated as causative (Table 6–3).

Descriptions of the clinical symptoms of PTA in the period after emergence from coma until the phase of focal memory deficits are essentially descriptions of delirium. This is a period of "confusion, restlessness, perplexity, irritability, aggression, withdrawal, and frank psychosis" (Grant and Alves 1987) and of "restlessness, agitation, combativeness, confusion, hallucinations and other disturbed perceptions, disorientation, depression, paranoid ideation, hypomania, and confabulation" (Fisher 1985). These clinical descriptions

Table 6–2.	Other neuropsychiatric symptoms and features of delirium

Change in mood
Disorganized thinking
Psychotic symptoms
Perceptual disturbances
Language disturbances
Psychomotor changes
Sleep-wake cycle disturbances
Abrupt onset
Fluctuating course
Usually reversible

highlight the hyperactive variant of delirium, which may be more common in TBI or may be more easily recognized by staff. Ewert et al. (1989) described PTA as the "initial stage of recovery from TBI after emergence from coma and characterized by anterograde and retrograde amnesia, disorientation, and rapid forgetting," but not necessarily accompanied by attentional deficits, confusion, and changes in behavior. This latter description focuses on impaired memory and downplays other cognitive and behavioral symptoms of delirium. Wechsler Adult Intelligence Scale (WAIS) test results have revealed diffuse cognitive deficits in PTA (abstraction, comprehension, attention, general information, visuomotor skill, and vocabulary) and performance scores that were somewhat worse than verbal scores; scores improved after resolution of the PTA (Mandleberg 1975).

Causes of Delirium

Delirium, by definition, is caused by underlying physical problems or perturbations of the body that affect the brain directly or indirectly. Table 6–4 summarizes categories and common etiologies for delirium. The most common causes include drug intoxication and

---

Table 6–3.   DSM-IV diagnostic criteria for delirium due to a general medical condition

---

A. Disturbance of consciousness (i.e., reduced clarity of awareness of the environment) with reduced ability to focus, sustain, or shift attention.

B. A change in cognition (e.g., memory deficit, disorientation, language disturbance) or the development of a perceptual disturbance that is not better accounted for by a preexisting, established, or evolving dementia.

C. The disturbance develops over a short period of time (usually hours to days) and tends to fluctuate during the course of the day.

D. There is evidence from the history, physical examination, or laboratory findings that the disturbance is caused by the direct physiological consequences of a general medical condition.

Source. From American Psychiatric Association: *Diagnostic and Statistical Manual of Mental Disorders,* 4th Edition. Washington, DC, American Psychiatric Association, 1994. Used with permission.

withdrawal (often in the setting of polypharmacy when drug inter-actions or accumulations can unexpectedly lead to crossing of the blood-brain barrier), metabolic problems, cardiovascular-related problems, and infections. Often, more than one etiology exists. The first step in the management of delirium is the diagnosis and treat-ment of these underlying etiologic factors.

Table 6–5 lists etiologies of delirium that are more specific to the TBI population, although any of the problems listed in Table 6–4 also need to be considered. Delirium in TBI can be caused by both direct effects on the brain (in concussion, subdural hematoma, and contusion) and by extracranial injuries such as multiple trauma, hypoxemia from chest trauma or a compromised airway, and shock. TBI patients with systemic hypoxia or hypertension have an increased mortality (Gentleman and Jennett 1990). Increased in-tracranial pressure has been associated with a greatly increased

Table 6–4.   Etiologies for delirium in any population

Drug intoxication	Anticholinergics, digoxin, histamine antagonists, antiarrythmics, phenytoin, opioids, and others
Drug withdrawal	Alcohol, benzodiazepine, barbiturate
Metabolic	Hepatic or renal insufficiency, change in pH, hyper- or hypoglycemia, hypothermia, hyponatremia, hypercalcemia, vitamin deficiency, dehydration
Infection	Any systemic type, encephalitis, meningitis, abscess, tertiary syphilis
Endocrine	Hypothyroidism, hypo- or hypercortisolism, hyperparathyroidism
Seizures	Ictal and postictal states
Cancer	Metastases, brain tumor, carcinomatous meningitis, remote effects
Vascular	Stroke, transient ischemic attack, hypoperfusion, hypoxemia, subdural hematoma, shock, increased intracranial pressure, acute hypertension, pulmonary embolus, cardiac arrythmia, myocardial infarction, vasculitis
Environmental/ physical	Heat stroke, radiation, toxins, heavy metals (lead, mercury), industrial solvents, pesticides, electrocution, burns, carbon monoxide

mortality in TBI and strategies such as hyperventilation and barbiturate coma have been used to reduce acute brain swelling and metabolic rate (Lobato et al. 1988). These treatments, however, as well as these TBI complications, may cause delirium (see below, discussion of cerebral blood flow).

Risk Factors

Factors that increase the risk of delirium are listed in Table 6–6. Low serum albumin is an important risk factor that has been elucidated in a number of different patient samples and indicates not only poor nutrition (Levkoff et al. 1988; Trzepacz and Francis 1990): change in pharmacokinetics with increased free serum levels of drugs and consequent increased potential for CNS toxicity is one of several mechanisms proposed. Elderly patients are more vulnerable to delirium (Francis et al. 1990) and are a sometimes forgotten population susceptible to head trauma (Galbraith 1987). Unfortunately, patients who are traditionally considered to have a higher risk for delirium are nearly always excluded from PTA studies—especially alcoholic patients, elderly patients, those with prior psychiatric and neurological histories, and those with prior brain injury.

Table 6–5.   Causes of delirium in patients with traumatic brain injury

Mechanical effects (acceleration or deceleration, contusion, and others)
Cerebral edema
Hemorrhage
Infection
Subdural hematoma
Seizure
Hypoxia (cardiopulmonary or local ischemia)
Increased intracranial pressure
Alcohol intoxication or withdrawal; Wernicke's encephalopathy
Illicit drug intoxication or withdrawal
Reduced hemoperfusion related to multiple trauma
Fat embolism
Change in pH
Electrolyte imbalance
Medications (barbiturates, steroids, opioids, and anticholinergics)

Rating Scales

Various rating scales have been used to study PTA. These include the Glasgow Coma Scale (Teasdale and Jennett 1974), the Galveston Orientation and Amnesia Test (Levin et al. 1979a), the Rancho Los Amigos Cognitive Scale, and the Neurobehavioral Rating Scale (Levin et al. 1987). Although these scales have been used to characterize, follow the clinical course of, or assess the outcome of PTA, each scale has drawbacks and none of them adequately assesses delirium.

The Glasgow Coma Scale (see Chapter 1, Table 1–2) was devised to assess the depth and duration of impaired consciousness and coma by measuring three axes, each on a separately scored subscale, consisting of motor responsiveness, verbal performance, and eye opening. Although this scale has some utility in quantifying some clinical symptoms of coma, it does not assess delirium. The Glasgow Coma Scale has been used to rate TBI patients on admission to the hospital and then to compare various outcome measures; it has also been used to select study samples of TBI patients, depending on certain cutoff scores, to indicate initial severity of TBI (Changriss et al. 1987). Its simplicity makes it ideal for non-researchers (e.g., ward nurses) to do ratings.

The Galveston Orientation and Amnesia Test (see Chapter 4, Table 4–1) was developed for serial use in assessing cognitive status after TBI, and it specifically focuses on orientation and ability to remember events preceding and following the injury. It does not address the other cognitive deficits present in delirium, nor does it

Table 6–6. Risk factors predisposing toward delirium

Low serum albumin
Geriatric age, with or without dementia
Brain damage or central nervous system disease
Prior episode of delirium
Serious medical disease
Polypharmacy
Basal ganglia lesions on magnetic resonance imaging
Cerebral atrophy with right-hemisphere focal lesions

rate behavioral symptoms of delirium (e.g., mood, sleep, psycho-motor, psychotic, perceptual, and others). Delirious patients can become oriented before other symptoms have resolved (Gronwall and Wrightson 1980). A cutoff score of 75 out of 100 points has been used as an indicator that PTA has resolved (Ewert et al. 1989); however, given the nature of the questions, 75 is probably too low and too many false negative deliria may occur using this criterion. The Galveston Orientation and Amnesia Test would not be expected to be a sensitive or specific instrument to assess the presence or severity of delirium.

The Rancho Los Amigos Cognitive Scale (see Chapter 3, Table 3–3) is an 8-point scale describing the patient's behavior along a continuum from coma to a state close to normal, but often with persistent cognitive deficits. It is often used for rating chronic TBI patients who are in long-term rehabilitation settings. Levels IV and V include delirium symptoms, whereas level III corresponds more closely to stupor, and levels I and II correspond to coma.

Early attempts were made to address broader psychiatric symptoms of PTA (Levin and Grossman 1978; Levin et al. 1979b) using the Brief Psychiatric Rating Scale, which is usually used to rate psychotic patients, in particular patients with schizophrenia. This was an important step in recognizing other psychiatric symptoms of TBI delirium. The Neurobehavioral Rating Scale (see Chapter 3, Table 3–5) was developed by incorporating parts of the Brief Psychiatric Rating Scale and adding a number of other psychiatric symptoms considered to be relevant to the evaluation of TBI patients. This scale is more comprehensive than the Galveston Orientation and Amnesia Test or the Glasgow Coma Scale, with 27 clinician-rated items, each scored on a 7-point severity scale. Items include disorientation, inattention, anxiety, disinhibition, guilt, agitation, poor insight, depressed mood, fatigability, hallucinations, blunted affect, speech articulation deficit, and so on. The problem with its use for delirium is its great breadth and lack of focus on delirium, as it mentions most symptoms seen in nearly any psychiatric disorder. Its main utility might be as a screening tool to increase clinical detection of various psychiatric disorders occurring after TBI.

The Delirium Rating Scale specifically rates the severity of symptoms of delirium and differentiates patients with delirium from patients with psychosis and dementia (Trzepacz et al. 1988a). Each item is scored (trained clinician-rated) for severity and total scores above 12 or 15 points have been used to indicate delirium of varying severity (see Table 6–7). One of the items rates the degree of cognitive dysfunction and depends on specific testing of cognition. Detection of subclinical delirium (a score between 8 and 12 points) is enhanced by concurrent use of bedside cognitive screening tests. This rating scale has not yet been used in TBI populations, but could be expected to more crisply differentiate delirium from other disorders or from amnestic syndrome.

A commonly used cognitive screening test is the Mini-Mental State Exam (MMSE; Folstein et al. 1975), which covers areas of orientation, attention, concentration, short-term verbal memory, visuoconstructional ability, comprehension, naming, repetition, and writing (see Table 6–8). Scores below 24 indicate cognitive dysfunction, but do not specifically indicate delirium. The MMSE is also relatively insensitive and should be supplemented by more sensitive tests, like the Trail Making Tests. The Trail Making Tests, parts A and B, are useful as an adjunct to the MMSE because they are more sensitive to organic brain disease. They assess psychomotor speed, concentration, visuospatial ability, and switching of mental sets. Scores above 35 seconds for part A and 89 seconds for part B are abnormal for patients up to age 65 (Lezak 1983).

Other Features of TBI Delirium

Severity and Location of Injury

It is believed that more severe brain injuries result in more prolonged coma and PTA (Williams et al. 1990). PTA may persist for weeks or months, although it is not known whether this indicates a continuing delirium, a subclinical delirium, a dementia, or another process. A variety of brain lesions, especially those in the brain

Table 6–7.   Delirium Rating Scale

Item 1: Temporal onset of symptoms

This item addresses the time course over which symptoms appear; the maximum rating is for the most abrupt onset of symptoms—a common pattern for delirium. Dementia is usually more gradual in onset. Other psychiatric disorders, such as affective disorders, might be scored with 1 or 2 points on this item. Sometimes delirium can be chronic (e.g., in geriatric nursing home patients), and unfortunately only 1 or 2 points would be assessed in that situation.

   0 No significant change from longstanding behavior, essentially a chronic or chronic-recurrent disorder
   1 Gradual onset of symptoms, occurring within a 6-month period
   2 Acute change in behavior or personality occurring over a month
   3 Abrupt change in behavior, usually occurring over a 1- to 3-day period

Item 2: Perceptual disturbances

This item rates most highly the extreme inability to perceive differences between internal and external reality, while intermittent misperceptions such as illusions are given 2 points. Depersonalization and derealization can be seen in other organic mental disorders like temporal lobe epilepsy, in severe depression, and in borderline personality disorder and thus are given only 1 point.

   0 None evident by history or observation
   1 Feelings of depersonalization or derealization
   2 Visual illusions or misperceptions including macropsia, micropsia (e.g., may urinate in wastebasket or mistake bedclothes for something else)
   3 Evidence that the patient is markedly confused about external reality (e.g., not discriminating between dreams and reality)

Item 3: Hallucination type

The presence of any type of hallucination is rated. Auditory hallucinations alone are rated with less weight because of their common occurrence in primary psychiatric disorders. Visual hallucinations are generally associated with organic mental syndromes, although not exclusively, and are given 2 points. Tactile hallucinations are classically described in delirium, particularly due to anticholinergic toxicity, and are given the most points.

   0 Hallucinations not present
   1 Auditory hallucinations only
   2 Visual hallucinations present by patient's history or inferred by observation, with or without auditory hallucinations
   3 Tactile, olfactory, or gustatory hallucinations with or without visual or auditory hallucinations

Item 4: Delusions

Delusions can be present in many different psychiatric disorders, but tend to be better organized and more fixed in nondelirious disorders and thus are given

Table 6–7. Delirium Rating Scale *(continued)*

less weight. Chronic fixed delusions are probably most prevalent in schizophrenic disorders. New delusions may indicate affective and schizophrenic disorders, dementia, or substance intoxication but should also alert the clinician to possible delirium and are given 2 points. Poorly formed delusions, often of a paranoid nature, are typical of delirium.

- 0 Not present
- 1 Delusions are systematized, i.e., well organized and persistent
- 2 Delusions are new and not part of a preexisting primary psychiatric disorder
- 3 Delusions are not well circumscribed, are transient, poorly organized, and mostly in response to misperceived environmental cues (e.g., are paranoid and involve persons who are in reality caregivers, loved ones, hospital staff, etc.)

Item 5: Psychomotor behavior

This item describes degrees of severity of altered psychomotor behavior. Maximum points can be given for severe agitation or severe withdrawal to reflect either the hyperactive or the hypoactive variant of delirium.

- 0 No significant retardation or agitation
- 1 Mild restlessness, tremulousness, or anxiety evident by observation and a change from patient's usual behavior
- 2 Moderate agitation with pacing, removing iv's, etc.
- 3 Severe agitation, needs to be restrained, may be combative; or has significant withdrawal from the environment, but not due to major depression or schizophrenic catatonia

Item 6: Cognitive status during formal testing

Information from the cognitive portion of a routine mental status examination is needed to rate this item. The maximum rating of 4 points is given for severe cognitive deficits while only 1 point is given or mild inattention which could be attributed to pain and fatigue seen in medically ill persons. Two points are given for a relatively isolated cognitive deficit, such as memory impairment, which could be due to dementia or organic amnestic syndrome as well as to early delirium.

- 0 No cognitive deficits, or deficits which can be alternatively explained by lack of education or prior mental retardation
- 1 Very mild cognitive deficits which might be attributed to inattention due to acute pain, fatigue, depression, or anxiety associated with having a medical illness
- 2 Cognitive deficit largely in one major area tested, e.g., memory, but otherwise intact
- 3 Significant cognitive deficits which are diffuse, i.e., affecting many different areas tested; must include periods of disorientation to time or place at least once each 24-hour period; registration and/or recall are abnormal; concentration is reduced

Table 6–7. Delirium Rating Scale *(continued)*

    4 Severe cognitive deficits, including motor or verbal perseverations, confabulations, disorientation to person, remote and recent memory deficits, and inability to cooperate with formal mental status testing

Item 7: Physical disorder

Maximum points are given when a specific lesion or physiological disturbance can be temporally associated with the altered behavior. Dementias are often not found to have a specific underlying medical cause, while delirium usually has at least one identifiable physical cause.

    0 None present or active
    1 Presence of any physical disorder which might affect mental state
    2 Specific drug, infection, metabolic, central nervous system lesion, or other medical problem which can be temporally implicated in causing the altered behavior or mental status

Item 8: Sleep-wake cycle disturbance

Disruption of the sleep-wake cycle is typical in delirium, with persons with dementia generally having significant sleep disturbances much later in their course. Severe delirium is on a continuum with stupor and coma, and persons with a resolving coma are likely to be delirious temporarily.

    0 Not present; awake and alert during the day, and sleeps without significant disruption at night
    1 Occasional drowsiness during day and mild sleep continuity disturbance at night; may have nightmares, but can readily distinguish from reality
    2 Frequent napping and unable to sleep at night, constituting a significant disruption of or a reversal of the usual sleep-wake cycle
    3 Drowsiness prominent, difficulty staying alert during interview, loss of self-control over alertness and somnolence
    4 Drifts into stuporous or comatose periods

Item 9: Lability of mood

Rapid shifts in mood can occur in various organic mental syndromes, perhaps due to a disinhibition of one's normal control. The patient may be aware of this lack of emotional control and may behave inappropriately relative to the situation or to his or her thinking state (e.g., crying for no apparent reason). Delirious patients may score points on any of these items depending upon the severity of the delirium and upon how their underlying psychological state "colors" their delirious presentation. Patients with borderline personality disorder might score 1 or 2 points on this item.

    0 Not present; mood stable
    1 Affect/mood somewhat altered and changes over the course of hours; patient states that mood changes are not under self-control
    2 Significant mood changes which are inappropriate to situation, including fear, anger, or tearfulness; rapid shifts of emotion, even over several minutes

Table 6–7.   Delirium Rating Scale *(continued)*

3 Severe disinhibition of emotions, including temper outbursts,
   uncontrolled inappropriate laughter, or crying

Item 10: Variability of symptoms

The hallmark of delirium is the waxing and waning of symptoms, which is given
4 points on this item. Dementia, as well as delirium, patients who become more
confused at night when environmental cues are decreased, could score 2 points.

   0 Symptoms stable and mostly present during daytime
   2 Symptoms worsen at night
   4 Fluctuating intensity of symptoms, such that they wax and wane
        during a 24-hour period

                                                        Total score _____

Source. Reprinted from Trzepacz PT, Baker RW, Greenhouse JB: "A Symptom Rating Scale
for Delirium." *Psychiatry Research* 23:89–97, 1988. Copyright P. T. Trzepacz (1986). Used
with permission of Elsevier Science Publishing, New York.

stem, have been associated with protracted coma and PTA (Jellinger and Seitelberger 1970). Deeper brain lesions were associated with more severe brain injury (Ommaya and Gennarelli 1974) and deeper brain lesions resulted in longer duration and degree of coma and/or PTA (Katz et al. 1989; Levin et al. 1988a; Ommaya and Gennarelli 1974). The degree of mechanical shearing caused by acceleration/deceleration forces may determine the depth of lesion, along a continuum from the surface of the cortex to the brain stem (Ommaya and Gennarelli 1974). Basal ganglia (Katz et al. 1989) and basal forebrain lesions (Salazar et al. 1986) were more associated with unconsciousness than more superficial lesions. The severity of impaired consciousness did not differ among lesions located in frontal and temporal lobes, however (Levin et al. 1988a). Hemispheric lateralization of lesions was not related to behavioral sequelae (Levin and Grossman 1978), but left-sided lesions were associated with longer duration of PTA than right-sided lesions (Levin et al. 1989). Severe TBI cases had more symptoms consistent with delirium (conceptual disorganization, unusual thought content, excitement, and disorientation), even though patients were studied after the most severe confusional symptoms had resolved (Levin and Grossman 1978).

Table 6–8.   Mini-Mental State Exam (add points for each correct response)

		Score	Points
Orientation			
1. What is the	Year?		1
	Season?		1
	Date?		1
	Day?		1
	Month?		1
2. Where are we?	State?		1
	County?		1
	Town or city?		1
	Hospital?		1
	Floor?		1
Registration			
3. Name three objects, taking one second to say each. Then ask the patient all three after you have said them. Give 1 point for each correct answer. Repeat the answers until patient learns all three.			3
Attention and calculation			
4. Serial 7s. Give 1 point for each correct answer. Stop after five answers. Alternate: Spell WORLD backward.			5
Recall			
5. Ask for names of three objects learned in question 3. Give 1 point for each correct answer.			3
Language			
6. Point to a pencil and a watch. Have the patient name them as you point.			2
7. Have the patient repeat "No ifs, ands, or buts."			1
8. Have the patient follow a three-stage command: Take a paper in your right hand. Fold the paper in half. Put the paper on the floor.			3
9. Have the patient read and obey the following: CLOSE YOUR EYES (Write it in large letters.)			1
10. Have the patient write a sentence of his or her choice. (The sentence should contain a subject and an object and should make sense. Ignore spelling errors when scoring.)			1
11. Enlarge the design printed below to 1.5 cm per side, and have the patient copy it. (Give 1 point if all sides and angles are preserved and if the intersecting sides form a quadrangle.)			1

_____ = Total
(30 maximum)

Source.   Reprinted from Folstein MF, Folstein SE, McHugh PR: "Mini-Mental State: A Practical Method for Grading the Cognitive State of Patients for the Clinician." *Journal of Psychiatric Research* 12:189–198, 1975. Used with permission from Pergamon Press, New

Agitation

Motoric agitation is common after acute brain injury and includes combativeness, truncal rocking, and arm thrashing (Levin and Grossman 1978). In this study, such agitation was more common in younger patients, although the duration of coma was shorter (less than 24 hours) in patients who were agitated than in those who were not (Levin and Grossman 1978). Also agitation was not related to focal neurological signs, focal frontotemporal injury, or [inferred] mesencephalic injury, but was associated with visual and auditory hallucinations and delusions. Interestingly, Reyes et al. (1981) showed that patients with restlessness and agitation at the time of hospital discharge eventually had better recovery of premorbid physical and cognitive functions, but with a greater need for psychological intervention.

Memory

Memory studies have been performed in PTA, although the complexity of the tests suggests that these patients were not severely delirious. Both declarative and procedural long-term memory have been studied in TBI (Ewert et al. 1989; Levin et al. 1985). Disoriented PTA patients had poorer recall of autobiographical information as compared with their recall after PTA resolution (Levin et al. 1985). In this same study both retrograde and anterograde memory deficits occurred in PTA patients. In a test of visual memory, PTA patients had more difficulty in acquisition of material and forgot at a faster rate than did recovered PTA patients (Levin et al. 1988b). In a group of patients with frontal lobe lesions, procedural memory improved over the course of PTA, whereas declarative memory deficits remained stable (Ewert et al. 1989). Thus delirium in TBI involves an alteration of both declarative and procedural memory.

This is interesting because procedural memory remains relatively intact in amnestic patients, is implicit, and is not affected by the temporal lobe–diencephalon areas of the brain (Squire 1986). In contrast, declarative memory is impaired in amnestic syndrome, is "explicit" (conscious), is subserved by the medial temporal lobe, hippocampus, diencephalon, and ventromedial frontal lobe, and consolidates over time (Squire 1986). This suggests a neuroanatomical difference between amnestic syndrome and delirium.

PTA and Outcome

Several features of PTA are related to outcome after TBI (Katz et al. 1989; Levin et al. 1979b). Residual medical, cognitive, behavioral, linguistic, and psychosocial problems all may impede recovery to premorbid levels. The relationship between duration of coma or duration of PTA to outcome varies in different studies (Smith 1961). Although increased duration of coma correlates with poorer outcome, and duration of PTA increases with longer coma, duration of PTA may or may not correlate with outcome. Smith (1961) found that after excluding patients with focal injuries, duration of PTA correlated better with outcome; also longer duration of PTA was associated with a higher incidence of seizures.

Pathophysiology of Delirium in TBI

Delirium is considered to be a syndrome, that is, a constellation of signs and symptoms that result from a variety of different causes and culminate to a common presentation. At what point these various etiologies converge neurophysiologically to form this syndrome is unknown. In this section, attempts to study PTA will be compared to what is known about the pathophysiology of delirium in general.

Electroencephalography

A diagnosis of delirium is supported by an objective finding of generalized slowing on electroencephalography (EEG), particularly of the dominant posterior rhythm (Engel and Romano 1959; Trzepacz et al. 1988b). Most cases of delirium will be associated with EEG slowing, except for some cases of alcohol or sedative-hypnotic withdrawal (increased fast wave activity), partial complex status epilepticus (epileptiform complexes), or superimposed focal brain lesions (focal abnormalities).

Studies of PTA to date seem consistent with the usual finding of diffuse slowing in delirium (Levin and Grossman 1978). Focal findings are appropriately indicative of a focal lesion, such as contusion, ischemic injury, hemorrhage, or hematoma. Diffuse slowing occurs during "psychosis with amnesia" in TBI and may not resolve for weeks; focal lesions are also common and tend to normalize within several months, persisting longer in patients with traumatic epilepsy (Koufen and Hagel 1987). These abnormal foci have been associated with focal neurological signs and skull fractures. Abnormal sleep EEG with sleep spindles preceded the more classical generalized slowing phase (Koufen and Hagel 1987). Computed tomography scans showed evidence of cerebral edema associated with EEG slowing (Koufen and Hagel 1987). Interpretation of EEGs may be affected by barbiturates and other medications. The degree and type of EEG abnormality is correlated with prognosis during traumatic coma, showing reactivity (i.e., changes in the EEG pattern in response to various maneuvers such as eye opening, alerting, or hyperventilation) to be as important as the background activity (Synek 1988, 1990).

Somatosensory evoked potentials show delayed conduction in traumatic coma and PTA; conduction times improve as the PTA clears (Houlden et al. 1990; Hume and Cant 1981). The degree of abnormality correlates with outcome when performed within the first $3\frac{1}{2}$ days after injury (Hume and Cant 1981). Damage to subcortical areas, including the medial lemniscus, has been hypothesized in TBI, in addition to cortical factors (Hume and Cant 1981; Lindsay et al. 1981). These findings are consistent with the slowed conduction of somatosensory evoked potentials in delirious patients with hepatic insufficiency, wherein a subcortical, as well as a cortical, pathophysiology was considered (Trzepacz et al. 1989b).

Computed Tomography Scans

Computed tomography scans are useful in evaluating TBI delirium to diagnose structural lesions such as hemorrhage, subdural hematoma, stroke, and contusions (Feuerman et al. 1988). Cerebral atrophy (perhaps preexisting) usually suggests a brain that is more vulnerable to delirium. In addition, evidence of cerebral edema from compression of the third ventricle and basal cisterns correlates closely with increased intracranial pressure (Teasdale et al. 1984), a known cause of delirium and coma in TBI.

Cerebral Blood Flow Studies

Cerebral blood flow (CBF) studies using Xenon-SPECT (single photon emission computed tomography) scans have been performed in TBI patients who are in coma or emerging from coma, in an effort to better understand the underlying physiology of brain damage (Deutsch and Eisenberg 1987; Jaggi et al. 1990; Obrist et al. 1984). Under most circumstances, CBF is coupled to metabolism in essentially a 1:1 relationship (Raichle et al. 1976), except for acute vascular events such as stroke when luxury perfusion of an ischemic area is much higher than the actual metabolic demand, and CBF does not accurately reflect physiological needs (Lassen 1966). A reduction of frontal CBF as compared to the normal resting pattern (i.e., a reversal of the normal anteroposterior gradient) was noted in comatose patients after TBI (Deutsch and Eisenberg 1987); with increased global blood flow (hyperemia), this pattern was more exaggerated, but upon regaining consciousness, this frontal defect normalized.

Acute brain trauma is another condition in which metabolism and CBF are not tightly coupled (Obrist et al. 1984). Xenon-SPECT scan quantitative CBF measures were compared to arteriojugular venous oxygen differences in two groups of TBI coma patients, hyperemic and reduced CBF, and cerebral metabolism for oxygen was estimated (Obrist et al. 1984). Metabolism was reduced in all TBI coma patients as a consequence of normal metabolic coupling between CBF and metabolism; uncoupling occurred only in the hyperemic cases. Hyperemia was often associated with intracranial hypertension and was believed to result in luxury perfusion, perhaps related to cerebrospinal fluid (CSF) lactic acidosis or failure of CBF autoregulation (Obrist et al. 1984). Hyperventilation of reduced

CBF patients was cautioned as risking ischemia from vasoconstriction (Obrist et al. 1984), which would increase susceptibility to delirium. Lower levels of cerebral oxygen metabolism are related to poorer outcome, and when hyperemic patients are excluded, lower CBF also predicts a poorer outcome (Jaggi et al. 1990). Upon recovery, CBF and presumably metabolism increase. Although not yet directly studied, it may be hypothesized that CBF progresses toward normal during delirium.

Treatment

Treatment of delirium after TBI is essentially the same as that for other patient samples (Lipowski 1990). It involves a work-up for etiology(ies), treatment of the underlying etiology when possible, manipulation of the environment, and medication (Table 6–9).

Search for Underlying Causes

The search for underlying causes can be guided by considering the many possible etiologies as outlined above and as listed in Tables 6–1 and 6–2, individualized according to each patient's needs. The clinician must reduce polypharmacy, discontinuing or replacing medications that produce delirium. Laboratory tests, CSF examination, computed tomography or magnetic resonance imaging brain scans, arterial blood gases, intracranial pressure monitoring, electrocardiogram, blood cultures, and so on, can all be performed as needed to investigate various potential causes. If the diagnosis of delirium is uncertain, use of a specific delirium symptom rating scale can be used along with EEG and bedside cognitive tests. The

Table 6–9.   Principles for treatment of delirium

1. Search for underlying cause(s)
2. Treat or reverse underlying causes(s)
3. Environmental manipulations
4. Medication

EEG shows the usual pattern of diffuse background slowing (Engel and Romano 1959; Koufen and Hagel 1987), sometimes with the presence of sleep spindles (Koufen and Hagel 1987). Bedside cognitive tests, such as the MMSE, Trail Making Tests (Trzepacz et al. 1988b), and specific attentional, visuoconstructional, and abstraction tasks (see Chapter 4) are useful in determining the degree of diffuse cognitive dysfunction, and can be followed over time.

Environmental Manipulations

Traditionally, efforts are made to help familiarize and structure the delirious patient's environment (Table 6–10). The delirious patient requires external structure to compensate for a disorganized and cognitively impaired internal mental state. When the patient is so confused or frightened that physical harm might inadvertently happen, or uncooperativeness with medical treatment occurs, then physical restraints may be appropriate. Restraints must never be used to replace good nursing observation, only to supplement other treatment efforts. However, some have expressed opinions about the negative aspects of using restraints in TBI patients (Berrol 1988; DeChancie et al. 1987), although not based on controlled studies. The increased use of restraints in TBI patients has been associated with alcohol use, but not with a lower level of consciousness (Edlund et al. 1991); these restrained patients also had longer lengths of stay, more combativeness and aggression, and more alcohol withdrawal, but very few were seen in consultation by a

Table 6–10. Environmental manipulations in the treatment of delirium

1. Familiarize the environment	Put family pictures nearby
2. Structure the environment	Clock in full view; large calendar on wall, with days marked off; nightlight; reorient patient frequently; have natural window light to assist day-night biorhythms
3. Adjust sensory stimulation level:	Minimize loud noises, do not remove all stimulation
4. Assure safety	Use a sitter

psychiatrist. The use of sitters can often reduce the need for restraints while assisting with observations and reassurance of the confused patient.

One view is that instead of medication ("too sedating") and restraints ("increases agitation") for agitated delirious TBI patients, a portable, Naugahyde padded room enclosure should be used to allow freer movement (DeChancie et al. 1987). This is essentially a seclusion room, a comfortable room with a mattress and devoid of objects, which is well known to psychiatrists and has been used for decades to reduce distracting sensory stimulation and provide safety. Although this may be a useful adjunct (no controlled studies), it should not preclude appropriate use of antidelirium medication, because changing the environment will not by itself alter the pathophysiology of delirium. In addition, a balance must be struck between minimizing excessive or confusing sounds and providing enough environmental structure (e.g., family photos) to reduce anxiety from disorientation and cognitive deficits that contribute to agitation. Deafness, blindness, and other causes of sensory deprivation actually increase the risk for delirium (Lipowski 1990).

Medication

Appropriately chosen and monitored medication for reducing the cognitive, behavioral, and psychotic symptoms of delirium is the clinical standard of care (see Table 6–11). Neuroleptic medication is the treatment of choice for TBI delirium (Cassidy 1990; Gualtieri 1991; Lipowski 1985), specifically haloperidol, because of its safety profile in medically ill patients and its convenience for route of administration. It can be given orally, intramuscularly, or intravenously. Its sedating side effect can be used to the patient's benefit initially to enhance and consolidate nocturnal sleep by dosing at bedtime. This sedating effect is minimized by using lower doses than conventionally used for mania or schizophrenia and diminishes after several days. Further, haloperidol is not sedating to all patients. Those unfamiliar with psychopharmacology and its appropriate clinical use for delirium tend not to understand this point. In addition, delirium itself involves napping and drowsy periods.

Haloperidol is generally given in 0.5–1 mg doses at h.s. or bid initially, and titrated upward according to the patient's response (up to 5 mg total daily dose, or even to 20 mg in severe cases). At low doses, extrapyramidal side effects are uncommon, especially when given intravenously (Menza et al. 1987). Haloperidol can be safely given intravenously (Sos and Cassem 1980) without respiratory depression or significant cardiac side effects, even in very large doses (hundreds of mg per day) (Adams 1988), but this is neither routinely recommended nor necessary for most patients. Dystonic reactions tend to occur at the initiation of treatment and akathisia may increase restlessness. These are uncommon complications when haloperidol is used in low doses for brief periods of time. Neuroleptic malignant syndrome is even less common, but must be considered in the differential diagnosis of fever, increased confusion, and lead-pipe muscle rigidity (Guze and Baxter 1985). The response to haloperidol in delirium is often remarkable. By promptly reducing the symptoms of delirium, the patient becomes more aware and able to begin rehabilitation.

Neuroleptics should be tapered and discontinued after the delirium clears (Gualtieri 1991) and continued only if a psychotic disorder persists (or preexisted, such as mania or schizophrenia) into the rehabilitation phase. Some speculate that neuroleptics' anti-

---

Table 6–11.　Pharmacological management of delirium

1. Minimize polypharmacy, especially those drugs affecting the brain.
2. Avoid most psychoactive drugs, especially those with anticholinergic effects and sedative-hypnotics.
3. Administer haloperdiol in low doses for symptomatic relief:

   Begin with 0.5- to 1-mg doses po, im, or iv at bedtime or bid for mild delirium.

   Begin with higher doses (up to 5 mg) for more severe delirium, especially if patient is agitated.

   For rapid behavioral control, use intravenous route and give several doses one-half hour apart.
4. Avoid benzodiazepines except in patients with concurrent alcohol or benzodiazepine withdrawal, or in exceptional cases when insomnia has not responded to haloperidol.

dopaminergic effects may delay or interfere with the TBI patient's cognitive rehabilitation (Feeney et al. 1982; Gualtieri 1991) because dopaminergic medications have been shown to enhance memory (Gualtieri 1991) and even to arouse chronically comatose TBI patients (Cope 1990). The danger is in overstating these caveats, because assumptions have been made from motor cortex rat models about human cognition in TBI (Feeney et al. 1982) and from one phase of TBI recovery (coma or amnestic syndrome) about another's (delirium) neurochemical mechanisms. The brief duration of antidelirium treatment and the morbidity and mortality associated with delirium argue for careful use of neuroleptics in TBI delirium.

Benzodiazepines can worsen delirium and further impair cognition, and therefore are usually avoided unless specifically indicated. Most clinicians reserve benzodiazepines as an adjunct to haloperidol only for complicating conditions of alcohol (or other sedative-hypnotic drug) withdrawal (Edlund et al. 1991). Benzodiazepines are the safest of the sedative class of drugs and can be used if the sleep-wake cycle disturbance does not normalize after adjusting the dose of haloperidol, or if extreme agitation is not responsive to haloperidol, although this is usually not necessary. The choice depends on the need—lorazepam has a shorter half-life than diazepam. Unlike most benzodiazepines, lorazepam can be effectively administered intramuscularly because it is well absorbed with that route. Longer-acting agents may be helpful in treating alcohol withdrawal. The use of barbiturates during TBI suggests more caution when subsequently using benzodiazepines; also, the use of barbiturates may delay the onset of alcohol withdrawal symptoms, which generally peak 3–5 days after cessation of drinking.

Summary and Need For Further Studies

There is a need for nomenclature clarification in the TBI literature in order for research on the features, risk factors, duration, prognosis, and outcome of delirium after TBI to proceed in a meaningful way.

The adoption of published psychiatric diagnostic criteria for delirium and the use of rating scales and cognitive tests that assess the whole range of behavioral symptoms of delirium is necessary. Delirium after TBI must be differentiated from coma and amnestic syndrome.

The exclusion of certain patients from most TBI PTA studies has unfortunately excluded some of the patients at greatest risk for TBI, namely those who abuse alcohol (Honkanen and Smith 1991; Yates et al. 1987) and other substances, and those with antisocial personality disorder, mania, schizophrenia, suicidal depression, and so on. Whether these psychiatrically impaired persons have a higher risk for delirium is unknown but could be hypothesized for at least some of them (alcoholic patients). Neurologically impaired persons are also excluded from TBI PTA studies, yet they are at higher risk for delirium. A person with impaired cognition or prior brain injury that alters personality (e.g., aggressive) or frontal lobe executive functions (e.g., judgment and abstraction) may be at increased risk for recurrent TBI from fighting or falling, for example, and would likely have an increased risk for delirium after TBI. Elderly patients, with or without dementia, have diminished brain reserve and reduced ability to withstand effects of TBI (Galbraith 1987), probably also with increased TBI delirium.

References

Adams F: Emergency intravenous sedation of the delirious, medically ill patient. J Clin Psychiatry 49:22–26, 1988

Artiola D, Fortuny I, Briggs M, et al: Measuring the duration of post traumatic amnesia. J Neurol Neurosurg Psychiatry 40:377–379, 1980

Berrol S: Risks of restraints in head injury. Arch Phys Med Rehabil 69:537–538, 1988

Cassidy JW: Pharmacological treatment of post-traumatic behavioral disorders: aggression and disorders of mood, in Neurobehavioural Sequelae of Traumatic Brain Injury. Edited by Wood RL. New York, Taylor and Francis, 1990, pp 227–229

Changriss DG, McGraw CP, Richardson JD, et al: Correlation of cerebral perfusion pressure and Glasgow coma scale. J Trauma 27:1007–1013, 1987

Cope DN: Pharmacology for behavioral deficits: disorders of cognition and affect, in Neurobehavioural Sequelae of Traumatic Brain Injury. Edited by Wood RL. Taylor and Francis, New York, 1990, p 255

DeChancie H, Walsh JM, Kessler LA: An enclosure for the disoriented head-injured patient. J Neurosci Nurs 19:341, 1987

Deutsch G, Eisenberg HM: Frontal blood flow changes in recovery from coma. J Cereb Blood Flow Metab 7:29–34, 1987

Edlund MJ, Goldberg RJ, Morris PLP: The use of physical restraint in patients with cerebral contusion. Int J Psychiatry Med 21:173–182, 1991

Engel G, Romano J: Delirium: a syndrome of cerebral insufficiency. Journal of Chronic Disease 9:260–277, 1959

Ewert J, Levin HS, Watson MG, Kalinsky Z: Procedural memory during posttraumatic amnesia in survivors of severe closed head injury: implications for rehabilitation. Arch Neurol 46:911–916, 1989

Feeney DM, Gonzalez A, Law WA: Amphetamine, haloperidol, and experience interact to affect rate of recovery after motor cortex injury. Science 217:855–857, 1982

Feuerman T, Wackym PA, Gade GF, et al: Value of skull radiography, head computed tomographic scanning, and admission for observation in cases of minor head injury. Neurosurgery 22:449–453, 1988

Fisher JM: Cognitive and behavioral consequences of closed head injury. Semin Neurol 5:197–204, 1985

Folstein MF, Folstein SE, McHugh PR: Mini-Mental State: a practical method for grading the cognitive state of patients for the clinician. J Psychiatr Res 12:189–198, 1975

Francis J, Martin D, Kapoor W: A prospective study of delirium in hospitalized elderly. JAMA 263:1097–1101, 1990

Galbraith S: Head injuries in the elderly. Lancet 1:325, 1987

Gentleman D, Jennett B: Audit of transfer of unconscious head-injured patients to a neurosurgical unit. Lancet 1:330–334, 1990

Grant I, Alves W: Psychiatric and psychosocial disturbances in head injury, in Neurobehavioral Recovery From Head Injury, edited by Levin HS, Grafman J, Eisenberg HM. New York, Oxford University Press, 1987, pp 234–235

Gronwall D, Wrightson P: Duration of post-traumatic amnesia after mild head injury. Journal of Clinical Neuropsychology 2:51–60, 1980

Gualtieri CT: Neuropsychiatry and Behavioral Pharmacology. New York, Springer-Verlag, 1991

Guze BH, Baxter LR: Neuroleptic malignant syndrome. N Engl J Med 313:463–466, 1985

Honkanen R, Smith G: Impact of acute alcohol intoxication on patterns of non-fatal trauma: cause-specific analysis of head injury effect. Injury 22:225–229, 1991

Houlden DA, Li C, Schwartz ML, et al: Median nerve somatosensory evoked potentials and the Glasgow Coma Scale as predictors of outcome in comatose patients with head injuries. Neurosurgery 27:701–708, 1990

Hume AL, Cant BR: Central somatosensory conduction after head injury. Ann Neurol 10:411–419, 1981

Jaggi JL, Obrist WD, Gennarelli TA, et al: Relationship of early cerebral blood flow and metabolism to outcome in acute head injury. J Neurosurg 72:176–182, 1990

Jellinger K, Seitelberger F: Protracted post-traumatic encephalopathy: pathology, pathogenesis and clinical implications. J Neurol Sci 10:51–94, 1970

Katz DI, Alexander MP, Seliger GM, et al: Traumatic basal ganglia hemorrhage: clinicopathologic features and outcome. Neurology 39:897–904, 1989

Koufen H, Hagel K-H: Systematic EEG follow-up study of traumatic psychosis. Eur Arch Psychiatry Neurol Sci 237:2–7, 1987

Lassen NA: The luxury-perfusion syndrome and its possible relation to acute metabolic acidosis localized within the brain. Lancet 2:1113–1115, 1966

Levin HS, Grossman RG: Behavioral sequelae of closed head injury: a quantitative study. Arch Neurol 35:720–727, 1978

Levin HS, O'Donnell VM, Grossman RG: The Galveston Orientation and Amnesia Test: a practical scale to assess cognition after head injury. J Nerv Ment Dis 167:675–684, 1979a

Levin HS, Grossman RG, Rose JE, et al: Long-term neuropsychological outcome of closed head injury. J Neurosurg 50:412–422, 1979b

Levin HS, High WM, Meyers CA, et al: Impairment of remote memory after closed head injury. J Neurol Neurosurg Psychiatry 48:556–563, 1985

Levin HS, High WM, Goethe KE, et al: The Neurobehavioral Rating Scale: assessment of the behavioral sequelae of head injury by the clinician. J Neurol Neurosurg Psychiatry 50:183–193, 1987

Levin HS, Williams D, Crofford MJ, et al: Relationship of depth of brain lesions to consciousness and outcome after closed head injury. J Neurosurg 69:861–866, 1988a

Levin HS, High WM, Eisenberg HM: Learning and forgetting during posttraumatic amnesia in head-injured patients. J Neurol Neurosurg Psychiatry 51:14–20, 1988b

Levin HS, Gary HE, Eisenberg HM: Duration of impaired consciousness in relation to side of lesion after severe head injury. Lancet 1:1001–1003, 1989

Levkoff SE, Safran C, Cleary PD, et al: Identification of factors associated with the diagnosis of delirium in elderly hospitalized patients. J Am Geriatr Soc 36:1099–1104, 1988

Lezak MD: Neuropsychological Assessment. New York, Oxford University Press, 1983

Lindsay KW, Carlin J, Kennedy I, et al: Evoked potentials in severe head injury—analysis and relation to outcome. J Neurol Neurosurg Psychiatry 44:796–802, 1981

Lipowski ZJ: Delirium (acute confusional state), in Handbook of Clinical Neurology. Edited by Vinken PJ, Bruyn GW, Klawans HL. New York, Elsevier Science Publishing Co., 1985, pp 523–559

Lipowski ZJ: Delirium. New York, Oxford University Press, 1990, pp 399–401

Lobato RD, Sarabia R, Cordobes F, et al: Posttraumatic cerebral hemispheric swelling: Analysis of 55 cases studied with computerized tomography. J Neurosurg 68:417–423, 1988

Mandleberg IA: Cognitive recovery after severe head injury: WAIS during post-traumatic amnesia. J Neurol Neurosurg Psychiatry 38:1127–1132, 1975

Menza MA, Murray GB, Holmes VF, et al: Decreased extrapyramidal symptoms with intravenous haloperidol. J Clin Psychiatry 48:278–280, 1987

Obrist WD, Langfitt TW, Jaggi JL, et al: Cerebral blood flow and metabolism in comatose patients with acute head injury: relationship to intracranial hypertension. J Neurosurg 61:241–253, 1984

Ommaya AK, Gennarelli TA: Cerebral concussion and traumatic unconsciousness. Brain 97:633–654, 1974

Raichle ME, Grubb RL, Gado MH, et al: Correlation between regional cerebral blood flow and oxidative metabolism: in vivo studies in man. Arch Neurol 33:523–526, 1976

Reyes RL, Bhattacharyya AK, Heller D: Traumatic head injury: restlessness and agitation as prognosticators of physical and psychological improvement in patients. Arch Phys Med Rehabil 62:20–23, 1981

Russell WR, Smith A: Post-traumatic amnesia in closed head injury. Arch Neurol 5:4–17, 1961

Salazar AM, Grafman JH, Vance SC, et al: Consciousness and amnesia after penetrating head injury: neurology and anatomy. Neurology 36:178–187, 1986

Smith A: Duration of impaired consciousness as an index of severity in closed head injuries: a review. Diseases of the Nervous System 22:70–74, 1961

Smith LW, Dimsdale J: Postcardiotomy delirium: conclusions after 25 years. Am J Psychiatry 146:452–458, 1989

Sos J, Cassem NH: Intravenous use of haloperidol for acute delirium in intensive care settings, in Psychic and Neurological Dysfunctions After Open Heart Surgery. Edited by Speidel H, Rodewald G. Stuttgart, Georg Thieme Verlag, 1980, pp 196–199

Squire LR: Mechanisms of memory. Science 232:1612–1619, 1986

Synek VM: EEG abnormality grades and subdivisions of prognostic importance in traumatic and anoxic coma in adults. Clin Electroencephalogr 19:160–166, 1988

Synek VM: Value of a revised EEG coma scale for prognosis after cerebral anoxia and diffuse head injury. Clin Electroencephalogr 21:25–30, 1990

Teasdale G, Jennett B: Assessment of coma and impaired consciousness: a practical scale. Lancet 2:81–84, 1974

Teasdale E, Cardosos E, Galbraith S, et al: CT scan in severe diffuse head injury: physiological and clinical correlations. J Neurol Neurosurg Psychiatry 47:600–603, 1984

Trzepacz PT, Francis J: Low serum albumin and risk of delirium. Am J Psychiatry 147:675, 1990

Trzepacz PT, Baker RW, Greenhouse JB: A symptom rating scale for delirium. Psychiatry Res 23:89–97, 1988a

Trzepacz PT, Brenner R, Coffman G, et al: Delirium in liver transplantation candidates: discriminant analysis of multiple test variables. Biol Psychiatry 24:3–14, 1988b

Trzepacz PT, Brenner R, Van Thiel DH: A psychiatric study of 247 liver transplant candidates. Psychosomatics 30:147–153, 1989a

Trzepacz PT, Sclabassi RJ, Van Thiel DH: Delirium: a subcortical phenomenon? J Neuropsychiatry Clin Neurosci 1:283–290, 1989b

Williams MA, Campbell EB, Raynor WJ, et al: Reducing acute confusional states in elderly patients with hip fractures. Res Nurs Health 8:329–337, 1985

Williams MA, Levin HS, Eisenberg HM: Mild head injury classification. Neurosurgery 27:422–428, 1990

Yates DW, Hadfield JM, Peters K: Alcohol consumption of patients attending two accident and emergency departments in north-west England. Journal of the Royal Society of Medicine 80:486–489, 1987

Chapter 7

Mood Disorders

Robert G. Robinson, M.D.
Ricardo Jorge, M.D.

Associations between traumatic brain injury (TBI) and a variety of neuropsychiatric disorders have been reported in the medical literature for many years. Adolf Meyer (1904), for example, identified a number of disorders that he referred to as the "traumatic insanities" and proposed that there might be associations between these disorders and specific lesion locations. Lishman (1968), in his classical study on the Oxford collection of head injury records, analyzed potential etiologic factors involved in the development of psychiatric disturbances following TBI. These studies stressed the importance of biological variables such as the extent of brain damage, lesion location, and the presence of posttraumatic epilepsy in determining the type and duration of psychiatric disorder.

Quantification of severity of TBI by Teasdale and Jennett (1974), using the Glasgow Coma Scale (GSC), led to a large number of studies that analyzed behavioral and emotional consequences of brain injury, as well as different prognostic factors related to long-term outcome (Alexander et al. 1983; Livingston et al. 1985; Teas-

This work was supported in part by the following National Institutes of Health and National Institute of Mental Health Grants: Research Scientist Award (MH000163) (to RGR), MH40355, and NS151178.

dale et al. 1979). However, there have been relatively few studies that have examined the prevalence of mood disorders associated with TBI and their effect on outcome variables. Issues such as the prevalence of major depressive disorder following TBI, clinical variables that predict the development of major depression, the natural course of post-TBI major depression, and the influence of mood disorders on the longitudinal evolution of post-TBI physical and intellectual impairments are largely unexplored and deserve further research endeavor.

In this chapter, we review our findings, as well as those of other investigators, concerning the frequency, course, and clinical correlates of mood disorders. We also examine the interesting issue of whether depressive symptoms are specific for depression in patients with acute brain injury or are nonspecific effects of an acute medical illness.

Depression

Prevalence

As previously indicated, there have been relatively few systematic studies of the prevalence of depression following TBI. In addition, most of the studies have relied on cutoff points on rating scales (e.g., The Minnesota Multiphasic Personality Inventory [MMPI]) or relatives' reports, rather than on structured interviews and diagnostic criteria (e.g., DSM-IV; American Psychiatric Association 1994) to establish a diagnosis of depression (Silver et al. 1991). Perhaps because of this lack of uniformity in defining depression, the reported frequency of depressive disorders following TBI has varied from 6%–77% (Brooks et al. 1986; Levin and Grossman 1978; Rutherford et al. 1977; Schoenhuber and Gentili 1988; Varney et al. 1987). McKinlay et al. (1981) reported indirect evidence of a depressed mood in about half of their patients at 3, 6, or 12 months following severe brain injury. Kinsella et al. (1988) reported that in a series of 39 patients with severe brain injury, 33% were classified as depressed and 26% as suffering from anxiety, within two years postinjury. More recently, Gualtieri and Cox (1991) estimated that the frequency of major depression in TBI patients lies between 25%–50%.

We have reported on the in-hospital evaluation of 66 patients with acute TBI (Fedoroff et al. 1992). Severity of brain injury was determined using the 24-hour GCS scores (i.e., mild: GCS 12–15; moderate: GCS 8–11; or severe GCS: 3–7). In addition, patients with GCS scores in the 12–15 range but who had intracranial surgical procedures or focal lesions greater than 25 cc were considered to have moderate head injuries (Levin et al. 1987). The majority of the patients (68%) were categorized as having moderate head injuries, 17% with severe injuries, and 15% with mild. GCS scores ranged from 3 to 15, with a median of 10 and an interquartile range of 6.

Diagnoses of depression were based on a semistructured psychiatric interview (Wing et al. 1974) and DSM-III-R criteria (American Psychiatric Association 1987) for major or minor (dysthymic) depression (Robinson et al. 1983). The mean interval between TBI and the psychiatric interview was approximately 1 month (median = 31 days, interquartile range = 32). We found that major depression occurred in 17 patients (26%) and minor depression in 2 patients (3%) (Figure 7–1). We also analyzed data at a 3-, 6-, and 12-month follow-up (Jorge et al. 1993a). Of 54 patients reevaluated at 3 months, 12 patients (22%) had major depression and 4 patients (7%) had minor depression. Among the patients who were not depressed during the acute in-hospital period, major depression had occurred in 17% by 3 months after injury.

At 6 months posttrauma, 43 patients were reevaluated and 11 patients (26%) met DSM-III-R diagnostic criteria for either major or minor depression; 10 of them (23%) were diagnosed as major depression and 1 patient (2%) had minor depression. Among patients who were not depressed in the acute stage or at 3-month follow-up, the incidence of new onset major depression was 15%. Finally, of the original 66 patients, 43 were interviewed at 1-year follow-up. At that time, 11 patients (26%) met DSM-III-R criteria for either major or minor depression. There were 8 patients with major depression and 3 patients with minor depression. Among the patients who had not developed depressive disorders at the time of the preceding evaluations, the incidence of new onset major depression was 12%.

In summary, 15 patients developed delayed onset major or minor depression during the follow-up period. Of the 41 initially nondepressed patients seen at follow-up, 11 (26.8%) were later diagnosed with major depressive disorder and 4 with minor (dysthymic) depression. Of the 66 original patients, 42% developed major depression and 9% minor depression at some time during the 1-year follow-up period. Because some patients were improving while others were developing new depressions, the overall frequency of major depression remained relatively stable at about 25% throughout the first year following TBI (Figures 7–1 and 7–2).

Natural Course of Post-TBI Depression

In addition to the frequency of depressive disorders, another important aspect of post-TBI mood disorders is their duration. Affective disorders may be transient syndromes lasting for a few weeks or persistent disorders lasting for many months (Grant and Alves 1987). Previous investigators have suggested that transient disor-

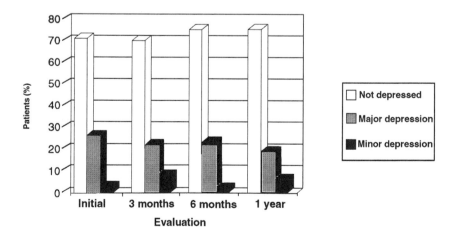

Figure 7–1. Prevalence of depression in traumatic brain injury, based on 66 patients evaluated in the hospital and at 3 months, 6 months, and 1 year after injury.

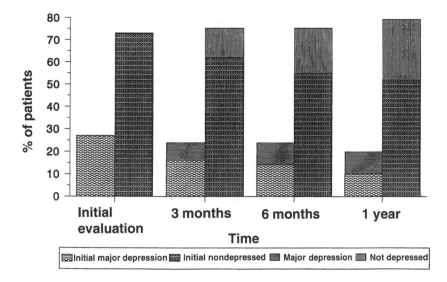

Figure 7–2. Percentage of patients with major depression or no depression evaluated at initial evaluation, at 3 months, at 6 months, and at 1 year. The percentage of patients who were depressed or nondepressed at the time of the initial evaluation is indicated as a portion of the total patients who were depressed or nondepressed at the 3-month, 6-month, and 1-year follow-up evaluations. Although the total percentage of major depression remains fairly stable at about 25% during the 1-year follow-up, some of the acutely depressed patients had recovered at each follow-up evaluation, whereas other initially nondepressed patients had developed delayed onset depressions at each time point.

ders may be associated with neurophysiological disturbances (e.g., neurochemical changes in the injured brain) whereas prolonged depressive disorders may be reactive psychological responses to physical or cognitive impairment (Lishman 1988; Prigatano 1987; Silver et al. 1991; Van Zomeren and Saan 1990).

We examined the duration of depression in the 17 patients diagnosed with major depression during the in-hospital evaluation. Although 1 patient dropped out by the time of the 3-month follow-up evaluation, there were 7 patients with an estimated duration of 8 weeks (i.e., they were no longer depressed at 3 months), 3 patients with an estimated duration of 4.5 months (i.e., at least 3 months but less than 6 months duration), and 6 patients with an estimated duration of 9 or 12 months (i.e., more than 6 up to 12 months duration). Thus patients who developed major depression during the acute period following TBI had an estimated mean duration of depression of 4.7 months, with a minimum of 1.5 months and a maximum of 12 months. Consistent with this finding, delayed onset major depressions also had an estimated mean duration of 4.0 months (Jorge et al. 1993b). Finally, we identified 2 patients with recurrent depressions who had major depression in-hospital, but were not depressed at the 3- or 6-month evaluation, only to become depressed again at 1-year follow-up. In summary, major depression appears to have a natural course of about 4 to 5 months following TBI. There may be groups of patients who develop transient major depressions of 6 or 8 weeks duration and others who have prolonged depressions lasting up to a year. We will discuss the differences between these groups later in this chapter.

Diagnosis

Although most of the previous studies of depressive disorders following TBI have used rating scale cutoff scores to determine the existence of these disorders, our studies have used a semistructured psychiatric interview (i.e., the Present State Examination) and DSM-III-R diagnostic criteria for major or minor (dysthymic) depression. However, if DSM-III-R criteria are to be used in a medically ill population such as patients with TBI, one of the basic issues that must be addressed is the specificity of these depressive symptoms and the validity of the diagnostic criteria. Symptoms of major depression such as sleep, appetite, or libido changes, may occur in patients with TBI as a consequence of brain injury or as a nonspecific consequence of an acute medical illness with hospitalization (e.g., hospital routine leading to insomnia). Thus symptoms used to diagnose depressive disorders could be independent of the associated mood disturbance. Consequently, major depressive disorders could be systematically overdiagnosed. On the other hand, patients might deny the presence of a depressed mood as part of a general unawareness deficit (Prigatano 1991a) or a denial syndrome. This would result in underdiagnosis of depression.

In a recent study, we longitudinally examined the specificity of symptoms of depression following TBI (Jorge et al. 1993c). Depressive symptoms were divided into "autonomic" and "psychologic" subtypes using the distinctions proposed by Davidson and Turnbull (1986). We then analyzed their frequency in patients who presented with a depressed mood compared to those without a depressed mood. In addition, we analyzed the relative frequency of depressive symptoms used in DSM-III-R diagnostic criteria for major depressive disorder (Table 7–1).

We found that the mean frequency of autonomic symptoms was 2.7 (SD = 1.4) and the mean frequency of psychological symptoms was 3.1 (SD = 1.9). This was more than three times the frequency of autonomic (0.8 [SD = 0.8]) and psychological (0.9 [SD = O.9]) symptoms in patients who denied having a depressed mood. The psychological symptoms that discriminated depressed from nondepressed patients at both the initial evaluation and at 1-year follow-up were symptoms related to changes in self-attitude (feelings of hopelessness, suicidal ideation, loss of interest, self-deprecation, lack of self-confidence). The only autonomic symptom that held up over 1 year was lack of energy (i.e., subjective anergia).

Anxiety symptoms were significantly associated with depression during the first 6 months following closed head trauma. At 1-year follow-up, however, their frequency was not significantly different in patients with or without depressed mood.

Autonomic symptoms such as decreased appetite and weight loss, difficulty falling asleep, and diurnal mood variation (with morning depression) appeared to be significantly associated with depression only during the initial or 3-month evaluation, not at 1-year follow-up. On the other hand, early morning awakening, loss of libido, difficulty concentrating, and inefficient thinking distinguished depressed from nondepressed patients only after 6 months or a year had elapsed. Finally, increased appetite, weight gain, and hypersomnia did not differentiate between depressed and nondepressed groups at any time.

The fact that the symptoms that are specific to depression

Table 7–1. Percentage of 66 traumatic brain injury patients with or without depressed mood presenting with DSM-III-R symptoms for major depressive disorder

DSM-III-R symptoms	Initial evaluation		6-month follow-up		1-year follow-up	
	Depressed	Non-depressed	Depressed	Non-depressed	Depressed	Non-depressed
Depressed mood	100	0[a]	100	0[a]	100	0[a]
Loss of interest/anhedonia	11	6	25	10	45	3[a]
Weight loss/loss of appetite	37	11[a]	17	6	18	3
Weight gain/increased appetite	5	7	8	3	18	0
Insomnia	53	26	67	16[a]	50	6[a]
Hypersomnia	32	34	17	23	190	
Psychomotor agitation	32	4[a]	8	11	20	4
Psychomotor retardation	11	9	8	7	20	0
Anergia	58	26[a]	50	13[a]	45	9[a]
Feelings of worthlessness	5	2	50	6[a]	55	0[a]
Guilt	37	11[a]	54	16[a]	18	0
Diminished ability to think or concentrate	84	60	58	23	55	6[a]
Suicidal ideation	16	0[a]	24	0[a]	27	0[a]

[a] $P < .05$.

changed over the course of the first year following TBI suggests that the nature of post-TBI depressions may change over time. Symptoms that are associated with depression during the acute period after TBI such as anxiety symptoms, initial insomnia, diurnal mood variation, and perhaps decreased appetite and weight loss may be clinical manifestations of a biologically determined depressive syndrome. On the other hand, terminal insomnia, loss of libido, and diminished ability to think or concentrate, which are significantly associated with depression only after 6 months post-TBI (Table 7–1), may be symptoms that emerge only after the acute effects (i.e., nonspecific effects) of TBI have subsided and some recovery has taken place.

Because there are depressive symptoms that are not *specific* to depression, the question arises whether existing DSM-III-R criteria for major depression should be modified to account for this finding. If we required the presence of at least three specific symptoms (including depressed mood) as a criterion for diagnosing major depression, standard DSM-III-R criteria would have a 100% sensitivity and 94% specificity at the initial evaluation, 88% sensitivity and 94% specificity at 3 months, 91% sensitivity and 96% specificity at 6 months, and 80% sensitivity and 100% specificity at 1-year follow-up. Thus the standard diagnostic criteria (DSM-III-R) have a high sensitivity and specificity for identifying depressed patients when compared with alternative specific *symptom* diagnostic criteria and may, therefore, be used for the diagnosis of depression in the TBI population. Finally, the frequency of possible masked depressions (i.e., patients who presented with at least three specific symptoms of depression but denied a depressed mood) was very low and occurred in only two patients at 1-year follow-up.

The use of DSM-III-R criteria for major and minor (dysthymic) depression provides valid and reliable operational constructs that are essential for conducting longitudinal studies and for designing effective therapeutic strategies. DSM-IV (American Psychiatric Association 1994) criteria characterize depressive disorders following brain injury by their syndromic features (i.e., major depression or dysthymia) and by the fact that they are the consequence of a medical illness (i.e., secondary), which, in turn, is specified by an

Axis III diagnosis. The differential diagnosis of post-TBI major depression includes adjustment disorder with depressed mood, emotional lability, apathy, and posttraumatic stress disorder. Patients with adjustment disorders develop short-lived and relatively mild emotional disturbances within 3 months of a stressful life event. Although these may include depressive symptoms, patients with adjustment disorders do not meet DSM-III-R criteria for major depression. Posttraumatic stress disorder occurs following an unusually severe distressing event. It is characterized by symptoms of reexperiencing the trauma ranging from transient flashbacks or vivid nightmares to more severe dissociative states in which the patient behaves as if he or she is actually living the traumatic event. In addition, patients typically avoid all those circumstances associated with the trauma and become withdrawn and emotionally blunted.

Emotional lability is characterized by the presence of sudden and uncontrollable affective outbursts (e.g., crying or laughing), which may be congruent or incongruent with the patient's mood and which occur either spontaneously or triggered by minor stimuli. It lacks the pervasive alteration of mood, as well as the specific vegetative symptoms associated with a major depressive episode. Emotional lability, however, may respond to treatment with antidepressants (Robinson et al. 1992).

Finally, TBI patients may present with apathetic syndromes that interfere with the rehabilitation process (Prigatano 1986). In our experience, apathy is frequently associated with psychomotor retardation and emotional blunting. Some patients, however, also have a depressed mood. Although apathy is frequently associated with frontal lobe damage, the relationship between apathy and the type, extent, and location of traumatic brain damage has not been systematically studied.

Premorbid Risk Factors for Depression

Previous clinical and epidemiological studies have stressed that several premorbid factors may influence patients' emotional response to acute TBI and may, therefore, be relevant to the etiology of depressive disorders following TBI (Lishman 1973). Moreover, it has been suggested that these premorbid factors (e.g., previous psychiatric disorder, disturbing life events) may predispose the individual to receive head injury (Selzer et al. 1968).

In our study of 66 patients with acute TBI (Fedoroff et al. 1992), there were no significant differences between the depressed and nondepressed groups in their demographic variables (i.e., age, sex, race, marital status, education, socioeconomic status) or in the frequency of family history of psychiatric disorders (Table 7–2). There was, however, a significantly greater frequency of previous personal history of psychiatric disorders (χ^2 = 4.379, df = 1, P = .03) in the major depressed group. If patients with a history of alcohol or other substance abuse are excluded, however, this significant difference is lost (χ^2 = 1.683, df = 1, P = .195). There was not, on the other hand, a significant difference between groups in the frequency of personal history of alcohol and/or other substance abuse (χ^2 = 2.1, df = 1, P = .14).

Table 7–2. Demographic data and history of psychiatric disorders in 64 patients with acute traumatic brain injury, for depressed and nondepressed subgroups

Variables	Major depression (n = 17)	Nondepressed (n = 47)
Age (mean, SD)	26.8 (5.8)	29.5 (10.7)
Sex (% male)	82.4	87.2
Race (% black)	29.4	23.4
Handedness (% left)	5.9	8.5
Education, in years (mean, SD)	12.4 (2.0)	12.3 (2.1)
Hollingshead socioeconomic status (% class IV or V)	75	72
Family history of psychiatric disorder (%)	47.0 (8/17)	48.9 (23/47)
Personal history of psychiatric disorder (%)[a]	70.6 (12/17)	37.0 (17/46)

[a]P < .05.

In addition, the major depressed group had significantly increased (i.e., more impaired) Social Functioning Examination (SFE) scores (Starr et al. 1983) (Table 7–3). The SFE, during the initial evaluation, measured satisfaction with social functioning during the period prior to brain injury. This suggests that patients with poor social adjustment and social dissatisfaction prior to the brain injury

Table 7–3. Psychiatric findings in the study group of 64 patients with acute traumatic brain injury, for depressed and nondepressed subgroups

Variable	Major depression mean scores (SD)	No depression mean scores (SD)	*F*	*P*
MMSE				
Initial	27.5 (2.3)	26.5 (3.1)	1.7	.1923
3-month follow-up	6.9 (2.5)	27.6 (2.7)	0.9	.3355
6-month follow-up	28.1 (1.6)	27.3 (3.5)	0.1	.8123
1-year follow-up	27.9 (1.6)	26.1 (3.2)	1.8	.1882
JHFI				
Initial	2.2 (3.3)	1.4 (1.8)	0.3	.5827
3-month follow-up	1.25 (1.4)	0.88 (1.1)	0.6	.4266
6-month follow-up	2.0 (2.4)	0.5 (0.9)	3.4	.0740
1-year follow-up	0.5 (1.1)	0.4 (1.0)	0.2	.6913
STC				
Initial	4.2 (1.2)	3.6 (1.5)	2.5	.1196
3-month follow-up	4.6 (1.1)	3.6 (1.7)	4.6	.0367
6-month follow-up	5.2 (1.8)	3.7 (1.5)	7.6	.0085
1-year follow-up	4.3 (1.8)	3.8 (1.9)	0.6	.4469
SFE				
Initial	.190 (.160)	.11 (.10)	4.9	.0302
3-month follow-up	.201 (.127)	.122 (.088)	4.5	.0397
6-month follow-up	.290 (.130)	.114 (.087)	17.5	.0002
1-year follow-up	.217 (.067)	.110 (.097)	11.4	.0016

Note. MMSE = Mini-Mental State Exam (Folstein et al. 1975); JHFI = Johns Hopkins Functional Inventory (Robinson and Szetela 1981); STC = Social Ties Checklist (Starr et al. 1983); SFE = Social Functioning Examination (Starr et al. 1983).

were more prone to develop depression following TBI.

In summary, our work, as well as that of other investigators, suggests that premorbid psychological (i.e., previous history of psychiatric disorder) and social impairments increase the risk of developing significant depressive disorders following TBI.

Biological Factors:
The Importance of Lesion Location

Although there appear to be significant premorbid psychological and social factors that influence the development of depression following TBI, biological variables may also play an important role in the pathogenesis of post-TBI depression.

Head injury has consistently been found to produce dynamic neurotransmitter and neurohormonal changes. Van Woerkom et al. (1977), for example, found that TBI patients with frontotemporal contusions had decreased levels of 5-hydroxyindoleacetic acid (5-HIAA) in their cerebrospinal fluid as compared to patients with diffuse traumatic injuries and evidence of brain stem dysfunction. Hamill et al. (1987) serially measured plasma epinephrine, norepinephrine, and dopamine levels in 33 TBI patients and proposed that highly elevated circulating catecholamines might be useful endogenous markers of the amount of brain damage, as well as predictors of long-term outcome. There is also evidence that the sympathetic response to brain injury may be modulated by the administration of clonidine, an α_2-adrenergic agonist (Payen et al. 1990).

Pretreatment with scopolamine influences the long-term motor and behavioral outcome following experimental brain injury in the rat (Lyeth et al. 1988); this finding suggests that acetylcholine may play a role in the pathophysiology of CNS trauma. In the same sense, there is evidence of a deleterious effect of endogenous opiates and of increased glutaminergic activity in acute TBI (Faden and Salzman 1992; Silver et al. 1991). There is also evidence of a pathophysiological role of certain neuropeptides. The administration of thyrotropin-releasing hormone or its pharmacological analogues appear to enhance recovery following CNS trauma (Faden and Salzman 1992). Corticotropin Releasing Factor is involved in adaptation to acute stress and may also be responsible for certain features of anxiety and depressive disorders (Nemeroff 1992). Prigatano (1987) hypothesized that changes in adrenocorticotropic hormone (ACTH) and cortisol levels that occur in patients with TBI may mediate changes in mood. However, the magnitude, regional distribution, and relationship of the temporal course of these neurochemical changes to depression remain largely unexplored and constitute an interesting field for further investigation.

TBI is characterized by the presence of diffuse and/or focal lesions that may be the direct result of traumatic strains or secondary to ischemic complications (Katz 1992). During the past several years, there have been significant advances in neuroimaging techniques that will certainly increase our understanding of the relationship between structural abnormalities and behavioral disturbances following TBI. Computed tomography (CT) and magnetic resonance imaging (MRI) have comparable sensitivity in the detection of hemorrhagic intra-axial lesions, as well as in the diagnosis of significant extradural and subdural hematomas. MRI, however, is more sensitive in detecting posttraumatic nonhemorraghic lesions (e.g., cortical contusions and deep white matter lesions) and in identifying small subdural collections. Thus CT scanning is the procedure of choice for the assessment of potential surgical lesions in the emergency setting whereas MRI scanning may prove to be more useful for classification of head injury, as well as the study of lesion correlates of neurobehavioral deficits (Wilson and Wyper 1992).

There is also some evidence that late MRI scanning may identify more functionally significant lesions than early MRI scans (Wilson et al. 1988). Positron-emission tomography (PET) and single photon emission computerized tomography (SPECT) studies may also provide functional information regarding metabolic and blood flow patterns, as well as regional distribution of specific neurotransmitter receptors. Roper et al. (1991) studied cerebral blood flow patterns in 15 patients with acute closed head injury using Tc-99m-HMPAO SPECT. They found focal disturbances that were not seen on CT scans and proposed a distinction between those contusions associated with a decreased cerebral blood flow and those without such a change.

Two recent SPECT studies analyzed the regional uptake of Tc-99m-HMPAO in 36 patients during the chronic stage of severe TBI. Impaired neuropsychological performance (i.e., memory and executive functions) was associated with reduced blood flow in thalamic regions rather than in the expected cortical regions (Goldenberg et al. 1992). On the other hand, disinhibited behavior was significantly correlated with lower frontal flow rates (Oder et al. 1992). These imaging techniques, however, have not been applied to the study of mood or anxiety disorders following TBI.

There is some empirical evidence supporting an association between post-TBI depression and specific lesion locations (Finset 1988). Lishman (1968) reported that several years after penetrating brain injury, depressive symptoms were more common among patients with right-hemisphere lesions. Depressive symptoms were also more frequent among patients with frontal and parietal lesions than among patients with other lesion locations. Grafman et al. (1986) also reported that several years following head injury, depressive symptoms were more frequently associated with penetrating injuries involving the right hemisphere (right orbitofrontal lesions) than with any other lesion location.

Of our 66 TBI patients, 42 (64%) had a diffuse pattern of brain injury on their CT scans and 24 (36%) presented with focal lesions. Among the 42 patients with diffuse injury, 11 (17% of total) had normal CT scans. Among the 24 patients with focal injury, the lesion was surgically evacuated in 12 patients (18% of total) (9 of these 12 patients had an acute subdural hematoma, 2 patients had an epidural hematoma, and 1 patient underwent a right temporal lobectomy; 6 of the 12 patients also had associated parenchymal contusions). The remaining 12 patients (18%) had brain contusions greater than 25 cc on their CT scans. In addition, 3 of these patients had associated small extraparenchymal hemorrhages (2 subdural and 1 epidural hematoma) that did not require surgery.

There were no significant differences between the major depressed and the nondepressed groups in the frequency of diffuse or focal patterns of injury. In addition, there were no significant between-group differences in the frequency of extraparenchymal hemorrhages, contusions, intracerebral or intraventricular hemorrhages, hydrocephalus, or CT findings suggestive of brain atrophy.

To analyze the relationship between lesion location and the presence of major depression, a logistic regression model included the following location variables: frontal, temporal, parieto-occipital, subcortical (i.e., lesions involving deep white matter, basal ganglia, brain stem, and cerebellum), and left anterior (i.e., lesions involving the left dorsolateral frontal cortex and/or left basal ganglia lesions). There was an overall significant association between lesion location and the development of major depression (χ^2 = 33.6, df = 12, P = .0008). A backward selection procedure was then performed in order to remove the nonsignificant variables (P > .05). The presence of left anterior lesions (Wald χ^2 = 12.9, df = 1, P = .0003) was the strongest correlate of major depression. On the other hand, the presence of frontal lesions (i.e., left, right, or bilateral frontal lesions, including orbitofrontal cortex) was associated with a lesser probability of developing major depression (Wald χ^2 = 6.6, df = 1, P = .01). We then examined whether lesion location might differentiate between patients with transient depressions (i.e., less than 3 months) and long-term depressions (i.e., greater than 3 months). The in-hospital transiently depressed group showed a significantly higher frequency of left frontodorsolateral and/or left basal ganglia lesions (Fischer Exact Test, P = .006). There was also a higher frequency of subcortical involvement (Fischer Exact Test, P = .006) in the patients with brief depressions. The transiently depressed group also showed a higher frequency of left dorsolateral frontal and/or left basal ganglia lesions than the prolonged depressed group (Fischer Exact Test, P = .002).

These results are consistent with our previous findings in stroke patients of an increased frequency of depression among patients with left dorsolateral cortical and left basal ganglia lesions (Starkstein et al. 1987). They are also consistent with a previous study in which patients with anterior left-hemisphere lesions were found to have more severe depressive symptoms than patients with left posterior hemisphere lesions in both stroke and TBI (Robinson and Szetela 1981).

Left dorsolateral frontal cortex and left basal ganglia may be strategic locations in the left hemisphere for the disruption of the ascending noradrenergic or serotonergic pathways and their related behavioral functions (Robinson et al. 1984). Our anatomical findings in patients with TBI and acute depression are consistent with this hypothesis. Thus although closed head injury is associated with widespread, diffuse neuropathological findings (e.g., multiple contusions and diffuse axonal injury), there seem to be specific brain lesion locations whose involvement is associated with a greater risk of developing depressive disorders. Cross-sectional analysis of our data at 3-, 6-, and 12-month follow-up periods, however, revealed that this relationship between major depression and lesion location was temporally bound. Left anterior lesions were significantly associated with depression during the acute posttrauma period, but by the 3-month follow-up there was no longer a significant correlation between depression and lesion location. This finding is in contrast to our results in patients with poststroke depression where the significant association between severity of depression and left anterior lesion location held up for 1 year (this association, however, was lost by the 2-year follow-up) (Robinson et al. 1987). It could also be hypothesized that the shorter time course of depression following left anterior TBI lesions compared with left anterior ischemic lesions was a result of the nature of the neuropathological findings. TBI is associated with diffuse shear axonal injury and contusing lesions, which have a greater potential for functional or structural restoration than large ischemic lesions. Reorganization of neuronal connections (e.g., pruning, reactive synaptogenesis, and regenerative sprouting) may be easier and more extensive following TBI.

Another contributing factor to this difference between stroke and TBI patients may be the age of the affected subjects. TBI involves a significantly younger population than stroke. It has been demonstrated that there is a greater potential for neuronal regeneration and relocalization of functional brain activity among young brains compared with old ones (Chollet et al. 1991; Steward 1989).

In summary, some acute onset depressions appear to be related to lesion characteristics and may have their etiology in biological responses of the injured brain such as neurochemical changes. Left dorsolateral frontal and left basal ganglia lesions are strongly associated with major depression during the initial in-hospital evaluation and may represent strategic lesion locations that elicit biochemical responses ultimately leading to the clinical manifestation of depression.

By the 3-month follow-up, however, the major correlates of depression were previous history of psychiatric disorder and impaired social functioning. Thus prolonged or delayed onset depressions may be mediated by psychosocial factors suggesting psychological reaction as a possible mechanism.

Relationship Between Depression and Impairment Variables

One of the most potentially important issues associated with post-TBI depression is its relationship to the degree of physical or cognitive impairment. Depressive disorders occurring in the chronic stage of TBI are generally considered to represent a psychological reaction to the associated impairments and to occur as a consequence of the patient's insight concerning his or her physical or cognitive deficits. Empirical studies, however, have reported conflicting findings with regard to this issue. Prigatano did not find an association between depression and the level of neuropsychological impairment (Prigatano 1986). On the other hand, Bornstein et al. (1989) found a positive relationship between the severity of neuropsychological deficits and emotional abnormality.

In our series, we found no significant association between major depression and the severity of intellectual impairment (as measured by the Mini-Mental State Exam [MMSE; Folstein et al. 1975]) or the severity of impairment in activities of daily living (as measured by the Johns Hopkins Functional Inventory [JHFI; Robinson and Szetela 1981]). This finding held true during the initial (in-hospital) evaluation, as well as at 3-, 6-, and 12-month follow-up. Social functioning (tested with the SFE) was the clinical variable with the most consistent relationship with depression throughout the whole follow-up period (Jorge et al. 1993a) (Table 7–3).

Although it is likely that a lack of social support after the brain injury contributed to depression, it is also conceivable that depression negatively influenced social functioning. The speculation that depression may have negatively influenced social functioning after the TBI is consistent with our finding that depression scores at the onset of depression were significantly correlated with SFE scores but not with the initial SFE scores (Jorge et al. 1993b). Head injury patients often have severe problems in regaining a productive life and maintaining satisfactory interpersonal relations; they may not be able to return to a previous work and they may become dependent and progressively isolated and withdrawn (Prigatano 1986). Emotional and motivational disturbances may also affect the rehabilitation process and may play an important role in determining final psychosocial adjustment, perhaps the most complex and relevant measure of outcome.

In summary, although severity of impairment may contribute to the development of depression in some patients, our findings suggest that depression is not simply a psychological response to the severity of physical or intellectual impairment. Depression, however, does appear to be related to impaired social functioning. Patients with poor social adjustment and social dissatisfaction prior to the brain injury had a high frequency of depression. In addition, after the brain injury, patients who continued to have impaired social functioning remained depressed and perhaps the social functioning of the depressed patients deteriorated. One might infer from these findings, therefore, that social intervention, as well as the treatment of depression, may be necessary to alleviate these severe and long-lasting mood disorders.

Treatment of Depression

To our knowledge, there have been no double-blind, placebo-controlled studies of the efficacy of pharmacologic treatments of depression in TBI patients.

Selection among competing antidepressants is usually guided by their side effect profiles. Mild anticholinergic activity, minimal lowering of seizure threshold, and low sedative effects are the most important factors to be considered in the choice of an antidepressant drug in this population (Silver et al. 1990).

Tricyclic antidepressants have important anticholinergic effects that may interfere with cognitive and memory functions (Lipsey et al. 1984). In addition, they may lower the seizure threshold. Fluoxetine, a serotonin reuptake inhibitor, is an antidepressant that appears to have a less adverse effect profile (Cassidy 1989). Initial dosing should be 20 mg/day given as a single morning dose. The dose may be increased up to 80 mg/day bid. The most common side effects include headache, gastrointestinal complaints, and insomnia.

Trazodone is an alternative antidepressant that also inhibits serotonin reuptake. Treatment is started at low doses (50–100 mg) at bedtime following a snack. Dose may be gradually increased every 3–4 days up to 400 mg. The most troublesome side effects are sedation and orthostatic hypotension (Zasler 1992).

There are case reports of successful treatments of post-TBI depression with psychostimulants (Gualtieri 1988). These include dextroamphetamine (8–60 mg/day), methylphenidate (10–60 mg/day), and pemoline (56.25 to 75 mg/day). They are given twice a day with the last dose at least 6 hours before sleep in order to prevent initial insomnia. Treatment is begun at lower doses, which are then gradually increased. Patients taking stimulants need close medical control to prevent abuse or toxic effects. The most common side effects are anxiety, dysphoria, headaches, irritability, anorexia, insomnia, cardiovascular symptoms, dyskinesias, or even psychotic symptoms (Zasler 1992).

Electroconvulsive therapy is not contraindicated in TBI patients and may be considered if other methods of treatment are unsuccessful. Buspirone—a drug that has an agonist effect on serotonin, subtype 1 (5-HT$_1$), receptors and an antagonist effect on dopamine, subtype 2 (D$_2$), receptors—has proved to be a safe and efficacious anxiolytic. Initial dosing is 15 mg/day given in three divided doses and it may be gradually increased (5 mg every 4 days) up to 60 mg/day. The most common side effects are dizziness and headaches (Gualtieri 1991; Zasler 1992).

Finally, we have already mentioned the role that social intervention and adequate psychotherapeutic support may play in the treatment of depression following TBI (Prigatano 1991b; Sbordone 1990). However, these psychological, as well as pharmacological, treatments need to be examined in controlled treatment trials.

Secondary Mania

Prevalence of Mania Following TBI: Associated Clinical Variables

Secondary manic and hypomanic states have been reported in a number of organic disorders such as thyroid disease (Corn and Checkley 1983; Zolese and Henryk-Gutt 1987), uremia (Thomas and Neale 1991), vitamin B_{12} deficiency (Goggans 1984), electrical trauma (Khanna et al. 1991), after a hyperbaric diving experiment (Stoudemire et al. 1984), and following open-heart surgery (Isles and Orrell 1991). Mania has also been associated with brain tumors (Jamieson and Wells 1979; Robinson et al. 1988), CNS infections (Thienhaus and Khosla 1984), stroke (Blackwell 1991; Cummings and Mendez 1984; Fawcett 1991; Robinson et al. 1988), and TBI (Bamrah and Johnson 1991; Shukla et al. 1987; Starkstein et al. 1990).

Shukla et al. (1987) reported on 20 patients who developed manic syndromes after closed head trauma. They found a significant association between mania and the presence of posttraumatic seizures, predominantly of the partial-complex ("temporal lobe epilepsy") type. They also found no association with a family history of bipolar disorder among 85 first-degree relatives. We have previously reported on 25 patients with manic syndromes secondary to cerebrovascular, traumatic, or neoplastic brain lesions (Robinson et al. 1988; Starkstein et al. 1990). We found that secondary manic patients had a significantly greater frequency of lesions involving the right hemisphere, particularly in specific limbic-related areas such as the basotemporal or orbitofrontal cortices, thalamus, or basal ganglia. In addition, both genetic vulnerability (as evidenced by an increased frequency of family history of mood disorder) and the presence of subcortical atrophy (as evidenced by increased ventricular-brain ratios) were identified as probable premorbid risk factors for the development of mania following brain injury (Robinson et al. 1988; Starkstein et al. 1988).

We have also studied the prevalence, clinical characteristics, and clinical correlates of manic syndromes diagnosed in the first year following TBI in our series of 66 closed head injury patients (Jorge et al. 1993d).

Of the 66 original patients, 6 patients met DSM-III-R criteria for major affective disorder, manic episode, at some time point during the 1-year follow-up period. One of them had a bipolar disorder. The manic episodes were short-lived, with an estimated duration of 2 months. The estimated duration of the presence of an elevated mood, however, was 5.7 months. In addition, 3 of the 6 secondary manic patients developed brief episodes of violent behavior at some point during the 1-year follow-up.

Aggressive behavior was significantly more frequent in the secondary mania group than in the group of patients who developed major depression (MD group, $n = 27$) or in the group of patients who did not experience an affective disorder (Non-AD group, $n = 26$) ($\chi^2 = 9.9$, df $= 2$, $P = .007$).

At the time the diagnosis of mania was established, two patients were receiving benzodiazepines (i.e., lorazepam) and one patient was receiving neuroleptics (i.e., haloperidol). Thus there may have been three patients who were receiving treatment for their manic symptoms. The duration of mania, however, did not appear to be significantly different in patients who were treated compared to those who were not treated. In addition, one patient was prescribed anticonvulsants (phenytoin), and one patient was prescribed triazolam for sleep disturbances. There were no significant between-group differences in sex, age, race, handedness, socioeconomic status, or educational level (Table 7–4).

There were also no significant between-group differences in the frequency of either family history of mood or other psychiatric disorders or personal history of alcohol or drug abuse. The three groups were not significantly different with regard to the frequency of mild, moderate, or severe head injury (Table 7–4).

Personal history of psychiatric disorder was, however, significantly more frequent among the major depressed group (χ^2 = 17.5 df = 2, P = .0002). Secondary manic patients did not have a greater frequency of personal history of psychiatric disorder than the non-affective disturbance (non-AD) group.

In summary, 6 out of 66 TBI patients (9%) developed secondary mania at some time during the 1-year follow-up period. One of these patients (17%) presented with a bipolar course. Secondary mania was not associated with the severity of brain injury, the degree of physical or cognitive impairment, a personal or family history of psychiatric disorder, the availability of social support, or social functioning level.

Table 7–4. Demographic data, history of psychiatric disorders, and severity of head injury in 59 patients with acute traumatic brain injury, for psychiatric subgroups

Characteristics	Secondary mania (*n* = 6)	Major depression (*n* = 27)	No organic affective disorder (*n* = 26)
SES (% of classes IV–V)	83	77	69
Race (% of black)	7	33	19
Sex (% of male)	100	78	85
Age (mean [SD])	30.3 (18.4)	27.7 (6.1)	29.6 (10)
Education (mean [SD])	12.8 (2.3)	11.5 (2.9)	12.5 (2.6)
Family history of mood disorders (%)	0	11	15
Personal history of psychiatric disorder (%)	17	74[a]	20
Personal history of alcohol or drug abuse (%)	0	33	12
Severe head injury (%)	17	30	9
Moderate head injury (%)	67	57	67
Mild head injury (%)	16	13	24

Note. SES = socioeconomic status.
[a]P < .05.

Biological Factors:
The Importance of Lesion Location

We have already mentioned that in our previous studies of secondary manic patients, we found that there was a significantly greater frequency of lesions involving specific limbic-related areas such as the temporal basopolar or orbitofrontal cortices, particularly in the right hemisphere. For example, Starkstein et al. (1990) reported a patient with a posttraumatic right frontal subcortical lesion who had a PET study during one of his recurrent manic episodes. The study revealed a significant hypometabolism of the right temporal basopolar area.

The cortical areas most frequently affected by closed head injury are the ventral aspects of frontal and temporal lobes. There is also frequent neuropathological evidence of damage to subcortical, diencephalic, and brain stem structures (Teasdale and Mendelow 1984).

We have compared the CT findings of the 6 secondary manic patients from our longitudinal study of 66 patients with those encountered in the major depression and the non-AD groups. There were no significant differences between the groups in the frequency of diffuse or focal patterns of brain injury. In addition, there were no significant differences in the frequency of extraparenchymal hemorrhages (i.e., epidural, subdural, or subarachnoid hemorrhages), intracerebral or intraventricular hemorrhages, contusions, hydrocephalus, or brain atrophy.

We also analyzed the relationship between lesion location and the presence of secondary mania using a logistic regression model. We first compared the manic group ($n = 6$) with the rest of the TBI patients ($n = 60$). There was an overall significant association between lesion location and the development of secondary mania ($\chi^2 = 28.2$, df = 12, $P = .0051$). A backward selection procedure was performed in order to remove the nonsignificant variables ($P > .05$). This procedure selected temporal basopolar location as the only location significantly associated with mania (Wald c2 = 12, df = 1, $P = .0005$). We then compared the manic group ($n = 6$) with the major depression ($n = 27$) group. There was also an overall significant association between lesion location and the development of secondary mania ($\chi^2 = 23.2$, df = 12, $P = .0260$). Once again, the presence of temporal basopolar lesions (Wald $\chi^2 = 8.72$, df = 1, $P = .003$) was associated with a greater risk of developing mania.

In summary, secondary manic syndromes occurred in almost 10% of a consecutive series of 66 TBI patients. The major correlate of mania was the presence of anterior temporal lesions. Factors such as personal history of mood disorders or posttraumatic epilepsy did not appear to significantly influence the frequency of secondary mania in this group of patients. The development of abnormal electrical activation patterns in limbic networks, functional changes in aminergic inhibitory systems, and the presence of aberrant regeneration pathways may play a role in the genesis of these syndromes (Stevens 1990; Csernansky et al. 1988). Future studies should look for specific risk factors for mania and effective methods for treatment of these disorders.

Treatment of Mania

There have been no systematic studies of the treatment of secondary mania. There are, however, several reports of potentially useful treatment modalities. Bakchine et al. (1989) conducted a double-blind, placebo-controlled study in a single patient with secondary mania following TBI. Clonidine (600 µg/day) was effective in reverting manic symptoms, carbamazepine (1200 mg/day) did not elicit mood changes, and l-dopa/benzeraside (375 mg/day) resulted in an increase of manic symptoms. Lithium (Starkstein et al. 1988), carbamazepine (Bouvy et al. 1988), and valproate (Pope et al. 1988) therapies have also been reported to be efficacious in individual cases.

Summary and Future Directions

In this chapter, we have reviewed the state of our knowledge about mood disorders following TBI. Although investigators are only beginning to identify depressive and manic disorders based on structured interviews and DSM-III-R diagnostic criteria, both major depression and mania appear to occur following TBI, in about 42% and 9% respectively of patients during 1 year following TBI. The frequency of major depression remained relatively constant throughout the first year following TBI, with some patients improving (average duration of depression 4 to 5 months) and other patients developing delayed onset depressions. Risk factors for depression included previous history of psychiatric disorder and poor social functioning. In addition, there appeared to be a group of transiently depressed patients who had depression based on injury to left dorsal lateral frontal or left basal ganglia structures. Similarly, manic patients were significantly more likely to have temporal basopolar lesions than were depressed or nondepressed patients.

The degree of physical or intellectual impairment did not appear to play a prominent role in the development of either mania or depression. However, subtle neuropsychological or physical deficits might have been overlooked by the instruments that were used in this study, and these may play a role in the development of depression.

There are many areas that are ripe for future research. Our findings utilized a patient population with traumatic injury restricted primarily to the brain, that is, without significant involvement of the other body systems. It is unclear whether these findings would be replicated in another population of patients with TBI. The most important elements of social functioning contributing to depression need to be explored, as well as the effect of social intervention. The role of antidepressant medications in treating patients with these depressive disorders has not been systematically explored and deserves study.

Finally, the mechanisms of these depressions, both those associated with psychosocial factors and those associated with neurobiological variables (e.g., strategic lesion locations), need to be investigated. It is only through the discovery of their mechanisms that we will ultimately be able to develop specific and rational treatment strategies for these disorders.

References

Alexander A, Colombo F, Nertempi P, et al: Cognitive outcome and early indices of severity of head injury. J Neurosurg 59:751–761, 1983

American Psychiatric Association: Diagnostic and Statistical Manual of Mental Disorders, 3rd Edition, Revised. Washington, DC, American Psychiatric Association, 1987

American Psychiatric Association: Diagnostic and Statistical Manual of Mental Disorders, 4th Edition. Washington, DC, American Psychiatric Association, 1994

Bamrah JS, Johnson J: Bipolar affective disorder following head injury. Br J Psychiatry 158:117–119, 1991

Bakchine S, Lacomblez L, Benoit N, et al: Manic like state after orbitofrontal and right temporoparietal injury: efficacy of clonidine. Neurology 39:777–781, 1989

Blackwell MJ: Rapid-cycling manic-depressive illness following subarachnoid hemorrhage. Br J Psychiatry 159:279–280, 1991

Bornstein RA, Miller HB, Van Schoor JT: Neuropsychological deficit and emotional disturbance in head injured patients. J Neurosurg 70:509–513, 1989

Bouvy PF, van de Wetering BJM, Meerwaldt JD, et al: A case of organic brain syndrome following head injury successfully treated with carbamazepine. Acta Psychiatr Scand 77:361–363, 1988

Brooks N, Campsie L, Symington C, et al: The five-year outcome of severe blunt head injury: a relative's view. J Neurol Neurosurg Psychiatry 49:764–770, 1986

Cassidy JW: Fluoxetine: a new serotonergically active antidepressant. Journal of Head Trauma Rehabilitation 4:67–69, 1989

Chollet F, Di Piero V, Wise RJS, et al: The functional anatomy of motor recovery after stroke in humans: a study with positron emission tomography. Ann Neurol 29:63–71, 1991

Corn TH, Checkley SA: A case of recurrent mania with recurrent hyperthyroidism. Br J Psychiatry 143:74–76, 1983

Csernansky JG, Mellentin J, Beauclair L, et al: Mesolimbic dopaminergic supersensitivity following electrical kindling of the amygdala. Biol Psychiatry 23:285–294, 1988

Cummings JL, Mendez MF: Secondary mania with focal cerebrovascular lesions. Am J Psychiatry 141:1084–1087, 1984

Davidson J, Turnbull CD: Diagnostic significance of vegetative symptoms in depression. Br J Psychiatry 148:442–446, 1986

Faden A, Salzman S: Pharmacological strategies in CNS trauma. Trends Pharmacol Sci 13:29–35, 1992

Fawcett RG: Cerebral infarct presenting as mania. J Clin Psychiatry 52:352–353, 1991

Fedoroff JP, Starkstein SE, Forrester AW, et al: Depression in patients with acute traumatic brain injury. Am J Psychiatry 149:918–923, 1992

Finset A: Depressed mood and reduced emotionality after right hemisphere brain damage, in Cerebral Hemisphere Function in Depression. Edited by Kinsbourne M. Washington, DC, American Psychiatric Press, 1988, pp 51–64

Folstein MF, Folstein SE, McHugh PR: MiniMental State: a practical method for grading the cognitive state of patients for the clinician. J Psychiatr Res 12:189–198, 1975

Goggans FC: A case of mania secondary to vitamin B12 deficiency. Am J Psychiatry 141:300–301, 1984

Goldenberg G, Oder W, Spatt J, et al: Cerebral correlates of disturbed executive function and memory in survivors of severe closed head injury: a SPECT study. J Neurol Neurosurg Psychiatry 55:362–368, 1992

Grant I, Alves W: Psychiatric and psychosocial disturbances in head injury, in Neurobehavioral Recovery from Head Injury. Edited by Levin HS, Grafman J, Eisenberg HM. Oxford, Oxford University Press, 1987, pp. 232–261

Grafman J, Vance SC, Swingartner H, et al: The effects of lateralized frontal lesions on mood regulation. Brain 109:1127–1148, 1986

Gualtieri CT: Pharmacotherapy and the neurobehavioral sequelae of traumatic brain injury. Brain Inj 2:101–129, 1988

Gualtieri CT: Buspirone: neuropsychiatric effects. Journal of Head Trauma Rehabilitation 6:90–92, 1991

Gualtieri CT, Cox DR: The delayed neurobehavioral sequelae of traumatic brain injury. Brain Inj 5:219–232, 1991

Hamill RW, Woolf PD, McDonald JV, et al: Catecholamines predict outcome in traumatic brain injury. Ann Neurol 21:438–443, 1987

Isles W, Orrell MW: Secondary mania after open-heart surgery. Br J Psychiatry 159:280–282, 1991

Jamieson RC, Wells CE: Manic psychosis in a patient with multiple metastatic brain tumors.Clin Psychiatry 40:280–283, 1979

Jorge RE, Robinson RG, Arndt SV, et al: Depression and traumatic brain injury: a longitudinal study. J Affect Dis 27:233–243, 1993a

Jorge RE, Robinson RG, Arndt SV, et al: Comparison between acute and delayed onset depression following traumatic brain injury. J Neuropsychiatry Clin Neurosci 5:43–49, 1993b

Jorge RE, Robinson RG, Arndt SV: Are depressive symptoms specific for a depressed mood in traumatic brain injury? J Nerv Ment Dis 181:91–99, 1993c

Jorge RE, Robinson RG, Starkstein SE, et al: Manic syndromes following traumatic brain injury. Am J Psychiatry 150:916–921, 1993d

Katz DI: Neuropathology and neurobehavioral recovery from closed head injury. Journal of Head Trauma Rehabilitation 7:1–15, 1992

Khanna R, Nizamie SH, Das A: Electrical trauma, nonictal EEG changes, and mania: a case report (letter). J Clin Psychiatry 52:280, 1991

Kinsella G, Moran C, Ford B, et al: Emotional disorder and its assessment within the severe head injured population. Psychol Med 18:57–63, 1988

Krauthammer C, Klerman GL: Secondary mania: manic syndromes associated with antecedent physical illness or drugs. Arch Gen Psychiatry 35:1333–1339, 1978 [AU: The above reference is not mentioned in your text; please mention it somewhere or delete it from this list.]

Levin HS, Grossman RG: Behavioral sequelae of closed head injury: a quantitative study. Arch Neurol 35:720–727, 1978

Levin HS, Amparo E, Eisenberg HM, et al: Magnetic resonance imaging and computerized tomography in relation to the neurobehavioral sequelae of mild and moderate head injuries. J Neurosurg 66:706–713, 1987

Lipsey JR, Robinson RG, Pearson GD, et al: Nortriptyline treatment of poststroke depression: a double-blind treatment trial. Lancet 1:297–300, 1984

Lishman WA: Brain damage in relation to psychiatric disability after head injury. Br J Psychiatry 114:373–410, 1968

Lishman WA: The psychiatric sequelae of head injury: a review. Psychol Med 3:304–318, 1973

Lishman WA: Physiogenesis and psychogenesis in the "post-concussional syndrome." Br J Psychiatry 153:460–469, 1988

Livingston MG, Brooks KN, Bond MR: Three months after severe head injury: psychiatric and social impact on relatives. J Neurol Neurosurg Psychiatry 48:870–875, 1985

Lyeth B, Dixon CE, Jenkins L, et al: Effects of scopolamine treatment on long-term behavioral deficits following concussive brain injury to the rat. Brain Res 452:39–48, 1988

McKinlay WW, Brooks DN, Bond MR, et al: The short-term outcome of severe blunt head injury as reported by the relatives of the head injury person. J Neurol Neurosurg Psychiatry 44:527–533, 1981

Meyer A: The anatomical facts and clinical varieties of traumatic insanity. American Journal of Insanity 60:373, 1904

Nemeroff CB: New vistas in neuropeptide research in neuropsychiatry: focus on corticotropin-releasing-factor. Neuropsychopharmacology 6:69–75, 1992

Oder W, Goldenberg G, Spatt J, et al: Behavioral and psychosocial sequelae of severe closed head injury and regional cerebral blood flow: a SPECT study. J Neurol Neurosurg Psychiatry 55:475–480, 1992

Payen D, Quintin L, Plaisance P, et al: Head injury: clonidine decreases plasma catecholamines. Critical Care Medicine 18:392–395, 1990

Pope HG, McElroy SL, Satlin A, et al: Head injury, bipolar disorder and response to valproate. Compr Psychiatry 29:34–38, 1988

Prigatano GP: Neuropsychological Rehabilitation After Brain Injury. Baltimore, MD, Johns Hopkins University Press, 1986

Prigatano GP: Psychiatric aspects of head injury: problem areas and suggested guidelines for research, in Neurobehavioral Recovery from Head Injury. Edited by Levin HS, Grafman J, Eisenberg HM. Oxford, Oxford University Press, 1987, pp 215–232

Prigatano GP: Disturbances of self-awareness of deficit after traumatic brain injury, in Awareness of Deficit After Brain Injury: Clinical and Theoretical Issues. Edited by Prigatano GP, Schacter DL. New York, Oxford University Press, 1991a

Prigatano GP: Disordered mind, wounded soul: The emerging role of psychotherapy in rehabilitation after brain injury. Journal of Head Trauma Rehabilitation 64:1–10, 1991b

Robinson RG, Szetela B: Mood change following left hemispheric brain injury. Ann Neurol 9:447–453, 1981

Robinson RG, Starr LB, Kubos TR: A two year longitudinal study of poststroke mood disorders: findings during the initial evaluation. Stroke 14:736–744, 1983

Robinson RG, Starr LB, Kubos KL, et al: Mood disorders in stroke patients: importance of location of lesion. Brain 107:81–93, 1984

Robinson RG, Bolduc P, Price TR: A two-year longitudinal study of poststroke depression: diagnosis and outcome at one- and two-year follow-up. Stroke 18:837–843, 1987

Robinson RG, Boston JD, Starkstein SE, et al: Comparison of mania with depression following brain injury: causal factors. Am J Psychiatry 145:172–178, 1988

Robinson RG, Parikh RM, Lipsey JR, et al: Pathological laughing and crying following stroke: validation of measurement scale and double-blind treatment study. Am J Psychiatry 150:286–293, 1992

Roper SN, Mena I, King WG, et al: An analysis of cerebral blood flow in acute closed head injury using technetiun-99m-HMPAO SPECT and computed tomography. J Nucl Med 32:1684–1687, 1991

Rutherford WH, Merrett JD, McDonald JR: Sequelae of concussion caused by minor head injuries. Lancet 1:1–4, 1977

Sbordone RJ: Psychotherapeutic treatment of the client with traumatic brain injury: a conceptual model, in Community Integration Following Traumatic Brain Injury. Edited by Kreutzer JS, Wehman P. Baltimore, MD, Paul H Brookes Publishing, 1990

Schoenhuber R, Gentili M: Anxiety and depression after mild head injury: a case control study. J Neurol Neurosurg Psychiatry 51:722–724, 1988

Selzer ML, Rogers JE, Kern S: Fatal accidents: the role of psychopathology, social stress, and acute disturbances. Am J Psychiatry 124:1028–1036, 1968

Shukla S, Cook BL, Mukherjee S, et al: Mania following head trauma. Am J Psychiatry 144:93–96, 1987

Silver JM, Hales RE, Yudofsky SC: Psychopharmacology of depression in neurologic disorders. J Clin Psychiatry 51:33–39, 1990

Silver JM, Yudofsky SC, Hales RE: Depression in traumatic brain injury. Neuropsychiatry, Neuropsychology, and Behavioral Neurology 4:12–23, 1991

Starkstein SE, Robinson RG, Price TR: Comparison of cortical and subcortical lesions in the production of poststroke mood disorders. Brain 110:1045–1059, 1987

Starkstein SE, Pearlson GD, Boston JD, et al: Mania after brain injury: a controlled study of causative factors. Arch Neurol 44:1069–1073, 1988

Starkstein SE, Mayberg HS, Berthier ML, et al: Secondary mania: neuroradiological and metabolic findings. Ann Neurol 27:652–659, 1990

Starr LB, Robinson RG, Price TR: Reliability, validity, and clinical utility of the social functioning exam in the assessment of stroke patients. Experimental Aging Research 9:101–106, 1983

Stevens JR: Psychiatric consequences of temporal lobectomy for intractable seizures. Psychol Med 20:529–545, 1990

Steward O: Reorganization of neuronal connections following CNS trauma: principles and experimental paradigms. J Neurotrauma 6:99–152, 1989

Stoudemire A, Miller J, Schmitt F, et al: Development of an organic affective syndrome during a hyperbaric diving experiment. Am J Psychiatry 141:1251–1254, 1984

Teasdale G, Jennett B: Assessment of coma and impaired consciousness: a practical scale. Lancet 2:81–84, 1974

Teasdale G, Mendelow D: Pathophysiology of head injuries, in Closed Head Injury: Psychological, Social and Family Consequences. Edited by Brooks N. Oxford, England, Oxford University Press, 1984, pp 4–36

Teasdale G, Parker L, Murray G, et al: Predicting the outcome of individual patients in the first week after severe head injury. Acta Neurochir Suppl 28:161–164, 1979

Thienhaus OJ, Khosla N: Meningeal cryptococosis misdiagnosed as a manic episode. Am J Psychiatry 141:1459–1460, 1984

Thomas CS, Neale TJ: Organic manic syndrome associated with advanced uraemia due to polycystic kidney disease. Br J Psychiatry 158:119–121, 1991

Van Woerkom TC, Teelken AW, Minderhoud JM: Difference in neurotransmitter metabolism in frontotemporal lobe contusion and diffuse cerebral contusion. Lancet 1:812–813, 1977

Van Zomeren AH, Saan RJ: Psychological and social sequelae of severe head injury, in Handbook of Clinical Neurology, Vol 13 (57): Head Injury. Edited by Braakman R. New York, Elsevier Science Publishers, 1990, pp 397–420

Varney NR, Martzke JS, Roberts RJ: Major depression in patients with closed head injury. Neuropsychology 1:7–9, 1987

Wilson JTL, Wiedmann KD, Hadley DM, et al: Early and late magnetic resonance imaging and neuropsychological outcome after head injury. J Neurol Neurosurg Psychiatry 51:391–396, 1988

Wilson JTL, Wyper D: Neuroimaging and neuropsychological functioning following closed head injury. Journal of Head Trauma Rehabilitation 7:29–39, 1992

Wing JK, Cooper E, Sartorius N: Measurement and Classification of Psychiatric Symptoms. Cambridge, MA, Cambridge University Press, 1974

Zasler ND: Advances in neuropharmacological rehabilitation for brain dysfunction. Brain Inj 6:1–14, 1992

Zolese G, Henryk-Gutt R: Mania induced by biochemical imbalance resulting from low-energy diet in a patient with undiagnosed myxoedema. BMJ 295:1026–1027, 1987

Psychotic Disorders

Donald J. Smeltzer, M.A.
Henry A. Nasrallah, M.D.
Shannon C. Miller, M.D.

Definition and Diagnostic Classification of Posttraumatic Psychoses

Posttraumatic psychosis is a generic term for psychotic illness in a person who has experienced brain trauma (i.e., a wound or injury of the brain). Because *posttraumatic* denotes a temporal rather than a causal relationship, all types of psychotic disorder are included.

Despite the apparent simplicity of this definition, the clinical and scientific literature on posttraumatic psychoses contains many diagnostic quandaries. One reason for inconsistency is that formal systems of psychiatric nomenclature differ in definition and classification of psychotic disorders. For example, such a diversity of approaches has been employed for diagnosing schizophrenia (Andreasen 1983; Bland and Kolada 1988; Carpenter and Strauss 1979) that this condition has sometimes been said to have "elastic boundaries."

DSM-III-R Definition and Classification

In this chapter we adhere strictly to DSM-III-R definitions (American Psychiatric Association 1987). The DSM-III-R "Glossary" defines *psychosis* as "gross impairment in reality testing and the creation of a new reality" (American Psychiatric Association 1987, p. 404). The definition further states that delusions or hallucinations (without insight into their pathological nature) are "direct" (i.e., *sufficient*) evidence of psychosis. However, neither of these symptoms is *necessary* for this designation because psychosis may also be inferred "when a person's behavior is so grossly disorganized that a reasonable inference can be made that reality testing is markedly disturbed" (American Psychiatric Association 1987, p. 404). Examples of such markedly disturbed behavior include significant catatonic symptoms (in nonorganic conditions) and markedly incoherent speech (without apparent awareness by the person that the speech is not understandable). The DSM-III-R mental disorders that are sometimes or always psychotic are listed in Table 8–1.

When determining the precise diagnosis for a patient who is psychotic and has a history of brain trauma, the clinician must consider the possible influence of the injury from two perspectives: as a neurobiological insult affecting the structure and function of brain tissue, and as a stressful experience having a psychosocial aftermath.

If neurobiological effects of brain injury or other specific *organic* factors are judged to be etiologically related to psychotic symptoms, the correct DSM-III-R diagnosis will include one or more of the organic mental disorders. This clinical judgment is most easily made when the interval of time between trauma and psychiatric symptoms is relatively brief. However, sometimes a past injury may logically be judged a significant organic factor in a psychiatric syndrome that develops many years later—for example, when the patient has shown intervening evidence of cerebral dysfunction, such as personality change or epilepsy.

When psychotic symptoms appear immediately after brain injury, or during emergence from posttraumatic coma, the first DSM-III-R diagnosis to consider is *delirium*. This syndrome is characterized by "reduced ability to maintain attention to external stimuli and to appropriately shift attention to new stimuli, [along with] disorganized thinking, as manifested by rambling, irrelevant, or incoherent speech" (American Psychiatric Association 1987, p. 100). Other key features of delirium include rapid onset, fluctuating course, impairment of consciousness, hallucinations and sensory misperceptions, disorientation, memory impairment, abnormalities of the sleep-wake cycle, and psychomotor agitation or retardation. Because this syndrome may encompass any combination of psychopathological manifestations, the presence of delirium usually precludes diagnosis of other psychiatric conditions. (Posttraumatic deliria are discussed in Chapter 6 of this volume and will not be further considered here.)

Other DSM-III-R organic mental syndromes that by definition

Table 8–1. DSM-III-R adult disorders in which psychotic symptoms may be present

Organic mental disorders

Primary degenerative dementia of the Alzheimer type[a]
Multi-infarct dementia[a]
Delirium[b]
Organic delusional disorder
Organic hallucinosis

Schizophrenia

Delusional (paranoid) disorder

Psychotic disorders not elsewhere classified

Brief reactive psychosis
Schizophreniform disorder
Schizoaffective disorder
Induced psychotic disorder
Psychotic disorder not otherwise specified

Mood disorders

Bipolar disorder[a]
Major depression[a]

---

[a]Psychotic features are not required for the diagnosis; their presence is indicated by a qualifying phrase and a fifth digit in the diagnostic code.
[b]Although psychotic features are common in delirium, their presence is neither required nor specified when recording this diagnosis.

are psychotic are *organic hallucinosis* and *organic delusional syndrome*. Diagnostic criteria for these conditions are similar: 1) prominent persistent or recurrent hallucinations, or prominent delusions; 2) a specific organic factor, such as brain injury, is judged to be etiologically involved; and 3) the symptoms do not occur exclusively during the course of delirium (American Psychiatric Association 1987, pp. 109–111). When either of these diagnoses is recorded, the specific organic factor(s) associated with the condition are noted on Axis III.

Thus, a schizophrenia-like psychosis in which brain trauma is judged to be a significant etiologic factor would be classified in DSM-III-R as organic delusional disorder or organic hallucinosis, depending on the relative prominence of delusions and hallucinations in the clinical picture. When both symptoms are prominent, both diagnoses should be recorded.

A psychotic disorder in a person who has previously experienced brain injury is diagnosed outside the organic mental disorders section of DSM-III-R when neurobiological effects of trauma and other organic factors are *not* considered etiologically relevant. This would happen, for example, when the clinician is unaware of the history of trauma and therefore is unable to evaluate its possible significance. Another possibility is that the trauma occurred many years before the onset of psychotic symptoms and the patient has been free for a long time from clinical signs of traumatic sequelae such as headaches, memory impairment, other cognitive disturbances, personality changes, neurodiagnostic abnormalities, and seizures. A third possibility is that the person had already experienced similar psychotic episodes prior to the brain injury. Finally, perhaps the trauma was of such minor degree—for example, causing no interruption of consciousness and no posttraumatic amnesia—that the clinician judges it to be an unlikely organic explanation for the subsequent onset of psychotic symptoms.

In these situations, a psychosis preceded by head trauma may be diagnosed as schizophrenia, schizophreniform disorder, or brief reactive psychosis (depending in part on the duration of the illness, including any prodromal and residual phases), as schizoaffective disorder, as delusional (paranoid) disorder, or as psychotic disorder

NOS (not otherwise specified). Complete descriptions of these conditions, lists of diagnostic criteria, and discussions of differential diagnosis can be found in DSM-III-R. (Psychotic features may also be present in posttraumatic mood disorders; these conditions are described in Chapter 7 and will not be directly discussed in this chapter.)

DSM-II and ICD-9 Definitions of Psychosis

The DSM-III-R concept of psychosis is more narrow and specific than definitions provided in other sources. DSM-II, the official nomenclature in the United States from 1968 to 1980, stated that "Patients are described as psychotic when their mental functioning is sufficiently impaired to interfere grossly with their capacity to meet the ordinary demands of life" (American Psychiatric Association 1968, p. 23). ICD-9, the Ninth Revision of the International Classification of Diseases (World Health Organization 1978), defines psychoses as "Mental disorders in which impairment of mental function has developed to a degree that interferes grossly with insight, ability to meet some ordinary demands of life or to maintain adequate contact with reality. It is not an exact or well defined term. Mental retardation is excluded" (quoted in American Psychiatric Association 1987, p. 444).

Employing one of the latter definitions, a psychiatrist may consider only the overall degree of functional impairment when deciding whether a condition is psychotic. A clinician unskilled in psychiatry might find even greater latitude for labeling puzzling or troublesome behavioral disturbances as psychotic disorders.

DSM-IV Classification

At the time of this writing, DSM-IV is still being finalized. Regarding the concept of organic mental disorders, DSM-IV states, "The term *organic mental disorder* is no longer used in DSM-IV because it incorrectly implies that "nonorganic" mental disorders do not have a biological basis" (American Psychiatric Association 1994, p. 123). The DSM-IV Options Book (American Psychiatric Association 1991) clarified that, "The accumulating knowledge about the numerous biological and physiological factors that contribute to a wide variety of traditionally 'nonorganic' mental disorders has made the organic-nonorganic dichotomy obsolete" (p. B:15). In DSM-IV, the category "organic mental syndromes and disorders" has been replaced by a new category of "delirium, dementia, and amnestic and other cognitive disorders." The remaining organic mental disorders from DSM-III-R are grouped under "mental disorders due to a general medical condition." For example, organic hallucinosis and organic delusional syndrome have been replaced by "psychotic disorder due to a general medical condition." A similar label, "catatonic disorder due to a general medical condition," is also included. Table 8–2 summarizes the classification of psychotic disorders in DSM-IV.

Research Literature on Posttraumatic Psychotic Disorders

Research reports on posttraumatic psychosis are meager and discrepant. Some reasons for the high degree of inconsistency among published studies are listed in Table 8–3.

Patients with traumatic brain injuries are clinically evaluated and managed by neurologists and neurosurgeons far more frequently than by psychiatrists, and many reports of research on posttraumatic behavioral abnormalities do not include psychiatrists among their authors. Most of these reports are not based on or consistent with DSM-III-R or any other psychiatric diagnostic system with sufficient reliability for research use. Further, many reports do not state what criteria were applied when judging that psychosis was present and do not describe the conditions studied in detail sufficient for readers to apply criteria retrospectively.

Regardless of how posttraumatic psychoses are defined, surprisingly little has been published about these conditions. By computer search and use of secondary sources, we sought recent reports on posttraumatic psychosis published in English. We found only two research reports since 1980 on this specific topic, both

Table 8–2.	DSM-IV adult disorders in which psychotic symptoms may be present

Cognitive impairment disorders

Delirium due to a general medical condition[a]

Substance intoxication delirium[a]

Substance withdrawal delirium[a]

Delirium due to multiple etiologies[a]

Delirium not otherwise specified[a]

Dementia of the Alzheimer's type[b]

Vascular dementia

Dementia due to other general medical conditions[b] (e.g., head trauma, human immunodeficiency virus [HIV] disease, Parkinson's disease, Huntington's disease, Pick's disease, and Creutzfeldt-Jakob disease)

Mental disorders due to a general medical condition

Catatonic disorder due to a general medical condition

Schizophrenia and other psychotic disorders

Schizophrenia

Schizophreniform disorder

Schizoaffective disorder

Delusional disorder

Brief psychotic disorder

Shared psychotic disorder

Substance-induced psychotic disorder

Psychotic disorder due to a general medical condition

Psychotic disorder not otherwise specified

Mood disorders

Major depressive disorder[b]

Depressive disorder not otherwise specified[b]

Bipolar I disorder[b]

Bipolar II disorder[b]

Bipolar disorder not otherwise specified[b]

Mood disorder due to a general medical condition[b]

Substance-induced mood disorder[b]

Mood disorder not otherwise specified [b]

[a]Although psychotic features are common in delirium, their presence is neither required nor specified when recording this diagnosis.

[b]Psychotic features are not required for the diagnosis; their presence is indicated by a qualifying phrase and a fifth digit in the diagnostic code.

Source. Based on DSM-IV criteria (American Psychiatric Association 1994).

authored by psychiatrists. We found many reports of research on behavioral disorders in patients with brain injury, but only five of these mentioned psychosis as an outcome in some cases. Four of these five reports did not include psychiatrists among their authors.

Table 8–4 lists case reports on posttraumatic psychosis published in English since 1980; all but one of these reports were authored by psychiatrists.

Although electroencephalography (EEG) and computed tomography (CT) findings were included in some recent reports, we found no research studies that used newer brain imaging technologies such as magnetic resonance imaging (MRI), brain electrical activity mapping (BEAM), positron-emission tomography (PET), or single photon emission computerized tomography (SPECT).

Epidemiology of Posttraumatic Psychosis

Incidence of Psychosis Among Brain Injury Patients

Widely varying estimates of the lifetime prevalence of posttraumatic psychosis have been reported. In any clinical series, the number of

Table 8–3. Some reasons for discrepancies in reported studies of posttraumatic psychosis

Imprecise descriptive terminology
Variations in diagnostic definitions
Failure to use reliable diagnostic criteria
Population differences
  Soldiers or civilians
  Adults or children
  Mental hospital patients or general hospital patients
Differences in types of head injuries
  Open or closed
  Severe or minor
  Blunt or penetrating
Varying durations of follow-up
Frequent use of retrospective data only

patients determined to be psychotic depends not only on character-istics of the population studied, but also on 1) the definition of psychosis, or whether any definition was used; 2) whether specific diagnostic criteria were employed and, if so, the reliability of those criteria; 3) the method of evaluating cases (e.g., from available records only, from direct examination of patients, from interviews of relatives) and by whom this was done (by psychiatrists or non-

Table 8–4.   Synopses of recent case reports on posttraumatic psychosis

Reference	Synopsis
Andy et al. 1981	Adolescent onset of schizophrenia-like psychosis
Bamrah and Johnson 1991	Distinct episodes of major depressive illness, schizophreniform disorder, mania, and focal epilepsy
Barnhill and Gualtieri 1989	Abrupt onset of psychosis 3 years after closed head injury
Bienenfeld and Brott 1989	Delusional misidentification of husband (Capgras syndrome)
Bouvy et al. 1988	Stress-related onset of psychosis treated with carbamazepine
Dolinar 1991	Delusions associated with posttraumatic headache
Filley and Jarvis 1987	Delusional misidentification of location
Isern 1987	Cyclically recurring Klüver-Bucy syndrome with psychotic features
Katz et al. 1989	Delusions with auditory and visual hallucinations in one of six patients with traumatic basal ganglia hemorrhage
Loyd and Tsuang 1981	Visual hallucinations of snakes
Mace and Trimble 1991	Six cases of psychosis following temporal lobe surgery for epilepsy
Nasrallah et al. 1981	Psychosis with a clinical course similar to chronic undifferentiated schizophrenia
O'Callaghan et al. 1988	Adolescent onset of schizophrenia-like psychosis
White et al. 1987	Compensation psychosis
Will et al. 1988	Posttraumatic Kleine-Levin syndrome with psychotic features

psychiatrists); 4) which categories of psychosis were included (organic delusional disorders, organic hallucinoses, schizophrenias and schizophreniform disorders, delusional or paranoid disorders, mood disorders, deliria) and whether any nonpsychotic conditions might also have been counted (e.g., amnestic disorders or uncomplicated dementias); 5) the duration of the follow-up period; and 6) the effectiveness of follow-up procedures.

Davison and Bagley (1969) tabulated eight reports of the prevalence of schizophrenia-like psychosis in large series of patients with brain injury. These studies had been conducted in diverse locales between 1917 and 1964 and likely were based on differing concepts and standards for diagnosis of schizophrenia. The types of patients ranged from civilians suffering concussions in peacetime accidents to soldiers injured in combat, and the average follow-up intervals ranged from 3 months to 20 years. The observed rates of psychosis ranged from 0.07%–9.8%, with a median of 1.35%. The two lowest rates came from the two studies with relatively brief follow-up periods (3 months and 2 years). Estimating the lifetime prevalence of schizophrenia in the general population as 0.8% during a period of risk of about 25 years, Davison and Bagley concluded that "the observed incidence over 10 to 20 year periods is 2 to 3 times the expected incidence."

In a study not included in Davison and Bagley's review, Lishman (1968) retrospectively searched extensive records of 670 British soldiers who had sustained penetrating head injuries during World War II. The patients had all been evaluated and treated at the same head-injury unit, and strong efforts had been made to follow all cases for 5 years after injury. Annual questionnaires had been sent to the patients, relatives, employers, general practitioners, and social service agencies.

He reported only five cases of "unequivocal psychoses" (0.7%) during a 4-year period of follow-up (from the second through the fifth years after injury). Although he provided no further information about the five cases found, it is clear that mood disorders, dementias, and amnestic disorders were not included because these conditions were counted separately.

In a prospective study of children followed for 27 months after head injuries, Brown et al. (1981) found one psychotic disorder (3.2%) in a group of 31 children whose severe brain injuries had caused at least 7 days of posttraumatic amnesia. No specific psychiatric diagnosis was stated. The patient's symptoms were described as "agitation, flight of ideas, ideas of reference, silly giggling, grimacing, a changed intonation in her speech, and the expression of various odd ideas." No cases of psychosis were found in control groups consisting of 29 children with mild head injuries and 28 children with hospital-treated orthopedic injuries.

Violon and De Mol (1987) defined posttraumatic psychoses as "regressive or chronic acquired delusional states appearing after a head injury in non-demented patients." Using this definition, they found 18 cases (3.4%) among records of 530 unselected head injury patients of a neurosurgical unit in a Belgian hospital who had been followed for 1 to 10 years. They mentioned that this figure included 6 cases (1.1%) of "posttraumatic schizophrenia." The remaining 12 cases evidently included paranoid disorders and mood disorders. None of the cases were fully described.

Thomsen (1984), a Danish neurologist, made follow-up visits to the residences of 40 patients who had suffered severe blunt head trauma 10 to 15 years previously. He reported that 8 patients (20%) had experienced "posttraumatic psychoses" since their injuries. He did not state a definition of psychosis or specific diagnostic criteria. His report includes brief descriptions that emphasize severe regression, impulsive aggressiveness, and other behavioral disturbances leading to psychiatric hospitalization. Hallucinations and delusions are not mentioned.

In addition, Thomsen found many patients with significant deficit symptoms present 10 to 15 years after their brain injuries. These symptoms and their frequencies included loss of social contact (68%), lack of interests (55%), aspontaneity (53%), slowness (53%), and various speech abnormalities not individually tabulated (subnormal rate of speaking, frequent pauses, use of many set phrases, and aposiopesis). Although these are not psychotic symptoms in the sense of DSM-III-R, they are included among the negative symptoms often found in schizophrenia. In the latter condition, negative symptoms are associated with chronicity or poor outcome, visual-motor deficits, structural brain abnormalities found by CT and MRI, and relatively poor response to neuroleptic treatment (Walker and Lewine 1988).

Frequency of Prior Brain Injury Among Psychotic Patients

Davison and Bagley (1969) reviewed five studies of the frequency of previous head injury among patients hospitalized with schizophrenia. These studies had been published between 1932 and 1961 and reported head-injury frequencies ranging from 1%–15%. The reviewers attributed the discrepancies among the five studies to "different definitions of head injury and/or the duration of latent interval regarded as significant." It seems likely that differences in standards for diagnosing schizophrenia were also important, and in any case these figures are difficult to interpret without comparable data on head injuries among control subjects or in the corresponding population.

In a more recent study, Wilcox and Nasrallah (1987) examined the hospital charts of 659 patients who had been admitted to a large university-based hospital between 1934 and 1944. Four groups of patients were studied: 200 persons with schizophrenia, 122 with mania, 203 with depressive illness, and 134 surgical controls. All psychiatric diagnoses conformed to research diagnostic criteria published by Feighner et al. (1972). The medical histories in the charts were quite extensive and considered of good quality.

While blinded to psychiatric diagnosis, the investigators searched each clinical history for reports of head trauma. They were especially interested in nontrivial childhood head injuries, which they defined as head traumas that occurred before age 10 and either resulted in loss of consciousness for at least one hour or else caused vomiting, confusion, or visual changes severe enough to warrant medical evaluation. They hypothesized that such injuries "were most likely to reflect disturbances of cortical organization during developmental years."

The investigators reported rates of childhood brain injuries among the four groups as follows: schizophrenic patients, 11.0%;

manic patients, 4.9%; depressive patients, 1.5%; and surgical control patients, 0.7%. The rate among schizophrenic patients was significantly greater than that among depressive patients ($P = .0001$) and surgical control patients ($P = .0001$), and also exceeded the rate among manic patients, but this difference was not statistically significant ($P = .06$). When all reported head injuries were tabulated without regard to age or severity, the rates were only slightly higher in each group and the pattern of differences did not change. The authors noted that these results agreed with previous reports that "head injury may lower the threshold for psychosis in some individuals."

This hypothesis is consistent with a "neurodevelopmental" theory of the pathogenesis of schizophrenia proposed by Weinberger (1986). In this model, "Schizophrenia is associated with a subtle, static structural brain lesion that involves a diffuse system of periventricular limbic and diencephalic nuclei and their connections to the dorsolateral prefrontal cortex" (Weinberger 1986, p. 405). The lesion is nonspecific and is presumed to originate early in development. It may be caused by diverse etiologies, including brain trauma. The time of onset of schizophrenia is related not to the time of occurrence of the lesion, but rather to the time that the lesioned structures reach physiological maturity.

An alternative hypothesis is that head injuries do not contribute to the etiology of schizophrenia but result from a shared risk factor (i.e., that a diathesis for schizophrenia in adulthood increases risk for injuries during childhood). Findings from prospective longitudinal studies of risk factors for schizophrenia support this hypothesis. Several studies showed that some children of schizophrenic parents show excessive "neurointegrative" or "pandysmaturational" defects involving attention deficits, impairment of motor development and coordination, and sensorimotor abnormalities, especially poor visual-motor coordination. These defects are present in early infancy and have been shown to be harbingers of adult onset of schizophrenia (Mednick and Silverton 1988). They could result from subtle effects of a brain lesion that is already present, as proposed by Weinberger (1986). Alternatively, they could increase the risk for accidental injuries during childhood.

Etiology of Posttraumatic Psychotic Disorders

The biopsychosocial model of disease (Engel 1977) is an apt paradigm for evaluating mental disorders associated with brain trauma. In a review of psychiatric sequelae of brain injury, Lishman (1973) commented, "The study of head-injured patients illustrates particularly well the complex interplay of many different factors, rebounding each upon the other, in contributing to the total clinical picture."

Lishman (1973, 1987) reviewed eight categories of etiologic factors leading to posttraumatic psychiatric disability: amount of brain tissue damage, location of brain tissue damage, development of epilepsy, response to intellectual impairment, environmental factors, compensation and litigation, emotional impact and emotional repercussions of injury, and premorbid personality and mental constitution. None of these categories seem disputable, but discernment of their relative importance in the illness of an individual patient may challenge the clinician's acumen. To illustrate more fully the range of variables to consider, Table 8–5 lists some biological, psychological, and social factors that may be influential in the clinical evolution of psychotic illness after brain injury.

Some of the variables listed in Table 8–5 are supported by scientific evidence, which varies in quantity and quality. Psychological and social variables are frequently mentioned in case reports but are seldom examined in scientifically rigorous fashion. The variables most thoroughly studied have been physical characteristics of the injury, such as the severity and anatomic location of brain damage, and physical sequelae such as posttraumatic epilepsy. Some studies have also examined the possible influence of constitutional endowment, especially preinjury personality traits and evidence of genetic risk for psychotic disorders.

Degree and Location of Brain Damage

In a retrospective study of records of 3,552 Finnish soldiers who suffered head injuries during active duty in World War II, Hillbom

(1960) found 1,071 (30.1%) who showed prominent posttraumatic psychiatric syndromes during an unspecified follow-up period. In a more thorough evaluation of 415 cases selected randomly from

---

Table 8–5.   A biopsychosocial list of possible etiological factors of psychotic illness after brain injury

---

Amount of brain tissue damaged

Location of brain tissue damage

Interaction with effects of previous brain insults

   Perinatal stress (e.g., from anoxia or abnormal delivery)

   Alcohol and other substance abuse

   Earlier traumas

   Other brain disease (e.g., tumors and cerebral palsy)

Development of epilepsy

Mental constitution, including genetic diathesis for various mental and neurological disorders (especially schizophrenia)

Preinjury character traits and functioning, especially schizophrenia spectrum disorders or traits (schizotypal, paranoid, schizoid) and episodes of psychosis

Emotional impact and repercussions of the injury

Environmental factors

   Peritraumatic: cause and circumstances of injury

   Posttraumatic: losses and other life changes resulting from injury

   Independence

   Mobility

   Occupational

   Marital, familial, and other relationships

   Financial

   Recreational

Legal issues

   Compensation

   Financial liability

   Criminal liability (e.g., for driving while intoxicated)

Response to intellectual impairments

Response to physical impairments and changes

   Sensory deficits (vision and hearing)

   Altered physical appearance

   Loss of motor function

Source. Adapted from Lishman 1987.

those having the most complete records, he identified 33 cases (7.95%) of posttraumatic psychosis.

He classified the psychotic cases into three groups: 10 epileptic paroxysmal psychic disturbances of short duration; 11 more chronic illnesses "which closest [sic] reminds one of schizophrenic paranoid-hallucinatory psychoses"; and 12 "depressive or hysteric or other episodic psychoses." He noted a tendency for the latter group to have slightly milder injuries in comparison with the first two groups. He also found that the rate of psychosis increased with the severity of injury: 2.8% of those with mild injuries, 7.2% of those with medium-severity injuries, and 14.8% of those with severe injuries had become psychotic.

Among patients whose injuries could be anatomically lateralized or localized, he found that 63% of the psychoses were associated with left-hemisphere lesions, 26% with right-hemisphere lesions, and 11% with bilateral injuries. The preponderance of left-hemisphere lesions was greater among the psychoses than in other categories of psychiatric disturbance. He also reported that 40% of the psychotic patients had temporal lobe lesions. Among psychotic cases this proportion was greater than for any other brain location analyzed, and the rate of temporal lobe injury was greater among patients with psychosis than among patients with other psychiatric conditions.

In another study based on World War II injuries, Lishman (1968) retrospectively analyzed records of 670 British soldiers who had suffered penetrating head injuries. He found that the retrospectively rated severity of psychiatric disability observed between 1 and 5 years after injury was significantly correlated with the severity of both focal brain damage (rated according to depth of tissue penetration, which he estimated from X-ray films and surgeons' operating notes) and diffuse brain damage (rated according to duration of posttraumatic amnesia). Left-hemisphere lesions were more closely related to psychiatric disability than right-hemisphere lesions, and temporal lobe lesions, especially on the left side, were more important than lesions in other locations. However, his series included only 5 cases of unequivocal psychosis out of 577 that had shown psychiatric disability during the follow-up period from 1 to 5 years after injury, and he did not contrast the psychotic patients with other groups.

Lishman reported that only about one-fifteenth of the variance in degree of psychiatric impairment could be attributed to the magnitude of brain tissue damage. He concluded (Lishman 1973) that "the strict anatamopathological model is inadequate because other aetiological factors are of as great or even greater importance where many posttraumatic disabilities are concerned. . . . "

Both of these studies suggested a link between left-hemisphere injury or dysfunction, especially involving the temporal lobe, and subsequent development of psychosis. However, the evidence is merely suggestive, not conclusive, and more recent studies have not diminished the uncertainty.

For example, in a prospective study of "traumatic psychosis with amnesia" in Germany, Koufen and Hagel (1987) followed a cohort of 100 patients from a cerebral trauma ward. They described their subjects in this way: "After excluding cerebral dysfunction independent of trauma, all patients up to 65 years of age who presented amnesia due to traumatically caused disturbance of consciousness lasting for longer than the 1st week, and in whose cases it was possible to record the EEG during psychosis within the 1st months and after the 1st year."

In this study, focal EEG abnormalities were used as criteria for neuroanatomical localization of cerebral dysfunction. A total of 1,004 EEG recordings were analyzed, and foci were found in 95 of the 100 patients (12 left unilateral, 13 right unilateral, and 70 bilateral). The authors concluded that "traumatic psychoses do not show the general pattern of left-sided preponderance because in the majority of cases they are concomitant with bilateral EEG foci." They also reported that "the concentration of EEG foci in the temporal region in the later stages . . . was confirmed as a tendency in our study."

However, the significance of these results is uncertain because the report does not define psychosis or explain how the condition was diagnosed. Only two sentences of behavioral description are included: "Most of the traumatic psychoses presented the classical sequence of coma, delirium, and Korsakow. In other cases simple lack of drive in combination with varying, sometimes purely euphoric, changes of affect were observed in place of delirious agitation." They further state that the duration of psychosis was measured by duration of amnesia. This description suggests that the conditions studied, in DSM-III-R terminology, may have been primarily deliria and amnestic syndromes.

Further evidence suggesting an association between posttraumatic psychosis and left-hemisphere or temporal lobe dysfunction comes from studies of other types of focal cerebral disease. For example, Davison (1983) concluded that schizophrenia-like psychosis in patients with brain tumors is associated more frequently with temporal lobe and hypophyseal tumors than with tumors in other locations. Davison and Bagley (1969) tabulated from the psychiatric literature a series of 150 cases of schizophrenia-like psychoses associated with a variety of CNS disorders having focal or generalized brain pathologies. By computing correlation coefficients between various symptoms of schizophrenia and sites of CNS lesions, they demonstrated significant associations with left-hemisphere and temporal lobe pathology for primary delusions and catatonic symptoms.

Cummings (1985) reviewed the literature and carefully examined 20 patients who had delusions associated with neurological disease, searching for relationships between the anatomic sites of CNS lesions and clinical characteristics of the associated delusions. Some of his "preliminary conclusions" are summarized in Table 8–6.

Posttraumatic Epilepsy

The most common form of seizures following closed head injury is temporal lobe seizures, and psychosis in epileptic patients is associated far more frequently with temporal lobe epilepsy than with other forms (Garyfallos et al. 1988; Lishman 1987; McKenna et al. 1985; Pincus and Tucker 1985). These observations are consistent with the hypothesis that development of epilepsy following brain injury is associated with increased likelihood of psychosis.

According to Lishman (1987), "post-traumatic epilepsy is known to develop in about 5% of closed head injuries and in over

30% when the dura mater has been penetrated." In his own research on penetrating head injuries, Lishman (1968) found that 45% of these patients developed epilepsy within 5 years of the injury, and that the development of epilepsy was positively correlated with the rated degree of psychiatric disability. This relationship was especially strong when seizures began within 1 year after the injury, and remained the same after controlling for differing amounts of brain damage associated with epileptic and nonepileptic outcomes.

Hillbom (1960) reported similar findings in his study of 415 Finnish soldiers who experienced head injuries in World War II. In his study, the incidence of posttraumatic epilepsy was 55.6% among cases showing significant psychiatric sequelae, and 57.5% in psychotic cases, compared with 31.8% among those with no psychiatric sequelae.

In psychotic disorders associated with epilepsy the mean interval between onset of seizures and onset of psychotic symptoms is about 14 years (Davison and Bagley 1969). Also, a significant proportion of posttraumatic seizure disorders begin 5 years or later after the injury (Lishman 1987). These long intervals demonstrate

Table 8–6.   Hypothesized relationships between neuroanatomic sites of lesions and types of associated delusions

Site of lesion(s)	Clinical characteristics of delusions
Diffuse lesions in cortical associationareas and hippocampus associated with dementia of Alzheimer type or multiinfarct dementia	Simple, loosely held persecutory beliefs that are often transient and that respond moderately well to treatment with neuroleptics
Subcortical (basal ganglia, thalamus, and rostral brain stem) and limbic lesions	Complex delusions that tend to be chronic and resistant to treatment Chronic schizophrenia-like delusional syndromes
Left-sided temporal lobe lesions	Short-lived hallucinatory delusional syndromes
Right-sided parietotemporal lesions	
Right-hemisphere lesions	Capgras syndrome and reduplicative paramnesia

Source. Adapted from Cummings 1985.

the importance of follow-up periods of at least 20 years in prospective studies of posttraumatic psychosis.

Several distinct types of epileptic psychoses have been described (McKenna et al. 1985). Brief psychotic episodes with clouded consciousness are typically associated with generalized EEG changes. These conditions are best understood as ictal or postictal confusional states; in DSM-III-R terminology they are classified as episodes of delirium.

Brief psychotic episodes in which normal consciousness is maintained are generally associated with an unchanged or even improved EEG. These episodes may last up to several weeks and often end in a convulsion. They are usually associated with temporal lobe epilepsy but their pathophysiology is not well understood.

Longer-lasting psychoses are also associated with epilepsy. Although often described as schizophrenia-like, these conditions frequently show "atypical" features (i.e., atypical for schizophrenia) such as frequent mood swings, visual hallucinations, mystical states, catatonic symptoms, and absence of negative symptoms. Some of these disorders would be better described as "pure delusional disorders" rather than as schizophrenia-like; others have prominent affective features suggestive of schizoaffective disorder or mood disorder with psychotic features. The clinical course is typically episodic and relatively benign, without cumulative deterioration or progression to a defect state (Garyfallos et al. 1988).

In their review of the clinical and scientific literature on psychotic syndromes in epilepsy, McKenna et al. (1985) concluded that the etiologic relationship between temporal lobe epilepsy and psychosis is complex. Factors that seem important include the actual seizure activity, subclinical electrical activity, and possibly other effects of the underlying temporal lobe lesions. One attractive hypothesis is that recurrent subconvulsive electrical discharge from a small lesion in the limbic system may initiate and maintain behavioral changes through the mechanism of limbic kindling (Mesulam 1985, pp. 304–305). Kindling has been shown, for example, to produce long-lasting changes in the function of dopamine, norepinephrine, and other neurotransmitters (McKenna et al. 1985). These changes suggest a neuropharmacological mechanism for development of psychosis. However, as Lishman (1987) points out, a seizure disorder also has psychogenic and socially disruptive effects that can lower self-esteem, hinder rehabilitation, and increase the difficulty of re-adapting to daily life. Therefore, the psychosocial consequences of seizures must also be considered as potential etiologic factors in the later onset of psychosis.

Constitutional Predisposition for Psychosis

Epidemiological data described above suggest that 1) the rate of psychotic illness occurring in persons with brain injury significantly exceeds the overall rate of psychosis in the general population, and 2) patients with schizophrenia have a high rate of brain injuries during childhood. These findings suggest that posttraumatic psychotic illnesses may occur in persons who were not otherwise predisposed to psychosis. However, an alternative hypothesis is that predisposition to psychosis is positively correlated with predisposition for brain injury.

Investigators who have looked for evidence of genetic or other predisposition in the etiology of posttraumatic psychosis have generally examined three variables: family history of psychosis, pretraumatic personality traits, and the clinical features of the psychotic syndrome itself. Each of these may be difficult to evaluate reliably, especially when the clinician is not a psychiatrist and when data are not available from a psychiatric evaluation of the patient prior to the brain injury.

Shapiro (1939) reported that out of 2,000 cases of dementia praecox (schizophrenia) comprising the resident population of a large public institution, he found "a large number . . . that showed some relationship to a severe head injury." He selected 21 cases "in which the connection between trauma and onset of mental symptoms could not well be discarded." In these cases the psychosis had begun within a few hours to at most 3 months after the injury.

Ten of the patients he selected had typical schizophrenic syndromes with no grossly obvious signs suggesting organic sequelae of trauma. (Sophisticated evaluations such as neuropsychological testing were, of course, not available.) In all of these cases he found evidence of predisposition to schizophrenia such as positive family histories and introverted premorbid personalities. He concluded that the trauma acted "simply as a precipitating factor" for the psychoses of these patients.

The other 11 patients showed not only symptoms typical of schizophrenia, but also symptoms that seemed connected to the head trauma, such as persistent headache, seizures, confusion, dizziness, disorientation, and memory impairment. In this group only 2 showed "hereditary tainting" and in 7 of them he judged the prepsychotic personalities to have been "well integrated." He argued that in this group the injuries had produced pathological changes in the brain that contributed to the etiology of psychosis.

Shapiro's conclusion that predisposition is a factor in some, but not all, cases of posttraumatic psychosis agrees with results of other investigators (summarized in Davison and Bagley 1969; Lishman 1987).

Recommendations

Prospective studies of posttraumatic psychosis are needed to resolve the enigmas described above. Important methodological features of these studies should include 1) use of precise diagnostic criteria of adequate reliability (e.g., from DSM-III-R or other published sources); 2) state-of-the-art neurobiological evaluation, including serial use of modern brain-imaging procedures; 3) thorough evaluation of subjects' family histories and premorbid functioning by procedures of adequate reliability; 4) evaluation of appropriate control subjects in parallel with subjects who have had a head injury; and 5) long follow-up periods (up to 25 years).

Prospective "high risk studies" of offspring of schizophrenic mothers (Mednick and Silverton 1988) should include attention to traumatic brain injury (TBI) so that these events can be evaluated as possible risk factors for later development of psychosis.

Another high-risk population that merits special scrutiny is homeless persons. Recent psychiatric surveys of persons entering or residing in public shelters in large U.S. cities have found very high rates of psychosis and other major mental disorders. For example, Koegel et al. (1988) reported a lifetime prevalence of 13.7% for schizophrenia and schizophreniform disorder among homeless persons in the Skid Row area of Los Angeles. Susser et al. (1989) found that 25% of homeless men entering public shelters in New York City for the first time may have psychotic illnesses.

Homeless persons may also have an elevated prevalence of traumatic brain injuries. On the one hand, the misfortune of being homeless likely increases exposure to risks such as assaults, fights, and accidents. On the other hand, having suffered a brain injury predisposes to cognitive impairment and other disabilities that may lead to unemployment, downward social mobility, and ultimately homelessness.

In their work with homeless mentally ill patients at Presbyterian Hospital in New York City, Silver et al. (1993) found that over 40% of homeless individuals with schizophrenia-like illness experienced traumatic brain injuries prior to the onset of psychosis. They argue that neuropsychiatric assessment of homeless persons is important not only for improving clinical care but also as a research strategy for identifying causes of homelessness. In addition, the homeless population may provide an important source of data for research on the neuropsychiatric consequences of TBI.

The evaluation of every psychotic patient should include inquiry about head injuries. When possible, questions should also be directed to family members and other informants because injuries may be forgotten if they were relatively minor or if they occurred at an early age or during intoxication. It is helpful to ask about each of the settings in which traumatic injuries may commonly occur: vehicle accidents, falls, fights and assaults, military activities, hazardous occupations, and recreational or athletic activities.

Knowledge that a psychotic patient has a history of head injury will assist in formulating a comprehensive differential diagnosis. It will often justify specialized neurodiagnostic procedures (neuropsychological testing, EEG, and brain imaging) that might otherwise not seem useful. It should alter the spectrum and priority of treatment options considered and may lead to more rapid discovery of the optimal treatment. It may make the patient eligible for special assistance that would otherwise not be available, such as workers' compensation or occupational retraining following an employment-related injury. Finally, a diagnosis of posttraumatic delusional disorder may be both less stigmatizing and more fully covered by medical insurance than a diagnosis of schizophrenia.

Pharmacological Treatment of Posttraumatic Psychoses

Optimal multidisciplinary treatment of posttraumatic psychotic disorders must be based on thorough biopsychosocial assessment of all possible factors of etiologic importance to the patient's symptoms (see Table 8–5). Therefore, initial evaluation of posttraumatic psychosis includes careful neuropsychiatric examination, mental status testing, and comprehensive review of the patient's medical status. The history of brain injury may indicate assessment by neurodiagnostic procedures such as electroencephalography or some form of brain imaging. It is especially advantageous to detect any evidence of seizure activity or kindling.

Preliminary Considerations

▮ **Rule out delirium.** Before initiating symptom-oriented treatment of psychosis, it is important to determine whether delirium is present and, if so, to identify all treatable causes that contribute to the mental abnormalities. Experienced clinicians will quickly suspect delirium when psychotic symptoms begin shortly after an injury or during emergence from posttraumatic coma. However, delirium may also begin after a latent period of days to months; in these cases it may not be immediately considered as a possible explanation for the onset of psychotic symptoms. Detailed information about evaluation and management of posttraumatic deliria may be found in Chapter 6.

A cause of delirium that should receive special consideration is medication toxicity. The patient's entire regimen should be reviewed. Blood levels of anticonvulsants should be checked. Drugs that are especially likely to cause or contribute to delirium include anticonvulsants, sedatives, and anticholinergics. Note that all psychotherapeutic drugs are included in these categories—even antipsychotic drugs can cause psychotic delirium (through their anticholinergic action).

▌ **Choice of treatment.** If delirium has been ruled out or if psychotic features persist after its remission, psychopharmacological interventions may be appropriate (Table 8–7).

We found no reports of controlled studies of treatments for psychotic symptoms in patients with TBI. The following recommendations are derived from case reports, descriptions of various authors' clinical experiences, and extrapolation from studies in other populations of patients with brain damage.

The absence of controlled studies makes it difficult to be certain about which treatment should be tried first for a particular patient. The priority indications shown in Table 8–7 are suggested as guidelines, but any of the treatments listed may be helpful for any patient; several should be systematically tried in treatment-resistant cases. For most patients, the first trial should be a standard neuroleptic (Table 8–8) or a psychotropic anticonvulsant (carbamazepine or valproic acid).

Neuroleptic Medication

▌ **Disadvantages.** Neuroleptics (Table 8–8) are drugs that ought to be avoided in patients with TBI, especially during the acute recovery period. Their spectrum of adverse effects includes the life-threatening neuroleptic malignant syndrome and several other conditions that are especially problematic for patients with brain injury (Table 8–9). It also includes a wide variety of other problems that patients find vexing and troublesome (Table 8–10).

Gualtieri (1991) argues that dopamine agonists may be useful in promoting recovery of neuronal function after brain injury, and that dopamine antagonists (i.e., neuroleptics) may impede recovery. At least one animal study supports these hypotheses. Feeney et al. (1982) found that amphetamine accelerated recovery of function by rats with brain lesions, that haloperidol retarded recovery, and that haloperidol blocked the beneficial effects of amphetamine. However, there are no analogous studies in humans, and the application of these findings to the clinical care of patients with brain injury remains uncertain.

Table 8–7. Psychopharmacological treatment options for nondelirious posttraumatic psychosis

Option	Priority indication(s)[a]
Any drug listed below	History of good result for this patient in a similar episode
Standard neuroleptic antipsychotics (Table 8–8)	Schizophrenia-like target symptoms (hallucinations, delusions, thought disorder), especially if accompanied by acute agitation or aggression
Nonstandard neuroleptic (pimozide)	Monosymptomatic delusional disorder
Nonneuroleptic antipsychotic (clozapine)	Schizophrenia-like psychosis with poor response to trials of standard neuroleptics
Psychotropic anticonvulsants (carbamazepine and valproic acid)	Possible complex partial epilepsy or limbic kindling; manic episode or prominent mood swings; episodic dyscontrol; poor response to neuroleptics or lithium
Clonazepam	Manic symptoms; alternative to carbamazepine and valproic acid for psychosis with epilepsy
Lithium	Manic syndrome; possible bipolar or schizoaffective disorder (see Chapter 7); also chronic aggressive or violent behavior (see Chapter 10)
β-Adrenergic receptor blockers (propranolol and others)	Chronic aggressive or violent behavior (see Chapter 10)

[a]Priority indications are those for which the treatment is a reasonable first choice. In treatment-resistant cases, each of the options listed may be considered.

▌ **Advantages.** In spite of these considerations, neuroleptic anti-psychotics are important options in the treatment of posttraumatic psychotic disorders because they are unsurpassed for alleviating certain psychotic target symptoms (delusions, hallucinations, loose

Table 8–8. Standard neuroleptic antipsychotics and their relative therapeutic potencies

Neuroleptic antipsychotic (by class)	Brand names	Approximate dosage (mg) that is therapeutically equipotent to 100 mg of chlorpromazine	Potency class[a]
Phenothiazines			
Aliphatic			
Chlorpromazine	Thorazine	100	Low
Piperidines			
Thioridazine	Mellaril	100	Low
Mesoridazine	Serentil	50–60	Low
Piperazines			
Perphenazine	Trilafon	9–10	Mid
Trifluoperazine	Stelazine	2–5	High
Fluphenazine[b]	Prolixin, Permitil	1–4	High
Thioxanthenes			
Chlorprothixene	Taractan	40–100	Low
Thiothixene	Navane	2–5	High
Butyrophenone			
Haloperidol[b]	Haldol	1–4	High
Dibenzoxazepine			
Loxapine	Loxitane, Daxolin	10–20	Mid
Dihydroindolone			
Molindone	Moban, Lidone	6–15	Mid

[a]Low-potency compounds are no more than 4 times as potent as chlorpromazine. High-potency compounds are at least 20 times as potent as chlorpromazine. Acute extrapyramidal side effects (bradykinesia, parkinsonism, akathisia, and dystonias) are more frequent with high-potency neuroleptics. Most other side effects (e.g., sedation, hypotension, and anticholinergic symptoms) are more frequent with low-potency neuroleptics.
[b]Fluphenazine and haloperidol are available in both short-acting (hours to days) and long-acting (weeks to months) preparations. Ordinarily only the short-acting forms should be considered for patients who have traumatic brain injury.
Source. Adapted from Gregory and Smeltzer 1983.

associations, other forms of disordered thinking, acute agitation, and acute aggressiveness) in schizophrenia, schizophreniform disorder, and delusional disorders. They are also effective against these symptoms in many other disorders, including psychotic mood disorders and organic delusional disorders and hallucinoses of diverse etiologies. Many psychotic patients will not obtain comparable benefit from any other form of treatment.

The key to optimal use of neuroleptics is to recognize those cases in which their superiority over alternative treatments justifies exposure to their special risks. A recommended strategy for use of neuroleptics is outlined in Table 8–11. Further discussion of neuroleptic management and side effects can be found in Chapter 19.

Other Psychopharmacological Regimens

When antipsychotic drugs are unduly toxic or insufficiently effective, other drugs that may be helpful in the treatment of posttraumatic

Table 8–9.   Adverse effects of neuroleptic antipsychotics that are especially problematic for patients with traumatic brain injuries

Adverse effects	Best drug choice to avoid this effect
Sedation	High-potency drugs
Lowered seizure threshold	Fluphenazine, molindone, pimozide
Potentiation of CNS depressants	High-potency drugs
Central anticholinergic toxicity (memory impairment and delirium)	High-potency drugs
Early or acute (reversible) extrapyramidal reactions (bradykinesia, parkinsonism, akathisia, and dystonias)	Low-potency drugs
Neuroleptic malignant syndrome	Low-potency drugs
Tardive dyskinesia (chronic, usually late-onset, potentially irreversible abnormal movement disorder)	None (minimize neuroleptic exposure)
Depressed mood	None (try a different drug)
Hypotension and orthostatic hypotension	High-potency drugs

psychosis include the psychotherapeutic anticonvulsants carbamazepine and valproic acid, the benzodiazepine anticonvulsant
clonazepam, b-adrenergic receptor antagonists such as proprano-

---

Table 8–10.　　Other adverse effects of neuroleptic antipsychotics

---

Peripheral anticholinergic effects (dry mouth, visual blurring due to
　paralysis of accommodation, constipation, paralytic ileus, decreased
　sweating, impaired micturition, pupillary changes, and narrow angle
　glaucoma)

Peripheral anti-adrenergic effects (tachycardia, quinidine-like
　electrocardiographic changes, and various arrhythmias)

Dermatologic (sensitivity to sunlight, maculopapular erythematous
　rashes,other rashes, and skin pigmentation change)

Sexual dysfunctions (changes in desire, erectile impairment, and ejaculatory
　abnormalities)

Endocrinologic changes (increased prolactin secretion, lactation,
　galactorrhea, breast enlargement, changes in fluid retention and
　glucose metabolism, and changes in laboratory measurements of various
　hormones)

Weight gain

Hematopoietic abnormalities (benign leukopenia, agranulocytosis, and other
　dyscrasias)

Obstructive jaundice, hepatitis, and elevated liver function tests

Ocular changes (pigmentary retinopathy, and corneal and lenticular
　opacities)

Changes in temperature regulation (hypothermia, hyperthermia,
　and poikilothermia)

Withdrawal symptoms after abrupt discontinuation (sleep disturbance,
　abnormal   movements similar to tardive dyskinesia, nausea,
　and abdominal distress)

Note. Most of these side effects are more frequent and more severe with low-potency
neuroleptics than with high-potency neuroleptics.

lol, and lithium compounds. Any of these may be prescribed alone or in combination with an antipsychotic, although it is best to avoid drug combinations until each agent has been tried independently. The use of these medications is discussed in Chapters 10 and 19.

Table 8–11.   Course of neuroleptic therapy for traumatic brain injury

---

1. Rule out delirium. (For treatment of delirium by neuroleptics or other approaches, see Chapter 6.)

2. Identify specific neuroleptic-responsive target symptoms.

3. Discuss the advantages and disadvantages of neuroleptic therapy, especially the risk of tardive dyskinesia, with patient and family; obtain written informed consent for neuroleptic treatment.

4. Select a specific neuroleptic on the basis of:

    a. Clinical history, if the patient has previously received neuroleptic treatment; or

    b. Side effects profile or the clinician's experience

5. Start with a very low daily dose, divided into 2 or 3 portions:

    a. If a low-potency neuroleptic is selected, or if the patient is medically unstable, in the acute recovery phase from brain injury, or younger than 18 or older than 60 years: no more than the equivalent of 25 mg of chlorpromazine per day

    b. Otherwise, no more than the equivalent of chlorpromazine 100 mg/day

6. Begin systematic examination for extrapyramidal changes (abnormal movements, parkinsonism, akathisia, and dystonia). Patient should be examined several times weekly during early stages of treatment; several times after each dosage increase; and several times yearly during long-term treatment.

7. Increase dosage slowly and in small increments; allow adequate time (up to 3 weeks) for each new dosage to achieve its full therapeutic potential.

8. After remission of psychotic symptoms, periodically try reducing the neuroleptic dosage in small increments; watch for break-through of psychotic symptoms.

9. After at most several months, begin slowly tapering the dosage down to zero, or until it becomes apparent that neuroleptic treatment is still needed.

10. If long-term treatment seems necessary, consider alternatives to neuroleptics (see Table 8–7).

References

American Psychiatric Association: Diagnostic and Statistical Manual of Mental Disorders, 2nd Edition. Washington, DC, American Psychiatric Association, 1968

American Psychiatric Association: Diagnostic and Statistical Manual of Mental Disorders, 3rd Edition, Revised. Washington, DC, American Psychiatric Association, 1987

American Psychiatric Association: Diagnostic and Statistical Manual of Mental Disorders, 4th Edition. Washington, DC, American Psychiatric Association, 1994

Andreasen NC: The clinical differentiation of affective and schizophrenic disorders, in Affective and Schizophrenic Disorders: New Approaches to Diagnosis and Treatment. Edited by Zales MR. New York, Brunner/Mazel, 1983, pp 29–52

Andy OJ, Webster JS, Carranza J: Frontal lobe lesions and behavior. South Med J 74:968–972, 1981

Bamrah JS, Johnson J: Bipolar affective disorder following head injury. Br J Psychiatry 158:117–119, 1991

Barnhill LJ, Gualtieri CT: Late-onset psychosis after closed head injury. Neuropsychiatry, Neuropsychology and Behavioral Neurology 2:211–218, 1989

Bienenfeld D, Brott T: Capgras' syndrome following minor head trauma. J Clin Psychiatry 50:68–69, 1989

Bland RC, Kolada J: Diagnostic issues and current criteria for schizophrenia, in Nosology, Epidemiology, and Genetics of Schizophrenia . Edited by Tsuang MT, Simpson JC. New York, Elsevier, 1988, pp 1–25

Bouvy PF, van de Wetering BJM, Meerwaldt JD, et al: A case of organic brain syndrome following head injury successfully treated with carbamazepine. Acta Psychiatr Scand 77:361–363, 1988

Brown G, Chadwick O, Shaffer D, et al: A prospective study of children with head injuries, III: pssychiatric sequelae. Psychol Med 11:63–78, 1981

Carpenter WT, Strauss JS: Diagnostic issues in schizophrenia, in Disorders of the Schizophrenic Syndrome. Edited by Bellak L. New York, Basic Books, 1979, pp 291–319

Cummings JL: Organic delusions: phenomenology, anatomical correlations, and review. Br J Psychiatry 146:184–197, 1985

Davison K: Schizophrenia-like psychoses associated with organic cerebral disorders: a review. Psychiatric Developments 1:1–34, 1983

Davison K, Bagley CR: Schizophrenia-like psychoses associated with organic disorders of the central nervous system: a review of the literature, in Current Problems in Neuropsychiatry: Schizophrenia, Epilepsy, the Temporal Lobe. Edited by Herrington RN. Br J Psychiatry [special publication no. 4], 1969, pp 113–184

Dolinar LJ: Delusions in a patient with post-traumatic headache. Psychosomatics 32:460–462, 1991

Engel GL: The need for a new medical model: a challenge for biomedicine. Science 196:129–136, 1977

Feeney DM, Gonzalez A, Law WA: Amphetamine, haloperidol, and experience interact to affect rate of recovery after motor cortex injury. Science 217:855–857, 1982

Feighner JP, Robins E, Guze SB, et al: Diagnostic criteria for use in psychiatric research. Arch Gen Psychiatry 26:57–63, 1972

Filley CM, Jarvis PE: Delayed reduplicative paramnesia. Neurology 37:701–703, 1987

Garyfallos G, Manos N, Adamopoulou A: Psychopathology and personality characteristics of epileptic patients: epilepsy, psychopathology, and personality. Acta Psychiatr Scand 78:87–95, 1988

Gregory I, Smeltzer DJ: Psychiatry: Essentials of Clinical Practice, 2nd Edition. Boston, MA, Little, Brown, 1983

Gualtieri CT: Neuropsychiatry and Behavioral Pharmacology. New York, Springer-Verlag, 1991

Hillbom E: After-effects of brain injuries. Acta Psychiatr Neurol Scand Suppl 142:1–195, 1960

Isern RD: Family violence and the Kluver-Bucy syndrome. South Med J 80:373–377, 1987

Katz DI, Alexander MP, Seliger GM, et al: Traumatic basal ganglia hemorrhage: clinicopathologic features and outcome. Neurology 39:897–904, 1989

Koegel P, Burnam A, Farr RK: The prevalence of specific psychiatric disorders among homeless individuals in the inner city of Los Angeles. Arch Gen Psychiatry 45:1085–1092, 1988

Koufen H, Hagel K-H: Systematic EEG follow-up study of traumatic psychosis. Eur Arch Psychiatry Neurol Sci 237:2–7, 1987

Lishman WA: Brain damage in relation to psychiatric disability after head injury. Br J Psychiatry 114:373–410, 1968

Lishman WA: The psychiatric sequelae of head injury: a review. Psychol Med 3:304–318, 1973

Lishman WA: Organic Psychiatry, The Psychiatric Consequences of Cerebral Disorder, 2nd Edition. Oxford, Blackwell Scientific Publications, 1987

Loyd DW, Tsuang MT: A snake lady: post-concussion syndrome manifesting visual hallucinations of snakes. J Clin Psychiatry 42:246–247, 1981

Mace CJ, Trimble MR: Psychosis following temporal lobe surgery: a report of six cases. J Neurol Neurosurg Psychiatry 54:639–644, 1991

McKenna PJ, Kane JM, Parrish K: Psychotic syndromes in epilepsy. Am J Psychiatry 142:895–904, 1985

Mednick SA, Silverton L: High-risk studies of the etiology of schizophrenia, in Nosology, Epidemiology, and Genetics of Schizophrenia (Handbook of Schizophrenia, Vol 3). Edited by Tsuang MT, Simpson JC. New York, Elsevier, 1988, pp 543–562

Mesulam M-M: Principles of Behavioral Neurology. Philadelphia, PA, Davis, 1985

Nasrallah HA, Fowler RC, Judd LL: Schizophrenia-like illness following head injury. Psychosomatics 22:359–361, 1981

O'Callaghan E, Larkin C, Redmond O, et al: "Early onset schizophrenia" after teenage head injury. Br J Psychiatry 153:394–396, 1988

Pincus JH, Tucker GJ: Behavioral Neurology, 3rd edition. New York, Oxford University Press, 1985

Shapiro LB: Schizophrenia-like psychosis following head injuries. Illinois Medical Journal 76:250–254, 1939

Silver JM, Caton CM, Shrout PE, et al: Traumatic brain injury and schizophrenia. New Research paper presented at the annual meeting of the American Psychiatric Association, San Francisco, CA, May 1993

Susser E, Struening EL, Conover S: Psychiatric problems in homeless men. Arch Gen Psychiatry 46:845–850, 1989

Thomsen IV: Late outcome of very severe blunt head trauma: A 10–15 year second follow-up. J Neurol Neurosurg Psychiatry 47:260–268, 1984

Violon A, De Mol J: Psychological sequelae after head trauma in adults. Acta Neurochir (Wien) 85:96–102, 1987

Walker E, Lewine RJ: The positive/negative symptom distinction in schizophrenia. Schizophrenia Research 1:315–328, 1988

Weinberger DR: The pathogenesis of schizophrenia: a neurodevelopmental theory, in The Neurology of Schizophrenia (Handbook of Schizophrenia, Vol 1). Edited by Nasrallah HA and Weinberger DR. New York, Elsevier, 1986, pp 397–406

White AC, Armstrong D, Rowan D: Compensation psychosis. Br J Psychiatry 150:692–694, 1987

Wilcox JA, Nasrallah HA: Childhood head trauma and psychosis. Psychiatry Res 21:303–306, 1987

Will RG, Young JPR, Thomas DJ: Kleine-Levin syndrome: report of two cases with onset of symptoms precipitated by head trauma. Br J Psychiatry 152:410–412, 1988

World Health Organization: Mental Disorders: Glossary and Guide to their Classification in Accordance with the Ninth Revision of the International Classification of Diseases. Geneva, World Health Organization, 1978

Chapter 9

Anxiety Disorders

Richard S. Epstein, M.D.
Robert J. Ursano, M.D.

M any patients with traumatic brain injury (TBI) have survived stressors of catastrophic proportions such as motor vehicle collisions, industrial accidents, and assaults. Subsequently, the patient with TBI must often face disorientation, confusion, memory loss, diminished cognitive function, neurological impairment, seizures, physical pain, marked dependency on others, diminished self-esteem, social isolation, job disability, and financial loss. Injury that affects the structure and function of the brain, the center of mental function, represents a "direct hit" to the individual's basic sense of awareness, identity, and existence. It is not surprising that as a result, clinical anxiety arises so frequently in TBI patients.

Whether anxiety is manifested in the florid catastrophic reactions of acutely confused brain injury patients (Goldstein 1952) or is the incipient type found in patients who have not begun to realize the full nature of their cognitive disabilities, it is important for all clinicians managing the care of TBI patients to be able to recognize and treat the various anxiety syndromes that may arise. An illustration of this issue is found in Ann Stewart's account of her effort to cope with severe anxiety after sustaining brain injury in a motor vehicle accident (Lipowski and Stewart 1973 [Copyright 1973, *Psychiatry in Medicine*, quoted with permission from the publisher]):

I was silenced by fear when he [the doctor] told me I had to be in that particular bed because of my seizure. I was incapable of further reaction beyond stark terror that I should be having seizures . . . all of these factors weighed heavily upon my return to a more conscious existence—my feeling of having been violated, my extreme fear of the seizures, an intense confusion that seemed incompatible with my intelligence, and a growing worry that I was emotionally inequipped to handle the situation . . . I felt much safer in the isolation of my room, where I wouldn't need to exhibit my impairments to everyone on the floor . . . my lack of comprehension would later sometimes result in a last minute panic over an event, necessitating the calling of a doctor to further explain something that had been gone over previously . . . my family was too much a source of a great deal of my anxiety and firmly closed to my expression of anxiety, eager to erase worry from my mind.

Frequency and Clinical Manifestations of Anxiety in TBI

A compilation of 12 studies (see Table 9–1), comprising a total of 1,199 patients from 1942 to 1990, revealed that approximately 29% of head injury patients were diagnosed with clinical anxiety following TBI. These studies varied quite considerably with regard to the severity and type of head injury, age, and method of selection. To date, we are unaware of any prospective studies that have estimated the incidence of specific anxiety syndromes according to present DSM-III-R categories (American Psychiatric Association 1987), using an unbiased population sample.

Although most clinical and psychometric studies of the psychiatric sequelae of brain injury address the problem of anxiety without further nosological subclassification, there are individual case reports and descriptive studies documenting a variety of syndromes resembling specific DSM-III-R anxiety disorders.

Generalized Anxiety States

Lewis and Rosenberg (1990) reported that the anxiety experienced by TBI patients is usually generalized and free floating, consisting of persistent tension, worry, and fearfulness, and experienced in an intense way but without much comprehension. TBI often impairs the ability of patients to understand or adapt to external and internal stimuli. As a result, they are less able to regulate anxiety or to use it as a signal to alert themselves to problems requiring an adaptive coping strategy. Lezak (1978) found that 76% of patients with TBI demonstrated perplexity, distractibility, and fatigue, which increased their risk for worry and depression. Perplexity in particular appears strongly related to the pathological worrying commonly seen in TBI patients. It reflects uncertainness about one's ability to

Table 9–1.   Incidence of anxiety disorder following head injury

Study	Total sample	Follow-up period	Anxiety (%)	Remarks
Lewis 1942	64	—	70	Compared with control group
Adler 1945	200	1–12 months	25	Consecutive admissions
Lishman 1968	144	5 years	28	Penetrating head wounds
Kay et al. 1971				
Sample 1	94	3–6 months	31	Minor head injury
Sample 2	61	3–6 months	18	Neurologically injured
Klonoff 1971				
Sample 1	100	1 year	11	Preschool age children
Sample 2	100	1 year	13	School age children
Merskey and Woodforde 1972	27	6 months–14 years	52	Initial exam
Rutherford 1977	145	6 weeks	19	Consecutive cases, mild head injury
McKinlay et al. 1981	55	1 year	58	Referral to secondary facility
Tyerman and Humphrey 1984	25	2–15 months	44	Unselected cases
Kinsella et al. 1988	39	0–2 years	26	Consecutive admissions
Schoenhuber et al. 1988	103	1 year	26	Minor head injury
Mureriwa 1990	42	10 months	60	Consecutive neurosurgical outpatients
Totals	1,199		29%	

rely on a previously well-mastered skill. A time-tested measure of one's self-appraisal has been called into doubt. Perplexity is manifested in hesitancy, self-doubt, and a need for assurance. Distractibility consists of the inability to screen out unwanted stimuli, such that the patient feels bombarded by sensations. The patient's "nerve endings seem more exposed" (Lezak 1978).

DiCesare et al. (1990) found that obsessive-compulsive behavior, interpersonal sensitivity, depression, and phobic anxiety were the most distressing symptoms experienced by their patients, whereas general anxiety, manifested by trembling, racing pulse, or free floating anxiety was not reported by patients above the average expected level. However, a number of other psychometric studies provide evidence that there is a generalized distress syndrome among patients with TBI. A test designed for patients with organic brain disease (OBD), the OBD-168, was administered to 23 TBI patients (Sbordone and Jennison 1983). The OBD-168 consists of 168 questions selected from the Minnesota Multiphasic Personality Inventory (MMPI; Hathaway and McKinley 1943) that have been simplified for the benefit of cognitively impaired patients. Although almost all of the patients denied experiencing emotional symptomatology in clinical interviews, their test scores revealed evidence for a distress syndrome consisting of depression, anxiety, tension, and nervousness. Sbordone and Jennison attributed the overt denial to the problem of anosognosia that is characteristic of right cerebral hemisphere impairment. Similarly, Dikmen and Reitan (1977) and Burton and Volpe (1988) found elevations in the Depression and Schizophrenia scales of the MMPI for patients with TBI. Composite scores indicated a distress syndrome consisting of depression, anxiety, and strange or unusual experiences.

A nonspecific anxiety state, frequently mixed with depression, may also be seen in patients following multiple trauma in which subtle effects of persisting cognitive deficits become masked by a chronic pain syndrome that is focused on orthopedic injuries (Anderson et al. 1990). Until proper diagnosis is made, the vicious cycle of a patient filled with uncertainty, worry, and preoccupation with somatic pain is continuously fueled by the inability of attending physicians to properly explain the symptomatology.

Panic States

Catastrophic panic and agitation is most commonly manifest in the acute phase of TBI, when the patient awakens to the terrifying reality of an impairment in his or her ability to interact with the environment. Fromm-Reichman (1959) hypothesized that catastrophic reactions resulted from a patient experiencing his or her personal inadequacy as a form of psychological death. Brain trauma that resulted in sudden cortical blindness precipitated severe agitation and anxiety in a number of pediatric cases when the children were unable to tell the treating physicians that they could not see (Woodward 1990). Aphasic patients may develop sudden severe anxiety when called upon to respond in tests of their communication skills (Strub and Black 1981). In the subacute phase, after the patient awakens from coma, some patients may become agitated and combative because of frightening illusions and hallucinations (O'Shanick 1986).

In a study comparing agitated versus nonagitated patients following TBI, Levin and Grossman (1978) found that individuals who evidenced screaming, combativeness, and other signs of sympathetic arousal in the acute confusional phase following TBI, displayed a significantly higher level of anxiety, depression, and thinking disturbance after stabilization or improvement in orientation. These symptoms did not appear related to the site of injury but did correlate with acute aphasia and the appearance of auditory or visual hallucinations.

Phobic Disorders

Lishman (1978) reported the case of a man who developed episodes of vertigo and nausea when he moved his head suddenly. These symptoms persisted for about a month after a mild TBI. He became quite phobic of being in a closed place or traveling. His phobic symptoms were later found to be a result of labyrinthine injury. Similarly, Roberts (1979) found that a number of his TBI patients who developed disabling anxiety, associated with mild memory deficit and a disturbance of equilibrium, evidenced phobic symptomatology related to their fear of falling. DiCesare et al. (1990) hypothesized that phobic anxiety resulted from diminished self-esteem that was associated with a loss of strength or mastery in males, and a loss of attractiveness in females. They also found that interpersonal sensitivity contributed to their patients' sense of social isolation. Phobic anxiety may also be precipitated by avoidance of the situation that caused the injury. This may include direct or symbolic reminders of a traumatic assault or accident.

Social phobia probably plays an important role in the ensuing morbidity and disability found in TBI patients. Johnson and Newton (1987) reported that high social anxiety was associated with low self-esteem and an impaired social adjustment. Social phobias in TBI patients often stem from negative changes in self-image and fears that other people will find them stupid or unattractive. Difficulty in attending to multiple simultaneous stimuli is often experienced at parties or other gatherings where more than one person is likely to be speaking at the same time. The patient is fearful of the profound embarrassment that could result if his or her cognitive difficulties are publicly exposed.

Posttraumatic Stress Disorder

In general, posttraumatic stress disorder (PTSD) can be difficult to diagnose (Epstein 1989). Avoidant symptoms tend to create a self-cloaking device around the patient's terrifying memories. This problem can be compounded in the brain injury patient. Confusion, impaired ability to deal with the environment, and changed self-perceptions are likely to promote even more difficulties in patients' ability to cope with the strange inner perceptions and arousal states that accompany the intrusive remembering of PTSD. Any significant anxiety disorder that arises following TBI should raise the suspicion of PTSD. Brain injury commonly occurs in association with multiple body trauma. Patients often experience fear of death or dismemberment at the time of the injury. They also report near-death and out-of-body experiences during the comatose state following the accident. Such stressors are severe enough to precipitate PTSD even without brain injury. PTSD by itself can cause impaired concentration, selective memory deficits, irritability, and other physiological changes that may overlap and interact with the effects of TBI. The subtle cognitive dysfunction seen following mild brain trauma often plays a synergistic role in the onset and maintenance of PTSD.

Although we are unaware of any accurate estimates of the frequency of PTSD following brain injury, there is evidence that it accounts for a sizable fraction of subsequent anxiety syndromes. Adler (1945) reported that 48 patients (24% of her sample of 200 consecutive admissions for TBI) developed posttraumatic anxiety neuroses, characterized by acoustic hypersensitivity, fatigue, sleep disturbance, anxiety dreams, and periodic irritability. She noted the onset of new traumatic dreams in 28 patients (14%) that were associated with episodes of perspiration, trembling, and regular awakening from their sleep. These dreams were similar in content to the dreams of patients in her study of the Cocoanut Grove nightclub fire (Adler 1943).

Epstein (1991) conducted a prospective study of 16 patients admitted to a hospital trauma center following severe accidental injury. He found that 3 out of 9 patients with closed head injury met DSM-III-R criteria for PTSD. Symptoms began almost immediately after admission. Three of the 7 patients whose injuries did not involve TBI also developed PTSD. In 2 of these cases the onset was delayed several months.

Theoretically, retrograde and anterograde amnesia would imply that the patient has no memory of the traumatic injury and that this should protect against the development of PTSD. Some TBI patients develop PTSD from the traumatic sequelae associated with the injury even if they have no direct memory of the event (McMillan 1991). Other patients may undergo traumatogenic out-of-body and near-death experiences while they are comatose or may experience psychogenic amnesia that is mistakenly assumed to be a result of concussive effects.

Case example.

A 40-year-old man fell asleep while driving his car, collided with a tree, and sustained a mild closed head injury. Because he could not recall the accident, it was believed that he had experienced retrograde amnesia, or that he was asleep at the time of impact. Shortly after admission to the hospital, he experienced vertiginous sensations that were attributed to possible labyrinthine damage. He later developed repeated panic attacks associated with tearfulness and suicidal feelings whenever he required treatment for other somatic injuries sustained in the accident. During follow-up psychiatric interviews, he finally remembered that he had actually awakened prior to impact and that he had struck a barrier that sent his vehicle careening into a second obstacle. It became possible to explore how his unconscious memories were stimulating and linking up with the spinning sensation associated with the accident. He began having dreams of his car crashing into the barrier, and felt as if the accident was recurring whenever he was a passenger in a vehicle that moved too close to another object.

It is not uncommon to see TBI patients who meet criteria for both PTSD and postconcussive syndrome. Patients who have brain injury with only brief loss of consciousness and no neurological sequelae will often report symptoms such as headache, dizziness, fatigue, decreased concentration, anxiety, irritability, memory deficits, insomnia, hypochondriacal concerns, photophobia, and increased sensitivity to noise (Goethe and Levin 1984; Lishman 1987, pp. 168–171). These symptoms usually resolve within several months, but sometimes persist longer. Six of the symptoms listed above are similar to some of the criteria for PTSD (see Table 9–2) and the overlap may confound diagnosis. Some postconcussive symptoms may be in response to an emotionally traumatizing experience, and others may be the result of subtle but potentially serious impairment in their ability to process information (Gronwall and Wrightson 1974; Hugenholtz et al. 1988; Leininger et al. 1990). Hugenholtz et al. (1988) found that the complex reaction time of concussed patients recovered gradually, but still remained slower than that of healthy control subjects after 3 months. Such cognitive impairment is likely to further complicate the pathophysiology of PTSD.

Kolb (1987) hypothesized that chronic stress has direct neurotoxic or neurosuppressive effects on cortical structures in the temporal-amygdaloid complex. He reasoned that suppression of normal cortical inhibition would lead to the symptomatic manifestations of PTSD through disinhibition of activated brain stem structures such as the locus ceruleus and the medial hypothalamic nuclei. If this mechanism is correct, one would expect that the

Table 9–2.   Symptoms of postconcussive syndrome and criteria for posttraumatic stress disorder

Posttraumatic stress disorder	Postconcussive syndrome
Re-experiencing trauma	
Recurrent intrusive recollections of traumatic event	
Recurrent distressing dreams of traumatic event	
Flashbacks of traumatic event	
Intense distress triggered by symbolic reminders[a]	
Physiological reactivity on exposure to events resembling trauma	Hypochondriacal concerns Headache Dizziness
Avoidance	
Efforts to avoid thoughts or feelings associated with event	
Efforts to avoid activities that arouse event	
Inability to recall aspect of event (psychogenic amnesia)[a]	Memory deficits[a]
Markedly diminished interest in activities	Fatigue
Feelings of detachment	
Restricted range of affect	
A sense of foreshortened future	
Increased arousal	Increased sensitivity to noise[a] Photophobia
Difficulty falling or staying asleep[a]	Insomnia[a]
Irritability or outbursts of anger[a]	Irritability[a]
Difficulty concentrating[a]	Decreased concentration[a]
Hypervigilance	
Exaggerated startle response[a]	Anxiety[a]

[a]Symptoms and criteria that overlap between postconcussive syndrome and posttraumatic stress disorder.
Source. Postconcussive syndrome symptoms are adapted from Goethe and Levin 1984 and Lishman 1987. Posttraumatic stress disorder symptoms are adapted from DSM-IV (American Psychiatric Association 1994).

coexistence of TBI and PTSD would lead to a synergistic exacerbation of the symptomatology of both conditions.

Obsessive-Compulsive Disorder

We have been able to find 36 reported instances of obsessive-compulsive (OC) symptomatology observed after TBI (see Table 9–3). In the five studies in which cases were sampled as part of a larger study population, the incidence of OC symptoms averaged 3.0%. Anderson's (1942) and Lewis's (1942) data, reviewed in Table 9–3, may not represent pure incidence following TBI, because it was unclear whether OC symptoms predated the injury in some of their cases. Milder cases of OC symptomatology may not be uncommon following TBI. Rigidity in thinking and ritualistic compulsiveness might be a direct result of perseveration, a compensation for perceived disability in organizing a confusing environment, or an unconscious effort to defend against severe anxiety in the face of impaired ability to regulate this emotion. Memory loss (DiCesare et al. 1990) and parietal lobe injuries (Hillbom 1960) have also been hypothesized to play a role in OC symptoms following TBI. As yet there is no conclusive evidence linking localization of brain lesion with the onset of OC symptoms. Studies linking obsessive-compulsive disorder (OCD) to hyperfunctionality of the orbital frontal cortex and caudate nucleus (Baxter et al. 1988; Benkelfat et al. 1990), findings that patients with OCD are more likely to show neurological soft signs suggestive of right-hemispheric deficits (Bihari et al. 1991; Hollander et al. 1990), and evidence suggesting that the right orbital cortex plays an important role in the regulation of anxiety (Grafman et al. 1986) are some of the recent findings that may provide important direction in future research regarding the onset of OC symptomatology following TBI. The psychic effects of trauma at the time of injury also may play a major etiological role. The prevalence of OCD was 10 times higher for subjects in a population of randomly sampled adults who also experienced PTSD (Breslau et al. 1991).

In six of the reported cases (Drummond and Gravestock 1988; Lewis and Rosenberg 1990; McKeon et al. 1984) the onset of OC symptoms was preceded by a state of free floating anxiety and hyperarousal. In Lewis and Rosenberg's (1990) case, a 23-year-old man developed hemiplegia, diminished inhibitory control over his emotions, and loss of recent memory. While in treatment at a rehabilitation hospital following his brain injury, he was overcome

Table 9–3. Reports of obsessive-compulsive symptoms following head injury

Study	Cases	% of study population	Remarks	Total sample
Lewis 1942	5	7.8	Onset not clearly specified	64
Anderson 1942	7	4.7	Onset not clearly specified	150
Adler 1945	1	0.5	New cases	200
Hillbom 1960	14	3.4	New cases	415
Lishman 1968	2	1.4	New cases	144
McKeon et al. 1984	4	—	Increased arousal, agitation or anxiety preceded onset of obsessive-compulsive disorder	—
Jenike and Brandon 1988	1	—	Immediate onset of obsessive-compulsive symptoms Fronto-temporal subdural hematoma Partial resection left temporal lobe Responded to phenelzine	—
Drummond and Gravestock 1988	1	—	Irritable state following injury Onset of obsessive-compulsive symptoms 6 months later Nonresponsive to behavior therapy	—
Lewis and Rosenberg 1990	1	—	Free floating anxiety preceded obsessive-compulsive symptoms Responded to psychoanalytic psychotherapy	—
Total cases with percentages reported	29	3.0		973
Total cases reported	36	—		

by free-floating anxiety. Subsequently he developed compulsive handwashing and an excessive neatness that was an exaggerated feature of his premorbid personality. His free floating anxiety state abated as his compulsiveness expanded to an insistently ritualized politeness and a rigid adherence to schedules. Work on these maladaptive defenses during psychotherapy helped him to relax them somewhat. Although he began to experience generalized anxiety again, efforts to help him to identify the useful signaling aspects of these feelings were successful in enabling him to identify and more adaptively cope with the events causing this anxiety.

Etiology of Anxiety Following TBI

Nosological Considerations

The diagnosis of anxiety disorder due to a general medical condition (DSM-IV; American Psychiatric Association 1994) should be used for an anxiety syndrome resembling panic disorder or generalized anxiety disorder that is caused by specific organic factors, such as metabolic disorders, brain tumor, or psychoactive substances. This syndrome would be based on prominent anxiety, panic attacks, obsessions, compulsions, or phobic symptoms, judged to be etiologically related to a general medical disturbance.

Although TBI is not included in the list of suggested causes outlined in DSM-III-R, Horvath et al. (1989) mentioned the anxiety related to postconcussion syndrome and the sudden ictal terror of a partial complex seizure emanating from the temporal lobe as causes of organic anxiety syndrome. The differential diagnosis depends on the degree to which the anxiety disturbance itself is related to the organic factor. For TBI, the clinical features of anxiety are rarely as clear-cut from an etiological point of view as they might be, for example, in a case of thyrotoxicosis.

The multiple interactions between anxiety and TBI are quite complex. As is evident from the large number of interacting factors, the relationship between the level of anxiety and the severity of brain injury is unlikely to be a simple one. There have been a number of studies supporting the role of various factors in the clinical manifestations of anxiety following TBI. For example, Fordyce et al. (1983) found that chronic TBI patients were likely to be more anxious, depressed, confused in their thinking, and socially withdrawn than acute patients. This difference was not related to increased cognitive impairment or duration of coma in the chronic group, and was felt by the authors to be a function of premorbid personality factors, and patients' increased awareness over time of their degree of impairment. Similarly, Van Zomeren and Van den Burg (1985) found no relationship between severity of head injury and the presence of anxiety at 2-year follow-up, although they did find an apparent association with depression. They reasoned that patients with milder TBI are likely to have chronic stress because they must adapt to subtle but significant deficits that receive less environmental acceptance. As a result, the summation of the effects of severity versus subtlety in correlations with anxiety would tend to cancel out in population samples. Hillbom (1960) suggested that the low visibility of impairment in milder TBI cases, combined with the patient's feeling of shame and secretiveness, resulted in a skeptical response from physicians examining them for compensation. The effect of multiple interacting variables may thus explain many of the conflicting findings in the literature from studies attempting to correlate either trauma severity or anatomical site of injury to the presence of anxiety.

Anatomical Specificity as an Etiological Factor in Anxiety Syndromes

In a study of 52 Vietnam veterans who sustained penetrating head wounds causing damage to the orbital frontal cortex, Grafman et al. (1986) found that patients with left and bilateral lesions showed no differences in mood states when compared with controls. Patients who had right-sided orbitofrontal lesions initially manifested anger that later gave way to panic, lassitude, general anxiety, and edginess. This was interpreted as suggesting a relatively large role for the right orbitofrontal cortex in the regulation of anxiety.

Lishman (1968) studied 144 cases of penetrating head trauma in World War II veterans. He found no evidence associating the development of anxiety with the severity of the patient's posttraumatic amnesia, total volume of brain tissue injury, or laterality of injury. There appeared to be some association between anxiety and left occipital injuries. Aside from the reactions seen in acute aphasia, Levin and Grossman (1978) found no association between overall psychiatric disturbances and the presence of hematoma, hemiparesis, focal frontotemporal injury, or mesencephalic impairment. Their patients with mesencephalic signs tended to manifest less evidence of anxiety and depression. Lezak (1983) found anxiety to be a common feature of left-hemisphere damage. It was manifest as excessive cautiousness, oversensitivity, impaired performance, and an exaggeration of disabilities. Left-sided injury is more likely to result in the sudden catastrophic reaction that can be observed when patients with brain damage become aware of their inability to perform a task. This is particularly prominent in patients with aphasia (Gainotti 1972; Lezak 1983; Strub and Black 1981). On the other hand, some brain lesions may result in the patient's appearing less anxious than would be clinically expected. For example, patients with right-hemisphere lesions are more prone to show an indifference reaction, are less likely to be dissatisfied with themselves, and more likely to deny their impairment particularly during the acute phase (Gainotti 1972; Lezak 1983). Sbordone and Jennison (1983) observed that patients with right-hemisphere lesions will commonly have anosognosia and be impaired in their ability to appreciate the magnitude of their deficits. Kwentus et al. (1985) cautioned that aprosodia may hamper the ability of patients with right-hemisphere deficits either to perceive or to express the affective tone reflecting their inner state. Some of these findings about severity of impairment and laterality have been confirmed by psychometric studies (Black 1975; Bornstein et al. 1989; Gass and Russell 1987).

Patients with complex partial seizures resulting from temporal lobe injury have reported ictal phenomena including uncanny experiences, feelings of impending disaster (Horvath et al. 1989; Wells and Duncan 1980), and peculiar apprehensions (Benson and Blumer 1982). Some patients with traumatically induced seizure disorders of any type become extremely anxious because they are worried that they might experience repeated seizures, lose their driver's license, lose their job, or have a humiliating loss of control such as bowel or bladder incontinence.

Treatment

General Considerations

Clinicians should base the treatment of anxiety in TBI on a thorough psychiatric and neuropsychological evaluation of the patient. Assessment should include a review of all factors that might play an important role in provoking or maintaining symptomatology. Some patients who initially report amnesia later remember traumatic aspects of the accident. One should look carefully for the effects of noncerebral injuries and explore the patient's memories about the period of physical convalescence and rehabilitation. It is important to inquire about the presence of chronic pain, orthopedic limitations, and motor or sensory loss. Patients with mild brain injury sometimes have subtle neurological deficits such as anosmia that are not reported spontaneously. The sense of smell and other sensory functions are an important part of maintaining connection with the environment. Impairment in sensory function may result in patients feeling they are "surrounded by a sheet of glass" (Gronwall 1986).

One should appraise the family's ability to be supportive to the patient, and the effect of family dynamics and psychiatric disturbance in its members as a result of the stress of caring for a TBI patient (see Chapter 17). In order to fully appreciate the source of the patient's anxiety, it is important to evaluate the patient's activities of daily living and functioning at work. Direct interviews with family members and employers provide important collateral information about the patient's emotional, interpersonal, financial, and legal stress.

Psychotherapy and Behavioral Treatment

By understanding the nature of any changes that have taken place in the patient's inner and outer worlds as a result of the injury, the clinician is in a better position to address the patient's sources of anxiety. Psychotherapeutic treatment should employ an empathic approach that helps the patient to appreciate and comprehend the changes that he or she has experienced, and to develop strategies for coping with them. Because of the adverse effects that anxiety can have on the rehabilitative process, treatment should be instituted as soon as possible.

The cornerstone of treatment for patients with mild brain injury is reassurance, education, support, and regular neuropsychological monitoring (Gronwall 1986). Reassurance is necessary to help patients cope with the commonly expressed fears of "going mad" that may accompany emotional lability, extreme fatigue, and feelings of sensory detachment. Because disturbed sleep cycles are common following TBI, patients may require increased sleep and nap times. This often helps decrease the irritability and emotional lability associated with fatigue. Social support and the use of structured meditation, hypnosis, or other relaxation techniques can help the patient interrupt the vicious cycle of anxiety's detrimental effects on impaired capacity to process information, and may be of use in increasing the patient's motivation in the overall rehabilitative effort (Crasilneck and Hall 1970; Morozov 1989). Follow-up monitoring can provide useful feedback that encourages the patient to identify the way problematic issues may be inhibiting recovery.

Lezak (1978) recommended that clinicians explain to their TBI patients that perplexity is a common symptom of brain injury and that they are not going insane. In cases where neuropsychological testing has shown the patient's first responses to have the highest probability of being correct, one should advise him or her to trust the first solution to a problem no matter how unsure he or she feels. Lezak believes that it is also valuable to encourage the perplexed patient not to withdraw or inhibit spontaneous reactions because of the fear of making errors. Distractibility can be managed by helping the patient and the family to reduce unnecessary stimuli in the environment, develop strategies for pacing the time and duration of social involvement, and schedule naps prior to events.

Psychotherapeutic methods for treating anxiety disorders with TBI can successfully employ standard interventions such as clarification, confrontation, and interpretation of unconscious conflicts. These must be modified in a way that is empathic with the patient's specific cognitive deficits. Communications should be less complex, more down to earth, and geared to helping the patient to identify specific deficits and develop strategies to compensate for lost functions (see Chapter 20 for a more detailed discussion).

Psychodynamic psychotherapy employed with appropriate supportive features can play a useful role in the treatment of TBI patients, particularly when anxiety interferes with rehabilitative efforts (Lewis 1991; Lewis and Rosenberg 1990; Morris and Bleiberg 1986). Levels of anxiety may increase over time, despite improvement in cognitive status (Lewis and Rosenberg 1990). Young adults whose TBI occurs at a time when they are just establishing independence from their parents may have severe anxiety as a result of renewed dependency. For many patients, the anxiety associated with the loss of mental or physical functioning will interfere with their ability to maximize their capacity for rehabilitation and return to functioning.

Initial transference issues will often center around the patient's anger and envy of the therapist for being undamaged. This may manifest as blaming and projection onto others, combined with a passive-dependent attitude. Countertransference reactions in the therapist are likely to center around denial and difficulty facing the fact that another human being can sustain permanent loss of mental powers that are so closely connected with one's self-concept. If the therapist identifies with the patient's perception of the TBI as a psychological death, but is unable to deal with his or her own anxiety connected with this perception, he or she may unwittingly communicate to the patient, "Your problem is so awful that even I can't bear to deal with it." Fromm-Reichman (1959) emphasized how important it is for therapists to accept their patients' realistic deficits without getting so carried away by them that they fail to deal with the pathological aspects of the patient's anxiety.

A psychotherapeutic approach that establishes a relational climate of security, fosters reality, interprets projected aggression, rebuilds clear boundaries between self and other, and helps patients to understand and use the signaling value of anxiety, is likely to be most helpful to the patient facing aborted developmental tasks and alterations in self-image (Lewis and Rosenberg 1990). It is important to explore the patient's traumatic memories concerning injuries or failures experienced in the past. Recollections of the traumatic event that caused the injury can also be a vehicle for the expression of fears of frightening events in the patient's present day life (Holloway and Ursano 1984). When memories intrude on the patient's life, it is important for the clinician to inquire into present fears that may be provoking their call.

Psychotherapy with brain injury patients can effectively approach anxiety as a form of emotional perception that alerts the individual to potential dangers and problems that must be anticipated. For example, Zencius and Wesolowski (1990) described the treatment of a 28-year-old woman who developed seizures following closed head injury in a motor vehicle accident. She eloped from residential treatment whenever she became agitated in her confused state. Because she was unaware of perceiving anxiety, it was necessary for the treatment staff to teach her to observe other behaviors that could serve as indicators of anxiety, such as the onset of muscle tension or an emotional outburst.

Psychotherapeutic and behavioral treatment for TBI patients with severe cognitive deficits is often administered in a multidisciplinary setting that combines physical therapy, cognitive rehabilitation, occupational counseling, behavior modification (Gloag 1985), therapeutic social skills groups (Johnson and Newton 1987), trauma support groups, and family counselling. Head trauma support groups can be very effective by providing information from other TBI patients who have been through similar experiences, such as how to cope with the uncertainty of seizures, manage social rejections, handle employment, or deal with financial issues. Observing the resourcefulness, sense of humor, and resiliency with which other group members have dealt with their brain damage can provide an individual with the opportunity to learn new ways to cope with the profound uncertainty, loss, and feeling of unacceptability so frequently experienced after TBI.

Pharmacotherapy

Psychopharmacologic agents should not be used to treat anxiety in TBI patients until after behavioral and psychotherapeutic methods have been tried. All drugs presently available have risks of adverse effects that may increase feelings of strangeness and detachment from the environment. Cope (1987) emphasized the fact that using any agent with the potential to diminish arousal will also produce the risk of adverse effects on patients with problems of impaired motivation and drive. Anxiolytic agents may increase the patient's feeling of impairment and paradoxically increase his or her anxiety.

Buspirone (BuSpar) appears to be one of the most promising agents for use in the treatment of anxiety for TBI patients, primarily because it appears to be free of addiction potential and it causes relatively little cognitive impairment. There have been isolated case reports of abnormal movement disorders using buspirone, but there is evidence that other factors may have been responsible, such as prior use of neuroleptics (Jann et al. 1990). Gualtieri (1991) treated seven patients with postconcussional syndrome with buspirone. Dosage was gradually increased from a starting dosage of 5 mg bid in 5 mg increments every 5 days, to a maximum daily dosage of 45 mg. He found that four patients responded quite dramatically, even though they had had symptoms for 6 months. Symptoms responding to buspirone included anxiety, depression, irritability, somatic preoccupation, inattention, and distractibility. Seven other patients with severe brain injury who were also given buspirone did not show an impressive response (Gualtieri 1991).

Benzodiazepines are commonly used to treat anxiety. They are problematic in that they can cause memory impairment (Preston et al. 1989), ataxia, and sedation. TBI patients have an increased risk of preexisting alcohol and substance abuse. For such patients, benzodiazepines are probably contraindicated for long-term use. Benzodiazepines have been reported to produce disinhibition on rare occasions (Dietch and Jennings 1988), and clinicians should be especially alert for this effect in TBI patients. For severe acute anxiety that is not responsive to behavioral or social support, Yudofsky and Silver (1985) recommended using short-acting benzodiazepines such as oxazepam or lorazepam to minimize the sedative and cognitive problems that may be associated with these compounds.

Propranolol may be used for the management of certain components of anxiety. Unlike the dosages of propranolol used in the treatment of pathological aggression following TBI, dosages of up to 80 mg bid are usually sufficient to control uncomplicated agitation and anxiety (Rose 1988). We are unaware of any studies of propranolol for social anxiety experienced by TBI patients, but clinicians should consider its use in such cases.

Anecdotal evidence (personal communication, C. Olsen, September 1991) suggests that the opioid antagonist naltrexone (Trexan) may be helpful in treating symptoms of panic and anxiety in patients with mild TBI who have prolonged postconcussive symptomatology. Reduction of anxiety may have been a result of the patient's improved cognitive functioning. Tennant (1987) reported that naltrexone at doses of 50–100 mg/day was successful in reversing much of the cognitive impairment seen in 2 postconcussive patients.

Although neuroleptics may be useful in the reduction of anxiety and tension (Cardenas 1987), we strongly believe that use of these agents should be avoided if possible. A number of potential problems related to neuroleptic use in TBI patients include the risk of reducing neuronal recovery in the patient with TBI (Cardenas 1987; Rose 1988), the increased potential for tardive dyskinesia (Haas 1987) and diaphragmatic dyskinesia, which may impair ventilation and increase fatigue (O'Shanick 1987), reduced arousal, and anticholinergic effects that can reduce memory function. Clinicians must also be alert to the effects of centrally acting dopamine antagonists that are commonly employed for nonpsychiatric purposes, such as prochlorperazine (Compazine), metoclopramide (Reglan) for nausea, and promethazine for potentiating analgesia (O'Shanick 1987).

The treatment of OCD following brain injury should begin with a trial of psychotherapy and cognitive rehabilitation for memory loss. Because it has been shown to be effective in OCD without brain injury, behavior therapy may also be helpful in TBI patients and should be considered. If pharmacotherapy becomes necessary, a trial of fluoxetine (Prozac), buspirone (BuSpar), or a combination of the two is probably the safest regimen. Experience with clomipramine (Anafranil) for OCD in brain injury patients has been limited but unfavorable (Drummond and Gravestock 1988; Rose 1988). The drowsiness and anticholinergic activity commonly encountered with clomipramine would serve to aggravate the memory problems that have been implicated in OCD following brain injury (DiCesare et al. 1990). Phenelzine was successfully used in a patient who developed OCD after a brain injury (Jenike and Brandon 1988). The dietary restrictions that are necessary for the safe use of phenelzine and other monoamine oxidase inhibitors could present special difficulties for TBI patients with significant cognitive impairments. Although no reports have appeared of its specific use in the treatment of OCD following TBI, fluoxetine at doses of 20 mg daily was well tolerated by TBI patients treated for depression (Cassidy 1989) and should therefore be considered for OCD following brain injury as well. The higher rate of seizure associated with clomipramine as compared with fluoxetine (Prozac) or phenelzine (Davidson 1989) should also be considered when choosing a drug treatment for a TBI patient with OCD. Wroblewski et al. (1992) reported that fluoxetine lowered the seizure threshold in a patient with TBI.

The psychopharmacologic treatment of PTSD involves agents such as antidepressants, buspirone, and benzodiazepines to help symptoms of hyperarousal and intrusive memories (Epstein 1989; Silver et al. 1990). Silver et al. (1990) recommended that the following agents be considered in the regimen for PTSD when patients have not responded favorably to more standard psychopharmacotherapy: For sleep disturbance—trazodone or benzodiazepines; for persistent anger, hypervigilance, or startle—clonidine or propranolol; for persistent anger outbursts or flashbacks—carbamazepine; and for refractory depression and anger—phenelzine or lithium. Anticholinergic effects and the decreased arousal that may result from some of these agents will often cause patients with TBI to complain of increased cognitive problems, and may produce paradoxical results. For this reason agents such as fluoxetine, buspirone, propranolol, and phenelzine are most likely to be effective for treating PTSD in TBI patients.

Summary

Anxiety syndromes are quite common following TBI and have a potential for serious impact on rehabilitation and treatment outcome. Approximately 30% of TBI patients have clinically measurable anxiety. Clinicians should be especially alert to anxiety, because it does not always present in an overt fashion. The interrelationships between anxiety and TBI are multifactorial, and the effect of specific tissue damage upon the nature of the symptomatology remains uncertain. It is important to perform a careful psychiatric evaluation of the patient that includes assessment of family and other environmental factors. Treatment should be initiated using behavioral and psychotherapeutic methods before considering medication. Careful attention should be paid to family dynamics and to the potential for family members to develop severe and potentially disruptive psychiatric symptomatology as a result of the severe stress of caring for the patient. If pharmacological treatment becomes necessary, agents with the lowest potential for adverse side effects should be chosen. Dosage must be titrated to minimize the potential for many drugs to exacerbate cognitive impairment.

References

Adler A: Neuropsychiatric complications in victims of Boston's Cocoanut Grove disaster. JAMA 123:1098–1101, 1943

Adler A: Mental symptoms following head injury: a statistical analysis of two hundred cases. Archives of Neurology and Psychiatry 53:34–43, 1945

American Psychiatric Association: Diagnostic and Statistical Manual of Mental Disorders, 3rd Edition, Revised. Washington, DC, American Psychiatric Association, 1987

American Psychiatric Association: Diagnostic and Statistical Manual of Mental Disorders, 4th Edition. Washington, DC, American Psychiatric Association, 1994

Anderson C: Chronic head cases. Lancet 2:1–4, 1942

Anderson JM, Kaplan MS, Felsenthal G: Brain injury obscured by chronic pain: a preliminary report. Arch Phys Med Rehabil 71:703–708, 1990

Baxter LR, Schwartz JM, Mazziotta JC, et al: Cerebral glucose metabolic rates in nondepressed patients with obsessive-compulsive disorder. Am J Psychiatry 145:1560–1563, 1988

Benkelfat C, Nordahl TE, Semple WE, et al: Local cerebral glucose metabolic rates in obsessive-compulsive disorder: patients treated with clomipramine. Arch Gen Psychiatry 47:840–848, 1990

Benson DF, Blumer D: Psychiatric Aspects of Neurologic Disease, Vol 2. New York, Grune and Stratton, 1982

Bihari K, Pato, MT, Hill JL, et al: Neurologic soft signs in obsessive-compulsive disorder. Arch Gen Psychiatry 48:278–279, 1991

Black FW: Unilateral brain lesions and MMPI performance: a preliminary study. Percept Mot Skills 40:87–93, 1975

Bornstein RA, Miller HB, Van Schoor JJ: Neuropsychological deficit and emotional disturbance in head-injured patients. J Neurosurg 70:509–513, 1989

Breslau N, Davis GC, Andreski P, et al: Traumatic events and posttraumatic stress disorder in an urban population of young adults. Arch Gen Psychiatry 48:216–222, 1991

Burton LA, Volpe BT: Sex differences in emotional status of traumatically brain injured patients. Journal of Neurological Rehabilitation 2(4):151–157, 1988

Cardenas DD: Antipsychotics and their use after traumatic brain injury. Journal of Head Trauma Rehabilitation 2(4):43–49, 1987

Cassidy JW: Fluoxetine: a new serotonergically active antidepressant. Journal of Head Trauma Rehabilitation 4(2):67–69, 1989

Cope DN: Psychopharmacologic considerations in the treatment of traumatic brain injury. J Head Trauma Rehabil 2(4):1–5, 1987

Crasilneck HB, Hall JA: The use of hypnosis in the rehabilitation of complicated vascular and post-traumatic neurological patients. Int J Clin Exper Hypnosis 18:145–159, 1970

Davidson J: Seizures and buproprion: a review. J Clin Psychiatry 50:256–261, 1989

DiCesare A, Parente R, Anderson-Parente J: Personality change after traumatic brain injury. Cognitive Rehabilitation 8:14–18, 1990

Dietch JT, Jennings RK: Aggressive dyscontrol in patients treated with benzodiazepines. J Clin Psychiatry 49:184–188, 1988

Dikmen S, Reitan RM: Emotional sequelae of head injury. Ann Neurol 2:492–494, 1977

Drummond LM, Gravestock S: Delayed emergence of obsessive-compulsive neurosis following head injury. Br J Psychiatry 153:839–842, 1988

Epstein R: Posttraumatic stress disorder: a review of diagnostic and treatment issues. Psychiatric Annals 19:556–563, 1989

Epstein R: Posttraumatic stress disorder following severe accidental injury: a nine-month prospective study. Paper presented at the Seventh Annual Convention of the International Society of Traumatic Stress Studies, Washington, DC, October 1991

Fordyce DJ, Roueche JR, Prigatano GP: Enhanced emotional reactions in chronic head trauma patients. J Neurol Neurosurg Psychiatry 46:620–624, 1983

Fromm-Reichman F: Psychiatric aspects of anxiety, in Psychoanalysis and Psychotherapy, Selected Papers. Chicago, IL, University of Chicago Press, 1959, pp 306–321

Gainotti G: Emotional behavior and hemispheric side of the lesion. Cortex 8:41–55, 1972

Gass CS, Russell EW: MMPI correlates of performance intellectual deficits in patients with right hemisphere lesions. J Clin Psychol 43:484–489, 1987

Gloag D: Rehabilitation after head injury, II: behaviour and emotional problems, long-term needs, and the requirements for services. BMJ 290:913–916, 1985

Goethe KE, Levin HS: Behavioral manifestations during the early and long term stages of recovery after closed head injury. Psychiatric Annals 14:540–546, 1984

Goldstein K: The effect of brain damage on the personality. Psychiatry 15:245–260, 1952

Grafman J, Vance SC, Weingartner H, et al: The effects of lateralized frontal lesions on mood regulation. Brain 109:1127–1148, 1986

Gronwall D: Rehabilitation programs for patients with mild head injury: components, problems and evaluation. Journal of Head Trauma Rehabilitation 1(2):53–62, 1986

Gronwall D, Wrightson P: Delayed recovery of intellectual function after minor head injury. Lancet 2:605–609, 1974

Gualtieri CT: Buspirone: neuropsychiatric effects. Journal of Head Trauma Rehabilitation 6(1):90–92, 1991

Haas JF: Ethical and legal aspects of psychotropic medications in brain injury. Journal of Head Trauma Rehabilitation 2(4):6–17, 1987

Hathaway SR, McKinley JC: Minnesota Multiphasic Personality Inventory. Minneapolis, MN, University of Minnesota, 1943

Hillbom E: Aftereffects of brain injuries. Acta Psychiatrica et Neurologica Scandinavica 35 (suppl 142):1–195, 1960

Hollander E, Schiffman A, Cohen B, et al: Signs of central nervous system dysfunction in obsessive-compulsive disorder. Arch Gen Psychiatry 47:27–32, 1990

Holloway H, Ursano RJ: The Viet Nam veteran: memory, social content, and metaphor. Psychiatry 47:103–108, 1984

Horvath TB, Siever LJ, Mohs RL, et al: Organic mental syndromes and disorders, in Comprehensive Textbook of Psychiatry, Vol V. Edited by Kaplin HI, Saddock BJ. Baltimore, MD, Williams and Wilkins, 1989, pp599–641

Hugenholtz H, Stuss DT, Stethem BA, et al: How long does it take to recover from a mild concussion? Neurosurgery 22:853–858, 1988

Jann MW, Froemming JH, Borison RL: Movement disorders and new azapirone anxiolytic drugs. Journal of the American Board of Family Practice 3:111–119, 1990

Jenike MA, Brandon AD: Obsessive-compulsive disorder and head trauma: a rare association. Journal of Anxiety Disorders 2:353–359, 1988

Johnson DA, Newton A: HIPSIG: a basis for social adjustment after head injury. British Journal of Occupational Therapy 50:47–52, 1987

Kay DWK, Kerr TA, Lassman LP: Brain trauma and the post-concussional syndrome. Lancet 2:1052–1055, 1971

Kinsella G, Moran C, Ponsford J: Emotional disorder and its assessment within the severe head injured population. Psychol Med 18:57–63, 1988

Klonoff H: Head injuries in children: predisposing factors, accident conditions, accident proneness and sequelae. Am J Public Health 61:2405–2417, 1971

Kolb LC: A neuropsychological hypothesis explaining posttraumatic stress disorders. Am J Psychiatry 144:989–995, 1987

Kwentus JA, Hart RP, Peck ET, et al: Psychiatric complications of closed head trauma. Psychosomatics 26:8–17, 1985

Leininger BE, Gramling SE, Farrell AD, et al: Neuropsychological deficits in symptomatic minor head injury patients after concussion and mild concussion. J Neurol Neurosurg Psychiatry 53:293–296, 1990

Levin HS, Grossman RE: Behavioral sequelae of closed head injury. Arch Neurol 35:720–727, 1978

Lewis A: Discussion on differential diagnosis and treatment of post-concussional states. Proceedings of the Royal Society of Medicine 35:607–614, 1942

Lewis L: A framework for developing a psychotherapy treatment plan with brain-injured patients. Journal of Head Trauma Rehabilitation 6:22–29, 1991

Lewis L, Rosenberg SJ: Psychoanalytic psychotherapy with brain-injured adult psychiatric patients. J Nerv Ment Dis 178:69–77, 1990

Lezak MD: Subtle sequelae of brain damage: perplexity, distractibility and fatigue. American Journal of Physical Medicine 57:9–15, 1978

Lezak MD: Neuropsychological Assessment, 2nd Edition. New York, Oxford University Press, 1983, pp 60–61

Lipowski ZJ, Stewart AM: Illness as subjective experience. Psychiatry in Medicine 4:155–171, 1973

Lishman WA: Brain damage in relation to psychiatric disability after head injury. Br J Psychiatry 114:373–410, 1968

Lishman WA: Psychiatric sequelae of head injuries. Journal of the Irish Medical Association 71:306–314, 1978

Lishman WA: Organic Psychiatry: The Psychological Consequences of Cerebral Disorder, 2nd Edition. Oxford, Blackwell Scientific Publications, 1987

McKeon J, McGuffin P, Robinson P: Obsessive-compulsive neurosis following head injury: a report of four cases. Br J Psychiatry 144:190–192, 1984

McKinlay WW, Brooks DN, Bond MR, et al: The short-term outcome of severe blunt head injury as reported by relatives of the injured persons. J Neurol Neurosurg Psychiatry 44:527–533, 1981

McMillan TM: Post-traumatic stress disorder and severe head injury. Br J Psychiatry 159:431–433, 1991

Merskey H, Woodforde JM: Psychiatric sequelae of minor head injury. Brain 95:521–528, 1972

Morozov AM: Psychotherapy of post-traumatic borderline neuropsychiatric disorders [Psikhoterapiia posttravmaticheskikh pogranichnykh nervno-psikhicheskikh rasstroistva]. Vrachebnoe Delo 2:88–90, 1989

Morris J, Bleiberg J: Neuropsychological rehabilitation and traditional psychotherapy. International Journal of Clinical Neuropsychology 8:133–135, 1986

Mureriwa J: Head injury and compensation: a preliminary investigation of the postconcussional syndrome in Harare. Central African Journal of Medicine 36:315–318, 1990

O'Shanick GJ: Neuropsychiatric complications in head injury. Advances in Psychosomatic Medicine 16:173–193, 1986

O'Shanick GJ: Clinical aspects of psychopharmacologic treatment in head-injured patients. Journal of Head Trauma Rehabilitation 2(4):59–67, 1987

Preston GC, Ward CE, Broks P, et al: Effects of lorazepam on memory attention and sedation in man: antagonism by Ro 15-1788. Psychopharmacology 97:222–227, 1989

Roberts AH: Severe Accidental Head Injury. London, Macmillan, 1979

Rose M: The place of drugs in the management of behavior disorders after traumatic brain injury. Journal of Head Trauma Rehabilitation 3(3):7–13, 1988

Rutherford WH: Sequelae of concussion caused by minor head injuries. Lancet 1:1–4, 1977

Sbordone RJ, Jennison JH: A comparison of the OBD-168 and MMPI to assess the emotional adjustment of traumatic brain injured inpatients to their cognitive deficits. Clinical Neuropsychology 5:87–88, 1983

Schoenhuber R, Gentilini M, Orlando A: Prognostic value of auditory brain-stem responses for late postconcussion symptoms following minor head injury. J Neurosurg 68:742–744, 1988

Silver, JM, Sanberg DP, Hales RE: New approaches in the pharmacotherapy of posttraumatic stress disorder. J Clin Psychiatry 5 (Suppl):33–38, 1990

Strub RL, Black FW: Organic Brain Syndromes: An Introduction to Neurobehavioral Disorders. Philadelphia, PA, FA Davis Co., 1981

Tennant FS: Naltrexone treatment for postconcussional syndrome. Am J Psychiatry 144:813–814, 1987

Tyerman A, Humphrey M: Changes in self-concept following severe head injury. International Journal of Rehabilitation Research 7:11–23, 1984

Van Zomeren AH, Van Den Burg W: Residual complaints of patients two years after severe head injury. J Neurol Neurosurg Psychiatry 48:21–28, 1985

Wells CE, Duncan GW: Neurology for Psychiatrists. Philadelphia, PA, FA Davis, 1980, pp 120–122

Woodward, GA: Posttraumatic cortical blindness: are we missing the diagnosis in children? Pediatric Emergency Care 6:289–292, 1990

Wroblewski BA, Guidos A, Leary J, et al: Control of depression with fluoxetine and antiseizure medication in a brain-injured patient (letter). Am J Psychiatry 149:273, 1992

Yudofsky SC, Silver JM: Psychiatric aspects of brain injury trauma, stroke and tumor, in Psychiatric Update, American Psychiatric Association Annual Review, Vol 4. Edited by Hales RE, Frances AJ. Washington, DC, American Psychiatric Press, 1985, pp 142–158

Zencius A, Wesolowski MD: Brief report: using stress management to decrease inappropriate behavior in a brain injured adult. Behavioral Residential Treatment 5:61–64, 1990

Chapter 10

Aggressive Disorders

Jonathan M. Silver, M.D.
Stuart C. Yudofsky, M.D.

E xplosive and violent behavior has long been associated with focal brain lesions, as well as with diffuse damage to the central nervous system (CNS) (Elliott 1992). Irritability and/or aggressiveness is a major source of disability to brain injury patients and a source of stress to their families. Agitation that occurs during the acute stages of recovery from brain injury can endanger the safety of the patients and their caregivers. Subsequently, patients may develop low frustration tolerance and explosive behavior that can be set off by minimal provocation or occur without warning. These episodes range in severity from irritability to outbursts that result in damage to property or assaults on others. In severe cases, affected individuals cannot remain in the community or with their families, and often are referred to long-term psychiatric or neurobehavioral facilities. Therefore, it is essential that all psychiatrists be aware of this condition and its assessment and treatment, to provide effective care to patients with organically induced aggression and to their families.

Prevalence

It has been reported that during the acute recovery period, 35%–96% of patients with brain injury exhibit agitated behavior (Levin and Grossman 1978; Rao et al. 1985) (Table 10–1). After the acute recovery phase, irritability or bad temper is common. There has been only one prospective study of the occurrence of agitation and restlessness that has been monitored by an objective rating instru-

Table 10–1. Prevalence of aggression after traumatic brain injury

Studies (by type of occurrence)	Severity	N	Follow-up	Irritability or temper	Agita-tion
Acute					
Levin and Grossman 1978	All	62	Acute	—	35%
Rao et al. 1985	Severe	26	Acute	—	96%
Brooke et al. 1992	Severe	100	Acute	35% restless	11%
Chronic					
Rao et al. 1985	Severe	—	Rehabilitation	—	42%
McKinlay et al.1981	Severe	55	1 year	71%	67%
Brooks et al. 1986[a]	Severe	42	5 years	64%	64%
Oddy et al. 1985	Severe	44	7 years	43%	31%
Thomsen 1984	Severe	40	2–5 years	38%	—
Thomsen 1984	Severe	—	10–15 years	48%	—
Van Zomeren and Van Den Berg 1985	Severe	57	2 years	39%	—
Levin et al. 1979	Severe	27	1 year	37%	—
McMillan and Glucksman 1987[b]	Moderate	24	—	64%	—
Schoenhuber et al. 1988	Mild	—	1 year	54%	—
Dikmen et al. 1986[c]	Mild	20	1 month/ 1 year	70%	40%
Rutherford et al. 1977	Mild	131	1 year	5%	—

[a]Same patients as McKinlay et al. 1981; only 42 participated in the 5-year follow-up evaluation.
[b]Sixteen percent were orthopedic control subjects.
[c]Control subject: 45% irritability, 30% temper; NS.

ment, the Overt Aggression Scale (Brooke et al. 1992). These authors found that out of 100 patients with severe traumatic brain injury (TBI) (Glasgow Coma Scale score less than 8, more than 1 hour of coma, and greater than 1 week of hospitalization), only 11 patients exhibited agitated behavior. Only 3 patients manifested these behaviors for more than 1 week. However, 35 patients were observed to be restless, but not agitated. In follow-up periods ranging from 1 to 15 years after injury, these behaviors occurred in 31%–71% of patients who experienced severe TBI. Studies of mild TBI have evaluated patients for much briefer periods of time: 1-year estimates from these studies range from 5%–70%. Carlsson et al. (1987) examined the relationship between the number of traumatic brain injuries associated with loss of consciousness and various symptoms, and demonstrated that irritability increased with subsequent injuries. Of those men who did not have head injuries with loss of consciousness, 21% reported irritability, whereas 31% of men with one injury with loss of consciousness and 33% of men with two or more injuries with loss of consciousness admitted to this symptom ($P = .0001$).

Organic Aggressive Syndrome

In the acute phase after brain injury, patients often experience a period of agitation and confusion, which may last from days to months. In rehabilitation facilities, these patients are described as "Confused, Agitated" (a Rancho Los Amigos Scale score of 4), and have characteristics similar to patients with delirium (see Chapter 6). Brooke et al. (1992) suggest that agitation usually appears in the first 2 weeks of hospitalization and resolves within 2 weeks. Restlessness may appear after 2 months and may persist for 4 to 6 weeks. In our clinical experience, after the acute recovery phase has resolved, continuing aggressive outbursts have typical characteristics (Table 10–2). These episodes may occur in the presence of other emotional changes or neurological disorders that occur secondary to brain injury, such as mood lability or seizures.

Certain behavioral syndromes have been related to damage to specific areas of the frontal lobe (Auerbach 1986). The orbitofrontal syndrome is associated with behavioral excesses (e.g., impulsivity, disinhibition, hyperactivity, distractibility, and mood lability). Outbursts of rage and violent behavior occur after damage to the inferior orbital surface of the frontal lobe and anterior temporal lobes.

The DSM-III-R classification of aggression associated with brain injury was "organic personality syndrome—explosive type" (American Psychiatric Association 1987) (Table 10–3). Unfortunately, this was a "catch basket" diagnosis that in the clinical setting was over-inclusive. Specifically, this classification included many changes that may not occur concurrently with aggressive behavior, such as apathy, impaired social judgment, and suspiciousness.

The current diagnostic category in DSM-IV is "personality change due to a general medical condition" (American Psychiatric Association 1994) (Table 10–4). Patients with aggressive behavior would be specified as "aggressive type," whereas those with mood lability would be specified as "labile type." We believe that it is no less egregious to categorize the presence of rage outbursts as a "personality change" than to categorize psychotic and affective symptomatologies as personality changes. Because of the high prevalence and significant disability associated with this syndrome, we proposed a specific diagnostic category of organic aggressive

Table 10–2. Characteristic features of organic aggression syndrome

Reactive	Triggered by modest or trivial stimuli
Nonreflective	Usually does not involve premeditation or planning
Nonpurposeful	Aggression serves no obvious longterm aims or goals
Explosive	Buildup is NOT gradual
Periodic	Brief outbursts of rage and aggression; punctuated by long periods of relative calm
Ego-dystonic	After outbursts, patients are upset, concerned, and/or embarrassed, as opposed to blaming others or justifying behavior

Source. Reprinted from Yudofsky SC, Silver JM, Hales RE: "Pharmacologic Management of Aggression in the Elderly." *Journal of Clinical Psychiatry* 51 (Suppl. 10):22–28, 1990. Copyright 1990, Physicians Postgraduate Press. Used with permission.

syndrome (Table 10–5) (Silver and Yudofsky 1987; Yudofsky and Silver 1985; Yudofsky et al. 1989). The specific category of organic aggressive syndrome gives appropriate credence to the true specificity of this disorder, and would result in accurate diagnosis, specific treatment, and increased research in this condition. Future work in this area should document symptoms that often may occur concurrently with aggressive behavior. For example, many patients have both organic aggression and mood lability, with frequent episodes of tearfulness and irritability. In other patients, there is significant overlap with depression and with alcohol abuse.

Pathophysiology of Aggression

Neuroanatomy of Aggression

Many areas of the brain are involved in the production and mediation of aggressive behavior, and lesions at different levels of neuro-

---

Table 10–3.   Diagnostic criteria for organic personality syndrome, explosive type

A. Persistent personality disturbance, either life-long or representing a change or accentuation of a previously characteristic trait, involving at least one of the following:
  1. Affective instability, e.g., marked shifts from normal mood to depression, irritability, or anxiety
  2. Recurrent outbursts of aggression or rage that are grossly out of proportion to any precipitating psychosocial stressors
  3. Markedly impaired social judgment, e.g., sexual indiscretion
  4. Marked apathy and indifference
  5. Suspiciousness or paranoid ideation.
B. There is evidence from the history, physical examination, or laboratory tests of a specific organic factor (or factors) judged to be etiologically related to the disturbance.

Specify explosive type if outbursts of aggression or rage are the predominant feature.

Source. Adapted from DSM-III-R (American Psychiatric Association 1987).

nal organization can elicit specific types of aggressive behavior (Ovsiew and Yudofsky 1993). According to Valzelli (1981), several anatomic areas of the brain are important in the production (or lack of suppression) of "irritative aggression," that is, feelings of irritability with occasional explosions (Table 10–6).

Table 10–7 summarizes the roles of key regions of the brain in mediating aggression. The regulation of the neuroendocrine and autonomic responses is controlled by the hypothalamus, which is involved in "flight or fight" reactions. Investigations in animals have shown that lesions in the ventromedial hypothalamus result in

---

Table 10–4.   DSM-IV criteria for personality change due to a general medical condition

A.   A persistent personality disturbance that represents a change from the individual's previous characteristic personality pattern.

B.   There is evidence from the history, physical examination, or laboratory findings that the disturbance is the direct physiological consequence of a general medical condition.

C.   The disturbance is not better accounted by another mental disorder (including other mental disorders due to a general medical condition).

D.   The disturbance does not occur exclusively during delirium and does not meet criteria for a dementia.

E.   The disturbance causes clinically significant distress or impairment in social, occupational, or other important areas of functioning.

Specify type:

Labile type: if the predominant feature is affective lability

Disinhibited type: if the predominant feature is poor impulse control as evidenced by sexual indiscretions, etc.

Aggressive type: if the predominant feature is aggressive behavior

Apathetic type: if the predominant feature is marked apathy and indifference

Paranoid type: if the predominant feature is suspiciousness or paranoid ideation

Other type: if the predominant feature is not one of the above, (e.g., personality changes associated with a seizure disorder)

Combined type: if more than one feature predominates in the clinical picture

Unspecified

Source.   Reprinted from American Psychiatric Association: Diagnostic and Statistical Manual of Mental Disorders, 4th Edition. Washington, DC, American Psychiatric Association, 1994. Used with permission.

Table 10–5. Diagnostic criteria for proposed organic aggressive syndrome

Persistent or recurrent aggressive outbursts, whether of a verbal or physical nature.

The outbursts are out of proportion to the precipitating stress or provocation.

Evidence from history, physical examination, or laboratory tests of a specific organic factor that is judged to be etiologically related to the disturbance.

The outbursts are not primarily related to the following disorders: paranoia, mania, schizophrenia, narcissistic personality disorder, borderline disorder, conduct disorder, or antisocial personality disorder.

Source. Reprinted from Yudofsky SC, Silver JM, Yudofsky B: "Organic Personality Disorder, Explosive Type," in *Treatment of Psychiatric Disorders: A Task Force Report of the American Psychiatric Association.* Washington, DC, American Psychiatric Association, 1989, pp. 839–852. Used with permission.

nondirected rage with stereotypic behavior (i.e., scratching and biting). This area of the brain may be vulnerable to injury from diffuse axonal injury, and therefore would be associated with other deficits, such as cognitive slowing and slurred speech.

The limbic system, especially the amygdala, is responsible for mediating impulses from the prefrontal cortex and hypothalamus, and it adds emotional content to cognition and associating biological drives to specific stimuli (e.g., searching for food when hungry) (Halgren 1992). Activation of the amygdala, which can occur in seizure-like states or in kindling, may result in enhanced emotional reactions, such as outrage at personal slights. Damage to the amygdaloid area has resulted in violent behavior (Tonkonogy 1991). Injury to the anterior temporal lobe, which is a common site for contusions, has been associated with the "dyscontrol syndrome." Some patients with temporal lobe epilepsy exhibit emotional lability, impairment of impulse control, and suspiciousness (Garyfallos et al. 1988).

The most recent region of the brain to evolve, the neocortex, coordinates timing and observation of social cues, often prior to the expression of associated emotions. Due to the location of prominent bony protuberances in the base of the skull, this area of the brain is highly vulnerable to traumatic injury. Lesions in this area give rise to disinhibited anger after minimal provocation characterized by an individual showing little regard for the consequences of the affect or behavior. Patients with violent behavior have been found to have a high frequency of frontal lobe lesions (Heinrichs 1989). Frontal lesions may result in the sudden discharge of limbic and/or amygdala-generated affects—affects that are no longer modulated, processed, or inhibited by the frontal lobe. In this condition, the patient overreacts with rage and/or aggression upon thoughts or feelings that would have ordinarily been modulated, inhibited, or suppressed. In summary, prefrontal damage may cause aggression by a secondary process involving lack of inhibition of the limbic areas.

Neurotransmitters in Aggression

Many neurotransmitters are involved in the mediation of aggression, and this area has been reviewed in detail by Eichelman (1987). Among the neurotransmitter systems, serotonin, norepinephrine, dopamine, acetylcholine, and the γ-aminobutyric acid (GABA) systems have prominent roles in influencing aggressive behavior. It is often difficult to translate studies of aggression in various species of animals to a complex human behavior. Multiple neurotransmitter

Table 10–6. Areas of the brain that mediate aggressive behaviors

Triggers	Suppressors
Medial hypothalamus	Frontal lobes
Posteromedial hypothalamus	Septal nuclei
Thalamic center median	Cerebellar lobes
Thalamic lamella medialis	Cerebeller fastigium
Dorsomedial thalamus	
Anterior cingulum	
Anterior (ventral) hypothalamus	
Centromedial amygdala	

systems may be altered simultaneously by an injury that affects diffuse areas of the brain, and it may not be possible to relate any one neurotransmitter change to a specific behavior, such as aggression. In addition, different transmitters affect one another, and frequently the critical factor is the relationship among the neurotransmitters. However, in reviewing the available research data, we can advance certain generalizations that have merit in helping to understand the neurobiology of aggression and to guide treatment.

The major norepinephrine tracts in the brain start in the locus coeruleus and the lateral tegmental system and course to the forebrain, and are thus vulnerable to traumatic injury (Cooper et al. 1991). Interestingly, β_1-adrenergic receptors are located in the limbic forebrain and cerebral cortex, areas known to be involved in the mediation of aggressive behavior (Alexander et al. 1979). In patients who have sustained TBI, elevations of plasma norepinephrine have been documented (Clifton et al. 1981; Hamill et al. 1987). Animal studies suggest that norepinephrine enhances aggressive behavior, including sham-rage, affective aggression, and shock-

Table 10–7. Neuropathology of aggression

Locus	Activity
Hypothalamus	Orchestrates neuroendocrine response via sympathetic arousal
	Monitors internal status
Limbic system	
Amygdala	Activates and/or suppresses hypothalmus
	Input from neocortex
Temporal cortex	Associated with aggression in both ictal and interictal status
Frontal Neocortex	Modulates limbic and hypothalamic activity
	Associated with social and judgment aspects of aggression

Source. Reprinted from Silver JM, Hales RE, Yudofsky SC: "Neuropsychiatric Aspects of Traumatic Brain Injury," in *The American Psychiatric Press Textbook of Neuropsychiatry,* 2nd Edition. Edited by Yudofsky SC, Hales RE. Washington, DC, American Psychiatric Press, 1992, pp. 363–395. Used with permission.

induced fighting (Eichelman 1987). Higley et al. (1992) found an association between aggression in free-ranging Rhesus monkeys and norepinephrine in cerebrospinal fluid (CSF). Humans who exhibit aggressive or impulsive behavior have been shown to have increased levels of the norepinephrine metabolite 3-methoxy-4-hydroxyphenylglycol (MHPG) (G. L. Brown et al. 1979).

Serotonergic neurons originate in the raphe located in the pons and upper brain stem and project to the frontal cortex. Olivier et al. (1990) suggest that serotonin-specific drugs with putative anti-aggressive properties bind to the 5-hydroxytryptamine, subtype 1B (5-HT_{1B}), serotonin receptor, which can be found in the neocortex and hypothalamus, among other brain regions. Changes in serotonin activity have been found in patients who have sustained TBI, although these findings have been inconsistent (Bareggi et al. 1975; Van Woerkom et al. 1977; Vecht et al. 1975). Concentrations of CSF 5-hydroxyindoleacetic acid (5-HIAA) are correlated with the concentration of 5-HIAA in the frontal lobe (Knott et al. 1989; Stanley et al. 1985). Lowered levels of serotonergic activity have been associated with increased aggression in a number of studies, including studies of predatory aggression and shock-induced fighting in rats (Eichelman 1987) and in a study of free-ranging Rhesus monkeys (Higley et al. 1992). Clinical studies have confirmed the role of decreased serotonin in the expression of aggressiveness and impulsivity in humans (Kruesi et al. 1992; Linnoila and Virkkunen 1992)—particularly as it applies to self-destructive acts.

Dopamine systems are prominent in both mesolimbic and mesocortical regions. Although some investigators have found decreased levels of lumbar CSF homovanillic acid (HVA) levels, the metabolite of brain dopamine, in patients after severe TBI (Bareggi et al. 1975; Vecht et al. 1975). Porta et al. (1975) reported that ventricular CSF HVA was elevated. Hamill et al. (1987) reported elevated serum dopamine levels that correlated with the severity of the injury and with poorer outcome. Increases in dopamine may lead to aggression in several animal models (Eichelman 1987), and agitation is a common symptom in schizophrenia, often treated with antidopaminergic medications.

A cholinergic complex is found in the basal forebrain and the pontomesencephalotegmental area (Cooper et al. 1991). Elevated acetylcholine levels have been found in fluid obtained from intraventricular catheters or lumbar puncture in patients after TBI (Grossman et al. 1975). Acetylcholine has been reported to increase aggressive behaviors (Eichelman 1987).

GABA is an inhibitory neurotransmitter found throughout the brain. Although no studies have examined GABA levels after brain injury, it would be expected that injured neurons would produce less GABA. Increasing GABA, via benzodiazepines, results in reduced aggressive behavior in animals (Eichelman 1987), and GABA agonists such as the benzodiazepines have been reported to be associated with paradoxical rage attacks (Salzman et al. 1974).

Physiology of Aggression

Aggressive behavior may result from neuronal excitability of limbic system structures. For example, subconvulsive stimulation (i.e., kindling) of the amygdala leads to permanent changes in neuronal excitability (Post et al. 1982). Epileptogenic lesions in the hippocampus in cats, induced by the injection of the excitotoxic substance kainic acid, result in interictal defensive rage reactions (Engel et al. 1991). During periods that the cat experiences partial seizures, the animal exhibits heightened emotional reactivity and lability. In addition, defensive reactions can be elicited by excitatory injections to the midbrain periacqueductal gray region. Hypothalamus-induced rage reactions can be modulated by amygdaloid kindling.

Assessment of Aggression in Patients With TBI

Differential Diagnosis

Patients who exhibit aggressive behavior after sustaining TBI require a thorough assessment. Multiple factors may play a significant role in the production of aggressive behaviors in these patients. During the time period of emergence from coma, agitated behaviors can occur as the result of delirium. The usual clinical picture is one of restlessness, confusion, and disorientation. (The assessment and treatment of delirium are discussed in Chapter 6.) For patients who become aggressive after TBI, it is important to systematically assess the presence of concurrent neuropsychiatric disorders, because this may guide subsequent treatment. Thus the clinician must diagnose psychosis, depression, mania, mood lability, anxiety, seizure disorders, and other concurrent neurological conditions.

When aggressive behavior occurs during later stages of recovery, after confusion and posttraumatic amnesia have resolved, it must be determined whether or not the aggressivity and impulsivity of the individual antedated, was caused by, or was aggravated by the brain injury. Many patients with TBI have had a prior history of neuropsychiatric problems including learning disabilities, attentional deficits, behavioral problems, personality disorders, and/or drug and alcohol use. Because previous impulse dyscontrol and lability is exacerbated by brain injury, traits will intensify after damage to the prefrontal areas and other brain regions that inhibit preexisting aggressive impulses. Many patients are able to differentiate between the aggressivity exhibited before brain injury and their current dyscontrol. One patient stated "Before the accident, I engaged in hostile behavior when I wanted to and when it served my purpose; now I have no control over when I explode."

Drug effects and side effects commonly result in disinhibition or irritability (Table 10–8). By far the most common drug associated with aggression is alcohol, during both intoxication and withdrawal. Patients who were using alcohol when they incurred a brain injury exhibit longer durations of agitation when compared to patients with TBI with no detectable blood alcohol level at the time of hospitalization (Sparadeo and Gill 1989). Stimulating drugs, such as cocaine and amphetamines, as well as the stimulating antidepressants, commonly produce severe anxiety and agitation in patients with or without brain lesions. Because patients with TBI are highly likely to have concomitant alcohol or substance abuse, the clinician must consider the effects of illicit substances in all TBI patients with irritability. Antipsychotic medications often increase agitation through anticholinergic side effects, and agitation and irritability usually accompany severe akathisia. Many other drugs may produce confusional states, especially anticholinergic medications that cause agitated delirium (Beresin 1988). Drugs such as the tricyclic antidepressants (e.g., amitriptyline, imipramine, and doxepin) and the aliphatic phenothiazine antipsychotic drugs (e.g., chlorpromazine and thioridazine) are well known to have potent anticholinergic effects. However, other drugs have anticholinergic properties that are usually not considered to have these effects. These drugs include digoxin, ranitidine, cimetidine, theophylline, nifedipine, codeine, and furosemide (Tune et al. 1992).

Patients with TBI are susceptible to developing other disorders that may increase aggressive behaviors (Table 10–9), and comorbidity must always be considered in the TBI patient who is agitated. The clinician should not, a priori, assume that the brain injury, per se, is the cause of the aggressivity, but should assess the patient for the presence of other common etiologies of aggression. Because patients with neurological disorders are more susceptible to accidents, falls, and other sources of brain disorders, a neurological disorder may be the "underlying condition" that leads to the trau-

---

Table 10–8.   Medications and drugs associated with aggression

A. Alcohol: intoxication and withdrawal states

B. Hypnotic and antianxiety agents (barbiturates and benzodiazepines): intoxication and withdrawal states

C. Analgesics (opiates and other narcotics): intoxication and withdrawal states

D. Steroids (prednisone, cortisone, and anabolic steroids)

E. Antidepressants: especially in initial phases of treatment

F. Amphetamines and cocaine: aggression associated with manic excitement in early stages of abuse and secondary to paranoid ideation in later stages of use

G. Antipsychotics: high potency agents that lead to akathisia

H. Anticholinergic drugs (including over-the-counter sedatives) associated with delirium and central anticholinergic syndrome

---

Source. Reprinted from Yudofsky SC, Silver JM, Hales RE: "Pharmacologic Management of Aggression in the Elderly." *Journal of Clinical Psychiatry* 51 (Suppl. 10):22–28, 1990. Copyright 1990, Physicians Postgraduate Press. Used with permission.

matic injury. In addition, when there are exacerbations or recurrences of aggressive behavior in a patient who has been in good control, an investigation must be completed to search for other etiologies, such as medication effects, infections, pain, or changes in social circumstances.

Studies of the emotional and psychiatric syndromes associated with epilepsy have documented an increase in hostility, irritability, and aggression interictally (Mendez et al. 1986; Robertson et al. 1987). Weiger and Bear (1988) describe interictal aggression in patients with temporal lobe epilepsy. They have observed that interictal aggression is characterized by behavior that is justified on moral or ethical grounds and may develop over protracted periods of time. This aggressive behavior is distinguished from the violent behavior that occurs during the ictal or postictal period, which is characterized by its nondirected quality and the presence of an altered level of consciousness. Even in patients with temporal lobe epilepsy, there are many factors that influence aggression. In a

---

Table 10–9.   Common etiologies of organically induced aggression

A. Traumatic brain injury

B. Stroke and other cerebrovascular disease

C. Medications, alcohol and other abused substances, and over-the-counter drugs

D. Delirium (hypoxia, electrolyte imbalance, anesthesia and surgery, uremia, and so on)

E. Alzheimer's disease

F. Chronic neurological disorders: Huntington's disease, Wilson's disease, Parkinson's disease, multiple sclerosis, and systemic lupus erythematosis

G. Brain tumors

H. Infections diseases (encephalitis and meningitis)

I. Epilepsy (ictal, postictal, and interictal)

J. Metabolic disorders: hyperthyroidism or hypothyroidism, hypoglycemia, vitamin deficiencies and porphyria

---

Source. Reprinted from Yudofsky SC, Silver JM, Hales RE: "Pharmacologic Management of Aggression in the Elderly." *Journal of Clinical Psychiatry* 51 (Suppl. 10):22–28, 1990. Copyright 1990, Physicians Postgraduate Press. Used with permission.

retrospective survey of aggressive and nonaggressive patients with temporal lobe epilepsy, Herzberg and Fenwick (1988) found that aggressive behavior was associated with early onset of seizures, a long duration of behavioral problems, and the male gender. There was no significant correlation of aggression with electroencephalogram (EEG) or computed tomography scan abnormalities or a history of psychosis. These findings are consistent with those of Stevens and Hermann (1981), who critically examined the scientific literature on the association between temporal lobe epilepsy and violent behavior. They concluded that the significant factor predisposing to violence is the site of the lesion: particularly damage or dysfunction in the limbic areas of the brain.

Psychosocial factors are important in the expression of aggressive behavior. Patients with TBI may be acutely sensitive to changes in their environment or to variations in emotional support. Social conditions and support networks that existed before the injury affect the symptoms and course of recovery (G. Brown et al. 1981). Factors such as higher levels of education, income, and socioeconomic status positively affect a person's ability to return to work after minor head injury (Rimel et al. 1981).

Certain brain injury patients become aggressive only in specific circumstances, such as in the presence of particular family members. This suggests that the patient maintains some level of control over aggressive behaviors, and that the level of control may be modified by behavioral therapeutic techniques. Most families require professional support to adjust to the impulsive behavior of a violent relative with organic dyscontrol of aggression. Frequently, efforts to avoid triggering a rageful or violent episode often lead families to withdraw from a patient. This can result in the paradox that a way that the patient learns to gain attention is by being aggressive. Thus the unwanted behavior is unwittingly reinforced by familial withdrawal.

Documentation of Aggressive Behavior

Before therapeutic intervention is initiated to treat violent behavior, the clinician should document the baseline frequency of these behaviors. There are spontaneous day-to-day and week-to-week fluctuations in aggression that cannot be validly interpreted without prospective documentation. In our study of over 4,000 aggressive episodes in chronically hospitalized patients, hospital records failed to document 50%–75% of episodes (Silver and Yudofsky 1987, 1991). This study and others also indicated that aggression—like certain mood disorders—may have cyclic exacerbations. It is essential that the clinician establish a treatment plan, using objective documentation of aggressive episodes to monitor the efficacy of interventions and to designate specific time frames for the initiation and discontinuation of pharmacotherapy of acute episodes and for the initiation of pharmacotherapy for chronic aggressive behavior.

Many of the scales designed to measure rage, anger, and violence are self-report questionnaires of angry feelings, violent thoughts, or reactions to anger-provoking situations (Buss and Durkee 1957; Novaco 1976). However, patients whose cognitive abilities and/or frustration tolerance are impaired by brain injury cannot reliably complete questionnaires. Further, many patients have impaired insight into their behavior, and thus do not reliably recall or admit to past violent events.

There are few objective scales that may be used in rating aggressive behaviors. The Nurses' Observation Scale for Inpatient Evaluation (NOSIE; Honigfeld et al. 1965) and the Brief Psychiatric Rating Scale (BPRS; Overall and Gorham 1962) have a few items that rate aggressiveness, but these scales do not differentiate mild aggressive behaviors from more severe ones. Further, these scales lack the capacity to document the number or describe the types of aggressive behaviors. Other scales focus on a specific patient sample, require highly trained raters, and/or contain a large number of items to be completed (Ostrov et al. 1980; Rojahn 1984).

The Overt Aggression Scale is an operationalized instrument of proven reliability and validity that can be used to easily and effectively rate aggressive behavior in patients with a wide range of disorders (Silver and Yudofsky 1987, 1991; Yudofsky et al. 1986) (Figure 10–1). The scale comprises items that assess verbal aggression, physical aggression against objects, physical aggression against self, or physical aggression against others. Each category of

OVERT AGGRESSION SCALE (OAS)
Stuart Yudofsky, M.D., Jonathan Silver, M.D., Wynn Jackson, M.D., and Jean Endicott, Ph.D.
IDENTIFYING DATA

Name of Patient	Name of Rater
Sex of Patient: 1 Male 2 Female	Date / / (mo/da/yr) Shift: 1 Night 2 Day 3 Evening

☐ No aggressive incident(s) (verbal or physical) against self, others, or objects during the shift. (check here)

AGGRESSIVE BEHAVIOR (Check all that apply)

VERBAL AGGRESSION	PHYSICAL AGGRESSION AGAINST SELF
☐ Makes loud noises, shouts angrily ☐ Yells mild personal insults, e.g., "You're stupid!" ☐ Curses viciously, uses foul language in anger, makes moderate threats to others or self ☐ Makes clear threats of violence toward others or self (I'm going to kill you.) or requests to help to control self	☐ Picks or scratches skin, hits self, pulls hair, (with no or minor injury only) ☐ Bangs head, hits fist into objects, throws self onto floor or into objects (hurts self without serious injury) ☐ Small cuts or bruises, minor burns ☐ Mutilates self, makes deep cuts, bites that bleed, internal injury fracture, loss of consciousness, loss of teeth

PHYSICAL AGGRESSION AGAINST OBJECTS	PHYSICAL AGGRESSION AGAINST OTHER PEOPLE
☐ Slams door, scatters clothing, makes a mess ☐ Throws objects down, kicks furniture without breaking it, marks the wall ☐ Break objects, smashes windows ☐ Sets fires, throws objects dangerously	☐ Makes threatening gesture, swings at people, grabs at clothes ☐ Strikes, kicks, pushes, pulls hair (without injury to them) ☐ Attacks others causing mild–moderate physical injury (bruises, sprain, welts) ☐ Attacks others causing severe physical injury (broken bones, deep lacerations, internal injury)

Time incident began: _ _ : _ _ AM/PM	Duration of incident: _ _ : _ _ (hours/minutes)

INTERVENTION (check all that apply)

☐ None ☐ Talking to patient ☐ Closer observation ☐ Holding patient	☐ Immediate medication given by mouth ☐ Immediate medication given by injection ☐ Isolation without seclusion (time out) ☐ Seclusion	☐ Use of restraints ☐ Injury requires immediate medical treatment for patient ☐ Injury requires immediate treatment for other person

COMMENTS

Figure 10–1. The Overt Aggression Scale.
Source. Reprinted from Yudofsky SC, Silver JM, Jackson W, et al: "The Overt Aggression Scale for the Objective Rating of Verbal and Physical Aggression." *American Journal of Psychiatry* 143:35–39, 1986. Used with permission.

aggression has four levels of severity that are defined by objective criteria. An aggression score can be derived, which equals the sum of the most severe ratings of each type of aggressive behavior over a particular time course. Aggressive behavior can be monitored by staff or family members using the Overt Aggression Scale.

Treatment

Aggressive and agitated behaviors may be treated in a variety of settings, ranging from the acute brain injury unit in a general hospital, to a "neurobehavioral" unit in a rehabilitation facility, to outpatient environments including the home setting. A multifactorial, multidisciplinary, collaborative approach to treatment is necessary in most cases. The continuation of family treatments, psychopharmacologic interventions, and insight-oriented psychotherapeutic approaches are often required.

Although there is no medication that is approved by the FDA specifically for the treatment of aggression, medications are widely used (and commonly misused) in the management of patients with acute or chronic aggression. After diagnosis and treatment of underlying causes of aggression (e.g., brain tumor), and evaluation and documentation of aggressive behaviors, the use of pharmacological interventions can be considered in two categories: 1) the use of the sedating effects of medications, as required in acute situations, so that the patient does not harm himself or herself or others; and 2) the use of nonsedating antiaggressive medications for the treatment, when necessary, for chronic aggression. The clinician must be aware that patients may not respond to just one medication, but may require combination treatment, similar to the pharmacotherapeutic treatment for refractory depression.

Pharmacotherapy for Acute Aggression and Agitation

Agitation, irritability, rage, and/or violence may occur during the early phases of recovery after TBI. In the treatment of agitation and for treating acute episodes of aggressive behavior, medications that are sedating may be indicated. However, because these drugs are not specific in their ability to inhibit aggressive behaviors, there may be detrimental effects on arousal and cognitive function. Therefore, the use of sedation-producing medications must be time-limited to avoid the emergence of seriously disabling side effects ranging from oversedation to tardive dyskinesia. Some clinicians have suggested the use of amantadine, a dopamine agonist drug, or clonidine, an α-adrenergic agonist, as specific treatments of acute agitation beyond these drugs' sedating effects. We will also review this work.

∎ **Antipsychotic drugs.** Antipsychotic drugs are the most commonly used medications in the treatment of aggression. Although these agents are appropriate and effective when aggression is related to active psychosis, the use of neuroleptic agents to treat chronic aggression, especially secondary to organic brain injury, is often ineffective and entails significant risks that the patient will develop serious complications. Usually, it is the sedative side effects rather than the antipsychotic properties of antipsychotics that are used (i.e., misused) to "treat" (i.e., mask) the aggression. Often, patients develop tolerance to the sedative effects of the neuroleptics and, therefore, require increasing doses. As a result, extrapyramidal and anticholinergic-related side effects occur. Paradoxically (and frequently), because of the development of akathisia, the patient may become more agitated and restless as the dose of neuroleptic is increased, especially when a high potency antipsychotic such as haloperidol (Haldol) is administered. The akathisia is often mistaken for increased irritability and agitation, and a "vicious cycle" of increasing neuroleptics and worsening akathisias occurs. Herrera et al. (1988) demonstrated that there was a marked increase in violent behavior when patients with schizophrenia were treated with haloperidol (doses up to 60 mg/day) when compared with the behaviors that occurred during treatment with chlorpromazine (1800 mg/day) or clozapine (900 mg/day), two drugs that are associated with less akathisia than is haloperidol.

There is some evidence, from studies of injury to motor neurons in animals, that haloperidol has a detrimental effect on recovery.

This effect was seen only when animals actively participated in a behavioral task, not when they were restrained after drug administration (Feeney et al. 1982). It is possible that the effect of decreasing dopamine and inhibiting neuronal function, which may be the mechanism of action to treat aggression, may have other detrimental effects on recovery. Whether this finding is generalizable to recovery in brain injury remains unclear. However, the finding raises important potential risk-benefit issues that must be considered before antipsychotics are used to treat aggressive behavior.

Although other investigators have recommended antipsychotic drugs such as haloperidol for the treatment of agitation with closed head injury (Rao et al. 1985), we recommend the use of antipsychotic agents only for the management of aggression stemming from psychotic ideation or for the intermittent management of brief aggressive events related to organic dyscontrol (due to the sedative effects of neuroleptics). Table 10–10 summarizes the most disabling side effects that occur when neuroleptics are used to treat aggression in patients with TBI. Table 10–11 summarizes our prescribing regimen with haloperidol for the management of acute aggression.

■ **Sedatives and hypnotics.** The literature is inconsistent with regard to the effects of the benzodiazepines in the treatment of

---

Table 10–10. Common side effects of neuroleptics when used to treat patients with chronic aggression

---

Oversedation

Hypotension (falls)

Confusion

Neuroleptic malignant syndrome

Parkinsonian side effects

Akathisia

Dystonia

Tardive dyskinesia

Source. Reprinted from Yudofsky SC, Silver JM, Hales RE: "Pharmacologic Management of Aggression in the Elderly." *Journal of Clinical Psychiatry* 51 (Suppl. 10):22–28, 1990. Copyright 1990, Physicians Postgraduate Press. Used with permission.

Table 10–11.	Use of haloperidol in the management of aggression.

A. At first, 1 mg po or 0.5 mg iv or im every hour until control of aggression is achieved.

B. Then, haloperidol 2 mg po or 1 mg iv or im every 8 hours.

C. When patient is not agitated or violent for a period of 48 hours, taper at rate of 25% of highest daily dose.

D. If violent behavior reemerges on tapering drug, reassess etiology and consider changing to a more specific medication to manage chronic aggression.

E. Do not maintain patient on haloperidol for more than 6 weeks—except for aggression secondary to psychosis.

Source. Reprinted from Yudofsky SC, Silver JM, Hales RE: "Pharmacologic Management of Aggression in the Elderly." *Journal of Clinical Psychiatry* 51 (Suppl. 10):22–28, 1990. Copyright 1990, Physicians Postgraduate Press. Used with permission.

aggression. The sedative properties of benzodiazepines are especially helpful in the acute management of agitation and aggression (Silver and Yudofsky 1988; Yudofsky et al. 1987). Most likely, this is due to the effect of benzodiazepines on increasing the inhibitory neurotransmitter GABA. Several studies report increased hostility and aggression and the paradoxical induction of rage in patients treated with benzodiazepines (Silver and Yudofsky 1988; Yudofsky et al. 1987). However, these reports are balanced by the observation that this phenomenon is rare (Dietch and Jennings 1988). Table 10–12 summarizes the side effects associated with the use of benzodiazepines in patients with brain injury.

Benzodiazepines can produce amnesia (Angus and Romney 1984; Lucki et al. 1986; Roth et al. 1980). Preexisting memory dysfunctions or those associated with TBI can be exacerbated following the administration of benzodiazepines. Brain injury patients may also experience increased problems in coordination and balance with benzodiazepine use.

If sedation is necessary in the management of acute aggression, medications such as paraldehyde, chloral hydrate, or diphenhydramine may be preferable to sedative antipsychotic agents. Intramuscular lorazepam has been suggested as an effective medication in the emergency treatment of the violent patient (Bick and Hannah

1986). Lorazepam in 1 or 2 mg doses, administered either orally or by injection, may be administered, if necessary, in combination with a neuroleptic medication (haloperidol, 2 to 5 mg). Table 10–13 summarizes our use of lorazepam to treat acute aggression.

■ **Other medications.** Because of the potential detrimental effects of the antipsychotic medications and benzodiazepines, other agents have been used to treat acute agitation and aggression in patients with TBI. Gualtieri et al. (1989) reported that amantadine, a dopamine agonist drug, decreased aggressive behavior in a number of patients who were "severely agitated" in "coma recovery." Dosages used were 50 to 400 mg/day, and response was usually noted within days at a specific dosage. The hypothesized mechanism is through stimulation of striatal and cortical dopamine neurons. We have noted that several patients with severe TBI and poor arousal developed seizures after treatment with amantadine. Although this effect has not been reported to occur frequently, we believe that the clinician should be aware of this possible reaction.

There have been anecdotal reports of the use of the α-adrenergic agonist clonidine to treat acute agitation (J. W. Cassidy, personal communication, 1992). Clonidine acutely inhibits the activity of the locus ceruleus and decreases adrenergic transmission. It expectedly decreases blood pressure, and is also highly sedating. Patients should be started on low dosages (0.05 mg tid) with careful monitoring of blood pressure.

Table 10–12. Common side effects of benzodiazepines when used to treat patients with chronic aggression

---

Oversedation
Motor disturbances (poor coordination)
Mood disturbances
Memory impairment, confusion
Dependency, overdoses, withdrawal syndromes
Paradoxical violence

Source. Reprinted from Yudofsky SC, Silver JM, Hales RE: "Pharmacologic Management of Aggression in the Elderly." *Journal of Clinical Psychiatry* 51 (Suppl. 10):22–28, 1990. Copyright 1990, Physicians Postgraduate Press. Used with permission.

Table 10–13.   Use of lorazepam in the acute management of aggression

---

A.   Lorazepam 1–2 mg po or im.

B.   Repeat every hour until patient is calm.

C.   Once patient is no longer violent or agitated, maintain at maximum of 2 mg po or im tid.

D.   When patient is not agitated or violent for 48 hours, taper at rate of 10% of highest total daily dose.

E.   If violent behavior reemerges on tapering drug, reassess etiology and consider changing to a more specific medication to manage chronic aggression.

F.   If, after 6 weeks, lorazepam cannot be tapered without reemergence of aggression, reevaluate and revise treatment plan to include a more specific medication to manage chronic aggression.

Source.   Adapted from Yudofsky et al. 1990. Used with permission.

Propranolol, although more often used for the treatment of chronic aggression, has been used to treat acute aggressive behavior after traumatic or hypoxic brain injury (Elliott 1977). Unfortunately, this work has not been repeated to substantiate this early and encouraging report.

Pharmacotherapy for Treatment of Chronic Aggression

If a patient continues to exhibit periods of agitation or aggression beyond several weeks, the use of specific antiaggressive medications should be initiated to prevent these episodes from occurring. The choice of medication may be guided by the underlying hypothesized mechanism of action (e.g., effects on serotonin system, adrenergic system, and kindling), or in consideration of the predominant clinical features. Given that no medication has been approved by the FDA for treatment of aggression, the clinician must use medications that may be antiaggressive but may have been approved for other uses (e.g., for seizure disorders, depression, and hypertension).

∎ **Antipsychotic medications.** The use of antipsychotic medication has been previously discussed. If, after thorough clinical evaluation, it is determined that the aggressive episodes result from psychosis, such as paranoid delusions or command hallucinations, then antipsychotic medications will be the treatment of choice. (Guidelines for the use of antipsychotic medications in patients with brain injury are found in Chapters 8 and 19.) Clozapine may have greater antiaggressive effects than do other antipsychotic medications (Ratey et al. 1993; Volavka et al. 1993).

∎ **Anticonvulsive medications.** The anticonvulsant carbamazepine has proven effective for the treatment of bipolar disorders and has also been advocated for the control of aggression in both epileptic and nonepileptic populations (Yudofsky et al. 1987). The mechanism of action of anticonvulsants in the treatment of organic aggression may be through their effect on inhibiting kindling. Several noncontrolled studies have indicated that carbamazepine may be effective in decreasing aggressive behavior associated with dementia (Gleason and Schneider 1990; Leibovici and Tariot 1988), developmental disabilities (Folks et al. 1982; Tunks and Dermer 1973; Yatham and McHale 1988), and schizophrenia (Hakoloa and Laulumaa 1982; Luchins 1983), as well as a variety of other organic brain disorders (Mattes 1988). Carbamazepine can be a highly effective medication to treat aggression in patients with brain injury, and we believe it is the drug of choice for those patients who have aggressive episodes with concomitant seizures or epileptic foci. Reports also indicate that the antiaggressive response can be found in patients with (Hakoloa and Laulumaa 1982; Stone et al. 1986; Tunks and Dermer 1973; Yatham and McHale 1988) and without (Luchins 1983; Mattes 1988, 1990) EEG abnormalities.

Although a specific antiaggressive response to carbamazepine has not yet been demonstrated according to the most strict scientific criteria, a vast amount of clinical experience strongly suggests the efficacy of carbamazepine. However, the clinician should also be aware of the potential risks associated with carbamazepine treatment, particularly bone marrow suppression (including aplastic anemia) and hepatotoxicity. Complete blood counts and liver function tests should be appropriately monitored (Silver and Yudofsky 1988). Hematologic monitoring (complete blood count and platelet count) should be obtained every 2 weeks for the first 2 months of treatment, and every 3 months thereafter. Liver function monitoring (serum glutamic-oxaloacetic transaminase [SGOT], serum glutamic-pyruvic transaminase [SGPT], lactate dehydrogenase [LDH], alkaline phosphatase) should be obtained every month for the first 2 months of treatment, and every 3 months thereafter. In our experience and that of others (Giakas et al. 1990), the anticonvulsant valproic acid may also be helpful to some patients with organically induced aggression (Mattes 1992). For those patients with aggression and epilepsy whose seizures are being treated with anticonvulsant drugs such as phenytoin and phenobarbital, switching to carbamazepine or to valproic acid may treat both conditions.

▌ **Lithium carbonate.** Although lithium is known to be effective in controlling aggression related to manic excitement, many studies suggest that it may also have a role in the treatment of aggression in selected, nonbipolar patient populations (Yudofsky et al. 1987). These include patients with TBI (Haas and Cope 1985), patients with mental retardation who exhibit self-injurious (Luchins and Dojka 1989) or aggressive behavior (Craft et al. 1987; Dale 1980; Dostal and Zvolsky 1970; Worrall et al. 1975), children and adolescents with behavioral disorders (Campbell et al. 1972; Vetro et al. 1985), prison inmates (Sheard et al. 1976; Tupin et al. 1973), and patients with other organic brain syndromes (Williams and Goldstein 1979). Primary antiaggressive effects may be due to lithium's effect on the serotonergic system, although lithium also affects other important neuronal systems, such as inositol phosphate metabolism and kindling (Berrige et al. 1989).

Patients with brain injury have increased sensitivity to the neurotoxic effects of lithium (Hornstein and Seliger 1989; Moskowitz and Altshuler 1991). Because of lithium's potential for neurotoxicity and its relative lack of efficacy in many patients with aggression secondary to brain injury, we recommend the use of lithium in those patients whose aggression is related to manic effects or recurrent irritability related to cyclic mood disorders.

▮ **Antidepressants.** Antidepressants may have effects on serotonin, norepinephrine, and other neurotransmitter systems. The antidepressants reported to control aggressive behavior have been
those acting preferentially (amitriptyline) or specifically (trazodone
and fluoxetine) on serotonin. In open studies, Mysiw et al. (1988)
and Jackson et al. (1985) reported that amitriptyline (maximum
dose 150 mg/day) was effective in the treatment of patients with
recent severe brain injury whose agitation had not responded to
behavioral techniques. Szlabowicz and Stewart (1990) successfully
treated a 43-year-old man with aggressive behavior subsequent to
anoxic encephalopathy with amitriptyline 75 mg at bedtime.
Trazodone has also been reportedly effective in treating aggression
occurring with organic mental disorders (Greenwald et al. 1986;
Pinner and Rich 1988; Simpson and Foster 1986; Zubieta and Alessi
1992). Gedye (1991) reported that a 17-year-old mentally handicapped and autistic boy with aggressive and self-injurious behavior
had a favorable response after treatment with trazodone. Preliminary reports have been published on the use of fluoxetine, a potent
serotonergic antidepressant, in the treatment of aggressive behavior
in a patient with brain injury (Sobin et al. 1989), as well as patients
with personality disorders (Coccaro et al. 1990) and depression
(Fava et al. 1993). There have also been reports on the therapeutic
effect of fluoxetine in adolescents with mental retardation and self-
injurious behavior (Bass and Beltis 1991; King 1991). We have used
fluoxetine with considerable success in aggressive patients with
brain lesions. The dosage may be started with 10 mg/day, and
increased to 20 mg after 1 week. Cassidy (1989) reported on an
open trial using fluoxetine with 8 patients with severe TBI and
associated depression. Interestingly, half the patients experienced
sedative side effects, and 3 of them reported an increase in the
levels of anxiety.

Patients with emotional lability may also experience episodes of
aggressive behavior. Ross and Rush (1981) reported the case of a
38-year-old woman who had a TBI with loss of consciousness
extending 2 to 3 weeks after the accident. The authors examined
the patient 2 years later to discover that she was irritable and
exhibited pathologic laughing and crying, weight gain, and perva-

sive feelings of sadness and helplessness. The results of a head cerebral tomographic scan revealed bilateral prefrontal atrophy. Nonetheless, she had a "remarkable improvement in her behavior, with total resolution of her dysphoria" after treatment with nortriptyline at a dose of 100 mg/day.

We have evaluated and treated many patients with emotional lability characterized by frequent episodes of tearfulness and irritability, and the full symptomatic picture of organic aggressive syndrome (see Table 10–2). These patients, who would be diagnosed under DSM-IV as having personality change due to a general medical condition, labile type (Table 10–5), have responded well to antidepressants, consistent with the reports of Schiffer et al. (1985), who used amitriptyline for patients with multiple sclerosis, and Seliger et al. (1992) and Sloan et al. (1992), who used fluoxetine to treat patients after brain injury, stroke, or multiple sclerosis. In addition, it appears that sertraline, a new specific serotonin-reuptake inhibitor, is effective as well. It is usually necessary to administer these medications at standard antidepressant dosages to obtain full therapeutic effects.

▌ **Antianxiety medications.** As discussed earlier, serotonin appears to be a critical neurotransmitter in the modulation of aggressive behavior. In preliminary reports, buspirone, a 5-HT$_{1A}$ agonist, has been reported to be effective in the management of aggression and agitation in patients with head injury (Gualtieri 1991a, 1991b; Levine 1988; Ratey et al. 1992a), dementia (Colenda 1988; Tiller et al. 1988), and in the developmentally disabled and autistic (Ratey et al. 1989; Realmuto et al. 1989). We have also noted that some patients become more aggressive when treated with buspirone. Therefore, buspirone should be initiated at low dosages (i.e., 5 mg bid) and increased by 5 mg every 3–5 days. Dosages of 45–60 mg per day may be required before there is improvement in aggressive behavior.

Clonazepam may be effective in the long-term management of aggression, although controlled, double-blind studies have not been conducted. Freinhar and Alvarez (1986) found that clonazepam decreased agitation in 3 elderly patients with organic brain syndromes. Keats and Mukherjee (1988) reported antiaggressive effects of clonazepam in a patient with schizophrenia and seizures. We use clonazepam when pronounced aggression and anxiety occur together, or when aggression occurs in association with neurologically induced tics and similarly disinhibited motor behaviors. Doses should be initiated at 0.5 mg bid. Sedation and ataxia are frequent side effects.

■ **Antihypertensive medications (beta-blockers).** Since the first report of the use of β-adrenergic receptor blockers in the treatment of acute aggression in 1977, over 25 papers have appeared in the neurological and psychiatric literature reporting experience in using beta-blockers with over 200 patients with aggression (Silver and Yudofsky 1988; Yudofsky et al. 1987). Most of these patients had been unsuccessfully treated with antipsychotics, minor tranquilizers, lithium, and/or anticonvulsants before treatment with beta-blockers. The beta-blockers that have been investigated in controlled prospective studies include propranolol (a lipid-soluble, nonselective receptor antagonist) (Greendyke et al. 1986; Mattes 1988), nadolol (a water-soluble, nonselective receptor antagonist) (Alpert et al. 1990; Ratey et al. 1992b), and pindolol (a lipid-soluble, nonselective β-adrenergic receptor antagonist with partial sympathomimetic activity) (Greendyke and Kantor 1986; Greendyke et al. 1984, 1989). A list of beta-blockers and their pharmacologic properties is shown in Table 10–14. All beta-blockers are β_1-adrenergic antagonists. A growing body of preliminary evidence suggests that β-adrenergic receptor blockers are effective agents for the treatment of aggressive and violent behaviors, particularly those related to organic brain syndrome. Guidelines for the use of propranolol are listed in Table 10–15. When a patient requires the use of a once-a-day medication because of compliance difficulties, long-acting propranolol (Inderal LA) or nadolol (Corgard) can be utilized in once-a-day regimens. When patients develop bradycardia that prevents prescribing therapeutic dosages of propranolol, pindolol (Visken) can be substituted, using one-tenth the dosage of propranolol. Pindolol's intrinsic sympathomimetic activity stimulates the β-adrenergic receptor and restricts the development of bradycardia.

Table 10–14. Pharmacological characteristics of β-adrenergic receptor antagonists

Drug name (by receptor selectivity)	Trade name	Potency[a]	Local anesthetic activity	Intrinsic sympathominetic activity	Lipid soluble	Plasma half-life
Nonselective						
(β$_1$ and β$_2$) antagonists						
Alprenolol	Aptine	0.3–1	+	++	++	2–3
Nadolol	Corgard	0.5	0	0	0	14–18
Pindolol	Visken	5–10	+/–	++	+	3–4
Propranolol	Inderal	1.0	++	0	++	3–5
Sotalol	Sotalex	0.3	0	0	0	5–12
Timolol	Blockadren	5–10	0	+/–	0	4
Selective						
(β$_1$) antagonists						
Acebutalol	Sectral	0.3	+	+	0	3
Atenolol	Tenormin	1.0	0	0	0	6–8
Metoprolol	Lopressor	0.5–2	+/–	0	+	3–4

Note. 0 = none; +/– = questionable; + = intermediate; ++ = significant.
[a]Propranolol = 1.
Source. Data from Hoffman and Lefkowitz 1990 and American Medical Association Division of Drugs 1986.

The mechanism of action of beta-blockers in the treatment of aggression is not known. Although some investigators have hypothesized a peripheral (i.e., nonbrain) site of action secondary to decreased afferent input to the brain (Ratey et al. 1992b), even "non–lipid-soluble" β-adrenergic antagonists, when used over several days, gain access to the CNS (Gengo et al. 1988). Considering the presence of β-adrenergic receptors in the CNS, as well as the fact that these agents have antiaggressive effects when they are administered to animals intraventricularly (Leavitt et al. 1989), we

---

Table 10–15. Clinical use of propranolol

1. Conduct a thorough medical evaluation.

2. Exclude patients with the following disorders: bronchial asthma, chronic obstructive pulmonary disease, insulin-dependent diabetes mellitus, congestive heart failure, persistent angina, significant peripheral vascular disease, and hyperthyroidism.

3. Avoid sudden discontinuation of propranolol (particularly in patients with hypertension).

4. Begin with a single test-dose of 20 mg/day in patients for whom there are clinical concerns with hypotension or bradycardia. Increase dose of propranolol by 20 mg/day every 3 days.

5. Initiate propranolol on a 20 mg tid schedule for patients without cardiovascular or cardiopulmonary disorder.

6. Increase the dosage of propranolol by 60 mg/day every 3 days.

7. Increase medication unless the pulse rate is reduced below 50 bpm, or systolic blood pressure is less than 90 mmHg.

8. Do not administer medication if severe dizziness, ataxia, or wheezing occurs. Reduce or discontinue propranolol if such symptoms persist.

9. Increase dose to 12 mg/kg body weight or until aggressive behavior is under control.

10. Doses of greater than 800 mg are not usually required to control aggressive behavior.

11. Maintain the patient on the highest dose of propranolol for at least 8 weeks before concluding that the patient is not responding to the medication. Some patients, however, may respond rapidly to propranolol.

12. Use concurrent medications with caution. Monitor plasma levels of all antipsychotic and anticonvulsive medications.

Source. Reprinted from Yudofsky SC, Silver JM, Schneider SE: "Pharmacologic Treatment of Aggression." *Psychiatric Annals* 17:397–407, 1987. Used with permission.

believe that there is a central site of action.

The major side effects of beta-blockers when used to treat aggression are reduced blood pressure and pulse rate. Because peripheral β-adrenergic receptors are fully inhibited after doses of 300–400 mg/day are administered, further decreases in these parameters usually do not occur even when doses are increased to much higher levels. Despite reports of depression with the use of beta-blockers, controlled trials and our experience indicate that it is a rare occurrence (Yudofsky 1992). Because the use of propranolol is associated with significant increases in plasma levels of thioridazine, which has an absolute dosage ceiling of 800 mg/day, the combination of these two medications should be avoided whenever possible (Silver et al. 1986).

Table 10–16 summarizes our recommendations for the utilization of various classes of medication in the treatment of aggressive disorders. In treating aggression, the clinician, where possible, should diagnose and treat underlying disorders, and utilize, where possible, antiaggressive agents specific for those disorders. When there is partial response after a therapeutic trial with a specific medication, adjunctive treatment using a medication with a different mechanism of action should be instituted. For example, a patient with partial response to beta-blockers may show more improvement with the addition of an anticonvulsant or a serotonergic antidepressant.

Behavioral Treatment

It is clear that aggression can be caused and influenced by a combination of environmental and biological factors. Because of the dangerous and unpredictable nature of aggression, caregivers, both in institutions and at home, have intense and sometimes injudicious reactions to aggression when it occurs. Behavioral treatments have been shown to be highly effective in treating patients with organic aggression and may be useful when combined with pharmacotherapy. (A discussion of behavioral treatment is found in Chapter 22; for a review article see Corrigan et al. 1993.)

Conclusions

Aggressive behavior after brain injury is common and can be highly disabling. Aggression often significantly impedes appropriate rehabilitation and reintegration into the community. There are many neurobiological factors that can lead to aggressive behavior after injury. After appropriate evaluation and assessment of possible etiologies, treatment begins with the documentation of the aggressive episodes. Psychopharmacologic strategies differ according to whether the medication is for the treatment of acute aggression or the need to prevent episodes in the patient with chronic aggression. Although the treatment of acute aggression involves the judicious use of sedation, the treatment of chronic aggression is guided by underlying diagnoses and symptomatologies. Behavioral strategies remain an important component in the comprehensive treatment of aggression. In this manner, aggression can be controlled with minimal cognitive adverse sequelae.

Table 10–16. Psychopharmacological treatment of chronic aggression

Agent	Indications	Special clinical considerations
Antipsychotics	Psychotic symptoms	Oversedation and multiple side effects
Benzodiazepines	Anxiety symptoms	Paradoxical rage
Anticonvulsants		
Carbamazepine (CBZ)	Seizure disorder	Bone marrow suppression
Valproic acid (VPA)		(CBZ) and hepatoxicity (CBZ and VPA)
Lithium	Manic excitement or bipolar disorder	Neurotoxicity and confusion
Buspirone	Persistent, underlying anxiety and/or depression	Delayed onset of action
Propranolol (and other beta-blockers)	Chronic or recurrent aggression	Latency of 4–6 weeks
Serotonergic antidepressants	Depression or mood lability with irritability	May need usual clinical doses

Source. Adapted from Yudofsky et al. 1987. Used with permission.

References

Alexander RW, Davis JN, Lefkowitz RJ: Direct identification and characterization of β-adrenergic receptors in rat brain. Nature 258:437–440, 1979

Alpert M, Allan ER, Citrome L, et al: A double-blind, placebo-controlled study of adjunctive nadolol in the management of violent psychiatric patients. Psychopharmacol Bull 28:367–371, 1990

American Medical Association Division of Drugs: AMA Drug Evaluations, 6th Edition. Chicago, IL, American Medical Association, 1986

American Psychiatric Association: Diagnostic and Statistical Manual of Mental Disorders, 3rd Edition, Revised. Washington, DC, American Psychiatric Association, 1987

American Psychiatric Association: Diagnostic and Statistical Manual of Mental Disorders, 4th Edition. Washington, DC, American Psychiatric Association, 1994

Angus WR, Romney DM: The effect of diazepam on patients' memory. J Clin Psychopharmacol 4:203–206, 1984

Auerbach SH: Neuroanatomical correlates of attention and memory disorders in traumatic brain injury: an application of neurobehavioral subtypes. Journal of Head Trauma Rehabilitation 1:1–12, 1986

Bareggi SR, Porta M, Selenati A, et al: Homovanillic acid and 5-hydroxyindole-acetic acid in the CSF of patients after a severe head injury, I: lumbar CSF concentration in chronic brain post-traumatic syndromes. Eur Neurol 13:528–544, 1975

Bass JN, Beltis J: Therapeutic effect of fluoxetine on naltrexone-resistant self-injurious behavior in an adolescent with mental retardation. Journal of Child and Adolescent Psychopharmacology 1:331–340, 1991

Beresin E: Delirium in the elderly. J Geriatr Psychiatry Neurol 1:127–143, 1988

Berrige MJ, Downes CP, Hanley MR: Neural and developmental actions of lithium: a unifying hypothesis. Cell 59:411–419, 1989

Bick PA, Hannah AL: Intramuscular lorazepam to restrain violent patients. Lancet 1:206, 1986

Brooke MM, Questad KA, Patterson DR, et al: Agitation and restlessness after closed head injury: a prospective study of 100 consecutive admissions. Arch Phys Med Rehabil 73:320–323, 1992

Brooks N, Campsie L, Symington C, et al: The five-year outcome of severe blunt head injury: a relative's view. J Neurol Neurosurg Psychiatry 49:764–770, 1986

Brown G, Chadwick O, Shaffer D, et al: A prospective study of children with head injuries, III: psychiatric sequelae. Psychol Med 11:63–78, 1981

Brown GL, Goodwin FK, Ballenger JC, et al: Aggression in humans correlates with cerebrospinal fluid amine metabolites. Psychiatry Res 1:131–139, 1979

Buss AH, Durkee A: An inventory for assessing different kinds of hostility. J Consult Psychol 21:343–349, 1957

Carlsson GS, Svardsudd K, Welin L: Long-term effects of head injuries sustained during life in three male populations. J Neurosurg 67:197–205, 1987

Cambell M, Fishe B, Korein J, et al: Lithium and chlorpromazine: a controlled crossover study of hyperactive severely disturbed young children. Journal of Autism and Childhood Schizophrenia 2:234–263, 1972

Cassidy JW: Fluoxetine: a new serotonergically active antidepressant. Journal of Head Trauma Rehabilitation 4:67–69, 1989

Clifton GL, Ziegler MG, Grossman RG: Circulating catecholamines and sympathetic activity after head injury. Neurosurgery 8:10–14, 1981

Coccaro EF, Astill JL, Herbert JL, et al: Fluoxetine treatment of impulsive aggression in DSM-III-R personality disorder patients. J Clin Psychopharmacol 10:373–375, 1990

Colenda CC: Buspirone in treatment of agitated demented patient. Lancet 1:1169, 1988

Cooper JR, Bloom FE, Roth RH: The Biochemical Basis of Neuropharmacology, 6th Edition. New York, Oxford University Press, 1991

Corrigan PW, Yudofsky SC, Silver JM: Pharmacological and behavioral treatments for aggressive psychiatric inpatients. Hosp Comm Psychiatry 44:125–133, 1993

Craft M, Ismail IA, Krishnamurti D, et al: Lithium in the treatment of aggression in mentally handicapped patients: a double-blind trial. Br J Clin Psychiatry 150:685–689, 1987

Dale PG: Lithium therapy in aggressive mentally subnormal patients. Br J Psychiatry 137:469–474, 1980

Dietch JT, Jennings RK: Aggressive dyscontrol in patients treated with benzodiazepines. J Clin Psychiatry 49:184–189, 1988

Dikmen S, McLean A, Termkin N: Neuropsychological and psychosocial consequences of minor head injury. J Neurol Neurosurg Psychiatry 49:1227–1232, 1986

Dostal T, Zvolsky P: Antiaggressive effects of lithium salts in severe mentally retarded adolescents. International Pharmacopsychiatry 5:203–207, 1970

Eichelman B: Neurochemical and psychopharmacologic aspects of aggressive behavior, in Psychopharmacology: The Third Generation of Progress. Edited by Meltzer HY. New York, Raven Press, 1987, pp 697–704

Elliott FA: Propranolol for the control of belligerent behavior following acute brain damage. Ann Neurol 5:489–491, 1977

Elliott FA: Violence: The neurologic contribution: an overview. Arch Neurol 49:595–603, 1992

Engel Jr J, Bandler R, Griffith NC, et al: Neurobiological evidence for epilepsy-induced interictal disturbances, in Advances in Neurology, Vol 55: Neurobehavioral Problems in Epilepsy. Edited by Smith D, Treiman D, Trimble M. New York, Raven, 1991, pp 97–111

Fava M, Rosenbaum JF, Pava JA, et al: Anger attacks in unipolar depression, I: clinical correlates and response to fluoxetine treatment. Am J Psychiatry 150:1158–1163, 1993

Feeney DM, Gonzalez A, Law WA: Amphetamine, haloperidol, and experience interact to affect rate of recovery after motor cortex injury. Science 217:855–857, 1982

Folks DG, King LD, Dowdy SB, et al: Carbamazepine treatment of selective affectively disordered inpatients. Am J Psychiatry 139:115–117, 1982

Freinhar JP, Alvarez WA: Clonazepam treatment of organic brain syndromes in three elderly patients. J Clin Psychiatry 47:525–526, 1986

Garyfallos G, Manos N, Adamopoulou A: Psychopathology and personality characteristics of epileptic patients: epilepsy, psychopathology and personality. Acta Psychiatr Scand 78:87–95, 1988

Gedye A: Trazodone reduced aggressive and self-injurious movements in a mentally handicapped male patient with autism. J Clin Psychopharmacol 11:275–276, 1991

Gengo FM, Fagan SC, de Padova A, et al: The effect of β-blockers on mental performance in older hypertensive patients. Arch Intern Med 148:779–784, 1988

Giakas WJ, Seibyl JP, Mazure CM: Valproate in the treatment of temper outbursts (letter). J Clin Psychiatry 51:525, 1990

Gleason RP, Schneider LS: Carbamazepine treatment of agitation in Alzheimer's outpatients refractory to neuroleptics. J Clin Psychiatry 51:115–118, 1990

Greendyke RM, Kanter DR: Therapeutic effects of pindolol on behavioral disturbances associated with organic brain disease: a double-blind study. J Clin Psychiatry 47:423–426, 1986

Greendyke RM, Schuster DB, Wooton JA: Propranolol in the treatment of assaultive patients with organic brain disease. J Clin Psychopharmacol 4:282–285, 1984

Greendyke RM, Kanter DR, Schuster DB, et al: Propranolol treatment of assaultive patients with organic brain disease: a double-blind crossover, placebo-controlled study. J Nerv Ment Dis 174:290–294, 1986

Greendyke RM, Berkner JP, Webster JC, et al: Treatment of behavioral problems with pindolol. Psychosomatics 30:161–165, 1989

Greenwald BS, Marin DB, Silverman SM: Serotonergic treatment of screaming and banging in dementia. Lancet 2:1464–1465, 1986

Grossman R, Beyer C, Kelly P, et al: Acetylcholine and related enzymes in human ventricular and subarachnoid fluids following brain injury (abstract). Proceedings of the 5th Annual Meeting for Neuroscience 76:3:506, 1975

Gualtieri CT, Chandler M, Coons TB, et al: Amantadine: a new clinical profile for traumatic brain injury. Clin Neuropharmacol 12:258–270, 1989

Gualtieri CT: Buspirone: neuropsychiatric effects. Journal of Head Trauma Rehabilitation 6:90–92, 1991a

Gualtieri CT: Buspirone for the behavior problems of patients with organic brain disorders. J Clin Psychopharmacol 11:280–281, 1991b

Haas JF, Cope N: Neuropharmacologic management of behavior sequelae in head injury: a case report. Arch Phys Med Rehabil 66:472–474, 1985

Hakoloa HP, Laulumaa VA: Carbamazepine in treatment of violent schizophrenics (letter). Lancet 1:1358, 1982

Halgren E: Emotional neurophysiology of the amygdala within the context of human cognition, in The Amygdala: Neurobiological Aspects of Emotion, Memory, and Mental Dysfunction. New York, Wiley-Liss, Inc., 1992, pp 191–228

Hamill RW, Woolf PD, McDonald JV, et al: Catecholamines predict outcome in traumatic brain injury. Ann Neurol 21:438–443, 1987

Heinrichs RW: Frontal cerebral lesions and violent incidents in chronic neuropsychiatric patients. Biol Psychiatry 25:174–178, 1989

Herrera JN, Sramek JJ, Costa JF, et al: High potency neuroleptics and violence in schizophrenics. J Nerv Ment Dis 176:558–561, 1988

Herzberg JL, Fenwick PBC: The aetiology of aggression in temporal-lobe epilepsy. Br J Psychiatry 153:50–55, 1988

Higley JD, Mehlman PT, Taum DM, et al: Cerebrospinal fluid monoamine and adrenal correlates of aggression in free-ranging Rhesus monkeys. Arch Gen Psychiatry 49:436–441, 1992

Hoffman BB, Lefkowitz RJ: Adrenergic receptor antagonists, in Goodwin and Gilman's The Pharmacological Basis of Therapeutics, 8th Edition. Edited by Gilman AG, Rall TW, Neiw AS, et al. New York, Pergamon Press, 1990, 221–243

Honigfeld G, Gillis RD, Klett CJ: Nurses' Observation Scale for Inpatient Evaluation: a new scale for measuring improvement in chronic schizophrenia. J Clin Psychol 21:65–71, 1965

Hornstein A, Seliger G: Cognitive side effects of lithium in closed head injury (letter). J Neuropsychiatry Clin Neurosci 1:446–447, 1989

Jackson RD, Corrigan JD, Arnett JA: Amitriptyline for agitation in head injury. Arch Phys Med Rehabil 66:180–181, 1985

Kafantaris V, Campbell M, Padron-Gayol MV, et al: Carbamazepine in hospitalized aggressive conduct disorder children: an open pilot study. Psychopharmacol Bull 28:193–199, 1992

Keats MM, Mukherjee S: Antiaggressive effect of adjunctive clonazepam in schizophrenia associated with seizure disorder. J Clin Psychiatry 49:117–118, 1988

King BH: Fluoxetine reduced self-injurious behavior in an adolescent with mental retardation. Journal of Child and Adolescent Psychopharmacology 1:321–329, 1991

Knott P, Haroutunian V, Bierer L, et al: Correlations post-mortem between ventricular CSF and cortical tissue concentrations of MHPG, 5-HIAA, and HVA in Alzheimer's disease. Biol Psychiatry 25:112A, 1989

Kruesi MJP, Hibbs ED, Zahn TP, et al: A 2-year prospective follow-up study of children and adolescents with disruptive behavior disorders: prediction by cerebrospinal fluid 5-hydroxyindoleacetic acid, homovanillic acid, and autonomic measures? Arch Gen Psychiatry 49:429–435, 1992

Leavitt ML, Yudofsky SC, Maroon JC, et al: Effect of introventricular nadolol infusion on shock-induced aggression in 6-OHDA lesioned rats. Journal of Neuropsychiatry and Clinical Neuroscience 1:167–172, 1989

Leibovici A, Tariot PN: Carbamazepine treatment of agitation associated with dementia. J Geriatr Psychiatry Neurol 1:110–112, 1988

Levin HS, Grossman RG: Behavioral sequelae of closed head injury: a quantitative study. Arch Neurol 35:720–727, 1978

Levin HS, Grossman RG, Rose JE, et al: Long-term neuropsychological outcome of closed head injury. J Neurosurg 50:412–422, 1979

Levine AM: Buspirone and agitation in head injury. Brain Inj 2:165–167, 1988

Linnoila VMI, Virkkunen M: Aggression, suicidality, and serotonin. J Clin Psychiatry 53 (Suppl 10):46–51, 1992

Luchins DJ: Carbamazepine for the violent psychiatric patient (letter). Lancet 2:755, 1983

Luchins DJ, Dojka D: Lithium and propranolol in aggression and self-injurious behavior in the mentally retarded. Psychopharmacol Bull 25:372–375, 1989

Lucki I, Rickels K, Geller AM: Chronic use of benzodiazepines and psychomotor and cognitive test performance. Psychopharmacol 88:426–433, 1986

Mattes JA: Carbamazepine vs propranolol for rage outbursts. Psychopharmacol Bull 24:179–182, 1988

Mattes JA: Comparative effectiveness of carbamazepine and propranolol for rage outbursts. J Neuropsychiatry Clin Neurosci 2:159–164, 1990

Mattes JA: Valproic acid for nonaffective aggression in the mentally retarded. J Nerv Ment Dis 180:601–602, 1992

McKinlay WW, Brooks DN, Bond MR, et al: The short-term outcome of severe blunt head injury as reported by the relatives of the injured person. J Neurol Neurosurg Psychiatry 44:527–533, 1981

McMillan TM, Glucksman EE: The neuropsychology of moderate head injury. J Neurol Neurosurg Psychiatry 50:393–397, 1987

Mendez MF, Cummings JL, Benson DF: Depression in epilepsy: significance and phenomenology. Arch Neurol 43:766–770, 1986

Moskowitz AS, Altshuler L: Increased sensitivity to lithium-induced neurotoxicity after stroke: a case report. J Clin Psychopharmacol 11:272–273, 1991

Mysiw WJ, Jackson RD, Corrigan JD: Amitriptyline for post-traumatic agitation. Am J Phys Med Rehabil 67:29–33, 1988

Novaco RW: Anger Control: The Development and Evaluation of an Experimental Treatment. Lexington, MA, Lexington Books, 1976

Oddy M, Coughlan T, Tyerman A, et al: Social adjustment after closed head injury: a further follow-up seven years after injury. J Neurol Neurosurg Psychiatry 48:564–568, 1985

Olivier B, Mos J, Rasmussen DL: Behavioural pharmacology of the serenic, eltoprazine. Drug Metabolism and Drug Interactions 8:31–38, 1990

Ostrov E, Marohn RC, Offer D, et al: The adolescent antisocial behavior checklist. J Clin Psychol 36:594–601, 1980

Overall JE, Gorham DR: The Brief Psychiatric Rating Scale. Psychol Rep 10:799–812, 1962

Ovsiew F, Yudofsky SC: Aggression: a neuropsychiatric perspective, in Rage, Power, and Aggression. Edited by Roose S, Glick RD. New Haven, CT, Yale University Press, 1993, pp 213–230

Pinner E, Rich CL: Effects of trazodone on aggressive behavior in seven patients with organic mental disorders. Am J Psychiatry 145:1295–1296, 1988

Porta M, Bareggi SR, Collice M, et al. Homovanillic acid and 5-hydroxyindole-acetic acid in the CSF of patients after a severe head injury, II: ventricular CSF concentrations in acute brain post-traumatic syndromes. Eur Neurol 13:545–554, 1975

Post RM, Uhde TW, Putnam FE, et al: Kindling and carbamazepine in affective illness. J Nerv Ment Dis 170:717–731, 1982

Rao N, Jellinek HM, Woolston DC: Agitation in closed head injury: haloperidol effects on rehabilitation outcome. Arch Phys Med Rehabil 66:30–34, 1985

Ratey JJ, Sovner R, Mikkelsen E, et al: Buspirone therapy for maladaptive behavior and anxiety in developmentally disabled persons. J Clin Psychiatry 50:382–384, 1989

Ratey JJ, Leveroni CL, Miller AC, et al: Low-dose buspirone to treat agitation and maladaptive behavior in brain-injured patients: two case reports. J Clin Psychopharmacol 12:362–364, 1992a

Ratey JJ, Sorgi P, O'Driscoll GA, et al: Nadolol to treat aggression and psychiatric symptomatology in chronic psychiatric inpatients: a double-blind, placebo-controlled study. J Clin Psychiatry 53:41–46, 1992b

Ratey JJ Leveroni C, Kilmer D, et al: The effects of clozapine on severely aggressive psychiatric inpatients in a state hospital. J Clin Psychiatry 54:219–223, 1993

Realmuto FM, August GJ, Garfinkel BD: Clinical effect of buspirone in autistic children. J Clin Psychopharmacol 9:122–124, 1989

Rimel RW, Giordani B, Barth JT, et al: Disability caused by minor head injury. Neurosurgery 9:221–228, 1981

Robertson MM, Trimble MR, Townsend HRA: Phenomenology of depression in epilepsy. Epilepsia 28:364–372, 1987

Rojahn J: Self-injurious behavior in institutionalized severely profoundly retarded adults—prevalence data and staff agreement. Journal of Behavioral Assessment 6:13–26, 1984

Ross ED, Rush J: Diagnosis and neuroanatomical correlates of depression in brain-damaged patients. Arch Gen Psychiatry 38:1344–1354, 1981

Roth T, Hartse KM, Saab PG, et al: The effects of flurazepam, lorazepam, and triazolam on sleep and memory. Psychopharmacology 70:231–237, 1980

Rutherford WH, Merrett JD, McDonald JR: Sequelae of concussion caused by minor head injuries. Lancet 1:1–4, 1977

Salzman C, Kochansky GE, Shader RI, et al: Chloridazepoxide-induced hostility in a small group setting. Arch Gen Psychiatry 31:401–405, 1974

Schiffer RB, Herndon RM, Rudick RA: Treatment of pathologic laughing and weeping with amitriptyline. New Engl J Med 312:1480–1482, 1985

Schoenhuber R, Gentili M: Anxiety and depression after mild head injury: a case control study. J Neurol Neurosurg Psychiatry 51:722–724, 1988

Seliger GM, Hornstein A, Flax J, et al: Fluoxetine improves emotional incontinence. Brain Inj 6:267–270, 1992

Sheard MH, Marini JL, Bridges C, et al: The effects of lithium in impulsive aggressive behavior in man. Am J Psychiatry 133:1409–1413, 1976

Silver JM, Yudofsky SC: Documentation of aggression in the assessment of the violent patient. Psychiatric Annals 17:375–384, 1987

Silver JM, Yudofsky SC: The Overt Aggression Scale: overview and clinical guidelines. J Neuropsychiatry Clin Neurosc 3 (suppl):S22–S29, 1991

Silver JM, Yudofsky SC: Psychopharmacology and electroconvulsive therapy, in The American Psychiatric Press Textbook of Psychiatry. Edited by Talbott JA, Hales RE, Yudofsky SC. Washington, DC, American Psychiatric Press, 1988, pp 767–853

Silver, JM, Yudofsky SC, Kogan M, et al: Elevation of thioridazine plasma levels by propranolol. Am J Psychiatry 143:1290–1292, 1986

Silver JM, Hales RE, Yudofsky SC: Neuropsychiatric aspects of traumatic brain injury, in The American Psychiatric Press Textbook of Neuropsychiatry, 2nd Edition. Edited by Yudofsky SC, Hales RE. Washington, DC, American Psychiatric Press, 1992, pp 363–395

Simpson DM, Foster D: Improvement in organically disturbed behavior with trazodone treatment. J Clin Psychiatry 47:191–193, 1986

Sloan RL, Brown KW, Pentland B: Fluoxetine as a treatment for emotional lability after brain injury. Brain Inj 6:315–319, 1992

Sobin P, Schneider L, McDermott H: Fluoxetine in the treatment of agitated dementia (letter). Am J Psychiatry 146:1636, 1989

Sparadeo FR, Gill D: Effects of prior alcohol use on head injury recovery. Journal of Head Trauma Rehabilitation 4:75–82, 1989

Stanley M, Traskman-Bendz L, Dorovini-Zis K: Correlations between aminergic metabolites simultaneously obtained from human CSF and brain. Life Sci 37:1279–1286, 1985

Stevens JR, Hermann BP: Temporal lobe epilepsy, psychopathology, and violence: the state of the evidence. Neurology 31:1127–1132, 1981

Stone JL, McDaniel KD, Hughes JR, et al: Episodic dyscontrol disorder and paroxysmal EEG abnormalities: successful treatment with carbamazepine. Biol Psychiatry 21:208–212, 1986

Szlabowicz JW, Stewart JT: Amitriptyline treatment of agitation associated with anoxic encephalopathy. Arch Phys Med Rehabil 71:612–613, 1990

Thomsen IV: Late outcome of very severe blunt head trauma: a 10–15 year second follow-up. J Neurol Neurosurg Psychiatry 47:260–268, 1984

Tiller JWG, Dakis JA, Shaw JM: Short-term buspirone treatment in disinhibition with dementia (letter). Lancet 2:510, 1988

Tonkonogy TM: Violence and temporal lobes lesion: head CT and MRI data. Journal of Neuropsychiatry and Clinical Neuroscience 3:189–196, 1991

Tune L, Carr S, Hoag E, et al: Anticholinergic effects of drugs commonly prescribed for the elderly: potential means for assessing risk of delirium. Am J Psychiatry 149:1393–1394, 1992

Tunks ER, Dermer SW: Carbamazepine in the dyscontrol syndrome associated with limbic dysfunction. J Nerv Ment Dis 14:311–317, 1973

Tupin JP, Smith DB, Clanon TL, et al: Long-term use of lithium in aggressive prisoners. Compr Psychiatry 14:311–317, 1973

Valzelli L: Psychobiology of Aggression and Violence. New York, Raven Press, 1981

Van Woerkom TCAM, Teelken AW, Minderhoud JM: Difference in neurotransmitter metabolism in frontotemporal-lobe contusion and diffuse cerebral contusion. Lancet 1:812–813, 1977

Van Zomeren A, Van Den Burg W: Residual complaints of patients two years after severe head injury. J Neurol Neurosurg Psychiatry 48:21–28, 1985

Vecht CJ, Van Woerkom TCAM, Teelken AW, et al: Homovanillic acid and 5-hydroxyindoleacetic acid cerebrospinal fluid levels. Arch Neurol 32:792–797, 1975

Vetro A, Szentistvanyi L, Pallag M, et al: Therapeutic experience with lithium in childhood aggressivity. Pharmacopsychiatry 14:121–127, 1985

Volavka J, Zito JM, Vitrai J, et al: Clozapine effects on hostility and aggression in schizophrenia. J Clin Psychopharmacol 13:287–289, 1993

Weiger WA, Bear DM: An approach to the neurology of aggression. J Psychiatr Res 22:85–98, 1988

Williams KH, Goldstein G: Cognitive and affective responses to lithium in patients with organic brain syndrome. Am J Psychiatry 136:800–803, 1979

Wong MK, Lee S: Nadol in the treatment of aggression in chronic psychiatric inpatients. J Clin Psychiatry 54:235, 1993

Worrall EP, Moody JP, Naylor GT: Lithium in non-manic depressives: Antiaggressive effect and red blood cell lithium values. Br J Psychiatry 126:464–468, 1975

Yatham LN, McHale PA: Carbamazepine in the treatment of aggression: a case report and a review of the literature. Acta Psychiatr Scand 78:188–190, 1988

Yudofsky SC: β-blockers and depression: the clinician's dilemma. JAMA 267:1826–1827, 1992

Yudofsky SC, Silver JM: Psychiatric aspects of brain injury: Trauma, stroke, and tumor, in Psychiatry Update 1985. Washington, DC, American Psychiatric Press, 1985, pp 142–158

Yudofsky SC, Silver JM, Jackson W, et al: The Overt Aggression Scale for the objective rating of verbal and physical aggression. Am J Psychiatry 143:35–39, 1986

Yudofsky SC, Silver JM, Schneider SE: Pharmacologic treatment of aggression. Psychiatric Annals 17:397–407, 1987

Yudofsky SC, Silver J, Yudofsky B: Organic personality disorder, explosive type, in Treatment of Psychiatric Disorders: A Task Force Report of the American Psychiatric Association. Washington, DC, American Psychiatric Association, 1989, pp 839–852

Yudofsky SC, Silver JM, Hales RE: Pharmacologic management of aggression in the elderly. J Clin Psychiatry 51 (suppl 10):22–28, 1990

Zubieta JK, Alessi NE: Acute and chronic administration of trazodone in the treatment of disruptive behavior disorders in children. J Clin Psychopharmacol 12:346–351, 1992

Special Populations

Chapter 11

Mild Traumatic Brain Injury and the Postconcussive Syndrome

Thomas W. McAllister, M.D.

Severity of brain injury exists along a broad continuum both clinically and pathophysiologically. Clinical measures such as the duration of unconsciousness, the length of posttraumatic amnesia, or the initial Glasgow Coma Score (GCS; Teasdale and Jennett 1974)—a 3- to 15-point scale measuring visual, verbal, and motor function)—typically are used to quantify the severity of brain injury. Neither the magnitude of the forces causing injury nor the long-term sequelae of the injury factor explicitly into these measures.

Most clinicians and researchers follow the guidelines of the GCS and assign injury severity to one of three categories. GCS scores of 3–8 indicate a severe brain injury. Clinically this is often associated with prolonged (longer than 24 hours) periods of unconsciousness and poor outcomes (Levin et al. 1990). Abnormal motor posturing and ocular reflexes when present suggest a poorer prognosis as well (Mack and Horne 1989). Moderate brain injury is associated with GCS scores of 9–12, periods of unconsciousness of several hours, to a day or more, and periods of posttraumatic amnesia of 1 to 2 weeks or more. Outcomes are typically better than with severe head injury, but are still associated with significant degrees of disability (Rimel et al. 1982; Williams et al. 1990). Outcome measures in both of these categories are negatively influenced by the presence of focal lesions such as subdural hematomas (Rimel et al. 1982).

There is no universally accepted definition of *mild brain injury* (Table 11–1). Injuries in which loss of consciousness was less than 20 minutes and certainly less than 1 hour and for which GCS scores are 13 or greater are usually considered consistent with mild brain injury. When initially seen, these patients may be confused or disoriented, and appear lethargic. The prognosis for this group clearly is better than for the moderate and severe injury groups (Levin et al. 1990; Rimel et al. 1982; Williams et al. 1990). However, there is controversy about the nature, severity, and etiology of short- and long-term sequelae in these patients (Williams et al. 1990). This may reflect the inadequacy of the measures used to assess both severity and outcome. In a careful study, Williams et al. (1990) suggested that GCS scores alone may be insufficient predictors of outcome in certain patients with mild brain injury. In their study, patients with GCS scores in the mild range (13–15) with or without focal brain lesions, depressed skull fractures, or both,

Table 11–1.　Indicators of mild brain injury

Duration of loss of consciousness	None to 20 minutes
Posttraumatic amnesia	Minutes to 24 hours (can be longer)
Glasgow Coma Scale[a] score	13–15
Clinical condition	May appear stunned or dazed
	May appear drowsy or indifferent
	May be disoriented or have trouble with complex commands
	May complain of headache or nausea or vomit
	If hospitalized, generally < 48 hours

[a]See Teasdale and Jennett 1974.

were compared to patients with moderate brain injury. The group with mild injury and associated focal lesions or depressed skull fractures were similar to the moderate injury group in terms of neuropsychological and outcome measures. Thus the combination of clinical signs and symptoms shortly after injury and radiological findings may be a better scheme for predicting outcome. In terms of the literature to be reviewed, "mild traumatic brain injury [TBI]" is used in this chapter to signify injury with brief (less than 20 minutes) or no loss of consciousness and with GCS scores, when available, of 13–15. Typically the duration of posttraumatic amnesia is in the range of 1 to 24 hours, and many groups eliminate patients hospitalized for more than 48 hours.

Epidemiology

There are relatively few good epidemiological studies on the incidence of mild brain injury, especially given the magnitude of the problem, the age groups affected, and the potential for significant sequelae. In a careful study of all head injuries occurring in San Diego County, California, in 1981, Kraus and Nourjah (1988) found that mild brain injury accounted for 82% of all patients hospitalized with TBI; 75% of this group had GCS scores of 15. These figures are similar to those reported by Whitman et al. (1984) in two Chicago area communities and somewhat higher than those reported by Annegers et al. (1980) and Rimel (1981), who found that mild brain injury accounted for 60% and 49% of all head injuries, respectively. As Kraus and Nourjah (1989) noted, differences in definition of *mild brain injury,* time periods over which the data were collected, and patient referral source may account for the discrepancies. Conservatively, mild brain injury accounts for one-half to three-quarters of all patients hospitalized with a brain injury. Using data from Kraus and Nourjah's San Diego County study, hospitalization for mild brain injury occurs at a rate of 131 per 100,000 population or between 300,000 and 400,000 people per year in the United States. Probably four to five mild brain injuries occur for each one that results in hospitalization (Department of Health and Human Services 1989) (Table 11–2).

Mirroring the demographic profile of TBI in general, mild injury occurs twice as frequently in males, with a peak age distribution of 15–24 years (Kraus and Nourjah 1988). Causes of mild brain injury are also similar to those of brain injury in general with motor vehicle accidents, falls, assaults, and sports or recreation accidents accounting for 40–50%, 20%–25%, 15%–20%, and 10%–15%, respectively (Dacey and Dikmen 1987; Kraus and Nourjah 1988). Assaults account for a higher percentage in some areas, especially large urban centers (Sorenson and Kraus 1991). It is also probably true that the vast majority of sports-related mild brain injuries go unreported. Falls account for a larger percentage in children under 10 and people over 65 (Luerssen et al. 1988).

Kraus and Nourjah (1988) estimated the cost of hospitalized mild brain injury alone at well over a billion dollars per year. This does not include the nonhospitalized cases, nor does it include costs of ongoing care for patients. Of some interest given the known neuropsychiatric sequelae of mild brain injury, only 15 of 2,435 mild brain injury patients in the San Diego County study were discharged with planned medical follow-up.

Thus in many respects, "mild" brain injury is a misnomer. Sequelae include problems in cognition, behavior, the constellation of symptoms that make up "postconcussive syndrome," other psychopathology, and a surprisingly high rate of disability. Though

Table 11–2. Epidemiology of minor brain injury

Incidence (United States)	130–150 per 100,000 hospitalized patients (perhaps 4–5 this number treated as outpatients)
Age distribution (years)	15–24 (peak range)
Sex distribution	2:1 (M:F) (peak for females age > 75 years)
Etiology	Motor vehicle accidents: 40%–45%
	Falls: 20%–25%
	Assaults: 10%–15%
	Sports and recreation: 10%–15%
Treatment costs	Probably more than $1 billion/year

Source. See Kraus and Nourjah 1989.

the initial clinical picture may be minor relative to the spectrum of possible neuropathological and functional outcomes, the extent of the problem and frequency and intensity of certain predictable sequelae make minor brain injury anything but a minor problem.

Pathophysiology

The structural concomitants of mild brain injury have been a subject of some discussion. The alteration in level of consciousness, even if brief, suggests widespread neuronal dysfunction (Gennarelli 1987; Peerless and Rewcastle 1967). There is evidence that structural neuronal damage can accompany even very mild brain injury (Oppenheimer 1968). For example, Oppenheimer (1968) reported finding destruction of myelin, axonal retraction bulbs (bead-like structures at the proximal end of a ruptured axon), and aggregates of small reactive glial cells (indicating recent tissue injury) in a variety of brain regions in five patients with minor or trivial injuries. One such patient had been knocked down by a motor scooter, had no loss of consciousness, but was described as "stunned." Posttraumatic amnesia lasted approximately 20 minutes. Clinical description of the other four patients was not given, nor is it clear what percentage of total mild brain injury cases these five patients represent.

Animal models of brain injury using the fluid percussion model in cats (Povlishock and Coburn 1989) and controlled angular acceleration devices in nonhuman primates (Jane et al. 1985) strongly suggest that mild brain injury is often associated with evidence of axonal injury. Axonal dysfunction with disruption of axoplasmic transport, edema, and eventual separation of the proximal and distal portion of the axon can occur in the absence of an overt tear at the time of injury. Wallerian degeneration (with bead-like swelling and eventual degeneration of the distal axon and its terminals) can occur. Secondary deafferentation (structural changes and sometimes neuronal death due to loss of synaptic input) in target areas of the afflicted axon can follow (Povlishock and Coburn 1989). These changes in axon structure evolve over a 12- to 24-hour period in the cat model and can be seen in the absence of structural damage to neighboring supportive or vascular tissue. The Wallerian changes in this same model took place over the subsequent 2–60 days (Povlishock and Coburn 1989). Identification of the molecular mechanisms involved may eventually suggest interventions to block or reduce neuronal damage (see Chapter 23). This group also observed regenerative activity (including sprouting and enlarged axonal areas at the tip of growing axons) over a period of weeks to several months subsequent to the trauma, perhaps mirroring the recovery process observed in humans (Povlishock and Coburn 1989).

Injury does not always occur at the axonal level alone. Although cerebral concussion was the diagnosis in 80% of patients with mild brain injury in the San Diego County study (Kraus and Nourjah 1988), almost 5% had cerebral contusions, about 1% had intracerebral hemorrhages, and 14% had some other form of intracranial lesion. In Williams et al.'s study (1990) of 155 consecutive patients with mild brain injury, 32 had parenchymal contusions or hemorrhages (20%), and 27 (17%) had subdural or epidural hematomas.

The above suggests that brain injury considered trivial on the basis of the degree and duration of altered consciousness has demonstrable neuropathological effects, starting at the moment of impact and evolving over several hours to days and longer (Table 11–3). The types of injury seen, both macroscopically and microscopically, are similar in quality and location to those seen with moderate and severe degrees of brain injury.

Neurodiagnostic Findings

Neuroimaging

Abnormalities on neuroimaging studies vary as a function of the severity of injury, the interval between the injury and the study

(Wilson et al. 1988), and the imaging modality used (Wilson 1990). Computed tomography (CT) abnormalities are seen infrequently in mild brain injury, in approximately one-quarter of the cases of moderate brain injury (Rimel et al. 1982), and in about 90% of cases of severe brain injury (Lobato et al. 1986).

The location of abnormalities has been consistent with neuro-

Table 11–3. Mild traumatic brain injury (TBI): neurodiagnostic findings

Method	Findings
Neuropathology	
Animal models	
Fluid percussion model in cats (Povlishock and Coburn 1989)	Similar to more severe injuries with
	1) Disruption of axoplasmic transport
Controlled angular acceleration in primates (Jane et al. 1985)	2) Edema and separation of damaged axons
	3) Secondary deafferentation changes in affected target areas
Human data (Oppenheimer 1968)	Damaged axons with neuropathological changes similar to more severe injury reported in five patients with mild TBI.
Neurophysiology	
Standard electroencephalography (Schoenhuber and Gentilini 1989)	About 10% of mild TBI patients will have persistent abnormalities.
Evoked potentials (Schoenhuber and Gentilini 1989)	Poor correlation with postconcussive symptoms
Neuroimaging	
Computed tomography (CT) (Wilson 1990)	Often normal, though contusions and hemorrhages can be seen.
Magnetic resonance imaging (MRI) (Eisenberg and Levin 1989; Wilson 1990)	Abnormalities seen more frequently than with CT. Location and resolution of abnormalities correlate with neuropsychological findings.
Functional imaging[a] (Humayun et al. 1989)	May show regional abnormalities even when CT and MRI results are normal. Still largely experimental.

[a]Positron-emission tomography (PET) and single positron emission computed tomography (SPECT).

pathological findings. Thus cortical abnormalities are found primarily with milder injury, and injury to progressively deeper structures are seen with progressive degrees of severity, particularly with longer periods of unconsciousness (Eisenberg and Levin 1989; Levin et al. 1987a; Wilson et al. 1988).

Recent CT studies and studies comparing CT and magnetic resonance imaging (MRI) suggest that structural abnormalities are more common in mild brain injury than originally thought. Jenkins et al. (1986) found MRI abnormalities in all 8 patients with minor brain injuries (no loss of consciousness in 4, GCS scores of 15 in the other 4) in their study of mild and severe brain injuries. Levin and colleagues (Eisenberg and Levin 1989; Levin et al. 1987a) compared CT and MRI in 11 patients with mild (GCS 13–15) and 9 patients with moderate (GCS 9–12) brain injury. Only 3 of the patients had no abnormality on either scan. They did not specify in which group these 3 patients were, but this indicates that at least 8 of the 11 patients with mild head injury had demonstrable lesions (predominantly frontal and temporal cortical contusions) on MRI. Overall, MRI showed 44 more intracranial lesions than did CT scanning, volumetric estimates of lesion size were larger on MRI, and there tended to be correspondence between lesion location, size, and neuropsychological performance. Follow-up measures on a smaller sample of these patients at 1 and 3 months suggested that marked diminution of lesion volume occurred in association with significant improvement in the neuropsychological measures.

Methods of functional neuroimaging such as single photon emission computed tomography (SPECT) and positron-emission tomography (PET) eventually may play a significant role in the evaluation of minor brain injury. Humayun et al. (1989) studied regional glucose utilization with PET in three patients with mild head injury and persisting cognitive deficits. All three had normal MRI and CT scans. Compared with three control subjects, the patients had abnormal glucose utilization in several frontal and temporal regions and the left caudate nucleus. It is likely that areas of abnormal brain function will be detected in patients who have "minor" TBI and normal CT and MRI studies. However, PET and SPECT are largely clinical research tools at this time.

Two points should be highlighted from the above. The first is that clear evidence of brain injury can be seen in many patients with a history of seemingly minor brain injury. This is more likely to be visualized by MRI, and may be less evident with time. The preliminary data suggest that the findings on MRI correlate at least to some degree with functional deficits on neuropsychological measures. In addition many patients with a history of "minor" brain injury will not have abnormalities on even MRI, yet can manifest clear evidence of functional impairment on neuropsychological measures. It is possible that PET and SPECT may in the future help to clarify this situation. At this time, the presence of a normal CT or MRI scan cannot be equated with unequivocal absence of brain injury.

Neurophysiological Measures

There has not been much research performed on the use of the standard EEG or other neurophysiological measures in the evaluation of patients with mild brain injury. This is particularly surprising given the nature of many of the common cognitive and somatic complaints associated with mild brain injury. In a recent review of this topic, Schoenhuber and Gentilini (1989) suggest that with both standard EEGs and certain evoked potentials, about 10% of patients with mild brain injury will have persistent abnormalities. The abnormalities are nonspecific, such as mild disorganization of the background rhythms or a mild excess of slow wave frequencies. In their study of auditory brain stem responses in 165 patients with mild brain injury (GCS 13–15, loss of consciousness less than 20 minutes), about 10% of patients had at least one prolonged interpeak latency (Schoenhuber and Gentilini 1986). However, these abnormalities did not correlate with the presence or absence of relevant postconcussion symptoms. Pratrap-Chand et al. (1988) found increased P300 latencies in a group of 20 mild brain injury patients compared to healthy controls when tested within 4 days after the injury. The latencies were normal upon retesting 30–250 days subsequent to initial testing. Only 2 of these patients were complaining of any postconcussive symptoms. Abd Al-Hady et al.

(1990) also found prolongation of certain interpeak latencies in auditory brain stem responses in their group of 30 mild brain injury patients. It was not clear whether these findings correlated with any subjective complaints. Topographic brain electrical activity mapping can occasionally demonstrate abnormalities not shown on routine EEG or evoked potential studies, although this is not always the case (Garber et al. 1989). Thatcher et al. (1989) studied measures of EEG power spectral analyses in 608 patients with mild brain injury defined by GCS scores of 13–15 and loss of consciousness less than 20 minutes. They were able to develop a discriminate function that separated mild brain injury patients from age-matched controls with surprising accuracy. The location of the EEG abnormalities (frontal and frontotemporal, as well as changes in anterior-posterior patterns) were consistent with predictable areas of brain injury. Of note is that the patients were referred largely because of persistent complaints, and thus may not be representative of all patients with a mild brain injury. It does suggest that computerized EEG techniques may prove to be more valuable in the assessment of complaints following mild brain injury than standard EEGs.

Cognitive Sequelae

The evaluation of cognitive deficits subsequent to mild brain injury is a complex task. Until recently, most groups used different criteria for mild brain injury, tested patients at different times, and used different tests to assess cognitive functions. This makes comparison of study results difficult and generalization to clinical situations hazardous. Initial attempts to assess cognition used general measures of intellectual function such as the Wechsler Adult Intelligence Scale (Wechsler 1981), or general batteries designed more for discernment of focal neurological illness such as the Halstead-Reitan battery (Reitan 1979).

With better definition of the mild brain injury population and more consistent use of tests to probe attention, speed of information processing, and memory, several factors have become clear (Table 11–4).

Short-Term Effects

Most investigators now agree that mild brain injury patients can be distinguished from healthy controls on measures of speed of information processing, selected tests of attention and memory, and performance consistency in the first week or so subsequent to the injury (Gentilini et al. 1989; Gronwall 1989; McMillan and Glucksman 1987; Ruff et al. 1989; Stuss et al. 1989). The usual course of recovery is fairly rapid. Studies of cognitive testing at 1 month and 3 months subsequent to injury tend to show progressive diminution of the cognitive deficits, although when differences persist they are usually in the same three areas (Dikman et al. 1986; Gentilini et al. 1989; Gronwall 1989; Ruff et al. 1989). The more recent study by Williams et al. (1990) suggests that even within the mild brain injury group, those patients with complications such as depressed skull fractures, contusions, and subdural or epidural hematomas may be those who are more likely to have persistent deficits in speed of information processing, verbal and recognition memory, and verbal fluency.

Table 11–4. Cognitive sequelae of minor traumatic brain injury

Study	Cognitive function	Representative tests
Gronwall 1989	Speed of information processing	Choice reaction time Paced Auditory Serial Addition Task (PASAT; Gronwall and Sampson 1974)
Gentilini et al. 1989	Attention and concentration	Distributed attention test Divided attention test
Ruff et al. 1989	Memory	Mattis-Kovner Verbal Learning and Memory Test (Mattis and Kovner 1978) Benton Visual Retention Test (Benton 1974)

Long-Term Effects

The long-term cognitive sequelae of minor brain injury is a controversial area. In a careful study of 20 subjects with minor injury
(GCS $\geq$ 12, loss of consciousness $\leq$ 1 hour) compared with 20
uninjured friends on a variety of neuropsychological measures
taken largely from the Halstead-Reitan battery, Dikmen et al.
(1986) were unable to find significant differences between the two
groups 12 months after the injury. Leininger et al. (1990), however,
found significant impairment on four of eight neuropsychological
tests (Category Test, Paced Auditory Serial Addition Test–Revised,
Auditory Verbal Learning Test, Complex Figure-copy) in a group
of symptomatic patients with mild brain injury (GCS $\geq$ 13, loss of
consciousness less than 20 minutes) tested an average of 6 to 8
months after the injury. In this study 53 patients with mild TBI who
noted persistent complaints were compared with matched friends
and relatives of TBI patients. Patients with a prior history of TBI
were excluded. Of note is that a significant minority of the patients
(40%) had no history of loss of consciousness, having sustained
"dazing" injuries or mild concussions. Tests assessing information
processing, reasoning, and verbal learning were significantly different from those for the control group. There were no significant
differences between those who did or did not lose consciousness,
those tested before or after 3 months after the injury, or those who
were or were not pursuing compensation claims.

The impression from the work to date is that mild brain injury
results in measurable deficits in speed of information processing,
attention, and memory in the immediate postinjury period. Recovery from these deficits is the rule, occurring over a variable period
ranging from 4 to 12 weeks. For a minority, recovery may occur
much more slowly, or remain incomplete. Certain factors appear to
predict a poorer prognosis. Barth et al. (1983) and Rimel et al.
(1981) found significantly poorer outcomes in their studies that
included a large percentage of patients with a prior history of brain
injury, compared to studies (such as Dikman et al. 1986) in which
patients with a prior history of TBI were excluded. In the study by
Leininger et al. (1990) of symptomatic mild brain injury, the study

population was older than the "typical" brain injury population, perhaps consistent with the observation that age negatively influences a variety of outcome measures. Furthermore, it seems that more difficult or novel cognitive tasks, or tasks performed under mild degrees of physiological stress, can negatively influence the performance of patients with mild injury (Ewing et al. 1980; Gentilini et al. 1989; Gronwall 1989; Hugenholtz et al. 1988). It is important to note that excluding patients with a prior mild brain injury, history of alcohol abuse, or psychiatric illness is a double-edged sword; it makes it possible to better evaluate the pure contribution of the brain injury, and yet may not be easily generalizable to the mild brain injury population, most of whom will have a history of one or more of these factors (Dicker 1989).

Behavioral Sequelae of Mild Head Injury

In addition to the cognitive sequelae described above, a variety of significant behavioral sequelae are associated with mild brain injury.

Postconcussive Syndrome

Postconcussive syndrome refers to a constellation of symptoms described subsequent to brain injury (see Table 11–5). The symptoms can be grouped into three categories: cognitive complaints (decreased memory, attention, and concentration), somatic complaints (headache, fatigue, insomnia, dizziness, tinnitus, sensitivity to noise or light), and affective complaints (depression, irritability, and anxiety). The symptoms are commonly reported subsequent to brain injury of varying severity and should not be considered synonymous with mild brain injury (Hinkeldey and Corrigan 1990; McKinlay et al. 1981; Van Zomeren and Van Den Burg 1985).

In the immediate postinjury period, anywhere from 80%–100% of mild brain injury patients will describe one or more of the above symptoms (Levin et al. 1987b). Studies of the resolution of these symptoms over time are fairly unanimous in suggesting that a significant number of patients will be symptom-free at 1 month. By 3 months and certainly by 12 months, the majority of patients will be free of complaint.

These studies also are clear that this is not the case for all mild brain injury patients. McLean et al. (1983) found that 65% of their 20 patients complained of persistent fatigue, 40% of decreased memory, and 45% of decreased concentration at 1 month subsequent to their mild brain injury. Forty-five percent of these patients had not returned to their previous major daily activities and rated their overall level of function as significantly more impaired than controls. Rimel et al. (1981), in a widely quoted study of 424 patients with mild brain injury (GCS ≥ 13, loss of consciousness less than 20 minutes) found that 78% of their patients complained of headache; 60% complained of decreased memory; and 50% and 25% complained of either decrease in financial status or were unemployed respectively at 3 months after their injury. Thirty-one percent of this population had a history of prior head injuries.

Table 11–5. Components of the postconcussive syndrome

Symptom	% of patients with persistent complaints at	
	1 month	3 months
Cognitive		
Impaired attention or concentration	40–45	NK
Impaired memory	50–55	59
Somatic		
Fatigue or decreased energy	65	20–25
Headache	55	45–78
Dizziness	40	20–25
Sensitivity to noise	50	NK
Insomnia	40	NK
Behavioral		
Irritability or loss of temper	65	NK
Anxiety	55	NK

Note. NK = not known.
Source. Dikmen et al. 1986; Levin et al. 1987b; Rimel et al. 1981.

Dikmen et al. (1986), in a study of 20 patients (GCS ≥ 12, loss of consciousness less than 1 hour) using age, sex, and educationally matched friends of patients as controls, and eliminating patients with a prior history of head injury, drug or alcohol abuse, or prior psychiatric illness, found a much more encouraging pattern of recovery. However, at 1 month 55% complained of headache, 65% of fatigue, 40% of dizziness, and 65% of irritability. Although these percentages did not differ significantly from those in the control group, the percentages were greater in each case for the mild brain injury patients. Furthermore, the study made no attempt to quantify the degree of distress but rather looked at whether the patients and controls simply endorsed any degree of the above symptoms. Three complaints—sensitivity to noise, insomnia, and decreased memory—were endorsed by a significantly greater number of patients than controls. Levin et al. (1987b) found that 82%–100% of their 57 patients with mild brain injury in a multicenter study endorsed postconcussive complaints immediately after and at 1 month subsequent to the injury. The most common complaints were headache, decreased energy, and dizziness. Even at the 3-month follow-up, 47%, 22%, and 22% respectively continued to complain of the above three symptoms. This was a carefully defined group with GCS of ≥ 13, loss of consciousness not exceeding 20 minutes, no focal neurological deficits, and without skull fracture or focal lesions on CT Scans.

Several studies have examined the impact of mild brain injury on measures of emotional distress using instruments such as the Minnesota Multiphasic Personality Inventory (MMPI). Diamond et al. (1988) examined MMPI scores in 50 patients 3 months after mild brain injury (not defined) and compared those scores with normative values for the general population and a control group with chronic neurological illness. They found high levels of emotional distress in the brain injury group remarkably similar in profile to the patients with chronic neurological illness. Fully half of the brain injury patients had at least two scales that were more than two standard deviations from the mean. Dikmen and Reitan (1977a, 1977b), although not examining mild head injury per se, found that increased measures of psychopathology on the MMPI correlated with increased neuropsychological impairment in 27 brain injury patients.

Several studies have attempted to address the role of compensation in the genesis of postconcussive symptoms (see Table 11–6). Miller (1961), based on 47 patients with "indubitably psychoneurotic complaints" (p. 5230) from his medical-legal referral practice, argued that many of the postconcussive symptoms, especially those of the more chronic variety, were linked to pending litigation and compensation cases. He observed an inverse relationship between severity of injury (primarily length of unconsciousness) and the severity of "psychoneurotic" symptoms. Forty-two percent of his patients without history of unconsciousness were felt to have "psychoneurotic" symptoms. He also reported that 45 of 50 patients showed "symptomatic recovery" after settlement and he attributed many postconcussive symptoms to malingering. However, his experience was drawn from a population referred to him for medicolegal assessment and defined only as having "indubitably psychoneurotic complaints." Although some of the case studies suggest that conversion symptoms or malingering may have been present in those examples, there are little data in terms of diagnostic criteria, outcome criteria, and symptom picture supplied. Unfortunately this view has become enshrined in the literature and clinical lore, such that some clinicians may even refuse to treat mild TBI patients until their claims are settled.

In a survey of 63 poorly defined "mild head injury" patients, Cook (1972) found that patients pursuing compensation claims showed a threefold increase in absence from work compared to those not pursuing claims. He argued that these findings confirmed Miller's view. However, less than half of the patients returned the survey, there was no specific definition of mild head injury given, the results were not based on clinical interview, and no attempt was made to look at other complications (such as orthopedic injury) that often accompany head injury and have been shown to play a role in associated disability (Dikmen et al. 1986).

Other studies have failed to confirm any significant linkage between compensation or litigation and frequency or severity of postconcussive symptoms. Merskey and Woodforde (1972) studied 27 patients with mild brain injury, 10 of whom were not seeking compensation and 17 of whom had already settled (favorably) their compensation claims. Thirty percent were either in a lower occupational status or unemployed. Even in the compensated group, symptoms persisted for over a year, and many were not fully recovered. Strauss and Savitsky (1934) cite several examples

Table 11–6.   Role of compensation/litigation in postconcussive syndrome—selected studies

Study	Findings	Comment
Miller (1961)	Series of 47 from medical-legal practice whose symptoms were "gross and unequivocally psychoneurotic."	Not representative of all patients with mild traumatic brain injury (TBI).
Cook (1972)	Survey of "mild head injury" admissions.	"Mild" not defined. Poor compliance rate.
	Those with claims had increased absence from work.	Not controlled for other complications.
Keshavan et al. (1981)	60 TBI admissions, mixed severity followed at 1.5 and 3 months. Compensation unrelated to outcome measures.	Does not address mild brain injury specifically.
Rimel et al. (1981)	424 consecutive minor TBI patients. Litigation and compensation claims unrelated to symptoms or return to work.	Argues strongly against role of compensation in genesis or maintenance of symptoms.
Others[a]		Numerous studies document similar symptoms in brain injuries of all severities, arguing against inverse relationship between severity of injury and severity of symptoms as suggested by Miller (1961).

[a]See Hinkeldey and Corrigan 1990; McKinlay et al. 1983; and Van Zomeren and Van Den Burg 1985.

of significant disability independent of compensation claims. In a study of predictors of physical, social, and behavioral outcome in 60 TBI patients of varying severity, Keshavan et al. (1981) were unable to find a link between compensation issues and any outcome measure. Rimel et al. (1981), in their study of disability related to mild TBI, with a population of 424 patients, found no link between pursuit of compensation and disability; in fact only 6 of their patients were involved in litigation at the time of follow-up. In his review of postconcussive symptoms, Binder (1986) concluded that there was no clear causal linkage between compensation or litigation claims and genesis, maintenance, or resolution of symptoms. Further, the observation that postconcussive symptoms occur in patients with varying degrees of severity (Hinkeldey and Corrigan 1990; McKinlay et al. 1983) suggests that compensation factors alone are not responsible for the genesis or maintenance of postconcussive symptoms.

Rutherford (1989) reported on a series of mild brain injury patients involved in litigation, which casts further doubt on many preconceptions about the relationship between compensation and symptoms. Over 40% of his group involved in litigation had no symptoms at the time of their medicolegal evaluation, approximately 1 year after the injury. About one-third of those who had symptoms at that time did not have symptoms at the time of settlement approximately 1 year later. Virtually all of the patients who were symptomatic at the time of settlement remained symptomatic 1 year later. Thus for many patients, improvement can occur before medicolegal evaluation, during the interval between evaluation and settlement, and symptoms, when present, can remain long after compensation issues have been settled.

It seems from the above studies that the constellation of symptoms labeled as the "postconcussive syndrome" is endorsed by virtually all patients within the immediate postinjury period, and that significant resolution of these symptoms occurs in about half of the patients by 1 month and in perhaps roughly two-thirds at 3 months. The etiology of these symptoms remains unknown. Several authors have suggested that "organic factors" are instrumental in the initial pathogenesis of the postconcussive symptoms and that in patients in whom these symptoms do not resolve within a 2 to 3-month period, psychological "issues" are felt to be involved in the maintenance and elaboration of the symptoms (Goethe and Levin 1984; Leigh 1979; Lishman 1973, 1988). However, there may be times when a patient's attorney gives clear encouragement to maintain symptoms when litigation extends over a period of several years. Although compensation and litigation may play a role in individual situations, there is virtually no evidence at this point to suggest that it is the primary factor in the overwhelming majority of patients with mild brain injury.

In addition to the postconcussive syndrome, a variety of major psychiatric sequelae have been reported in association with mild brain injury including psychotic episodes, major depressive episodes, mania, and various anxiety syndromes (Table 11–7).

Psychotic Syndromes

Psychotic syndromes similar in presentation to those seen in schizophrenia and the affective disorders do occur subsequent to brain injury. Both time-limited and chronic presentations are described (Davison and Bagley 1969; Kwentus et al. 1985; Lishman 1973; Nasrallah et al. 1981). Overall, psychotic syndromes are felt to be a fairly rare complication of brain injury occurring in 0.07%–9.8% of brain injury patients (Kwentus at al. 1985). In Lishman's study of penetrating brain injuries, only 5 of 144 cases of severe psychiatric disability were diagnosed with a psychotic disorder (Lishman 1968).

The observation that up to 15% of schizophrenia patients have a history of head injury (Nasrallah et al. 1981), coupled with the above observation, has led to the question of predisposing factors. Few studies have addressed this, and those that have suggest there is no clear linkage between a family history or genetic predisposition to schizophrenia and the development of a psychotic syndrome after a brain injury (Nasrallah et al. 1981). Most of the above reports deal with moderate or severe brain injury. Psychotic syndromes after mild brain injury would appear to be rare (Merskey and Woodforde 1972), though no one has formally studied this.

Depression

Depressive symptoms are a very common complication of mild brain injury. However, actual figures on the incidence of depressive illness are difficult to obtain. Merskey and Woodforde (1972), in their study of 27 mild brain injury patients, found that 7 patients had "endogenous" depressions, 9 others had a mixture of anxiety and depression, and another 4 had "reactive" depression in combination with a variety of other behavioral problems. Thus depressive symptoms of some form were a part of the clinical picture in 20 to 27 patients. Schoenhuber and Gentilini (1988) studied 48 patients with mild brain injury and matched controls drawn from friends and relatives (about 9 months after injury) with self-report anxiety and depression scales. The mild brain injury group had significantly elevated depression scores compared with controls.

Studies of emotional distress following brain injury of varying severity and using a variety of instruments suggest that scales or

Table 11–7.   Mild traumatic brain injury (TBI) and subsequent psychopathology

Syndrome	Comment
"Emotional distress"	General symptom inventories generally elevated in minor TBI.
	Mixed symptom picture.
Affective Disorders	
Depression	Depression scales generally elevated (Schoenhuber and Gentilini 1988).
	Mobayed and Dinan (1990) found 20% of sample met DSM-III criteria.
Mania	May occur after very mild TBI, even without loss of consciousness (Reiss et al. 1987; Bracken 1987; Nizamie et al. 1988; Pope et al. 1988).
Psychotic disorders	Relatively rare complication. Can be associated with TBI-induced affective disorders.
Anxiety disorders	Symptoms consistent with anxiety often endorsed, though may not be more frequent than general population (Schoenhuber and Gentilini 1988).
	Posttraumatic stress disorder can be seen; unclear how common.

clusters that access depressive symptoms are elevated (Burke et al. 1990; Fordyce et al. 1983; Hinkeldey and Corrigan 1990). Furthermore, many of the symptoms of the postconcussive syndrome such as subjective slowing, irritability, fatigue, and sleep disturbance can be consistent with a depressive syndrome, even when patients may not endorse explicit items such as "depressed mood."

Mobayed and Dinan (1990) recently reported that 30% of their 55 mild brain injury patients had evidence of an affective disorder on the Leeds scale (Hamilton et al. 1976). Full psychiatric assessment of these 16 patients showed that 11 (20%) met DSM-III criteria for major depression and had mean Hamilton Depression Scale scores (Hamilton 1960) of 27. Interestingly, these patients showed blunted prolactin responses to buspirone challenge, consistent with alteration in serotonin function. Saran (1985) studied 10 patients with depression following mild brain injury. Although the patients met DSM-III criteria for depression with melancholia, they differed from other patients with depression (but not brain injury), manifesting less diurnal variation, less anorexia or weight loss, and less psychomotor retardation or agitation. They did not differ with respect to the melancholic quality of depressed mood, presence of early morning awakening, and presence of excessive guilt.

Thus depressive symptoms are a significant contributor to psychiatric disability subsequent to mild brain injury whether as part of the postconcussive syndrome, or as a discrete major depressive episode. Patients with a prior history or family history of depression may be at greater risk to develop depressive symptoms subsequent to injury. The above studies suggest that this is not a necessary prerequisite, and the majority of depressive episodes arise in patients with no such vulnerabilities.

Mania

Mania occurs subsequent to a wide array of neurological and medical disorders (Krauthammer and Klerman 1978). Secondary mania has been reported to occur in association with TBI of varying severity (Shukla at al. 1987). Phenomenologically, these manic syndromes are similar to "idiopathic" mania, demonstrating changes in mood, sleep, and activation level, and often associated with psychotic symptoms (Shukla et al. 1987). The course of illness can be bipolar with both manic and depressed phases (Cohn et al. 1977; Hale and Donaldson 1982; Pope et al. 1988; Shukla et al. 1987; Stewart and Hemsath 1988), can be a rapid-cycling variant (Pope et al. 1988), and may be triggered by antidepressants (Stewart and Hemsath 1988).

However, TBI-related mania can differ somewhat from primary or idiopathic mania in having a higher rate of relapse (Hoff et al. 1988) and a higher percentage of irritable and assaultive behavior (Shukla et al. 1987). Quite commonly, patients have both an organic personality syndrome and a manic syndrome. The latter can present as a periodic worsening of the irritability and impulsivity characteristic of the former. This periodicity may be mistaken as an integral part of the organic personality syndrome and may account for the lower frequency of mania diagnosed in these patients (Hale and Donaldson 1982; Stewart and Hemsath 1988). Of note are several reports of manic syndromes occurring subsequent to quite mild brain injuries (Bracken 1987; Nizamie et al. 1988; Pope et al. 1988; Reiss et al. 1987), including some cases in whom there was no documented loss of consciousness.

It is not known whether these patients have an increased genetic vulnerability to bipolar illness. Most of the reports are small case series without adequate controls. One study (Shukla et al. 1987) failed to find bipolar illness in 85 first-degree relatives of 20 patients with TBI-related mania—although 30% of the patients had at least one relative with a history of depression. Studies of secondary mania with other underlying neurological causes suggest that genetic predisposition may be an important factor in the expression of manic syndromes (Robinson et al. 1988).

Anxiety and Posttraumatic Stress Disorder

Few studies have examined anxiety syndromes that occur after mild brain injury. As with depression, many symptoms often seen as part of a generalized anxiety disorder are frequently seen as part of the postconcussive syndrome. Thus complaints of headache, dizziness, blurred vision, irritability, and sensitivity to noise or light are endorsed by many patients after mild brain injury (Binder 1986; Dikmen et al. 1986; Levin et al. 1987b). It is less clear how many patients actually experience anxiety and how many have diagnosable anxiety disorders. Although 55% of Dikmen's group (Dikmen et al. 1986) of 20 mild brain injury patients complained of subjective anxiety, 45% of the matched controls had similar complaints (a statistically nonsignificant difference). Schoenhuber and Gentilini (1988) were unable to find a significant difference in mean anxiety scores in their study of 35 mild brain injury patients and matched controls. Thus although many postconcussive symptoms are similar to somatic complaints accompanying anxiety disorders, the relationship of the symptoms to subjective anxiety is not clear cut.

Even less has been written about the occurrence of posttraumatic stress disorder (PTSD) subsequent to mild (or severe) brain injury. Lishman (1973), in his review of the psychiatric sequelae of brain injury, refers to PTSD-like symptoms including "the circumstances of the accident may recur vividly in dreams, maintain states of anxiety, or become the focus for obsessional rumination or conversion hysteria." (p. 306). He goes on to suggest that these and other "neurotic disabilities" may be more likely to occur in milder degrees of injury especially in the absence of posttraumatic amnesia. However, McMillan (1991) recently described PTSD symptoms in a woman with a severe brain injury despite amnesia for the event itself, and a posttraumatic amnesia of some 6 weeks. Certainly it is not uncommon in clinical practice to see patients with a history of mild brain injury and signs and symptoms suggestive of PTSD. This may include sleep disturbance, recurrent nightmares, exaggerated startle responses, daytime flashbacks, and avoidant behaviors such as refusing to drive or leave home. However, the timing of the emergence and resolution of these symptoms and the prevalence of PTSD subsequent to mild brain injury are uncertain. In general, the symptoms of PTSD may become more evident over time and may have a delayed onset. Symptoms of the postconcussive syndrome start immediately after the injury and should improve over the subsequent several months. True PTSD is of course a distinct entity and should not be equated with the postconcussive syndrome, or what is sometimes referred to as the posttrauma syndrome in the older literature. Both PTSD and the postconcussive syndrome may occur in the same person, complicating the evaluation and treatment of both.

Disability

The overall disability caused by minor brain injury is not known. In the widely quoted study by Rimel et al. (1981), 34% of 310 patients gainfully employed before their mild brain injury were unemployed 3 months after the injury. Seventy-nine percent of these patients complained of persistent headaches, 59% of persistent memory deficits, and 15% noted difficulty with common household chores. This study has been criticized for including a high percentage of patients with a prior brain injury, although it may be more reflective of real life. Subsequent studies controlling for this variable and with more rigorous selection of control populations indicate that psychosocial disability at 1 month is significant across a wide range of variables, and although it is present in a small percentage of patients at 12 months, it is greatly reduced both in terms of the frequency of complaints and the degree of disability caused by the symptoms. For example, in their study of 20 patients with mild brain injury and matched controls drawn from a pool of acquaintances of the injured subjects, Dikmen et al. (1986) found significant impairment in many common daily activities such as work, sleep or rest, home management, and ambulation at 1 month after the injury. Only 4 of 19 subjects had returned to their major role (work, home management, studies) and leisure activities without limitations. Significant improvement in all of the above areas had occurred 12 months after the injury such that 15 of 19 had resumed their major activities without limitations. The presence of other system injury (such as orthopedic injuries) appeared to account for some of the above disability.

Thus it would seem that rates of overall disability mirror those of cognitive and behavioral dysfunction after minor brain injury, being quite high within the first 1–3 months and showing a significant drop over the subsequent 3–12 months. Again it must be noted, however, that a small percentage of patients continue to experience significant degrees of disability in various areas (cognitive, behavioral, psychosocial) at the 1-year mark and beyond.

Treatment Issues

Evaluation

Not surprisingly the foundation of any treatment approach to patients with minor brain injury is a proper evaluation. Significant effort must be expended to clarify premorbid history. In particular one must look for a prior history of brain injury, which can be seen in as many as 30% of patients (Rimel et al. 1981). The association of substance abuse with brain injury is well described (Sparadeo et al. 1990) and may contribute to postinjury sequelae. Interviews with significant others can be invaluable in gaining a clearer picture of these issues.

Signs and symptoms must be clearly defined, as well as any changes in symptom picture as a function of time from the injury. The profile of the injury itself must be outlined, including the type of injury, the presence or absence of loss of consciousness and its duration, and the presence, absence, and duration of any retrograde and anterograde amnesia. Corroborative information including accounts from observers, emergency medical technicians, ambulance and emergency room personnel, and inpatient hospital records can be invaluable. When evaluating these records, phrases such as "normal mental status" without sufficient documentation do not eliminate the possibility that there were cognitive changes. This is particularly true when the emergency team is distracted by other trauma such as injury to the spinal cord (Davidoff et al. 1985). The presence or absence and location of complications such as depressed skull fractures, cerebral contusions, and extradural hematomas should be noted because of the potential prognostic complications (Williams et al. 1990). The neurodiagnostic tests done and the timing in relation to the injury should be clarified, and the reports or actual studies obtained.

All of the above information can then be integrated with findings from the clinical interview to determine the consistency of the history and exam with the known sequelae of minor brain injury. This process should determine the presence or absence of one or more of the specific syndromes outlined above, including postconcussive syndrome, depression, mania, anxiety syndromes (including PTSD), and psychotic syndromes. Treatment should then follow rationally from this diagnostic scheme.

Medication Approaches

Several general principles should be borne in mind when prescribing psychotropic agents in this population. These patients seem to be more sensitive to common psychotropic side effects such as sedation, psychomotor slowing, and cognitive impairment (such as recent memory and attention). Although there are little actual data, most clinicians working with TBI patients note this tendency toward increased side effects and a resultant narrowing of the benefit to toxicity ratio. In general it is prudent to use lower starting and (often) final doses, and prolong the titration intervals (Cope 1987; Gualtieri 1988; McAllister 1992; McAllister and Price 1990; Silver et al. 1992).

Therapeutic efficacy studies are lacking in this group. The study by Saran (1985) of 10 patients with mild brain injury and depression suggests that some of these patients may be less responsive to antidepressants than patients without a brain injury. Hoff et al. (1988) reported a higher relapse rate in patients with CNS secondary mania, although these were not mild brain injury patients. The phenomenology of depressive and manic syndromes can also be altered by a brain injury (McAllister 1992; McAllister and Price 1990; Saran 1985; Shukla et al. 1987; Silver et al. 1991), resulting in a mixed and atypical clinical presentation. Thus psychotropic use is complicated by enhanced sensitivity to side effects, a mixed and atypical clinical picture (which can complicate assessment of target symptoms and drug response), and perhaps a reduced efficacy of certain standard agents, although the evidence for this is tentative.

The treatment of the postconcussive syndrome is even less clear-cut. Despite the presence of mixed depressive and anxiety features often seen, use of standard agents in the absence of a clear cut depressive or anxiety syndrome has not been too successful. For example, Saran (1988) treated depressed mild brain injury patients with headache with amitriptyline without success. Other agents, however, may hold more promise. Tennant and Wild (1987) successfully used naltrexone (50 mg/day and 100 mg/day) in two patients with postconcussive syndrome, one in a single-blind, the other in a double-blind design.

Stimulants, particularly those with dopaminergic agonist properties such as methylphenidate, amphetamine, and L-dopa, have been used successfully in some brain injury patients to treat a variety of problems, including attentional deficits, agitation, and other forms of impulse dyscontrol (Gualtieri 1988; Gualtieri et al. 1989; McAllister 1992). Amantadine, a dopamine agonist that probably acts both presynaptically and postsynaptically, has also been reported effective in some brain injury patients (Chandler et al. 1988), although its use has been primarily in patients with more severe injury (Gualtieri et al. 1989). There is an increasing literature on the use of buspirone—an azaperone, non-benzodiazepine anxiolytic—in the management of a variety of behavioral problems in neuropsychiatric patients, although its use in mild brain injury has been limited (Levine 1988; McAllister 1992). Further work is needed to define the role of various agents in both specific symptoms and the postconcussive syndrome. Treatment of PTSD symptoms is discussed in Chapter 9.

Psychoeducation

Often the most effective intervention in patients with active neurobehavioral sequelae is a careful explanation of the pathophysiology, typical sequelae, and time course of recovery associated with minor brain injury. Problems with slowing, attention, and memory, especially in the first 3 to 6 months, should be described. The potential for longer term difficulties should be mentioned. This should be done soon after the injury and is best done in the presence of family, friends, or significant others (see Wrightson 1989). The realistic setting of goals for return to major activities is a difficult process that must be individualized for each patient. Unfortunately, psychiatrists often are involved in the later stages of the process by which time there is frequently an unpleasant dynamic operating in which various individuals (including family, friends, employers, insurance carriers, and health care workers) are questioning the validity of complaints based on the seemingly "minor" nature of the injury and the patient's healthy appearance. Validating the complaints of the patient without undue fostering of illness behavior can be a difficult and lengthy process.

Medical-Legal Issues

Psychiatrists increasingly are involved in the assessment of patients with mild brain injury, often at the request of attorneys or insurance carriers. Typically, an opinion is requested about whether the nature of the patient's complaints, as well as their severity and duration, are consistent with what is known about the injury.

The evaluation of such cases is time consuming and requires procurement and perusal of all pertinent records including school and/or employment records, testing and evaluation, accident and emergency transport reports, and subsequent treatment records. When possible the clinician should interview the patient and others who knew the patient prior to the event.

Results of neurodiagnostic tests must be evaluated. If they have not been performed, an MRI, careful neuropsychological evaluation, EEG, and evoked potentials can be helpful in establishing the presence of brain injury. All of these studies, as previously noted, are not always abnormal in the presence of obvious brain injury.

Furthermore, even when abnormal, these studies may not reveal abnormalities that are pathognomonic for mild brain injury. Because few patients will have these tests both before and after their injury, it is difficult to be certain that such abnormalities were caused by the traumatic event in question. Thus the foundation of such evaluation remains the careful assessment of premorbid function, delineation of the type, location, and severity of the trauma, documentation of the profile and time course of subsequent changes in cognitive, behavioral, and somatic areas, and integration of this information with the appropriate neurodiagnostic studies. Many of the latter may not have been done until weeks to months after the injury, making the yield from such studies lower than if done within a week or so of the trauma. Thus even in the absence of positive neurodiagnostic findings, the history of a documented injury, with subsequent onset of the symptoms described above, which as Wrightson (1989) pointed out "constitute a syndrome as constant as any in clinical medicine" (p. 247), should enable a reasonable opinion to be given about the relationship between the injury and the current clinical picture.

Summary

Minor brain injury is a significant problem numerically and financially. It can result in an array of common neurobehavioral sequelae. Several points in this chapter are worth highlighting:

- 400,000–500,000 people are hospitalized in the United States each year with brain injuries. The majority of these are classifiable as "minor." Probably 4 or 5 patients sustain a minor brain injury for each patient hospitalized.
- Limited human data and more extensive animal data suggest that minor brain injury produces neuropathological changes to a lesser extent but similar in quality and location to those seen in more severe brain injury.
- Minor brain injury is associated, as is more severe brain injury,

with cognitive impairments in speed of information processing, attention, and memory. These deficits are most pronounced in the initial days to weeks subsequent to the injury. Most patients show a rapid, progressive improvement over the subsequent 1 to 3 months. A small percentage of patients will have demonstrable long-term sequelae.

- The constellation of cognitive, somatic, and behavioral complaints known as the "postconcussive syndrome" is seen subsequent to brain injury of all levels of severity. After minor brain injury, most patients show progressive resolution of these symptoms over the subsequent 1 to 3 months. A small but significant percentage will have persistent symptoms at 6 and 12 months, or longer. A history of prior head injury, increased age at time of injury, certain complications (such as depressed skull fracture, CT evidence of cerebral contusions or hemorrhages), injury to other body systems, and probably certain psychosocial factors may predict poorer outcomes. Compensation issues, though no doubt important factors in individual cases, are not consistently linked to the genesis or maintenance of symptoms.

- Minor brain injury has been associated with the new onset of discrete psychiatric disorders including depression, mania, psychotic, and anxiety disorders. The brain injury may result in atypical clinical presentations, heightened sensitivity to standard psychotropic agents, and a somewhat more refractory course, although these observations must be considered tentative.

- Treatment of the neuropsychiatric sequelae involves careful assessment of premorbid function, psychosocial context, and injury profile. Psychoeducational strategies, supportive psychotherapy, and judicious use of appropriate psychotropic agents can be beneficial.

References

Abd Al-Hady MR, Shehata O, El-Mously M, et al: Audiological findings following head trauma. J Laryngol Otol 104:927–936, 1990

Annegers JF, Grabow JD, Kurland LT, et al: The incidence, causes, and secular trends of head trauma in Olmsted County, Minnesota, 1935–1974. Neurology 30:912–919, 1980

Barth JT, Maccioccri SN, Giordani B, et al: Neuropsychological sequelae of minor head injury. Neurosurgery 13:529–533, 1983

Benton AL: The Revised Visual Retention Test: Clinical and Experimental Applications, 4th Edition. New York, Psychological Corp, 1974

Binder LM: Persisting symptoms after mild head injury: a review of the post-concussive syndrome. J Clin Exp Neuropsychol 8:323–346, 1986

Bracken P: Mania following head injury. Br J Psychiatry 150:690–692, 1987

Burke JM, Imhoff CL, Kerrigan JM: MMPI correlates among post-acute TBI patients. Brain Inj 4:223–231, 1990

Chandler MC, Barnhill JB, Gualtieri CT: Amantadine for the agitated head-injury patient. Brain Inj 2:309–311, 1988

Cohn CK, Wright JR, De Vaul RA: Post head trauma syndrome in an adolescent treated with lithium carbonate—case report. Diseases of the Nervous System 38:630–631, 1977

Cook JB: The post-concussional syndrome and factors influencing recovery after minor head injury admitted to hospital. Scandinavian Journal of Rehabilitation Medicine 4:27–30, 1972

Cope DN: Psychopharmacologic consideration in the treatment of traumatic brain injury. Journal of Head Trauma Rehabilitation 2(4):5, 1987

Dacey RG, Dikman SS: Mild head injury, in Head Injury, 2nd Edition. Edited by Cooper PR. Baltimore, MD, Williams and Wilkins, 1987, pp 125–140

Davidoff G, Morris J, Roth E, et al: Closed head injury in spinal cord injured patients: retrospective study of loss of consciousness and post-traumatic amnesia. Arch Phys Med Rehabil 66:41–43, 1985

Davison K, Bagley CR: Schizophrenia-like psychosis associated with organic disorders of the central nervous system. Br J Psychiatry 114 (suppl 4):113–184, 1969

Department of Health and Human Services: Interagency Head Injury Task Force Report. Washington, DC, US Department of Health and Human Services, 1989

Diamond R, Barth JT, Zillmer EA: Emotional correlates of mild closed head trauma: the role of the MMPI. International Journal of Clinical Neuropsychology 10:35–40, 1988

Dicker BG: Preinjury behavior and recovery after a minor head injury: a review of the literature. Journal of Head Trauma Rehabilitation 4(4):73–81, 1989

Dikmen S, Reitan RM: Emotional sequelae of head injury. Ann Neurol 2:492–494, 1977a

Dikmen S, Reitan RM: MMPI correlates of adaptive ability deficits in patients with brain lesions. J Nerv Ment Dis 165:247–254, 1977b

Dikmen S, McLean A, Temkin N: Neuropsychological and psychosocial consequences of minor head injury. J Neurol Neurosurg Psychiatry 49:1227–1232, 1986

Eisenberg HM, Levin HS: Computed tomography and magnetic resonance imaging in mild to moderate head injury, in Mild Head Injury. Edited by Levin HS, Eisenberg HM, Benton AL. New York, Oxford University Press, 1989, pp 133–141

Ewing R, McCarthy D, Gronwall D, et al: Persisting effects of minor head injury observable during hypoxic stress. Journal of Clinical Neuropsychology 2:147–155, 1980

Fordyce DJ, Roueche JR, Prigatano GP: Enhanced emotional reactions in chronic head trauma patients. J Neurol Neurosurg Psychiatry 46:620–624, 1983

Garber HJ, Weilburg JB, Duffy FH, et al: Clinical use of topographic brain electrical activity mapping in psychiatry. J Clin Psychiatry 50:205–211, 1989

Gennarelli TA: Cerebral concussion and diffuse brain injuries, in Head Injury, 2nd Edition. Edited by Cooper PR. Baltimore, MD, Williams and Wilkins, 1987, pp 108–124

Gentilini M, Nichelli P, Schoenhuber R: Assessment of attention in mild head injury, in Mild Head Injury. Edited by Levin HS, Eisenberg HM, Benton AL. New York, Oxford University Press, 1989, pp 163–175

Goethe KE, Levin HS: Behavioral manifestation during the early and long-term stages of recovery after closed head injury. Psychiatric Annals 14:540–546, 1984

Gronwall D: Cumulative and persisting effects of concussion on attention and cognition, in Mild Head Injury. Edited by Levin HS, Eisenberg HM, Benton AL. New York, Oxford University Press, 1989, pp 153–162

Gronwall D, Sampson H: The Psychological Effects of Concussion. Auckland, New Zealand, Auckland University Press, 1974

Gualtieri CT: Pharmacotherapy and the neurobehavioral sequelae of traumatic brain injury. Brain Inj 2:101–129, 1988

Gualtieri CT, Chandler M, Coons TB, et al: Amantadine: a new clinical profile for traumatic brain injury. Clin Neuropharmacol 12:258–270, 1989

Hale MS, Donaldson JO: Lithium carbonate in the treatment of organic brain syndrome. J Nerv Ment Dis 170:362–365, 1982

Hamilton MA: A rating scale for depressions. J Neurol Neurosurg Psychiatry 23:56–62, 1960

Hamilton MA, Snaith RP, Bridge GW: The Leeds scale for the self-assessment of anxiety and depression. Br J Psychiatry 128:156–165, 1976

Hinkeldey NS, Corrigan JD: The structure of head injured patients' neurobehavioral complaints: a preliminary study. Brain Inj 4:115–133, 1990

Hoff AL, Shukla S, Cook BL, et al: Cognitive function in manics with associated neurologic factors. J Affective Disord 14:251–255, 1988

Hugenholtz H, Stuss DT, Stethem LL, et al: How long does it take to recover from a mild concussion? Neurosurgery 22:853–858, 1988

Humayun MS, Presty SK, Lafrance ND, et al: Local cerebral glucose abnormalities in mild closed head injured patients with cognitive impairment. Nucl Med Commun 10:335–344, 1989

Jane JA, Steward O, Gennarelli TA: Axonal degeneration induced by experimental noninvasive minor head injury. J Neurosurg 62:96–100, 1985

Jenkins A, Hadley MDM, Teasdale G, et al: Brain lesions detected by magnetic resonance imaging in mild and severe head injuries. Lancet 2:445–446, 1986

Keshavan MS, Channabasavanna SM, Narahana Reddy GN: Post-traumatic psychiatric disturbances: patterns and predictors of outcome. Br J Psychiatry 138:157–160, 1981

Kraus JF, Nourjah P: The epidemiology of mild, uncomplicated brain injury. J Trauma 28:1637–1643, 1988

Kraus JF, Nourjah P: The epidemiology of mild head injury, in Mild Head Injury. Edited by Levin HS, Eisenberg HM, Benton AL. New York, Oxford University Press, 1989, pp 8–22

Krauthammer C, Klerman GL: Secondary mania. Arch Gen Psychiatry 35:1333–1339, 1978

Kwentus JA, Hart RP, Peck ET, et al: Psychiatric complications of closed head trauma. Psychosomatics 26:8–17, 1985

Leigh D: Psychiatric aspects of head injury. Journal of Clinical and Experimental Psychiatry 40:21–33, 1979

Leininger BE, Gramling SE, Farrell AD, et al: Neuropsychological deficits in symptomatic minor head injury patients after concussion and mild concussion. J Neurol Neurosurg Psychiatry 53:293–296, 1990

Levin HS, Amparo EG, Eisenberg HM, et al: Magnetic resonance imaging and computerized tomography in relation to the neurobehavioral sequelae of mild and moderate head injuries. J Neurosurg 66:706–713, 1987a

Levin HS, Mattis S, Ruff RM, et al: Neurobehavioral outcome following minor head injury: a three-center study. J Neurosurg 66:234–243, 1987b

Levin HS, Gary HE, Eisenberg HM, et al: Neurobehavioral outcome 1 year after severe head injury: experience of the traumatic coma data bank. J Neurosurg 73:699–709, 1990

Levine AM: Buspirone and agitation in head injury. Brain Inj 2:165–167, 1988

Lishman WA: Brain damage in relation to psychiatric disability after head injury. Br J Psychiatry 114:373–410, 1968

Lishman WA: The psychiatric sequelae of head injury: a review. Psychol Med 3:304–318, 1973

Lishman WA: Physiogenesis and psychogenesis in the "post-concussive syndrome." Br J Psychiatry 153:460–469, 1988

Lobato RD, Sarabra R, Rivas JJ, et al: Normal computerized tomography scans in severe head injury: prognostic and clinical management implication. J Neurosurg 65:784–789, 1986

Luerssen TG, Klauber MR, Marshall LF: Outcome from head injury related to patient's age: a longitudinal prospective study of adult and pediatric head injury. J Neurosurg 68:409–416, 1988

Mack A, Horn LJ: Functional prognosis in traumatic brain injury, in Physical Medicine and Rehabilitation State of the Art Reviews—Traumatic Brain Injury, Vol 3(1). Edited by Horn LJ, Cope DN. Philadelphia, PA, Hanley & Belfus, Inc, 1989, pp 13–26

Mattis S, Kovner R: Different patterns of mnemonic deficits in two organic amnestic syndromes. Brain Lang 6:179–191, 1978

McAllister TW: Neuropsychiatric sequelae of head injuries. Psychiatr Clin North Am 15(2):395–413, 1992

McAllister TW, Price TRP: Depression in the brain-injured: phenomenology and treatment, in Depression: New Directions in Theory, Research, and Practice. Edited by Endler NS, McCann CD. Toronto, Canada, Wall and Emerson, 1990, pp 361–387

McKinlay WW, Brooks DN, Bond MR, et al: The short-term outcome of severe blunt head injury as reported by relatives of the injured persons. J Neurol Neurosurg Psychiatry 44:527–533, 1981

McKinlay WW, Brooks DN, Bond MR: Post-concussional symptoms, financial compensation and outcome of severe blunt head injury. J Neurol Neurosurg Psychiatry 46:1084–1091, 1983

McLean A, Temkin N, Dikman S, et al: The behavioral sequelae of head injury. Journal of Clinical Neuropsychology 5:361–376, 1983

McMillan TM: Post-traumatic stress disorder and severe head injury. Br J Psychiatry 159:431–433, 1991

McMillan TM, Glucksman EE: The neuropsychology of moderate head injury. J Neurol Neurosurg Psychiatry 50:393–397, 1987

Merskey H, Woodforde JM: Psychiatric sequelae of minor head injury. Brain 95:521–528, 1972

Miller H: Accident neurosis. British Medical Journal 1:919–925, 992–998, 1961

Mobayed M, Dinan TG: Buspirone/prolactin response in post head injury depression. J Affect Disord 19:237–241, 1990

Nasrallah HA, Fowler RC, Judd LL: Schizophrenia-like illness following head injury. Psychosomatics 22:359–361, 1981

Nizamie SH, Nizamie A, Borde M, et al: Mania following head injury: case reports and neuropsychological findings. Acta Psychiatr Scand 77:637–639, 1988

Oppenheimer DR: Microscopic lesions in the brain following head injury. J Neurol Neurosurg Psychiatry 31:299–306, 1968

Peerless SJ, Rewcastle NW: Sheer injuries of the brain. Can Med Assoc J 96:577–582, 1967

Pope HG, McElroy SL, Satlin A, et al: Head injury, bipolar disorder, and response to valproate. Compr Psychiatry 29:34–38, 1988

Povlishock JT, Coburn TH: Morphopathological change associated with mild head injury, in Mild Head Injury. Edited by Levin HS, Eisenberg HM, Benton AL. New York, Oxford University Press, 1989, pp 37–53

Pratrap-Chand R, Sinniah M, Salem FA: Cognitive evoked potential (P300): a metric for cerebral concussion. Acta Neurol Scand 78:185–189, 1988

Reiss H, Schwartz CE, Klerman GL: Manic syndrome following head injury: another form of secondary mania. J Clin Psychiatry 48:29–30, 1987

Reitan RM: Halstead-Reitan Neuropsychological Test Battery. Tucson, AZ, Neuropsychology Laboratory, University of Arizona, 1979

Rimel RW: A prospective study of patients with central nervous system trauma. Journal of Neurosurgical Nursing 13:132–141, 1981

Rimel RW, Giordani B, Barth JT, et al: Disability caused by minor head injury. Neurosurgery 9:221–228, 1981

Rimel RW, Giordani B, Barth JT, et al: Moderate head injury: completing the clinical spectrum of brain trauma. Neurosurgery 11:344–351, 1982

Robinson RG, Boston JD, Starkstein SE, et al: Comparison of mania and depression after brain injury: causal factors. Am J Psychiatry 145:172–178, 1988

Ruff RM, Levin HS, Mather S, et al: Recovery of memory after mild head injury: a three-center study, in Mild Head Injury. Edited by Levin HS, Eisenberg HM, Benton AL. New York, Oxford Press, 1989, pp 176–188

Rutherford WH: Postconcussive symptoms: relationship to acute neurological indices, individual differences, and circumstances of injury, in Mild Head Injury. Edited by Levin HS, Eisenberg HM, Benton AL. New York, Oxford University Press, 1989, pp 217–228

Saran AS: Depression after minor closed head injury: role of dexametharone suppression test and antidepressants. J Clin Psychiatry 46:335–338, 1985

Saran A: Antidepressants not effective in headache associated with minor closed head injury. Int J Psychiatry Med 18:75–83, 1988

Schoenhuber R, Gentilini M: Auditory brain stem responses in the prognosis of late postconcussional symptoms and neuropsychological dysfunction after minor head injury. Neurosurgery 19:532–534, 1986

Schoenhuber R, Gentilini M: Anxiety and depression after mild head injury: a case control study. J Neurol Neurosurg Psychiatry 51:722–724, 1988

Schoenhuber R, Gentilini M: Neurophysiological assessment of mild head injury, in Mild Head Injury. Edited by Levin HS, Eisenberg HM, Benton AL. New York, Oxford Press, 1989, pp 142–150

Shukla S, Cook BL, Mukherjee S, et al: Mania following head trauma. Am J Psychiatry 144:93–96, 1987

Silver JM, Yudofsky SC, Hales RE: Depression in traumatic brain injury. Neuropsychiatry, Neuropsychology, and Behavioral Neurology 4:12–23, 1991

Silver JM, Hales RE, Yudofsky SC: Neuropsychiatric aspects of traumatic brain injury, in The American Psychiatric Press Textbook of Neuropsychiatry. Edited by Yudofsky SC, Hales RE. Washington, DC, American Psychiatric Press, Inc, 1992, pp 179–190

Sorenson SB, Kraus JF: Occurrence, severity, and outcome of brain injury. Journal of Head Trauma Rehabilitation 6:1–10, 1991

Sparadeo FR, Strauss D, Bartels JT: The incidence, impact, and treatment of substance abuse in head trauma rehabilitation. J Head Trauma Rehabil 5:1–8, 1990

Stewart JT, Hemsath RN: Bipolar illness following traumatic brain injury: treatment with lithium and carbamazepine. J Clin Psychiatry 49:74–75, 1988

Strauss J, Savitsky N: Head injury: neurologic and psychiatric aspects. Archives of Neurology and Psychiatry 31:893–955, 1934

Stuss DT, Stethem LL, Hugenholtz H, et al: Reaction time after head injury: fatigue, divided and focused attention, and consistency of performance. J Neurol Neurosurg Psychiatry 52:742–748, 1989

Teasdale G, Jennett B: Assessment of coma and impaired consciousness: a practical scale. Lancet 2:81–84, 1974

Tennant FS, Wild J: Naltrexone treatment for postconcussional syndrome. Am J Psychiatry 144:813–814, 1987

Thatcher RW, Walker RA, Gerson I, et al: EEG discriminant analyses of mild head trauma. Electroencephalogr Clin Neurophysiol 73:94–106, 1989

Van Zomeren AH, Van Den Burg W: Residual complaints of patients two years after severe head injury. J Neurol Neurosurg Psychiatry 48:21–28, 1985

Wechsler D: Wechsler Adult Intelligence Scale—Revised. San Antonio, TX, Psychological Corporation, 1981

Whitman S, Coonley-Hoganson R, Desai BT: Comparative head trauma experiences in two socioeconomically different Chicago area communities—a population study. Am J Epidemiol 119:570–580, 1984

Williams DH, Levin HS, Eisenberg HM: Mild head injury classification. Neurosurgery 27:422–428, 1990

Wilson JTL: The relationship between neuropsychological function and brain damage detected by neuroimaging after closed head injury. Brain Inj 4:349–363, 1990

Wilson JTL, Wiedmann KD, Hadley DM, et al: Early and late magnetic resonance imaging and neuropsychological outcome after head injury. J Neurol Neurosurg Psychiatry 51:391–396, 1988

Wrightson P: Management of disability and rehabilitation services after mild head injury, in Mild Head Injury. Edited by Levin HS, Eisenberg HM, Benton AL. New York, Oxford University Press, 1989, pp 245–256

Chapter 12

Children and Adolescents

Boris Birmaher, M.D.
Daniel T. Williams, M.D.

Accidents are the leading cause of death in children, and traumatic brain injury (TBI) accounts for a large proportion of these deaths (Silver et al. 1992). The spectrum of TBI, however, ranges from minor scalp laceration to devastating brain injury resulting in permanent and severe neurological disability. The initial evaluation and treatment of patients who have TBI is clearly the neurologist's responsibility, yet a significant proportion of these patients experience subtle or substantial neuropsychological and/or neuropsychiatric deficits that may bring them to psychiatric attention.

Epidemiology

Because the term *head trauma* is used to describe a wide range of severity and type of injury, statistics in this area vary greatly among

The authors wish to acknowledge Therese Deiseroth for her assistance with the manuscript preparation.

reported studies. It has been estimated that more than one million children per year sustain TBI in the United States and approximately one-sixth of these cases are admitted to the hospital (Eiben et al. 1984). The overall incidence of pediatric TBI per 100,000 is 270 in males and 116 in females, with the highest incidence in the 15–24 age range. The pediatric TBI mortality rate is approximately 10/100,000, which far exceeds the second major cause of death in pediatric patients, leukemia. Males are more likely to sustain brain injury at a ratio of 2:1, and they also tend to have more severe TBI (for a review, see Goldstein and Levin 1987).

TBI is more common in families who are exposed to psychosocial adversity and who live in congested areas of the city. In addition, TBI is more likely to occur in children who exhibit behavior disturbances before the accident, have a low IQ, or have a history of previous head injuries (Table 12–1) (Annegers et al. 1980; Backett and Johnston 1959; Brown et al. 1981; Chadwick et al. 1981; Craft et al. 1972; Klonoff 1971; Partington 1960).

Children are highly vulnerable to accidents such as pedestrian–motor vehicle accidents, falls, impacts from moving objects, and sports injuries. Falls constitute a major cause of TBI in children under 5 years old. Sports-related injuries, pedestrian–motor vehicle accidents, and bicycle accidents predominate in the 5–14 age range. Motor vehicle accidents are more prevalent among individuals who are 15 years and older (Annegers 1983; Annegers et al. 1980; Klauber et al. 1981).

There are no accurate data about the incidence of TBI in sports, but it is estimated that TBI occurs in 19% of American football players per year. Children are at high risk for bicycle-related injuries and deaths (Centers for Disease Control 1987). From 1984 through 1988, 62% of all bicycling deaths were caused by TBI. Forty-one percent of brain injury deaths and 76% of bicycle-related brain injuries occurred among children under age 15 (Sacks et al. 1991).

Child abuse is also an important cause of TBI, especially in infants under 2 years old, and may result in intracranial hemorrhage or other major cerebral complications (Billmire and Myers 1985; Koo and Lorogue 1977).

Etiology

Details of the neuropathology, pathophysiology, and neurological evaluation of TBI are discussed in Chapters 2 and 3. In this chapter, we consider briefly only those details pertinent to children and adolescents.

A change in the shape of the brain without a change in its volume is the most common type of TBI in children because their skulls are more easily deformed than those of adults. The most common brain lesions, as seen by magnetic resonance imaging (MRI), are small oval abnormalities in white matter tracts close to the cortical gray matter, or sometimes in the splenium of the corpus callosum. In general, brain damage following TBI is less common and less severe in infants and children than in adults, but it depends upon the extent of vascular injury and edema (Holbourn 1945; Stalhammar 1986).

More than 90% of major pediatric traumatic brain injuries are nonpenetrating and closed and are clinically manifested by alterations in consciousness. Linear fractures of the skull, most commonly in the parietal region, are associated with 7%–40% of mild head injuries. The presence or absence of a linear fracture does not change the clinical management; a TBI can be fatal in the absence of a fracture (Leonidas et al. 1982; Menkes and Till 1990).

Evaluation

As previously noted, acute evaluation of children and adolescents in the wake of TBI is the domain of the neurologist or pediatric neurologist, and this will not be reviewed here. It seems reasonable to suggest, however, that when a patient presents clinically after a TBI with persistent neuropsychiatric symptoms, a full reassessment should be pursued, addressing the preexisting neuropsychiatric disorder, nonspecific effects of hospitalization after trauma, and secondary emotional factors, including the possible effects of potential litigation and the family's reaction to the child's TBI. In addition to psychiatric and neurological reassessment, repeat electroencephalogram and neuroradiological reassessment are often advisable. Thus Levin et al. (1987a) reported that out of 16 consecutive admissions with minor or moderate closed head injury, 14 had abnormalities on MRI, although their prior CT scans were normal or showed fewer abnormalities. Similarly, an apparent decline in academic performance, emotional responsiveness, or behavioral appropriateness should prompt formal neuropsychological and psychiatric consultation with the above considerations in mind. If a patient shows no objective evidence of neurological or cognitive impairment on the various diagnostic parameters enumerated, a supportive psychotherapeutic strategy geared to reassuring both the patient and the family regarding a generally favorable prognosis, and avoiding the secondary gains of invalidism, is most judicious. Advising prompt settlement of any outstanding legal claims is often helpful in this regard.

If symptoms persist in the wake of thorough negative reevaluations in all of the areas noted above, one needs to consider the possibility of a somatoform disorder, a factitious disorder, or malingering (Williams and Hirsch, 1988). Furthermore, it should be noted that any of these entities may coexist even in the presence of documented organic pathology.

Neurological Sequelae

In the acute stage following TBI, severely injured children may display symptoms of delirium (Williams 1991). They often are confused, and exhibit cognitive and behavioral problems such as being mute, withdrawn, agitated, or disinhibited. These symptoms may be secondary to the brain injury, or may be the consequence of complications of the injury, such as inappropriate secretion of antidiuretic hormone, electrolyte disturbances, extradural and subdural hematomas, seizures, and other injuries unrelated to the brain injury (Levin et al. 1982).

With the exception of those patients seen during the acute phases of recovery from TBI, most patients seen by psychiatrists have been neurologically stabilized.By this time, patients may have cognitive and neurological deficits such as hemiparesis, aphasia, and others, and physical deformities that may by themselves cause emotional disturbances. The description of all complications of TBI is beyond the scope of this chapter; however, we will describe two of these, seizures and subdural hematoma, because they may induce new change in the patient's mental status.

Seizures

Seizures that can occur shortly after the injury or appear following an interval of days to years are more common in children than in adults. Late posttraumatic seizures generally develop within the first 2 years following the injury. Seventy-five percent of children with late posttraumatic seizures do not have neurological deficits at the time of the injury. The risk for posttraumatic seizures increases by twofold if there was penetration of the dura and if the patient had more than 24 hours of posttraumatic amnesia (PTA). In general the prognosis for posttraumatic seizures is good (Menkes and Till, 1990).

Subdural Hematoma

Subdural hematoma is a relatively frequent complication of TBI of childhood. It can be acute or chronic and, in both, symptoms of increased intracranial pressure predominate. Chronic hematomas are rare in small children and more frequent in adolescents. Chronic hematomas are manifested as a gradual change in personality and alertness, headaches, and ultimately seizures or loss of consciousness. There often is no history of antecedent brain trauma (which may have been missed by parents). The prognosis of subdural hematoma secondary to nonaccidental trauma, such as those induced by child abuse, is poor (Menkes and Till 1990).

Neuropsychiatric Sequelae

Relationship to Neurological Damage

Rutter et al. (1970) compared the psychiatric status of all school-age children living on the Isle of Wight known to have epilepsy or unequivocal brain damage, with children in the general population and children with a chronic physical illness and/or a handicap not involving the CNS. As assessed on both a teacher's questionnaire and a clinical psychiatric interview, children of normal intelligence with an organic brain condition were twice as likely as children with other physical handicaps (such as asthma, diabetes, and heart disease) to show nonspecific behavioral disturbances. Bilateral brain damage, seizures, brain lesions accompanied by abnormal EEGs, low IQ, reading difficulties, and adverse psychosocial situations were found to be associated with an even higher rate of psychiatric disturbances. After controlling for IQ and family adversity, this increased risk for psychiatric disturbances was still high. However, in this study children with neurological disorders were more likely to have visible physical disabilities than children with other physical handicaps, which could explain the difference in psychopathology. Seidel et al. (1975) addressed this issue. He compared 33 normally intelligent school-age children with brain disorders (mostly cerebral palsy) to 42 children with handicapping conditions that had pathology below the brain stem (e.g., polio, muscular dystrophy). The two groups were comparable in terms of visible physical handicaps, but psychiatric disorder was found twice as frequently in the group with brain damage. Breslau (1985) compared 304 children with cystic fibrosis, cerebral palsy, myelodysplasia, and multiple physical handicaps with 360 healthy children. Children with physical disabilities (with and without brain involvement) were at increased risk for psychiatric disturbances (mainly oppositional behaviors). Children with brain pathology had more severe psychiatric impairment. In these children, however, the psychiatric impairment varied directly with the level of mental retardation.

Relationship to Severity of TBI

Brown et al. (1981) followed a group of 28 children with severe brain injuries who had PTA of at least 7 days, a matched control group of children with orthopedic injuries, and 29 children with mild brain injuries who had PTA exceeding 1 hour but less than 1 week. Immediately after the accident, parents and teachers were interviewed to assess the children's preaccident behaviors and behaviors immediately after the accident; further assessments were done at 4 months, 1 year, and $2\frac{1}{4}$ years after the initial injury. Children with mild brain injuries did not differ from the orthopedic controls and showed no increase in behavioral difficulties. At $2\frac{1}{4}$ years after the initial injury, 50% of the subjects with severe brain injury showed development of new psychiatric disorders at a rate more than three times that found in the control group.

An important issue is to determine the severity of injury above which neuropsychiatric sequelae occur. Brown et al. (1981) determined that behavioral sequelae could be identified only with injuries associated with PTA lasting at least 1 week. Although psychiatric disorder was most frequent among the children showing persistent neurological abnormalities at the $2\frac{1}{4}$ year follow-up, the rate of new psychiatric disorder was still substantially raised in those children who had significant brain injury but normal IQ and no residual neurological abnormalities. Hence there is a need for clinical sensitivity in considering TBI as a potential source of psychiatric morbidity even in the absence of abnormal neurological findings.

In summary, the patterns of psychiatric disorder found in children with TBI are similar to those found in the general population of children coming to child psychiatric attention (Bijur et al. 1990; Brown et al. 1981; Shaffer 1985). One difference, however, is an increased incidence of socially disinhibited behavior, particularly after severe brain injuries. These children can be markedly outspoken, with general lack of regard for social convention, may ask embarrassing questions, and may undress in social situations. They show forgetfulness, overtalkativeness, poor hygiene, and impulsive behavior, symptoms compatible with the DSM-IV diagnosis of personality change due to a general medical condition (labile, disinhibited, or aggressive type) (American Psychiatric Association 1994). In addition, symptoms such as headaches, moodiness, dizziness, and somnolence have been reported after TBI (Farmer et al. 1987; Guilleminault 1983).

Relationship to Location of Lesion

The question of whether the locus of brain injury influences the type of psychiatric symptomatology in childhood was examined by Shaffer et al. (1975). They studied 98 children with localized head injuries and associated dural tear and gross brain substance damage confirmed by surgery. No association was found between the locus of the injury and the presence of either psychiatric disorder or intellectual impairment. However, patients in this study had incurred cortical rather than subcortical damage, and the latter has been associated with persistent aphasia in children and adults (Rutter 1981). Similar to adults (Lishman 1978), there was a tendency for depression to be most common when the lesions were in the right frontal or left parieto-occipital areas.

In a similar study, Solle and Kindlon (1987) reported that children with nondominant lesions showed more internalizing symptomatology (e.g., depressive and anxiety symptoms) and those with dominant lesions more externalizing disorders (e.g., behavior problems). Several cases of mania have been reported following brain injury, especially in those cases with damage in the right hemisphere or limbic system (Robinson et al. 1988; Solle and Kindlon 1987; Starkstein et al. 1987, 1988). Although further studies are clearly needed in this area, it seems reasonable to postulate, as has been suggested by studies involving adult brain injury (Robinson et al. 1988), that psychopathological features in brain injury patients are likely to be the product of an interaction between the extent and location of brain injury (more with bilateral and subcortical lesions), genetic factors, and other predisposing influences, such as preaccident behavior, intellectual level, and social disadvantage.

Relationship to Previous Psychiatric and Social History

Besides the effects of possible neurochemical changes in the brain (see Chapter 2), other factors involved in the development of psychiatric and/or cognitive disturbances are summarized in Table 12–1. The development of psychiatric symptoms and cognitive deficits after a TBI is influenced not only by the presence of neurological sequelae and severity of the TBI, but also by the child's premorbid psychiatric history and social disadvantage. In this domain, Brown et al. (1981) showed that the development of psychiatric symptoms was correlated with the child's preaccident behavior, intellectual level, and the psychosocial circumstances. Those children with persistent behavioral problems after the TBI frequently came from broken homes, families with marital disturbances, or parents with psychiatric problems. Chadwick et al. (1981) showed that in children with minor brain injuries, the impairment in cognitive function already existed before the trauma. In the same vein, Rutter et al. (1970) found that children with adverse psychological situations had a higher rate of psychiatric disturbances. Others have confirmed these findings (Backett and Johnston 1959; Casey et al. 1986; Craft et al. 1972; Manheimer and Mellinger 1967; Partington 1960; Shaffer et al. 1975).

Table 12–1.   Factors associated with the development of behavioral and cognitive sequelae in children and adolescent after traumatic brain injury

Severity of the trauma

Extension of lesion: bilateral greater than unilateral

Localization of lesion: right versus left hemisphere, subcortical versus cortical

Secondary complications such as seizures and subdural hematoma

Child's level of intelligence

Child's previous history of psychiatric disturbance

Family adversity

Family reaction to the trauma

Parental mental disorder

Cognitive Deficits

Chadwick et al. (1981), in the best systematic study so far published, followed three groups of school-age children for a period of $2\frac{1}{4}$ years: 31 children with severe brain injuries (PTA of at least 7 days duration), 28 with orthopedic injuries and minor TBI, defined as PTA lasting more than 1 hour but less than 1 week, and 29 children with minor TBI. Chadwick et al. found a strong "dose-response" relationship between duration of PTA and cognitive deficit. Thus of the 10 children with PTA of more than 3 weeks, all but 1 showed cognitive impairment, and in 6 cases it was persistent. In contrast, when the PTA was less than 2 weeks, no children showed persistent impairment and 3 showed transient cognitive deficits. In the group with severe TBI, there was also a positive correlation between the severity of the injury and the neurological deficits. Recovery in the severe TBI group occurred in the first months, mainly by the fourth month, but deficits were still noticeable at 1 year, and in some cases, even at 2 years after the injury.

Following the trauma, Chadwick found greater impairment of the visual-motor and visual-spatial functions than the verbal functions. However, after the first year of follow-up there were no differences between performance IQ and verbal IQ. Consistent with other investigations (Brink et al. 1970; Heiskanen and Koste 1974), Chadwick et al. (1981) found that the scholastic performance was persistently affected only after a very severe TBI.

Despite the differences in methodology among studies such as definition of mild and severe TBI, type of injury, and time of assessment, there is consensus that there is a dose-response correlation between the severity of the TBI and cognitive impairment (Brink et al. 1970; Fletcher et al. 1990; Heiskanen and Koste 1974; Levin and Eisenberg 1979a; Perrot et al. 1991; Ruijs et al. 1990).

The effects of minor TBI on cognition are more controversial. Chadwick et al. (1981) found that the minor TBI group had cognitive functioning below the controls, but it did not change during the evaluation period, suggesting that the cognitive impairment was present before the injury. Bijur et al. (1990) studied 114 children with mild TBI (as defined by the ICD-9 codes of concussion and head injury [World Health Organization 1978] and the fact that these children received either ambulatory treatment or hospitalization for only 1 night). These children were compared to a group of 601 children with limb fractures, 136 with burns, and 1,726 without injury. All were assessed at 1 year and 5 years after injury. There were no differences in cognitive assessment between children without injuries and those with mild brain injury. Children with lacerations and burns scored worse on tests of intelligence, math, reading, and aggression than children with mild brain injury.

In contrast with the above studies, other investigations (Bassett and Slater 1990; Gulbrandsen 1984; Klonoff 1971; Levin and Eisenberg 1979b) have shown that minor brain injuries might induce subtle cognitive disturbances, especially in tests of performance IQ. However, as shown by Chadwick et al. (1981) and Levin et al. (1987b), these abnormalities are transitory and tend to disappear a few months to a year after the TBI.

Recently, magnetic resonance imaging (MRI) and computed tomography (CT) have been used to evaluate patients with TBI. Kriel et al. (1988) followed 26 children who remained unconscious longer than 90 days after TBI. Children with the best recovery (defined as IQ greater than or equal to 70) were predicted by minimal cerebral atrophy demonstrated by CT performed 2 months after the injury. In subjects over 12 years old, minimal CT atrophy predicted a good outcome with 89% accuracy. CT may miss the brain lesion; for example, Wilson et al. (1988) followed 25 patients with closed head injury and found that deep lesions visualized by MRI at the end of 18 months were correlated with poor neuropsychological test performance. CT at the beginning or at the end of the 18-month follow-up period, or MRI at the beginning of the follow-up period, did not correlate with the neuropsychological testing.

In summary, cognition is affected after severe TBI. It improves gradually, especially during the first months after the injury, but continues to show improvement after 1 year and possibly 2 years postinjury. Although controversial, and depending on the definition, mild TBI, when controlled for cognitive functioning before the trauma, usually does not affect level of cognition.

Family Reactions to a Child's TBI

The study and treatment of the family reactions and dysfunction after pediatric TBI is very important because family factors may influence or (as in the case of minor brain injuries) may be one of the most important factors determining the psychiatric sequelae of the brain injury (Casey et al. 1986). Unfortunately, there are no systematic studies of families of children and adolescents with brain injury. Most of the information is derived from studies of families of adults with brain trauma and children with other disabilities or chronic diseases (for a review see Martin 1988). These investigations suggest that most of the families' reactions are similar to those described in bereavement. Families react first with shock, helplessness, and confusion. Changes in cognition and behavior after TBI have been identified as the greatest source of stress for children with brain injury and their families (Chadwick et al. 1981; Rosenthal and Geckler 1986). This stress increases when there is uncertainty about the child's prognosis.

The first stage of shock is often followed by denial. The denial may be more obvious in cases where the child has no neurological deficits or physical disabilities. If the denial is pervasive, it may prevent the family from responding to the child's needs and obstruct the child's rehabilitation. After the period of denial, a process of awareness and understanding of the child's disabilities begins, which can take from weeks to months. During this period, families usually feel depressed. This period may be followed by or mixed with feelings of anger toward the person who caused the accident, toward the staff in charge of the care of their child, or toward family members themselves.

Finally, a period of adaptation begins in which families become more realistic and accept the child's disabilities and prognosis. All of these stages are variable, do not always follow the above order, and can last for varying periods of time. Some stages may repeat when triggered by any challenge or change, such as puberty, school requirements, or social demands.

The process of adaptation to the new situation is a time-related process involving many interrelated factors. These factors include primarily the age of the child, the severity of disability, and the coping abilities of the child and the family. In addition, many environmental factors have been found to influence post-TBI adaptation. These include family participation in recreation and social activities outside of the home, access to and utilization of informal support networks (e.g., the National Head Injury Foundation), availability of rehabilitation and educational services, quality and quantity of information given by the health caregivers, ambiguity and uncertainty about prognosis, school support, number of siblings, degree of posttrauma child dependence, parents' marital relationships, financial resources, and family ethnicity and parents' educational and religious background (Bristol and Schropler 1984; Holaday 1984; McCubbin 1979; McCubbin et al. 1982; Martin 1988; Simeonsson and McHale 1981).

Treatment

In the absence of controlled studies demonstrating clear-cut efficacy of specific treatment interventions, a broad-based, multidisciplinary approach is most reasonable (Birmaher and Williams 1991). Insofar as the range of child psychopathology encountered in the wake of brain injury is representative of the spectrum of child psychopathology generally, those treatment strategies that would ordinarily apply would still pertain to specific psychopathology encountered in the wake of brain injury. We will address here only a few additional considerations that are particularly pertinent to the child with brain injury.

Psychopharmacological Treatment

In the psychopharmacological domain, the greater sensitivity of brain injury patients to the sedative and anticholinergic effects of various psychotropic medications leads to the advisory of starting with lower doses and raising these in small increments over time.

Similarly, because of the greater incidence of disinhibited, impulsive, and aggressive behavior documented in children with brain injury, it is important to avoid the indiscriminate use of neuroleptic drugs in such patients in the absence of documented psychosis (Silver et al. 1992). This is true not only because of the potential sedative and anticholinergic side effects noted and the dangers of tardive dyskinesia, but also because neuroleptics may lower the threshold for seizures, to which brain injury patients are particularly vulnerable.

There are no controlled studies of the use of stimulants (e.g., methylphenidate) for the treatment of children with attentional problems and hyperactivity after TBI. However, the literature suggests that the effects of stimulants on child behavior are nonspecific. Thus healthy children (Rapoport et al. 1980), mentally retarded children (Aman 1982), attention-deficit hyperactivity disorder (ADHD) children (Greenhill 1985), and autistic children (Birmaher et al. 1988) may all benefit symptomatically from stimulants. Therefore, if a child with TBI presents symptoms of hyperactivity and lack of concentration, it is worthwhile to try stimulants and titrate gradually in doses similar to the ones recommended for ADHD children (e.g., methylphenidate, 5 to 60 mg/day) (Greenhill 1985). Furthermore, if the TBI child has a premorbid history of ADHD, it is advisable to treat him or her with stimulants for ADHD symptoms after TBI, and in this way lower the risk for further TBI. When stimulants are given, the only caution to be observed is the potential hazard for facilitating seizure emergence in a vulnerable individual. Clear guidelines do not exist on this issue and a clinical judgment needs to be made based on how significant an impairment is generated for a given patient by the ADHD symptoms.

Carbamazepine has been used in increasing numbers of pediatric patients with a variety of neuropsychiatric disorders (Evans et al. 1987). There is some anecdotal support for the use of carbamazepine in children with disinhibited aggression, affective lability, and other psychopathological states in the wake of brain injury. This would be particularly justified if the patient's EEG demonstrated epileptiform abnormalities, despite the absence of clinical seizures. It should be noted, however, that growing clinical experience has recently expanded our awareness of the potentially untoward effects of carbamazepine, including worsening of irritability and aggressive behavior, as well as precipitation of mania (Pleak et al. 1988).

Propranolol, a β-adrenergic blocking medication, has been successfully used for the treatment of uncontrollable aggressive outbursts in patients with organic brain impairment (Williams et al. 1982). This can be done in conjunction with, or independent of, any concomitant anticonvulsant medication. Clinical experience to date, which requires controlled replication, suggests that a significant proportion of such patients demonstrate improved control of aggressivity and irritability after appropriate dose titration. Knowledge of appropriate monitoring and titration procedures is important, but easily mastered (Silver et al. 1992; Williams et al. 1982).

Psychosocial Treatment

Probably of equal importance to any psychopharmacological intervention are the behavioral and psychosocial measures that are widely used and of apparent benefit to a significant proportion of brain injury youngsters. These measures include parental counselling, individual and family supportive psychotherapy, speech therapy, associated rehabilitative therapies, academic tutoring, and psychoeducation. It is clearly important that such psychosocial interventions be undertaken by therapists who are familiar with the special characteristics of brain injury children and adolescents. Although systematic studies are undoubtedly desirable in this area, the many clinical variations within the broad spectrum of brain injury youngsters will continue to require individual tailoring of treatment plans to meet the unique needs of individual patients.

Prevention

Children less than 4 years old who are not restrained in safety seats are 11 times more likely to be killed in motor vehicle accidents

(National Safety Council 1985). Conversely, child safety seats have been found to be 80%–90% effective in the prevention of serious injuries to children. All 50 states in the United States and the District of Columbia have mandatory laws for child safety seats. In addition, Sacks et al. (1991) reported that the use of helmets by all bicyclists could prevent one death every day and one head injury every 4 minutes.

Public education to encourage compliance with these safety measures would clearly contribute to primary prevention of a large proportion of pediatric brain injuries caused by motor vehicle and bicycle accidents. More effective public health measures to curb child abuse, alcoholism (especially drunken driving), and preventable accidental and sport injuries would similarly be desirable.

Conclusions

Brain damage, after controlling for other variables such as IQ, socioeconomic factors, premorbid psychiatric symptoms, physical handicaps, and visible physical deformities, is clearly associated with a markedly increased risk of both intellectual impairment and psychiatric disorder. Intellectual impairment is directly associated with the severity of brain damage, especially bilateral damage. Psychiatric disorder is more likely to occur after severe damage, although it is not as clearly related to severity as intellectual impairment. Although controversy remains, it seems that minor TBI does not induce cognitive and/or behavioral impairment, and if it does, the behavioral and cognitive morbidity resolves in most cases within a few months.

References

Aman M: Stimulant drug effects in developmental disorders with hyperactivity—towards a resolution of disparate findings. J Autism Dev Disord, 12:385–398, 1982

American Psychiatric Association: Diagnostic and Statistical Manual of Mental Disorders, 4th Edition, Revised. Washington, DC, American Psychiatric Association, 1994

Annegers JF: The epidemiology of head trauma in children, in Pediatric Head Trauma. Edited by Shapiro K. Mont Kisko, NY, Futura, 1983, pp 1–10

Annegers JF, Grabow JD, Kurland LT, et al: The incidence, causes, and secular trends of head trauma in Olmsted County, Minnesota, 1935–1974. Neurology 30:912–919, 1980

Backett EM, Johnston AM: Social patterns of road accidents to children: some characteristics of vulnerable families. British Medical Journal 1: 409–413, 1959

Bassett SS, Slater E: Neuropsychological function in adolescents sustaining mild closed head injury. J Pediatr Psychol 15:225–237, 1990

Bijur PE, Haslum M, Golding J: Cognitive and behavioral sequela of mild head injury in children. Pediatrics 86:337–344, 1990

Billmire ME, Myers PA: Serious head injury in infants: accident or abuse. Pediatrics 75:340–342, 1985

Birmaher B, Williams DT: Acquired brain disorders, in Child and Adolescent Psychiatry: A Comprehensive Textbook. Edited by Lewis M. Baltimore, MD, Williams & Wilkins, 1991, pp 363–376

Birmaher B, Quintana, H, Greenhill L: Methylphenidate for the treatment of hyperactive autistic children. J Am Acad Child Adolesc Psychiatry 27:248–251, 1988

Breslau N: Psychiatric disorder in children with physical disabilities. Journal of the American Academy of Child Psychiatry 1:87–94, 1985

Brink JD, Garrett AL, Hale WR, et al: Recovery of motor and intellectual function in children sustaining severe head injuries. Dev Med Child Neurol 12:545–571, 1970

Bristol MM, Schropler E: A developmental prospective on stress and coping in families of autistic children, in Severely Handicapped Young Children and Their Families. Edited by Blacher J. San Francisco, CA, Academic Press, 1984, pp 91–141

Brown GL, Chadwick O, Shaffer D, et al: A prospective study of children with head injuries, III: psychiatric sequelae. Psychol Med 11:63–78, 1981

Casey R, Ludwing S, McCormick M: Morbidity following minor head trauma in children. Pediatrics 78:497–502, 1986

Centers for Disease Control: Bicycle-Related Injuries: National Electronic Injury Surveillance System. MMWR 36:269–271, 1987

Chadwick O, Rutter M, Brown G, et al: A prospective study of children with head injuries, II: cognitive sequelae. Psychol Med 11:49–61, 1981

Craft AW, Shaw DA, Cartlidge NE: Head injuries in children. British Medical Journal 3:200–203, 1972

Eiben CF, Anderson T, Lockman C, et al: Functional outcome of closed head injury in children and young adults. Arch Phys Med Rehabil 65:168–170, 1984

Evans RW, Clay TH, Gualtieri CT: Carbamazepine in pediatric psychiatry. J Am Acad Child Adolesc Psychiatry 26:2–8, 1987

Farmer MY, Singer HS, Mellits ED, et al: Neurobehavioral sequelae of minor head injuries in children. Pediatr Neurosci 13:304–308, 1987

Fletcher J, Ewing-Cobbs L, Miner M: Behavioral changes after closed head injury in children. J Consult Clin Psychol 58:93–98, 1990

Goldstein F, Levin HS: Epidemiology of pediatric closed head injury: incidence, clinical characteristics and risk factors. Journal of Learning Disabilities 20:518–525, 1987

Greenhill L: The hyperkinetic syndrome, in The Clinical Guide to Child Psychiatry. Edited by Shaffer D, Ehrhardt A, Greenhill L. New York, London, Free Press, 1985, pp 251–275

Guilleminault C, Faull, KF, Miles L, Van Den Hood J: Posttraumatic excessive daytime sleepiness: a review of 10 patients. Neurology 33:1584–1589, 1983

Gulbrandsen GB: Neuropsychological sequelae of light head injuries in older children 6 months after trauma. Journal of Clinical Neuropsychology 6:257–268, 1984

Heiskanen O, Koste M: Late prognosis of severe brain injury in children. Dev Med Child Neurol 16:11–14, 1974

Holaday B: Challenges of rearing a chronically ill child. Nurs Clin North Am 19:361–368, 1984

Holbourn AHS: The mechanics of brain injuries. Br Med Bull 3:147–151, 1945

Klauber MR, Barnett-Connor E, Marshall LF, et al: The epidemiology of head injury: a prospective study of an entire community—San Diego County, California, 1978. Am J Epidemiol 113:500–509, 1981

Klonoff H: Head injuries in children: predisposing factors, accident conditions, accident proneness, and sequelae. Am J Public Health 61:2405–2417, 1971

Koo AH, Lorogue RL: Evaluation of head trauma by computed tomography. Radiology 123:345–350, 1977

Kriel RL, Krach LE, Shean M: Pediatric closed head injury: Outcome following prolonged unconsciousness. Arch Phys Med Rehabil 69:678–681, 1988

Leonidas JC, Ting W, Binkiewicz A, et al: Mild head trauma in children: when is a roentgenogram necessary? Pediatrics 69:139–143, 1982

Levin HS, Eisenberg HM: Neuropsychological outcome of closed head injury in children and adolescents. Child's Brain 5:281–292, 1979a

Levin HS, Eisenberg HM: Neuropsychological impairment after closed head injury in children and adolescents. J Pediatr Psychol 4:389–402, 1979b

Levin HS, Benton AL, Grossman RG: Neurobehavioral Consequences of Closed Head Injury. New York, Oxford University Press, 1982

Levin HS, Gary HE, High WM, et al: Minor head injury and the post concussional syndrome: methodological issues in outcome studies, in Neurobehavioral Recovery From Head Injury. Edited by Levin HS, Grafman J, Eisenberg HM. New York, Oxford University Press, 1987a, 262–276

Levin HS, Mattis S, Ruff RM, et al: Neurobehavioral outcome following minor head injury: a three-center study. J Neurosurg 66:234–243, 1987b

Lishman WA: Organic Psychiatry. London, Blackwell Scientific Publications, 1978

Manheimer DI, Mellinger GD. Personality characteristics of the child accident repeater. Child Dev 38:491–513, 1967

Martin DA: Children and adolescents with traumatic brain injury: impact on the family. Journal of Learning Disabilities 21:464–470, 1988

McCubbin HI: Integrating coping behavior in family stress theory. Journal of Marriage and the Family 42:237–244, 1979

McCubbin HI, Cauble AE, Patterson JM: Family Stress, Coping and Social Support. Springfield, IL, Charles C Thomas, 1982

Menkes JH, Till K: Postnatal trauma and injuries by physical agents, in Textbook of Child Neurology, 4th Edition. Philadelphia, PA, Lea & Febiger, 1990, pp 462–496

National Safety Council: Acidents facts. Chicago, IL, National Safety Council, 1985

Partington MW. The importance of accident-proneness in the aetiology of head injuries in childhood. Arch Dis Child 35:215–223, 1960

Perrot S, Taylor HG, Montes JL: Neuropsychological sequela, familial stress, and environmental adaptation following pediatric head injury. Developmental Neuropsychology 7:69–86, 1991

Pleak R, Birmaher B, Gavrelescu A, et al: Mania and neuropsychiatric excitation following carbamazepine. J Am Acad Child Adolesc Psychiatry 27:500–503, 1988

Rapoport JL, Bushbaum MS, Weingartner H, et al: Dextroamphetamine: its cognitive and behavioral effects in normal and hyperactive boys and normal men. Arch Gen Psychiatry 37:933–943, 1980

Robinson RG, Boston JD, Starkstein SE, et al: Comparison of mania and depression after brain injury: causal factors. Am J Psychiatry, 145:172–178, 1988

Rosenthal M, Geckler C: Family therapy issues in neuropsychology, in The Neuropsychology Handbook. Edited by Wedding D, Horton AM, Webster J. New York, Springer, 1986, pp 325–344

Ruijs MBM, Keyser A, Gabreels FJM. Long-term sequela of brain damage from closed head injury in children and adolescents. Clin Neurol Neurosurg 92:323–328, 1990

Rutter M: Psychological sequelae of brain damage in children. Am J Psychiatry, 138:1533–1544, 1981

Rutter M, Graham P, Yule W: A neuropsychiatric study in childhood, in Clinics in Developmental Medicine 35/36. London, William Heinemann Medical Books/SIMP, 1970

Sacks JJ, Holmgreen P, Smith SM, et al: Bicycle-associated head injuries and deaths in the United States from 1984 through 1988. How many are preventable? JAMA 266:3016–3018, 1991

Seidel VP, Chadwick OFD, Rutter M: Psychological disorders in crippled children: a comparative study of children with and without brain damage. Dev Med Child Neurol 17:563–573, 1975

Shaffer D: Brain damage, in Child and Adolescent Psychiatry: Modern Approaches, 2nd Edition. Edited by Rutter M, Hersov L. Oxford, Blackwell, 1985, 129–151

Shaffer D, Chadwick O, Rutter M: Psychiatric outcome of localized head injury in children, in Outcome of Severe Damage to the Central Nervous System: Ciba Foundation Symposium 34. Edited by Porter R, Fitzsimons DW. Amsterdam, Elsevier/Excerpta Medica/North-Holland, 1975

Silver JM, Hales RE, Yudofsky SC: Neuropsychiatric aspects of traumatic brain injury, in The American Psychiatric Press Textbook of Neuropsychiatry, 2nd Edition. Edited by Hales RE, Yudofsky SC. Washington, DC, American Psychiatric Press, 1992

Simeonsson RJ, McHale S: Review: research on handicapped children in sibling relationships. Child Care, Health, and Development 7:153–171, 1981

Solle ND, Kindlon DJ: Lateralized brain injury and behavior problems in children. J Abnorm Child Psychol 15:479–491, 1987

Stalhammar D: Experimental models of head injury. Acta Neurochir Suppl (Wien) 36:33–40, 1986

Starkstein SE, Pearlson GD, Boston J, et al: Mania after brain injury: a controlled study of causative factors. Arch Neurol 44:1069–1073, 1987

Starkstein SE, Boston JD, Robinson RF: Mechanisms of mania after brain injury: 12 case reports and review of the literature. J Nerv Ment Dis 176:87–100, 1988

Williams D: Neuropsychiatric signs, symptoms, and syndrome, in Child and Adolescent Psychiatry: A Comprehensive Textbook. Edited by Lewis M. Baltimore, MD, Williams & Wilkins, 1991, pp 340–347

Williams D, Hirsh G: Somatoform disorders, factitions disorders and malingering, in Handbook of Clinical Assessment of Children and Adolescents. Edited by Kestenbaum C, Williams D. New York, New York University Press, 1988, pp 743–769

Williams D, Mehl R, Yudofsky S, et al: The effect of propranolol on uncontrolled rage outbursts in children and adolescents with organic brain dysfunction. Journal of the American Academy of Child Psychiatry 21:129–135, 1982

Wilson JT, Weidman KD, Hadley DM, et al: Early and late magnetic resonance imaging and neuropsychological outcome after head injury. J Neurol Neurosurg Psychiatry 51:391–396, 1988

World Health Organization: Mental Disorders: Glossary and Guide to their Classification in Accordance with the Ninth Revision of the International Classification of Diseases. Geneva, World Health Organization, 1978

Chapter 13

Elderly Patients

Barry S. Fogel, M.D.
James Duffy, M.D.

Although estimates of incidence vary from country to country, traumatic brain injury (TBI) may be as common in elderly people as it is in young adults (Hung et al. 1991; Jennett 1982; Kraus and Arzemanian 1989; Pentland et al. 1986). However, its causes, acute neurological complications, and delayed neurobehavioral consequences occur at different rates. Moreover, the medical and neurological comorbidities common in older people have important implications for treatment and rehabilitation. In this chapter we discuss aging-associated issues in TBI. General considerations in the assessment and management of TBI and its consequences are discussed elsewhere in this book; we will focus primarily on areas deserving special emphasis with older patients.

Influence of Age on TBI Outcome

There is overwhelming evidence that age is a negative prognostic factor in TBI. Mortality following severe brain injury (a Glasgow Coma Scale [GCS; Teasdale and Jennett 1974] score of less than 8) rises steadily with age, with death a virtual certainty after age 75

(Jennett 1982). Elderly patients with moderate brain injuries (GCS score between 8 and 12) also have a higher mortality rate (Pentland et al. 1986). Miller and Pentland (1989) found that in Edinburgh, the mortality rates of moderate and severe brain injuries were 20% and 77% in patients over 65, compared with 1% and less than 39% in patients under 65. In a large series at Allegheny General Hospital, Coffey (1992) found the mortality of severe brain injury to be 35% for adults age 25 to 54, and 65% for patients over 65. Even mild brain injury was associated with a mortality rate of 12% in patients aged 75 or older. Higher severity-adjusted mortality rates in older patients with TBI have been confirmed by recent studies in China (Hung et al. 1991), Germany (Meier et al. 1991), as well as the United States (Luerssen et al. 1988; Waxman et al. 1991).

In the fluid-percussion model of TBI in the rat, mortality rates are strongly influenced by the animal's age. Hamm et al. (1991) showed that "mild" experimental injury caused a 17% mortality rate in 3-month old rats, but a 50% mortality rate in 20-month old rats. "Moderate" experimental injury killed 20% of the young rats, but was lethal to all of the older rats.

Elderly patients are more likely than young TBI patients to develop traumatic mass lesions, including subdural hematomas and intracerebral hemorrhage, from mild to moderate injury (Jennett 1982; Miller and Pentland 1989; Moulton 1992). They are more likely to develop permanent disability as a result of their injuries (Miller and Pentland 1989; Oder et al. 1991; Pentland et al. 1986; Waxman et al. 1991). Survivors tend to have longer hospital stays (Miller and Pentland 1989).

Age is associated with a greater number of postconcussional symptoms at both 6 weeks and 1 year after injury (Rutherford et al. 1977, 1979). Elderly TBI patients also are at increased risk for showing the chronic neurobehavioral consequences of TBI (Adler 1945; Alexander 1982; Levin et al. 1982), including depression, apathy, irritability, and impulsive behavior. Furthermore, sexual dysfunction following recovery from TBI requiring hospitalization also has been shown to be associated with age (O'Carroll et al. 1991).

Causes of TBI in the Elderly

The most common cause of TBI in the elderly is falls (Baker et al. 1984; Pentland et al. 1986; Roy et al. 1987). Many of these falls are associated with concomitant fractures and soft tissue injuries. For example, Oster (1977) found that 10% of elderly patients admitted to hospital with a fractured femur or other bony fracture also had a subdural hematoma. The occurrence of mild TBI may go unappreciated in a conscious but confused elderly patient who presents with a fracture; the abnormal mental state either is not noted, or is attributed to other causes.

Motor vehicle accidents are the second most common cause of TBI and the predominant cause of severe and fatal injuries (Jennett 1982; Pentland et al. 1986). Pedestrian injuries comprise a larger proportion of motor vehicle accidents in the elderly than in younger adults. Rarer causes of TBI in the elderly include sports injuries, assaults, and industrial accidents. Though these do occur, the life-styles of older people render them less exposed to these causes of TBI.

Clinical Presentation

Several patterns of presentation of TBI are more common in elderly people than in young people, because of demographic differences, differences in causation, and differences in the prevalence of comorbidities. These are

1) Delayed presentation hours to days after TBI, with altered mental status. For example, an older person living alone may fall, lose consciousness, and not be brought to medical attention until he or she is discovered unconscious or confused or recovers enough to call for help. Another example is the patient who gradually develops a subdural hematoma after relatively trivial injury. This patient may present as long as 3 months after the onset of symptoms and even longer after the injury (Jennett 1982).

2) Presentation after a fall, with orthopedic or acute medical problems demanding urgent intervention. When the patient presents this way, there is a risk that the associated TBI may receive insufficient attention. Common situations include hip fracture plus TBI, and TBI from a fall precipitated by syncope due to an acute medical problem such as a cardiac arrhythmia or hypotension. Even when TBI is recognized in these situations, its severity may be difficult to assess, because the patient's medical problems may independently contribute to altered mental status, confounding the interpretation of the length of posttraumatic amnesia.

3) Presentation with chronic progressive debility and cognitive impairment. In this situation, patients are brought to medical attention by concerned family, neighbors, or police because of their inability to care for themselves, associated with impaired memory and cognition. Gait instability or physical evidence of trauma suggests that the patient may have had one or more falls, but is unable to provide details. In this situation, TBI or a complication of TBI should be suspected as a contributing or aggravating factor in the patient's dementia.

Differences in Pathophysiology

The most salient difference between older and younger TBI patients is the much greater likelihood of preexisting or coincident medical or neurological disease in the former (Miller and Pentland 1989). We discuss this in detail below. An equally important and well-established difference is the greater vulnerability of older patients to vascular complications. This is likely to be due, at least partially, to age-associated degenerative and atherosclerotic changes in blood vessels, making them more vulnerable to traumatic injury. Age-associated cortical atrophy, by increasing the distance to be crossed by the veins bridging the brain and the venous sinuses, may be relevant to the increased likelihood of subdural hematoma (Berrol 1989).

Four other mechanisms are likely to play a role, but their

precise roles have not yet been established. These factors are different neuroendocrine responses to stress in elderly people, catecholamine depletion, increased susceptibility to excitotoxic injury, and the likelihood of preexisting frontal lobe dysfunction.

Aged individuals show greater and more prolonged adrenal hypersecretion following stress (Sapolsky et al. 1986). Stress-associated vasopressin secretion may also be greater (Urban and Veldhuis 1988). Hypertensive responses to stress also may be greater for several reasons, including the above endocrine factors, reduced arterial compliance, and a higher prevalence of preexisting hypertension (Gualdoni and Sowers 1988). Metabolic consequences of the neuroendrocrine stress response can contribute to a more complicated and morbid clinical course. Hyponatremia, if it occurs, increases the risk of seizures and prolongs delirium. Hypertensive responses to stress increase the risk of both cardiac complications and intracerebral hemorrhage.

At the time of acute brain injury, there is a massive release of catecholamines. Following this release, levels of catecholamines and their metabolites fall. Diminished catecholamine reserves or decreased metabolism aggravate this process. Lower levels of catecholamines may be associated with a worse prognosis following TBI (Boyeson and Feeney 1990). It is known that in both humans and nonhuman primates, aging is associated with decreased catecholamines in associative cortex, including the prefrontal cortex (Carlsson 1981; Goldman-Rakic and Brown 1981). Loss of dopaminergic neurons in the substantia nigra is seen in virtually all aged brains coming to autopsy (Morgan and May 1990). Taken together, these facts suggest that the lower catecholamine reserves of older people may contribute to their worse prognosis following TBI. Monoamine depletion also may be relevant to the occurrence of late neurobehavioral complications of TBI. For example, it is tempting to associate apathy with dopamine depletion, as well as with anatomic frontal lobe injury.

In addition to inducing the release of catecholamines, TBI also releases excitatory amino acid neurotransmitters—glutamate and aspartate (Katayama et al. 1988). These substances can excessively stimulate neurons, leading to metabolic exhaustion, or to the formation of free radicals with toxic effects on the cell. Cell damage, with dendritic swelling and nuclear shrinkage, or frank cell death, can result (Faden et al. 1989). Meldrum (1992) suggests that the clinical relevance of this mechanism to TBI is supported by Jennett's finding of hippocampal damage in patients dying of TBI coma, who did not have parahippocampal gyrus necrosis (which would have suggested temporal lobe ischemia or contusion). The sector of the hippocampus damaged in the TBI death cases was the same as that damaged by experimental excitotoxic injury in animal models.

The greater vulnerability of aged people to excitotoxins is suggested by their differential mortality from blue mussel poisoning, which is thought to be mediated by an excitotoxin (Perl et al. 1990; Teitelbaum et al. 1990). Reasons for a greater vulnerability of aged brains to excitotoxic injury include decreased metabolic reserves, less effective detoxification of free radicals (Canada and Calabrese 1991), and a greater likelihood of ischemia (Meldrum 1992).

Cognitive and behavioral consequences of TBI in older patients may be potentiated by preexisting frontal lobe dysfunction. Frontal lobe blood flow and metabolism tend to be lower in aged people, even those without dementia or clinically evident cognitive deficits (Kuhl et al. 1982; Shaw et al. 1984; Smith 1984). TBI, particularly from closed head injury, tends to affect the prefrontal region and its connections. Traumatic effects superimposed on preexisting age-related changes might produce greater clinical deficits. Although this phenomenon may be regarded as one of comorbidity, the interaction suggested here is with normal age-associated changes, rather than age-associated *disease*.

Comorbidities

The clinical outcome of the elderly patient with TBI often is determined by other diseases the patient has, either existing prior to the head injury or acquired at the same time as the injury. We discuss below several common and relevant comorbidities (Table 13–1).

Dementia, which affects at least 5% of people over 65, implies that the cognitive deficits of TBI will add to preexisting intellectual impairment. Subclinical dementia may become clinically evident after TBI, or patients capable of independent living may lose that capacity. Preexisting dementia, if unknown to the clinician, poses obvious problems for the attribution of cognitive deficits to recent TBI. However, in one relatively common case, attribution is possible. Mild TBI, even with a postconcussional syndrome, produces deficits in memory and concentration, but does not cause significant deficits in higher cortical function, such as aphasia and

Table 13–1. Common comorbidities in older people with traumatic brain injury

Dementia
Frontal lobe dysfunction
    Pure frontal lobe degeneration
    Frontal lobe stroke
    White matter lesions affecting frontal lobe connections
    Basal ganglia diseases affecting frontal lobe inputs
    Prior traumatic brain injury
    Primary mental disorders
        Depression
        Bipolar disorder
        Schizophrenia
Cerebrovascular disease
Alcoholism
Prescription drug side effects
Sensory impairment
    Hearing
    Vision
    Position sense
Physical disability
    Arthritis
    Peripheral vascular disease
    Cardiovascular disease
    Pulmonary disease
    Other central nervous system diseases (e.g., Parkinson's disease
        and stroke)
Hip fracture

apraxia. Such findings, which suggest cortical dementia, should not be ascribed to a mild brain injury, particularly if brain imaging excludes complications such as cortical contusion or subdural hematoma.

Frontal lobe dysfunction, which, as noted above, can occur to some extent in normal aged people, can occur to a greater extent as a result of neurological disease, in the absence of generalized cognitive impairment. Causes include pure frontal lobe degeneration (Neary and Snowden 1991), frontal lobe stroke, and prior TBI. Such dysfunction renders the patient particularly vulnerable to changes in personality and behavior following TBI. A retrospective diagnosis of preexisting frontal lobe dysfunction should be considered when the patient has a history of impaired executive function (planning, judgment, impulse control, and decision-making capacity) antedating the injury.

Ischemic cardiovascular disease increases the risk that TBI, particularly if severe, will be complicated by cardiac arrhythmia or myocardial infarction. Acute brain injury causes autonomic changes and catecholamine release that may produce hypertension and electrocardiographic abnormalities even in patients with normal hearts (Miner 1988). A diseased heart is less able to withstand this stress (de Silva 1993).

Hip fracture, a frequent concomitant of TBI due to falls, has an outcome strongly dependent on mental status. Cognitively impaired patients are less likely to regain independent ambulation, and are less able to participate actively in rehabilitation. Moreover, deficits in balance or motor function associated with acquired brain injury interact with orthopedic problems to limit the return of ambulation.

Alcoholism is a frequent concomitant of TBI in elderly people, as it is in young people. Jennett (1982) reported alcohol to be involved in half of fall-related brain injuries in his elderly patients. Pentland et al. (1986) found alcohol to be implicated in approximately one-third of both elderly and young men with head injury. Miller and Pentland (1989) found alcohol to contribute to the injury in 54% of men and 12% of women over 65. Thus alcohol is less associated with TBI in elderly women. Alcoholism increases the rate of sequelae associated with TBI (Carlsson et al. 1987). Administration of alcohol before experimental brain injury in animals increases lesion size (Albin and Bunegin 1986).

Physical and sensory impairments of various kinds affect the majority of people over 65, but often do not affect physical activities of daily living (ADLs) or instrumental activities of daily living (IADLs) because those affected develop compensatory strategies, such as using assistive devices, modifying their environments, or doing tasks more slowly. TBI, if it causes confusion or even subtle frontal lobe dysfunction, can disrupt these compensatory strategies, and produce a level of functional disability far greater than would be expected in a patient without comorbidities. Moreover, impairments acquired from TBI or associated somatic injuries may overlap with or aggravate preexisting deficits. Vision may be further compromised by hemorrhage into the eye, and hearing loss can be aggravated by the trauma to the ear that is inevitable when the brain is injured (Bauer et al. 1991). Amacher and Bybee (1987) observed that few elderly patients who survive a moderate or severe brain injury ever return to independent living, and that over a quarter of those sustaining mild brain injury do not regain their premorbid functional status. Miller and Pentland (1989) found that of 28 elderly patients who were living alone prior to a mild TBI, only 21 were living by themselves 6 weeks after hospital discharge.

Relation of TBI to Dementia

The occurrence of a subcortical dementia with extrapyramidal features in professional boxers was first described by Martland in 1928. The association between repeated minor trauma and the development of a subcortical dementia, now well-established, gave rise to the notion that head trauma may be causally related to other primary degenerative disorders, specifically Alzheimer's disease and Parkinson's disease. The association with Alzheimer's disease was also suggested by the occurrence of neurofibrillary tangles in patients with dementia pugilistica (Corsallis 1978). However, other neuropathological features of dementia pugilistica, such as cerebellar degeneration and the absence of senile plaques, suggest that the pathological process is distinct (Jellinger and Seidelberger 1970; Lindenberg and Freytag 1960). The distinction between the neuropathology of multiple brain injury and the neuropathology of Alzheimer's disease does not, however, rule out a contributory role of TBI in the genesis of Alzheimer's disease, and perhaps other degenerative diseases as well. At least, it is quite likely that significant preexisting brain injury from any cause will make a dementing process become clinically manifest at an earlier stage, because there will be less cognitive reserve. The notion that trauma may set in motion a specific degenerative process, for example by releasing excitotoxins, is vastly more speculative.

The empirical evidence for an association between TBI and Alzheimer's disease is contradictory, and all retrospective data are confounded by recall bias (Chandra et al. 1987; Heyman et al. 1984; Mortimer et al. 1985; Nee et al. 1987; Sullivan et al. 1987). In the studies by Sullivan et al. and Chandra et al., patients with a previous history of brain injury presented at a younger age than controls without a history of brain injury. This finding is as compatible with additive deficits of TBI and a degenerative process, as it is with TBI being a causal factor.

A recent population-based case-control study (van Duijn et al. 1992) found that patients with probable Alzheimer's disease with onset before age 70 were more likely to have a history of TBI with loss of consciousness. The effect appeared stronger for men and for TBI within the previous 10 years. However, the 95% confidence limits of all their odds ratios included unity. Because of this, and possible recall bias, the authors concluded that prospective replication was needed before inferring a causal relationship. A recent Chinese case-control study (Li et al. 1992) showed no increase in the odds of Alzheimer's disease related to a history of TBI.

Data linking Parkinson's disease with brain trauma also are inconclusive (Factor and Weiner 1991; Williams et al. 1991). However, there are well-documented cases of acutely acquired hemiparkinsonism following TBI, associated with lateralized abnormalities on brain imaging or at postmortem (Lindenberg 1964; Nayenouri 1985; Takeda et al. 1991). Also dementia pugilistica may have parkinsonian features (Critchley 1957).

In summary, recent TBI can make a subclinical dementia manifest, and remote TBI can lower the baseline from which a dementing process begins. Although severe TBI can occasionally produce dementia as a sequel, trauma in itself is a rare cause of dementia (Marsden and Harrison 1972; Smith and Kiloh 1981). Evidence is insufficient to implicate brain injury as the inciting cause of any degenerative dementing process.

Guidelines for Assessment and Treatment

Acute Stage

Age-specific issues in the acute management of TBI include 1) particular vigilance regarding vascular complications, especially subdural hematoma; 2) identification and management of comorbidities; 3) "tracking" of neuropsychiatric issues if orthopedic or medical problems predominate; 4) functional assessment before discharge planning; 5) preventing reinjury in patients who regain ambulation; and 6) life-support decisions in severely injured patients (see Table 13–2).

Intracranial hematomas are virtually always detected by computed tomography (CT) scanning when the patient is symptomatic.

Table 13–2. Guidelines for assessment and treatment of traumatic brain injury in elderly patients: acute stage

1. Monitor carefully for subdural hematomas and hydrocephalus.
2. Identify and manage comorbidities.
3. "Track" neuropsychiatric issues if primary care is medical, surgical, or orthopedic.
4. Assess function before planning discharge.
5. Avoid immobilization.
6. Prevent reinjury.
7. Address life-support decisions if the patient is severely injured.

The risk of missing hemorrhagic complications arises when a CT scan is done and is normal shortly after the injury, and the complication develops subsequently. Because acute hematomas will develop within 24 to 48 hours of the injury, and will have manifest effects on neurological function, the crucial issue is to ensure adequate and regular observation of the patient with brain injury for that period even when the initial CT is normal. Patients with skull fractures are at particular risk. Observation in hospital is advisable if there is the slightest doubt about the availability of a responsible observer.

Chronic subdural hematomas can develop weeks to months after a relatively mild brain injury, and may present with a range of signs, including persistent headache, progressive personality change, or slowly developing hemiparesis (Jennett 1982). The susceptibility of elderly TBI patients to chronic subdural hematoma argues for regular check-ups for at least 3 months after even mild TBI, with a repeat CT scan to be carried out if new neurological signs appear, or if a new and persistent headache develops.

A similar issue exists regarding *hydrocephalus*. Although acute hydrocephalus is a well-known complication of severe TBI, particularly if accompanied by hemorrhage, relatively mild TBI can precipitate or aggravate chronic normal pressure hydrocephalus. The insidious development of progressive gait disturbance, new incontinence, or worsening of frontal lobe signs over several weeks following the TBI would suggest this diagnosis, and would warrant repeat brain imaging. Because hydrocephalus is treatable, its possible occurrence is another reason for careful, scheduled follow-up of mild TBI in elderly patients.

Identification of medical and surgical comorbidities, whether preexisting or correlated with the same event as the brain injury, is an obvious necessity for optimal care, but one that is occasionally neglected in a busy emergency setting. The neuropsychiatrist's role in addressing these problems is largely one of advocacy. On the other hand, identifying comorbid neurological and psychiatric disorders is a central task of the neuropsychiatrist. Eliciting a prior history of cognitive impairment is particularly important in assessing the severity of mild TBI and is useful in assessing patients with more severe TBI if and when they emerge from coma.

In the common situation of TBI with preexisting dementia, the history often can establish which cognitive defects preceded the injury. Neuropsychological tests sometimes can distinguish defects typical of cortical dementia from defects typical of TBI, but distinction between degenerative and traumatic deficits is difficult and sometimes impossible in cases of subcortical dementia or pure frontal lobe degeneration, or when there has been focal cortical contusion.

The identification of comorbid major psychopathology is equally important, because psychiatric disorders, particularly depression, may interfere with rehabilitation and aggravate cognitive and functional deficits. In particular, information that a patient suffered from a major depression prior to the TBI would argue for earlier institution of antidepressant drugs during recovery. Without that history, one might be more inclined to observe the patient longer, hoping that mood changes due to acute injury would resolve spontaneously. Identifying comorbid alcoholism or drug abuse leads to taking relevant precautions against withdrawal, and to the planning for substance abuse treatment if the patient recovers sufficiently to return to the community.

"Tracking" of neuropsychiatric issues is a particular problem for the consulting psychiatrist in the general hospital, when a patient is admitted to the orthopedic service with a fracture, or to the medical or surgical service for an acute comorbidity such as cardiac arrhythmia or a visceral injury. When this happens, mental status is rarely the primary concern of the general medical or surgical service, and the attending physician is subject to pressure to make a rapid disposition as soon as the patient is stabilized. Daily mental status examinations during the first few days postinjury will help detect the patient who will need reassessment and possibly repeat brain imaging for a possible acute complication of TBI. Formal, structured mental status scales are always superior to casual examination, because they are more likely to demonstrate change. The Mini-Mental State Exam (MMSE; Folstein et al. 1975) or equivalents such as the Cognitive Capacity Screening Examination (Schwamm et al. 1987) are appropriate for pa-

tients who are not too injured to cooperate with them. For those who are, a locally standardized protocol for recording orientation, responsiveness to stimuli, coherence of speech, and performance on a simple attentional task is a reasonable substitute.

After medical stabilization, a thorough neuropsychiatric assessment should be performed to identify treatable psychiatric complications, such as depression or psychosis, and to help establish the disposition most compatible with an optimal long-term outcome.

The predischarge assessment should always include a comprehensive review of ADLs and IADLs with direct observation of function in any areas that are doubtful from the history and the medical record. Assessment of IADLs (shopping, transportation, telephone use, medication-taking, and managing money) is particularly important because these functions can be impaired in individuals without gross intellectual impairment and without physical handicap. Individuals living alone are particularly at risk for trouble if a loss of an IADL has not been recognized, as are individuals who live with a spouse whom they are accustomed to dominating and who lack awareness of their loss of function.

In some cases, IADL assessment leads to recommendations for disposition, supervision, or restrictions on activities that the patient finds unacceptable. Although coercive measures are possible in some localities, particularly regarding driving, we recommend that clinicians first try careful assessment followed by patient and family education, temporizing maneuvers, and, in some cases, family therapy. In our experience, a legal showdown usually can be averted. In the case of the elderly patient who is truly unable to manage self-care yet totally lacking in insight, there may be no alternative to pursuing a formal guardianship.

In ambulatory patients, most of whom will have been injured by falls or in motor vehicle accidents, *preventing reinjury* is an obvious sequel to acute treatment. Pertinent assessment of opportunities to prevent reinjury often can begin during the initial hospitalization, or during the first few outpatient follow-up visits for milder injury.

The prevention of falls is a major theme in geriatric medicine, discussed in numerous books and articles on the subject (Lipsitz

1988; Tideiksaar 1989; Tinetti 1990). Potentially remediable causes of falls in elderly patients are listed in Table 13–3.

Several of the principles of fall prevention also are relevant to preventing motor vehicle accidents, including pedestrian accidents. An additional potentially remediable factor in motor vehicle accidents is hearing loss.

Additional interventions to prevent reinjury may be suggested by the circumstances of the injury. For example, the occurrence of a pedestrian accident at night may lead to the discovery of inadequate night vision, leading to the recommendation that the patient not walk alone outdoors at night.

Patients with severe TBI may require intensive medical and surgical intervention simply to survive, including respiratory support, neurosurgery, and interventions to reduce intracranial pressure. Given the expected poor outcome for the majority of elderly people with severe TBI, whether to treat the patient at all is a relevant consideration. Waxman et al. (1991) argue that all patients with severe brain injury should receive initial aggressive treatment, because outcome is poorly correlated with GCS scores on arrival at the hospital, and is better correlated with GCS scores 6 hours later. On the other hand, it is often more difficult to discontinue aggressive treatment once begun, than not to start it at all. The

---

Table 13–3. Potentially remediable causes of falls in elderly patients

1. Visual impairments
2. Medications that impair gait and balance, especially long-acting benzodiazepines
3. Orthopedic disorders affecting gait
4. Alcohol abuse
5. Orthostatic hypotension
6. Parkinson's disease and drug-induced parkinsonism
7. Lower-extremity sensory impairment (e.g., from B_{12} deficiency or cervical spondylosis)
8. General frailty, especially that due to poor nutrition or inadequate exercise
9. Lack of appropriate assistive devices for fixed motor impairments
10. Environmental hazards including poor lighting, lack of railings, and a cluttered environment

---

argument against treatment has its greatest force when the patient is known to have either substantial cognitive and functional impairments prior to the injury, or chronic, uncomfortable, and irreversible physical illness. Although the ethical and legal details of decisions not to treat are beyond the scope of this chapter, the question of withholding treatment for appropriately selected elderly patients with severe TBI deserves examination on any head injury service. Neuropsychiatrists, with their focus on long-term outcome and concern for ethical issues, are well-placed to initiate and participate in such prospective consideration of guidelines for withholding treatment.

Postacute Stage

Age-associated issues in the postacute stage include 1) selecting patients for formal rehabilitation; 2) managing functional deficits; 3) dealing with the patient's family; and 4) treating posttraumatic neurobehavioral complications, including depression, apathy, irritability, and impulsive or explosive behavior. For virtually all of these issues, existing literature has not focused exclusively on elderly patients, or on comparing these patients with younger populations with brain injury. For the most part, our recommendations represent informed opinion. We hope that further empirical research will eventually provide a firmer basis for decision making. Recommendations are summarized in Table 13–4.

Formal rehabilitation for the elderly TBI patient, implying intensive multidisciplinary intervention on either an inpatient or outpatient basis, should be focused mainly on those patients whose deficits are unlikely to improve without such intervention, but are not so overwhelming as to suggest a poor prognosis regardless of vigorous rehabilitative efforts. A good example of a patient deserving formal rehabilitation is the elderly person with a mild dementia, physical deconditioning, mild apathy, and a recent hip fracture occurring concomitantly with mild TBI. Because of the apathy and dementia, this person could not be expected to independently follow a program of exercise and safe, gradual return to ambulation. A formal rehabilitation program could provide physical therapy, gait training, nutritional support if necessary, and attention to any fall prevention issues not addressed during acute

Table 13–4. Guidelines for assessment and treatment of traumatic brain injury in elderly patients: postacute stage

1. Select patients for formal rehabilitation:
     Significant but not overwhelming disabilities.
     Multiple morbidities.
     Inadequate support for home-based care.
2. Approach functional deficits systematically:
     Assistance.
     Supervision.
     Cuing.
     Limited independence.
     Full independence.
3. Counsel the family:
     Address caregiver stress, loss, and depression.
     Offer behavioral management training.
     Observe patient-caregiver interactions.
     Realistically assess support needed for home care.
4. Treat neurobehavioral complications:
     Behavior therapy for milder syndromes, and as an adjunct in
       more severe cases.
     Pharmacological treatment emphasizes defined target symptoms,
       assessment of effects on physical and cognitive function, and
       definite duration of trials.
5. Choose psychotropics to increase benefit-to-risk ratio:
     Depression:
        Avoid strongly anticholinergic drugs.
        Obtain pretreatment electroencephalogram and give
          concomitant antiepileptic drugs to high-risk patients and
          those given bupropion.
        Avoid tricyclics and monoamine oxidase inhibitors in patients
          with fall-related injuries.
     Apathy:
        Consider stimulants or dopamine agonists.
     Irritability:
        Low-dose serotonin drugs.
     Explosiveness:
        Minimize use of benzodiazepines and neuroleptics.

care. Concurrently, the patient could be taught strategies for coping with memory loss, and the family could be educated on when and how to provide assistance.

In *addressing functional deficits* of elderly TBI patients, particularly IADLs, the key decision is whether the function must be carried out entirely by a formal or informal caregiver, or whether some form of cuing or supervision is more appropriate. For example, should a patient be given his or her medication, be asked to take it, or simply have a reminder note on the refrigerator or bathroom mirror?

Here, assessment by a neuropsychologist with an interest in rehabilitation, or by an occupational therapist with neuropsychological sophistication, is helpful. As a general strategy, gradual approaches to testing function and facilitating independence work best. The patient who appears ready to take his or her own medication is initially supervised, then verbally cued, then cued with a note, with each step contingent on the success of the prior stage. Also, if particular medicines are crucial for life support, or dangerous if taken incorrectly, they should continue to be given until the patient's ability to handle other medications independently is established. Similarly, for patients recovering the ability to use public transportation, the first trips should be short and accompanied; the length, complexity, and independence of future trips should be gradually increased if possible. When it is clear that the patient has reached a limit of independent function, the recommendation should be to wait a few months before trying again for a higher level of independence. Deficits persisting after 2 years are very likely to be permanent.

Once a patient has been stabilized at a level of function requiring supervision or cuing for one or more ADLs or IADLs, the issue must be faced as to whether it is better to provide supervision and cuing, or simply to do the task for the patient. This analysis involves an assessment of the effort involved for each of the two alternatives, but also the difference between the two for the particular patient's emotional well being and self-esteem. The level of dependency in the premorbid personality often is an important factor.

Some cuing and supervision tasks may eventually have technological solutions. Medication bottles are already available that make an audible signal when drugs are due to be taken, and alarms are available to detect when a stove has been left on too long. More sophisticated devices, such as electronic devices offering verbal cuing for specific daily activities, surely will be developed in the future.

Families of elderly TBI patients have in common with families of younger TBI patients the challenge of understanding and coping with personality changes, particularly those associated with frontal lobe damage. In addition to generic issues of emotional reaction to loss and trauma, specific feelings are evoked when a loved one suffers a loss of insight, judgment, goal-directed motivation, and impulse control. Understanding the linkage of these symptoms with frontal lobe damage is somewhat helpful, but certainly does not mitigate the pain of recurrently witnessing inappropriate behavior. O'Carroll et al. (1991) showed that 41% of the partners of 36 patients previously hospitalized for TBI had scores on the General Health Questionnaire (Goldberg 1972) suggesting psychiatric "caseness."

Work with a family should begin with education and advice. Relatives involved in daily caregiving should be explicitly trained in behavioral techniques, using written handouts and detailed exercises. The overall strategy for managing behavioral problems is to use intensive prompting and contingency management, gradually fading the frequency of these interventions if they are successful. Most patients with significant frontal lobe injury will do better with external cuing and frequent feedback than with completely "internal" strategies dependent on the patient's memory.

Education and training, however, often are insufficient to enable the family to cope with the patient's altered behavior. A particular problem in elderly patients arises when the primary caregiver is a spouse, child, or paid caregiver who historically has been in a subordinate position to the patient. The patient may have an exceedingly difficult time accepting limit-setting and supervision from such a person. Direct observation of the problematic interaction sometimes can help, with the clinician instructing the caregiver in the most tactful and subtle ways of addressing the patient's inappropriate behavior. For patients with more intact cognition and some preservation of insight, grieving for the loss of the dominant position in the family may be possible and helpful.

The decision to resort to institutional long-term care is more likely to arise with the elderly TBI patient, because of the worse prognosis and the frequent occurrence of other functional impairments. In equivocal cases, decision making is aided, and guilt minimized, by a detailed multidisciplinary assessment of the patient prior to the placement decision, with careful explanation to the family of cognitive test results and occupational therapy assessment. The options for coping with the patient's deficits are explored, always with explicit consideration of what realistically would be needed to keep the patient in the community.

When either the patient or the caregiver is clinically depressed, a situation that arises quite frequently, it is desirable whenever possible to treat all depressed parties before making permanent long-term care decisions. Respite care sometimes may be needed to facilitate the treatment of both the patient's and the caregiver's depression. The aged patient with impaired cognition may find it easier to obtain respite care than the younger TBI patient, because nursing homes and adult day care services may be willing to accept the former type of patient.

Treatment of Neurobehavioral Complications

As suggested above, behavior therapy interventions may be helpful for both deficient and inappropriate behaviors in TBI patients; parallel experiences with Alzheimer's disease specialty units suggest that neither age nor cognitive impairment rules out the efficacy of environmental and behavioral interventions. Eames and Wood (1985) demonstrated 75% reduction in explosive behaviors in TBI patients using formal behavior modification.

Notwithstanding the success of behavior modification with highly motivated families and generously endowed facilities, psychopharmacological treatment usually is considered for the major neurobehavioral complications of TBI. This is partly because behavioral therapies may be practically difficult to implement, and partly because some complications, such as profound apathy or the major depressive syndrome, usually are not responsive to nonpharmacological measures. In this section we will offer psychopharmacological advice for the treatment of posttraumatic depression, apathy, irritability, and explosive or impulsive behavior, and conclude with general recommendations for organizing drug trials in patients with sequelae of TBI.

Post-TBI depression in elderly patients generally should be treated as any other clinically significant geriatric depression. Antidepressant drugs should be started at low dosage and built up slowly, and psychotherapy should be offered to all patients whose cognitive status permits. Strongly anticholinergic antidepressants should be avoided because of their greater cognitive side effects.

Effects on seizure threshold are particularly relevant in elderly TBI patients, because brain trauma and its vascular complications produce seizure foci, and because unrecognized seizures may be the cause of falls and motor vehicle accidents leading to TBI. Prophylactic antiepileptic drugs should be considered when giving antidepressants to TBI patients if the patient has had a history of seizures, a penetrating injury, a definite contusion or hemorrhage, or if bupropion is to be used. For other patients, a pretreatment EEG should be considered if full-dose antidepressant treatment is contemplated. Patients with definite epileptiform features should receive prophylactic antiepileptic drugs.

In choosing and monitoring antidepressant drug therapy, considerations of fall prevention are relevant. If the brain injury resulted from a fall, and particularly if orthostatic hypotension was an issue, tricyclics and trazodone would be inferior to serotonin reuptake inhibitors or bupropion. If ataxia was implicated in the cause of falling, the patient should be rechecked for aggravation of ataxia after each increase in antidepressant dosage.

Apathy following TBI may respond to psychostimulants or dopamine agonists (Gualtieri 1991), although there have been no controlled clinical trials, let alone trials focusing on elderly patients. The distinction between apathy and depression should be made because stimulants are not drugs of choice for major depression. Marin (1990) delineates this distinction in detail: the non-depressed apathetic patient lacks interest and drive, but does not show the negative affects and cognitions typical of depressive disorders. A practical first step is to try methylphenidate 2.5 mg morning and noon, increasing gradually to a maximum of 10 mg tid if tolerated, and if smaller doses are ineffective. Contraindications are tachyarrhythmia, untreated hypertension, unstable angina, and paranoid psychosis. Dextroamphetamine, on a similar dosage schedule, is another option. Among the antiparkinson drugs, both amantadine and bromocriptine have been used to treat apathy subsequent to brain injury (Gualtieri 1991). The latter are given exactly as in treating early Parkinson's disease, with a "start low, go slow" dosage strategy.

Irritability, with or without psychomotor agitation, may respond to serotonergic agents. Options include buspirone, trazodone, and the serotonin reuptake inhibitors. With buspirone and the serotonin reuptake inhibitors, the potential problems are restlessness, anxiety, and agitation worsening or beginning when the drug is begun. To minimize these problems, we recommend starting buspirone at a dose no higher than 5 mg bid, fluoxetine at 5 mg/day, and sertraline at 12.5 mg/day. Sometimes, very small doses are adequate to treat the irritability. If they are not, dosage should be increased gradually, eventually reaching maximal recommended antianxiety or antidepressant levels if necessary.

Trazodone's major drawback in treating elderly patients with TBI is its propensity to cause ataxia and orthostatic hypotension, both of which put patients at risk for falls. If trazodone is used, we suggest starting at 25 mg qhs, and monitoring both orthostatic blood pressure and a standardized test of gait, such as the tandem walk, each time the dosage is titrated upward.

Explosive or impulsive behavior in a variety of organically impaired patients, including elderly patients and TBI patients, has been successfully treated with a wide range of agents, including β-adrenergic blockers, lithium, carbamazepine, tricyclics, buspirone, and even neuroleptics (Haas and Cope 1985; Jackson et al. 1985; Levine 1988; Rao et al. 1985; Ratey et al. 1989; Silver and Yudofsky 1985). The practical problem is which drugs to try in what order, how long to try each drug, and how to assess the outcome. All of these issues were addressed by Fogel (1991) in a systematic analysis of the treatment of agitation in elderly patients with non-neuroleptic agents. Schneider and Sobin (1991) offered a similar review focusing on the problem of agitation in dementia.

Our recommendations, based mainly on experience and opinion, are as follows:

- If irritability and negative affect are prominent, or if there is a long history of chronic depression or anxiety preceding the TBI, try serotonin drugs first.
- If an explosive patient requires an antiepileptic drug for neurological reasons, carbamazepine is the drug of choice, with valproate the second choice if carbamazepine is ineffective or not tolerated.
- If episodes of explosiveness are accompanied by gross autonomic arousal, and if there is no history of congestive heart failure, asthma, or chronic obstructive pulmonary disease, β-adrenergic blockers deserve a trial.
- Because lithium is often poorly tolerated by elderly people with brain injury, mood-stabilizing antiepileptic drugs usually should be tried first. If lithium is to be used, try a level between 0.5 and 1.0 mEq/L for at least 2 weeks before attempting a higher dosage. Watch for aggravation of ataxia, or the development of tremor or confusion.

Both neuroleptics and benzodiazepines often are used for acute management of explosive patients. Both have substantial disadvantages for the chronic treatment of elderly TBI patients. Neuroleptics aggravate apathy, may cause akathisia, and may impair ambulation by their extrapyramidal side effects. Benzodiazepines aggravate memory impairment, are a risk factor for falling, and occasionally may aggravate socially inappropriate behavior by causing disinhibition. Notwithstanding, both of these agents occasionally have helped patients in the long term. In our experience, low-dose neuroleptics have been most helpful for patients with psychotic features or paranoid attitudes, and benzodiazepines have been most helpful for patients who were long-term benzodiazepine users prior to their TBI. When neuroleptics are used in elderly patients with TBI, dosage should be kept low, and there should be a low threshold for prescribing concomitant anti-parkinson medication. When benzodiazepines are used in elderly TBI patients, the crucial issue is to monitor patients closely for changes in cognition, behavior, and gait as dosage is titrated upward. With short-acting agents such as lorazepam, check for confusion or ataxia at the peak of the dose, and for rebound anxiety or agitation as the dose wears off. With longer-acting agents, watch for slowly developing lethargy or ataxia as levels of active metabolites reach a steady state over several weeks.

In general, drugs that are tolerated should be tried for several weeks, because virtually all reports of psychotropic drug action suggest the possibility of delayed therapeutic effects. In assessing the value of a particular agent, one should not only consider target symptoms of behavior or mood, but should also consider overall function, including cognitive testing, ADLs, and IADLs. A drug that relieves depression but impairs ambulation may be less satisfactory than one that offers partial relief without compromising the patient's ability to walk. The trade-off between symptom relief and function is particularly evident with the neuroleptics and benzodiazepines, both of which can provide dramatic relief of agitation, but often do so at the expense of diminished independent functioning.

Conclusions

Older people have a worse prognosis after TBI, both because of comorbidities and because of age-associated changes in baseline brain function and in the capacity for recovery of function. In the longer term, the best hope for elderly TBI patients is likely to be some form of neuroprotective agent, given as soon as possible after the injury. At present, all elderly TBI patients can benefit from a holistic, functionally oriented approach to management that embodies the principles of geriatrics, especially secondary and tertiary prevention.

References

Alexander MP: Traumatic brain injury, in Psychiatric Aspects of Neurologic Disease, Vol II. Edited by Benson DF, Blumer D. New York, Grune & Stratton, 1982, pp 219–249

Adler A: Mental symptoms following head injury. Archives of Neurology and Psychiatry 53:34–43, 1945

Albin MS, Bunegin L: An experimental study of craniocerebral trauma during ethanol intoxication. Crit Care Med 14:841–846, 1986

Amacher AL, Bybee DE: Toleration of head injury by the elderly. Neurosurgery 20:954–958, 1987

Baker SP, O'Neill B, Karpf RS: The Injury Fact Book. Lexington, MA, Lexington Books, 1984

Bauer P, Korpert K, Neuberger M, et al: Risk factors for hearing loss at different frequencies in a population of 47,388 noise-exposed workers. J Acoust Soc Am 90:3086–3098, 1991

Berrol S: Other factors: age, alcohol, and multiple injuries, in Mild to Moderate Head Injury. Edited by Hoff JT, Anderson TE, Cole TM. Cambridge, MA, Blackwell Scientific, 1989, pp 135–142

Boyeson MG, Feeney DM: Intraventricular norepinephrine facilitates motor recovery following senorimotor cortex injury. Pharmacol Biochem Behav 35:497–501, 1990

Canada AT, Calabrese EJ: Free radicals, aging, and toxicology, in Aging and Environmental Toxicology: Biological and Behavioral Perspectives. Edited by Cooper RL, Goldman JM, Harbin TJ. Baltimore, MD, Johns Hopkins University Press, 1991, pp 31–55

Carlsson A: Aging and brain neurotransmitters, in Strategies for the Development of an Effective Treatment for Senile Dementia. Edited by Crook T, Gershon S. New Canaan, CT, Mark Powley Associates, 1981, pp 93–104

Carlsson GS, Svardsudd K, Welin L: Long-term effects of head injuries sustained during life in three male populations. J Neurosurg 67:197–205, 1987

Chandra V, Philipose RN, Bell PA, et al: Case-control study of late onset "probable Alzheimer's disease." Neurology 37:1295–1300, 1987

Coffey E: Traumatic brain injury in the elderly. Paper presented at British Neuropsychiatric Association Annual Meeting, Oxford, England, July 1992

Corsallis JAN: Post-traumatic dementia, in Aging. Edited by Katzman R, Terry RD, Bick KL. New York, Raven, 1978

Critchley M: Medical aspects of boxing. Br Med J 1:357–362, 1957

de Silva RA: Cardiac arrhythmias and sudden cardiac death, in Medical Psychiatric Practice, Vol 2. Edited by Stoudemire A, Fogel BS. Washington, DC, American Psychiatric Press, 1993, pp 199–236

Eames P, Wood R: Rehabilitation after severe brain injury in a follow-up study of a behavior modification approach. J Neurol Neurosurg Psychiatry 48:613–619,1985

Factor SA, Weiner WJ: Prior history of head trauma in Parkinson's disease. Mov Disord 6:225–229, 1991

Faden AI, Demediuk P, Panter S, et al: The role of excitatory amino acids and NMDA receptors in traumatic brain injury. Science 244:798–800, 1989

Fogel, BS: Beyond neuroleptics: the treatment of agitation, in The Elderly with Chronic Mental Illness. Edited by Light E, Lebowitz BD. New York, Springer, 1991, pp 167–190

Folstein MF, Folstein SE, McHugh PR: Mini-Mental State: a practical method for grading the cognitive state of patients for the clinician. J Psychiatr Res 12:189–198, 1975

Goldman-Rakic PS, Brown RM: Regional changes of monoamines in cerebral cortex and subcortical structures of aging mesus monkeys. Neuroscience 6:177–187, 1981

Goldberg DP: The Detection of Psychiatric Illness by Questionnaire (Maudsley Monograph No 21). London, Oxford University Press, 1972

Gualdoni SM, Sowers JR: Hypertension in the elderly, in Endocrinology of Aging. Edited by Sowers JR, Felicetta JV. New York, Raven, 1988, 251–277

Gualtieri CT: Neuropsychiatry and Behavioral Pharmacology. New York, Springer-Verlag, 1991

Haas JF, Cope N: Neuropharmacological management of behavior sequelae in head injury: a case report. Arch Phys Med Rehabil 66:472–474, 1985

Hamm RJ, Jenkins LW, Lyeth BG, et al: The effect of age on outcome following traumatic brain injury in rats. J Neurosurg 75:916–921, 1991

Heyman A, Wilkinson WE, Stafford JA, et al: Alzheimer's disease: a study of epidemiological aspects. Ann Neurol 15:335–341, 1984

Hung CC, Chiu WT, Tsai JC, et al: An epidemiological study of head injury in Haulien County Taiwan. Taiwan I Hsueh Hui Tsa Chih 90:1227–1233, 1991

Jackson RD, Corrigan JD, Arnett JA: Amitriptyline for agitation in head injury. Arch Phys Med Rehabil 66:280–282, 1985

Jellinger K, Seidelberger F: Protracted and post-traumatic encephalopathy. J Neurol Sci 10:51–94, 1970

Jennett B: Head injuries, in Neurological Disorders in the Elderly. Edited by Caird FI. Littleton, MA, John Wright & Sons, 1982, pp 202–211

Katayama Y, Cheung MK, Gorman L, et al: Increase in extracellular glutamate and associated massive ionic fluxes following concussive brain injury (abstract). Neuroscience Abstracts 14:1154, 1988

Kraus JF, Arzemanian S: Epidemiologic features of mild and moderate brain injury, in Mild to Moderate Head Injury. Edited by Hoff JT, Anderson TE, Cole TM. Cambridge, MA, Blackwell Scientific, 1989, pp 9–28

Kuhl DE, Metter EJ, Riege WH, et al: Effects of human aging on patterns of local cerebral glucose utilization determined by the [18F]fluorodeoxyglucose method. J Cereb Blood Flow Metab 2:163–171, 1982

Levin HS, Benston AL, Grossman RC: Neurobehavioral Consequences of Closed Head Injury. New York, Oxford University Press, 1982

Levine AM: Buspirone and agitation in head injury. Brain Inj 2:165–167, 1988

Li G, Shen YC, Li YT, et al: A case-control study of Alzheimer's disease in China. Neurology 42:1481–1488, 1992

Lindenberg R: Die Schadigungsmechanismen der Substantia nigra bei Hirntraumen und das Problem des posttraumatischen Parkinsonismus. Dtsch Z Nervenheilk 185:637–663, 1964

Lindenberg R, Freytag L: The mechanism of cerebral contusions:a pathologic-anatomic study. Archives of Pathology 69:440–469, 1960

Lipsitz LA: Falls and syncope, in Geriatric Medicine. Edited by Rowe JW, Besdine RW. Boston, MA, Little, Brown, 1988, pp 208–218

Luerssen TG, Klauber MR, Marshall LF: Outcome from head injury related to patient's age. A longitudinal prospective study of adult and pediatric head injury. J Neurosurg 68:409–416, 1988

Marin RS: Differential diagnosis and classification of apathy. Am J Psychiatry 147:22–33, 1990

Marsden CD, Harrison MJG: Outcome of investigation of patients with presenile dementia. BMJ 2:249–252, 1972

Martland HS: Punch drunk. JAMA 91:1103–1107, 1928

Meier U, Knopf W, Klotzer R, et al: Postoperative results following severe craniocerebral trauma. Zentralbl Chir 116:845–854, 1991

Meldrum B: Excitotoxicity and Head Injury. Paper presented at the British Neuropsychiatric Association Annual Meeting, Oxford England, July 1992

Miller JD, Pentland B: The factors of age, alcohol and multiple injury in patients with mild and moderate head injury, in Mild to Moderate Head Injury. Edited by Hoff JT, Anderson TE, Cole TM. Boston, MA, Blackwell Scientific, 1989, pp 125–133

Miner ME: Systemic effects of brain injury. Trauma 2:75–83, 1988

Morgan DG, May PC: Age-related changes in synaptic neurochemistry, in Handbook of the Biology of Aging. Edited by Schneider EL, Rowe JW. San Diego, CA, Academic Press, 1990, pp 219–254

Mortimer JA, French LR, Hutton JT, et al: Head injury as a risk factor for Alzheimer's disease. Neurology 35:264–267, 1985

Moulton RJ: Traumatic intracranial mass lesions: how soon for evacuation? Can J Surg 35:35–37, 1992

Nayenouri T: Posttraumatic parkinsonism. Surg Neurol 24:263–264, 1985

Neary D, Snowden J: Dementia of the frontal lobe type, in Frontal Lobe Function and Dysfunction. Edited by Levin HS, Eisenberg HM, Benton AL. New York, Oxford University Press, 1991, pp 304–317

Nee LE, Eldridge R, Sunderland T, et al: Dementia of the Alzheimer type: clinical and family study of 22 twin pairs. Neurology 37:359–166, 1987

O'Carroll RE, Woodrow J, Maroun F: Psychosexual and psychosocial sequelae of closed head injury. Brain Inj 5:303–313, 1991

Oder W, Goldenberg G, Deecke L: Prognostic factors in rehabilitation after severe craniocerebral injuries. Fortschr Neurol Psychiatr 59:376–385, 1991

Oster C: Signs of sensory deprivation versus cerebral injury in post-hip fracture patients. J Am Geriat Soc 25: 368–370, 1977

Pentland B, Jones PA, Roy CW, et al: Head injury in the elderly. Age Ageing 15:193–202, 1986

Perl TM, Bedard L, Kosatsky T, et al: An outbreak of toxic encephalopathy caused by eating mussels contaminated with domoic acid. N Engl J Med 322:1775–1780, 1990

Rao N, Jellinek HM, Woolston DC: Agitation in closed head injury: haloperidol effects on rehabilitation outcome. Arch Phys Med Rehabil 66:30–34, 1985

Ratey JJ, Sovner R, Mikkelson F, et al: Buspirone for maladaptive behavior and anxiety in developmentally disabled children. J Clin Psychiatry 50:382–384, 1989

Roy CW, Pentland B, Miller JD: The causes and consequences of minor head injury in the elderly. Injury 24:318–321, 1987

Rutherford WH, Merrett JD, McDonald JR: Sequelae of concussion caused by minor head injuries. Lancet 1:1–4, 1977

Rutherford WH, Merrett JD, McDonald JR: Symptoms at one year following concussion from minor head injuries. Injury 10:225–230, 1979

Sapolsky RM, Krey LC, McEwen BS: The neuroendocrinology of stress and ageing: the glucocorticoid cascade hypotheses. Endocr Rev 7:284–301, 1986

Schneider LS, Sobin PB: Non-neuroleptic medications in the management of agitation in Alzheimer's disease and other dementia: a selective review. International Journal of Geriatric Psychiatry 6:691–708, 1991

Schwamm LH, Van Dyke C, Kiernan RJ, et al: The neurobehavioral cognitive status examination: comparison with the cognitive capacity screening examination and the mini-mental state. Ann Intern Med 107:486–491, 1987

Shaw TG, Mortel KF, Meyer JS, et al: Cerebral blood flow changes in benign aging and cerebrovascular disease. Neurology 34:855–862, 1984

Silver JM, Yudofsky SC: Propanolol for aggression: literature review and clinical guidelines. International Drug Therapy Newsletter 20:9–12, 1985

Smith CB: Aging and changes in cerebral energy metabolism. Trends Neurosci 7:203–208, 1984

Smith JS, Kiloh LG: The investigation of dementia: results in 200 consecutive admissions. Lancet 1:824–827, 1981

Sullivan P, Pettiti D, Barbaccia J: Head trauma and age of onset of dementia of the Alzheimer type. JAMA 257:2289–2296, 1987

Takeda M, Okuda B, Tomino Y, et al: A case of posttraumatic parkinsonism. Rinsho Shinkeigaku 31:842–846, 1991

Teasdale G, Jennett B: Assessment of coma and impaired consciousness: a practical scale. Lancet 2:81–84, 1974

Teitelbaum JS, Zatorre RJ, Carpenter S, et al: Neurologic sequelae of domoic acid intoxication due to the ingestion of contaminated mussels. N Engl J Med 322:1781–1787, 1990

Tideiksaar R: Falling in Old Age: Its Prevention and Treatment. New York, Springer, 1989

Tinetti ME: Falls, in Geriatric Medicine, 2nd Edition. Edited by Cassel CK, Riesenberg DE, Sorensen LB, et al. New York, Springer-Verlag, 1990, pp 528–534

Urban RJ, Veldhuis JD: Hypothalamo-pituitary concomitants of aging, in Endocrinology of Aging. Edited by Sowers JR, Felicetta JV. New York, Raven, 1988, pp 41–74

van Duijn CM, Tanja TA, Haaxma R, et al: Head trauma and the risk of Alzheimer's disease. Am J Epidemiol 135:775–782, 1992

Waxman K, Sundine MJ, Young RF: Is early prediction of outcome in severe head injury possible? Arch Surg 126:1237–1241, 1991

Williams DB, Annegers JF, Kokmen E, et al: Brain injury and neurological sequelae: a cohort study of dementia, parkinsonism, and amyotrophic lateral sclerosis. Neurology 41:1554–1557, 1991

Chapter 14

Sexual Dysfunction

Nathan D. Zasler, M.D.

Traumatic brain injury (TBI) may adversely affect the expression of sexuality due to a variety of different factors. Alterations in physical, cognitive, and behavioral status, as well as communication skills, can all adversely impact expression of sexuality. Brain injury may produce sexual dysfunction at the genital level, as well as adversely affect expression of sexuality at the nongenital level. Ultimately the mediating factors in these functional alterations include disruption of neuroanatomical pathways and/or aberrations in neurophysiological function as a result of the TBI. To better comprehend the effect of brain injury on sexuality, one must understand the basic neuroanatomical pathways and neurophysiological mechanisms involved in the mediation of sexual function.

Appropriate neuromedical, psychiatric, and rehabilitative intervention should be available to this patient population to allow for maximal reintegration into preinjury sexual life-styles at the community, personal, and family levels. Professionals must address the area of sexuality as they do other functional areas of human "performance," including mobility, activities of daily living, and bowel and bladder function, in order to provide a comprehensive approach to the problem and minimize any resultant functional impairment. By providing appropriate early intervention following trauma, the professional allows for a smoother transition and accommodation to potential postinjury sexuality issues.

Sexual Neuroanatomy and Neurophysiology

In order to understand how sexual function and sexuality may be adversely affected by TBI, an appreciation of neuroanatomical, neurophysiological, and neurochemical correlates of sexual function is critical. By gaining a sense of the myriad of interactions required for "normal" sexual function, we can improve diagnosis and treatment when functional difficulties occur.

Sexual Neuroanatomy

Although exact neuroanatomical pathways responsible for normal sexual function have not been definitively elucidated, the multi-

Table 14–1. Sexual neuroanatomy: substructures and theoretical behavioral correlates

Neuroanatomical structure	Neuroanatomical substructure	Theorized behavioral correlate
Cortical	Piriform cortex	Modulation of
	Frontal lobes	drive, initiation,
	Temporal lobes	and sexual activation
Subcoritcal	Hippocampus	Modulation of
	Amygdala	sexual behaviors
	Septal complex	and genital responses
	Hypothalamus	
Brain stem	Reticular activating system	Maintenance of arousal and alertness
	Afferent input	and conduit for
	Efferent output	information
Peripheral nervous system	Autonomic	Genital sexual function
	Sympathetic	
	Parasympathetic	
	Somatic	

plicity of neural networks involved are believed to include structures in the peripheral nervous system (both autonomic and somatic), brain stem, subcortex, and cortex (Table 14–1). Given the propensity for frontotemporal focal cortical contusion and diffuse axonal injury, it is not surprising that sexual dysfunction commonly occurs after any significant brain insult (Horn and Zasler 1990).

Cortical structures, including the paralimbic cortex, are involved in the mediation of sexual function. Stimulation of cortical structures has produced genital hallucinations and erections (MacLean 1975). Certain cortical structures, such as the piriform cortex, are in intimate connection with more primitive "sexual" systems, including the olfactory system. Animal studies have shown that lesions in these areas may produce hypersexuality (Mesulam 1985). The frontal lobes are intimately involved with limbic and paralimbic structures via numerous neural connections. Frontal injury may result in various behavioral abnormalities. Inferomedial frontal injury may produce disinhibited and sexually inappropriate behavior, whereas dorsolateral frontal injury typically will result in impaired sexual initiation (Walker 1976). Clinical experience has revealed that certain patients with frontal injury demonstrate a compromised ability to fantasize that may impede masturbation. Observations derived from patients who have had strokes suggest that right brain injury results in a greater degree of sexual impairment (Coslett and Heilman 1986). However, frontal involvement rather than laterality may be the more significant factor (Horn and Zasler 1990). Research has demonstrated that lesions in the nondominant hemisphere may lead to a cornucopia of deficits that compromise expression of sexuality, including dysprosody, visuoperceptual problems, and anosognosia (Zasler 1991). Additionally, the nondominant temporal lobe has been theorized to be the sexual activation center for the brain (Cohen et al. 1976). Lesions in the dominant hemisphere may produce aphasias and apraxias, thereby compromising both communication and motor performance (Zasler 1991).

Subcortical structures, including the hippocampus, amygdala, septal complex, and hypothalamic nuclei play important roles in mediation of sexual function. MacLean hypothesized that penile tumescence is modulated by the hippocampus (MacLean 1975). The septal complex has been theorized to be involved in erection as well as pleasurable sexual sensations similar to orgasm (Heath 1964; Penfield and Rasmussen 1950). The amygdala has been studied quite extensively through ablation and stimulation studies. Among the classic studies were those involving removal of the anterior temporal lobes resulting in so-called Klüver-Bucy syndrome. The hypothalamus is thought to be one of the critical limbic structures relative to sexual behavior. The anterior hypothalamus is involved in endocrine activity and associated copulatory behaviors. The posterior hypothalamus has been linked functionally to copulatory behaviors and precocious puberty (Bauer 1959; Boller and Frank 1982). Thalamic relays from sensory afferents in the ventrolateral and intralaminar nuclei have also been postulated to play important roles in normal sexual functioning (Horn and Zasler 1990). Stimulation of ascending thalamic sensory inputs has been shown to produce erection (MacLean 1975; Walker 1976). Hypersexuality has also been reported as a sequela of thalamic lesion (Miller et al. 1986). Basal ganglia stimulation may produce complex forms of species specific ritualistic sexual behaviors (MacLean 1975).

Brain stem structures such as the catecholaminergically "driven" pontine and mesencephalic reticular activating systems are responsible for maintaining arousal and alertness. These systems innervate limbic and frontal structures responsible for many sexually oriented behaviors. The brain stem also serves as the conduit for sexual information carried by afferent and efferent fibers (Horn and Zasler 1990). Injury to brain stem pathways can result in decreased ability to prepare the organism for processing incoming information. This fact takes on additional importance given the evidence supporting the need for activation within certain limbic and cortical structures for normal libido and potency (Coslett and Heilman 1986; Miller et al. 1986).

The peripheral autonomic and somatic nervous systems comprise the remaining structures involved with sexual function. Autonomic activity is mediated through the sympathetic and parasympathetic nervous systems. Sympathetic fibers emanate from the T10 to L2 level and from the inferior mesenteric ganglion and merge to form the hypogastric plexus and provide innervation to the testes, prostate, seminal vesicles, and vas deferens. Parasympathetic innervation occurs via the nervi erigentes formed by the preganglionic fibers that originate in the intermediolateral nuclei of the sacral spinal cord between S2 and S4. These fibers innervate the penis, prostate, seminal vesicles, and vas deferens. An afferent parasympathetic system also exists via the posterior roots at the S2 to S4 level. The pudendal nerve, which arises from S2 to S4, carries somatic innervation in both sexes and provides motor innervation to pelvic floor musculature with the sensory dermatomes being supplied by S2 to S5. The pudendal nerve becomes the dorsal nerve distally in both the female and the male (Goutier-Smith 1986). In females, the sympathetic nerve supply is mixed; however, the parasympathetic nerve supply is through the pelvic nerves via the uterine and hypogastric plexi. Interestingly, the uterus and ovaries receive only sympathetic innervation, whereas other genital structures receive mixed autonomic innervation (Horn and Zasler 1990; Zasler 1991).

Sexual Neurophysiology

The major pituitary hormones involved in the regulation of sexual function include follicle-stimulating hormone (FSH), luteinizing hormone (LH), and prolactin (PRL). These glycoproteins regulate levels of gonadal hormones, specifically testosterone in males and estrogen in females. Testosterone secretion is stimulated by the effect of LH on the cells of Leydig in the testes. FSH acts on the seminiferous tubules complementing the effects of LH relative to spermatozoa maturation. FSH and LH in females are mainly involved with the control of the menstrual cycle. PRL levels are suppressed in the presence of hypothalamic portal system dopamine. PRL secretion is increased secondary to stress, in association with certain types of seizure disorders, and as a consequence of certain medications (mainly antidopaminergic drugs such as neuroleptics). Normally, increases in PRL exert an inhibitory effect on the hypothalamic-pituitary-gonadal axis (Horn and Zasler 1990).

Cells in the arcuate nucleus of the hypothalamus secrete gonadotropin-releasing hormone (GnRH) into the portal circulation and subsequently stimulate the release of both LH and FSH from the anterior pituitary. GnRH release is regulated by feedback from gonadal hormone levels, prolactin levels, and other extra-hypothalamic structures in the brain stem and limbic system.

Gonadal hormones play an integral role in normal sexual maturation and function. The principal male gonadal hormone is testosterone. Androgens, including testosterone, are secreted mainly by the cells of Leydig in the testes but also in smaller amounts by the ovary and adrenal glands. Testosterone is responsible for the development of the male sexual organs, secondary sexual characteristics, and behavioral patterns. Ovarian hormones consist principally of estrogens, progesterones, and small amounts of androgens, and are required for normal female sexual maturation, including sex organ development, secondary sexual characteristics, menstruation, and libido (Table 14–2).

In addition to neuroendocrine dysfunction, there are multiple neuroactive substances that may impact sexual behavior. In general, the following relationships have been found between neurotransmitter receptor status and sexual behavior: 1) serotonergic agonists decrease libido, 2) dopaminergic agonists increase libido

Table 14–2. Sexual neurophysiology: hormone source and effect

Hormone	Site of release	Physiological effect
GnRH	Hypothalamus	Stimulate release of LH/FSH
FSH	Pituitary	Sperm maturation
LH	Pituitary	Increase testosterone secretion
PRL	Pituitary	Inhibit HPG axis
Testosterone	Testes	Primary and secondary male sexual characteristics, and libido
Estrogen and progesterone	Ovaries	Primary and secondary female sexual characteristics, and libido

Note. GnRH = gonadotropin-releasing hormone; FSH = follicle stimulating hormone; LH = luteinizing hormone; PRL = prolactin; HPG = hypothalamic-pituitary-gonadal.

and sexual behaviors, 3) noradrenergic agonists facilitate sexual arousal, and 4) cholinergic agonists facilitate ejaculation and impede initiation of copulation. Neuropeptides such as opiates, adrenocorticotropic hormone, melanocyte stimulating hormone, prolactin, and oxytocin generally inhibit sexual behavior. The relationship of neurotransmitters and neuromodulators to sexual function is important also because certain pharmacotherapeutic agents may adversely affect sexual function, whereas others may be therapeutically beneficial (please refer to the "Treatment" section in this chapter) (Horn and Zasler 1990; Zasler 1991; Zasler and Horn 1990).

Review of Research Literature

There are very few clinical research studies examining specific issues related to sexual dysfunction in people following TBI. Most of the more methodologically sound studies examining sexuality issues have been performed in the last five years.

Bond (1976) examined issues of psychosocial changes arising from severe brain injury using interview assessments. He found that the level of sexual activity was not related to posttraumatic amnesia, level of physical disability, or level of cognitive impairment. Specific sexual function patterns were not examined.

Rosenbaum and Najenson (1976) interviewed wives of wartime patients with either brain or spinal cord injuries. Reduced sexual function and emotional distress were present more often in the brain injury group relative to a group of uninjured individuals. The greatest level of mood disturbance was found for the wives of men with brain injury when compared to the wives of the spinal cord injured group and the control group. There was no significant relationship between the locus of injury and the specific area of sexual dysfunction. In the same study, a secondary analysis using a 22-item mood inventory for wives assessed the relationship between mood disturbance and sexual activity level. Greater levels of mood disturbance in the wives were associated with decreased levels of sexual activity. Additionally, negative attitudes toward perceived sexual changes were associated with a lower mood level in the wives questioned.

Oddy et al. (1978) studied 50 adults with TBI who were at least 6 months postinjury and had a minimum of 24 hours of posttraumatic amnesia. Half of the 12 married patients reported an increase in sexual intercourse and half reported a decrease. In a subsequent study, Oddy and Humphrey (1980) investigated alterations in sexual behavior 1 year after injury. Slightly less than 50% of spouses reported that they were significantly less affectionate toward their injured partners.

Lezak (1978) reported that many patients demonstrated completely absent libido whereas others reported increases in sexual drive. Generally, altered sexual interest, as well as other commonly seen posttraumatic cognitive-behavioral problems, contributed to family and marital difficulties. Lezak theorized that spouses were sexually frustrated in part due to their spouses' poor interpersonal skills and diminished capacity for empathy.

Social adjustment 2 years after severe TBI was assessed by Weddell et al. (1980), who interviewed relatives of a group of patients after they completed a rehabilitation program. Although no direct inquiries were made regarding sexuality issues, personality changes were examined. Irritability was the most frequent behavioral alteration, followed by altered expression of affection. Other common "adverse" behavioral sequelae included childishness, disinhibition, and increased talkativeness. This study reinforced perceptions regarding the deleterious effects of poor interpersonal skills on community reentry and psychosocial reintegration commonly seen in survivors of significant TBI.

One of the best early studies on alterations in sexual function following brain injury was done by Kosteljanetz et al. (1981) on a group of 19 male patients who had experienced concussions. They found that a majority of patients (53%) reported reduced libido and that a lesser but still significant percentage (42%) reported erectile dysfunction. A positive correlation was noted between reports of sexual dysfunction and intellectual impairment.

A survey of 40 wives and mothers of male patients with brain injury (not necessarily after trauma) by Mauss-Clum and Ryan (1981) found that a large proportion (47%) of the respondents reported that the survivor was either disinterested in sex or preoccupied with it. Forty-two percent of wives also reported that they had no sexual outlet.

Miller et al. (1986) suggested that sexual behavior changes were related to injury neuropathology; specifically, medial basal-frontal or diencephalic injury was more highly correlated with hypersexuality, whereas limbic injury was more likely to result in altered sexual preference.

Kreutzer and Zasler (1989) developed the Psychosexual Assessment Questionnaire and administered it to 21 sexually active male patients following TBI. This 11-item questionnaire assesses changes in sexual behavior, affect, self-esteem, and heterosexual relationships. Kreutzer and Zasler (1989) reported that the majority of these patients reported negative changes in sexual behavior, including decreased libido, erectile dysfunction, and decreased frequency of intercourse. Common personality changes included depression and reduced self-esteem and sex appeal. There was no relationship between the level of mood change and altered sexual behavior. Interestingly, despite negative changes, there was evidence that the quality of the marital relationships was preserved.

Garden et al. (1990) studied 11 men and 4 women who had sustained TBI at least 2 months before the evaluation. Both the spouses and the patients completed a sexual history and function questionnaire. A variety of factors were assessed, including libido, intercourse frequency, time spent in foreplay, sexual attractiveness, and erectile, ejaculatory, and orgasmic capabilities, as well as marital adjustment. Only a few significant positive correlations were found. Intercourse frequency decreased for 75% of female patients whereas 55% of the male patients reported a decline. Interestingly, although male genital sexual dysfunction rarely was reported, female spouses reported a significant decline in their ability to achieve orgasm after their partner was injured.

In a recent article, O'Carroll et al. (1991) examined the psychosexual and psychosocial sequelae of TBI in a series of 36 patients followed for up to 4 years after injury. Using several previously validated scales, they assessed both patients and partners. Approximately half of all male patients scored within the dysfunctional range on the psychosexual profiles. The major psychosexual complaint was decreased frequency of sexual intimacy, including intercourse. A large number of patients demonstrated significant emotional distress and/or anxiety and/or depression (61%, 25%, and 22%, respectively). Of the partners evaluated, the percentages were 41%, 18%, and 6%, respectively. These findings did not seem to correlate with severity of neurological insult. There was a clear relationship noted between advancing patient age and psychosexual dysfunction. Time since injury was positively correlated with the degree of sexual dissatisfaction among male survivors of TBI.

There is a great deal of literature on temporal lobe epilepsy; however, the patient populations that formed the bases of these studies were typically quite heterogeneous. Herzog (1984) found that 40%–58% percent of males with temporal lobe epilepsy were impotent or hyposexual, and up to 40% of women had menstrual irregularities. Blumer (1970a) reported that 70% of patients with temporal lobe epilepsy reported sexual problems. The most chronic alteration in sexual behavior was hyposexuality indicative of a loss of libido. Anecdotal observations suggest that mesial temporal involvement may be correlated with libidinal alterations in temporal lobe epilepsy; however, no well-controlled studies have confirmed this finding (Blumer 1970b; Blumer and Walker 1967). Less commonly, hypersexuality (which may follow surgical intervention or be related to anticonvulsant medication), homosexual behavior, and ictal or postictal sexual arousal have been reported.

In summary, the literature is sparse in the area of sexuality and sexual dysfunction in patients with TBI. Few studies have focused specifically on sexual behavior and many of these have disparate results (Table 14–3). Many of the studies are anecdotal reports and do not provide empirical evidence to guide clinical decision making or relate information to patients and families. It is not surprising that alterations in sexuality as well as sexual function occur in patients with TBI. As of now, we have only a sense of the magnitude of this area of functional deficit, which is unfortunate given the importance of sexuality to most people, whether single or married.

Clinical Evaluation

Problems can occur after TBI from a number of factors, including nongenital and genital dysfunction. Genital dysfunction may result in erectile dysfunction, ejaculatory problems, orgasmic dysfunction, vaginal lubrication problems, and vaginismus. Nongenital problems that may adversely affect sexual intimacy include senso-

Table 14–3.   Research on sexual function following traumatic brain injury (TBI)

Study	Conclusions
Bond 1976	No association between level of impairment and level of sexual activity.
Rosenbaum and Najenson 1976	TBI > SCI relative to reduction in sexual function and emotional distress in relatives.
Oddy et al. 1978	50% decrease and 50% increase in sexual intercourse.
Oddy and Humphrey 1980	Approximately 50% of spouses less affectionate toward injured partner.
Lezak 1978	High frequency of altered libido.
Weddell et al. 1980	Behavioral changes were common affecting expression of affection.
Kosteljanetz et al. 1981	53% reduced libido, 42% erectile dysfunction.
Mauss-Clum and Ryan 1981	47% altered libido, 42% of wives with no sexual outlet.
Miller et al. 1986	Correlation between sexual behavior and neuropathology.
Kreutzer and Zasler 1989	Majority reported negative changes in sexual behavior.
Garden et al. 1990	Majority reported decline in intercourse frequency.
O'Carroll et al. 1991	Approximately 50% of male patients were dysfunctional.

Note.   SCI = spinal cord injury.

rimotor deficits, communication deficits, perceptual deficits, limited joint range of motion, neurogenic bowel and bladder dysfunction, dysphagia with or without problems controlling secretions, motor dyspraxias, posttraumatic behavioral deficits, as well as alterations in self-image and self-esteem (Zasler and Horn 1990).

A decreased serum testosterone level, in an otherwise healthy male, will often first manifest as a decrease in libido and later as impotence and infertility. There may also be loss of secondary sexual characteristics. Females with acquired hormonal dysregulation may present with oligomenorrhea or amenorrhea, infertility, and signs of relative androgen access, such as acne and hirsutism (Horn and Zasler 1990). It is critical that professionals treating patients after TBI recognize clinical presentations suggestive of neuroendocrine dysfunction.

Clinicians working with this patient population must have an appreciation for the appropriate assessment and management of this class of functional deficits. One protocol that has been proposed is the General Rehabilitation Assessment Sexuality Profile (GRASP), which divides assessment into the sexual history, sexual physical exam, and clinical diagnostic testing (Zasler and Horn 1990) (Table 14–4).

Sexual History

A thorough sexual history defines needs, expectations, and behavior. Additionally, it identifies problems, misconceptions, and areas for education, counseling, and reassurance in relation to sexuality issues. When possible, interviews should be conducted with both the patient and the sexual partner. The assessment should include demographic and personal information, as well as past medical history, to identify medical disorders that potentially affect sexual function. Questions pertaining to premorbid sexual functioning, practices, and relationships should be asked. Both partners should be questioned about genital function, as well as sexuality concerns, including birth control, fertility, genital dysfunction, libidinal alterations, and others. Sexuality issues may not be important for all patients and this fact must be recognized by treating professionals. Key points when interviewing include provision of a private atmosphere, not rushing the interview, being frank yet empathic, and using nonconfrontational techniques and appropriate vocabulary relative to the patient's educational and cultural background (e.g., "do you suffer from premature ejaculation?" versus "do you cum too quickly?"). The clinician should avoid putting the patient in conflict with religious or moral beliefs by, for example, advocating that a practicing Catholic use birth control. Lastly, the status of an individual's sexual preference should be clarified and discussed. Ultimately, the interview can serve as a foundation for demonstrating to the patient that he or she has a right to be sexual

---

Table 14–4. General Rehabilitation Assessment Sexuality Profile (GRASP)

Sexual history

Interview both patient and partner if possible.

Obtain information about preinjury medical and sexual status and performance.

Delineate sexuality concerns.

Provide a private room and take your time.

Use appropriate vocabulary.

Clarify sexual preference.

Sexual physical exam

Assess general mobility and activities of daily living.

Assess general hygiene.

Inspection and palpation of genitalia.

Neurourological assessment: rectal exam, sensory testing, lumbosacral reflex arc testing.

Clinical sexual diagnostic testing

Urodynamics.

Male: penile biothesiometry, dorsal nerve SSEP, NPT, and ICP.

Female: photoplethysmography, thermal clearance and heat electrode.

Neuroendocrine evaluation: FSH, LH, PRL with testosterone (male) and estradiol and dehydroepiandrosterone (female).

Note. SSEP = somatosensory potentials; NPT = nocturnal penile tumescence; ICP = intracavernosal pharmacotherapy; FSH = follicle-stimulating hormone; LH = luteinizing hormone; PRL = prolactin.
Source. Zasler and Horn 1990.

and that sexual expression resulting in intimacy, not necessarily vaginal intercourse, is the goal of the process (Zasler 1991).

Sexual Physical Examination

The sexual physical examination begins when the clinician first sees the patient. Mobility deficits may give clues as to physical limitations that may adversely impact sexuality and sexual function. Of particular importance are the flexibility of the hips and degree of adductor spasticity. The clinician should note the patient's general hygiene status and use of adaptive equipment. Obviously, ruling out other preexisting neurological or medical conditions that might contribute to sexual dysfunction is critical, as well as assessing for posttraumatic neuromedical sequelae, including epilepsy, neuroendocrine dysfunction, and affective disorders.

The genitals should be examined from both a neurological and non-neurological standpoint by a physician comfortable in these procedures. In the female, direct visualization of the genitalia followed by a bimanual examination is critical. The vaginal walls must be evaluated for tone and mucosal alterations. In the male, the clinician must palpate the penis to assess for plaques as found in Peyronie's Disease. Testicular presence in the scrotal sacs and size and consistency should all be evaluated. In both males and females, assessment of hair distribution in the genital region and in locations of secondary sexual hair growth is paramount to rule out possible endocrinopathies that could be either primary or secondary in nature. The neurological assessment of the genitalia includes a rectal exam, sensory testing, and assessment of lumbosacral reflex integrity. The skilled clinician can utilize the information from bedside testing to guide recommendations as well as prognosticate genital sexual function relative to the neurological insult in question (Zasler 1991; Zasler and Horn 1990).

Clinical Sexual Diagnostic Testing

Urodynamics can help obtain a better understanding of the integrity of genital innervation. Afferent neurological assessment can be done with penile biothesiometry and/or dorsal nerve somatosensory evoked potentials (DNSSEP). Penile biothesiometry, which measures the vibration perception threshold of the skin of the penis, is performed using a portable hand-held electromagnetic vibration device with a fixed frequency and variable amplitude. DNSSEP provides an objective physiological assessment of the entire pudendal nerve afferent pathway. Efferent neurological assessment, whether motor or autonomic, can be performed in a gross manner via nocturnal penile tumescence and/or response to intracavernosal pharmacotherapy (Padma-Nathan 1988).

Female sexual clinical assessment is less sophisticated and has been conducted with various techniques. Photoplethysmography, thermal clearance, and heat electrode techniques have been used to assess vaginal hemodynamics via indirect evaluation of vaginal wall blood flow parameters (Levin 1980). These techniques can be used to treat orgasmic and arousal deficits via biofeedback training (Levin 1980; Zasler 1991; Zasler and Horn 1990).

Initial laboratory evaluation should include assessment of FSH, LH, PRL, and free testosterone in males. Given the pulsatile cycle of the release of these hormones, it has been suggested that three samples be obtained approximately 20 minutes apart and then be combined for a single measurement. In females, the same hormones should be assessed, in addition to estradiol and dehydroepiandrosterone. Due to normal menstrual variations, the best time for this assessment is during the early follicular phase. An awareness of appropriate neuroendocrine tests relative to specific clinical presentations is paramount for any practitioner working with these patients (Table 14–5). Clinicians should keep in mind that other factors, such as medications or physiological stress in acute patients, may contribute to neuroendocrine abnormalities.

Clinical Management

The management of sexual dysfunction must take into consideration the many issues that may directly or indirectly contribute to

alterations in sexual function following TBI, including neuroendocrine, nongenital, and genital dysfunction. Clinicians should be
aware of how subjective complaints may provide clues to guiding
treatment (Figure 14–1). Additionally, adequate knowledge of the
potential benefits and side effects of pharmacological agents in this
patient population is critical in optimizing outcome (Table 14–6).
There are also multiple issues related to sexuality following TBI

Table 14–5.　Posttraumatic neuroendocrine dysfunction: clinical
presentation and appropriate laboratory evaluation

Clinical syndrome	Clinical presentation (possible symptoms)	Neuroendocrine evaluation
Male postpubertal sexual dysfunction	Decreased libido Impotence Ejaculatory dysfunction Infertility	FSH, LH, PRL, free testosterone Rule out associated medical condition
Female postpubertal sexual dysfunction	Oligomenorrhea Amenorrhea Virilization Galactorrhea Decreased libido Recurrent spontaneous abortions	FSH, LH, PRL, estradiol, and dihydroepiandrosterone Rule out associated medical condition
Male prepubertal sexual dysfunction	Delay in development of secondary sexual characteristics Precocious puberty	FSH, LH, PRL, free testosterone
Female prepubertal sexual dysfunction	Delay in development of secondary sexual characteristics Precocious puberty	FSH, LH, PRL, estradiol, and dihydroepian-drosterone
Sexual dysfunction associated with temporolimbic epilepsy	Male: impotence, decreased libido, and endocrine disturbances	Same as above
	Female: menstrual irregularities, endocrine disturbances, and polycystic ovarian syndrome	Same as above Rule out drug side effect

Note.　FSH = follicle-stimulating hormone; LH = luteinizing hormone; PRL = prolactin.

that require management through counseling interventions, including matters of birth control, sex education, competency to engage in sexual activity, sexual abuse, and sexual "release."

Neuroendocrine Dysfunction

Neuroendocrine dysfunction may occur following TBI; however, the general clinical experience has been that this phenomenon is relatively rare in the TBI population. In postpubertal females, cyclic administration of oral estrogen-progesterone preparations will restore the menstrual cycle, maintain secondary sexual characteristics, and reduce the risk for osteoporosis. In the postpubertal male, hypogonadism may be treated with intramuscular testosterone (200–400 mg) replacement, typically given every 2 to 4 weeks. In cases of delayed puberty, treatment should begin during adolescence; males are typically treated with human chorionic gonadotropin (500–1,000 USP units 3 times per week for the first 3 weeks, followed by 500 USP units 2 times per week for 1 to 2 years) and subsequently followed by maintenance testosterone therapy. In females, cyclic estrogen and progesterone therapy should be instituted to establish menses and secondary sexual characteristics (Zasler and Horn 1990).

Nongenital Dysfunction

Other areas of nongenital neurological impairment must also be assessed relative to treatment options, whether pharmacologic, surgical, or compensatory. Sensorimotor deficits, cognitive and behavioral deficits, language-based alterations, changes in libido, as well as neurogenic bowel and bladder dysfunction, can all be addressed by the clinician as they affect ability for sexual expression (Zasler and Horn 1990). Libidinal changes can be treated behaviorally and pharmacologically. Hormonal treatment and/or serotonergic agents can be utilized for hypersexuality. Medroxyprogesterone acetate has been used in varying doses to suppress both aggressive behavior and sexual arousal (100–200 mg per week typically preceded by a loading dose of 400 mg/week over

Table 14–6. Sexual pharmacology: drug class and clinical effect

Drug (by class)	Clinical effect
Anabolic steroids Methandrostenolone	Decreased libido
Anorexiants Amphetamines	Decreased libido, impotence, ejaculatory dysfunction, anorgasmia
Anticholinergics Oxybutynin Scopolamine	Inhibited erection and ejaculation, decreased libido
Anticonvulsants Carbamazepine Phenytoin	Impotence and decreased libido
Antidepressants Nortriptyline Doxepin	Decreased libido, delayed orgasm in women, ejaculatory and erectile dysfunction
Antihypertensives Beta-blockers Methyldopa Clonidine	Impotence, decreased libido, and ejaculatory dysfunction
Antiparkinsonian Levodopa Bromocriptine	Generally increase libido, may also improve erectile function
Antipsychotic Haloperidol	Impotence, decreased libido, ejaculatory dysfunction, priapism
Antispasticity Baclofen	Impotence, ejaculatory dysfunction, and menstrual irregularities
Diuretics Thiazides	Decreased libido and impotence
Estrogens	Decreased libido in both sexes
H$_2$-Antihistamines Ranitidine	Decreased libido, erectile dysfunction
Nonsteroidal **anti-inflammatory** Naproxen	Erectile problems and anejaculation
Noradrenergic agonists	Increased libido in both sexes
Phenoxybenzamine	Ejaculatory dysfunction
Progestins Medroxyprogesterone	Decreased libido, impotence
Serotonergic agonists Trazodone	In general, decreased libido; however, reports of increased libido in females

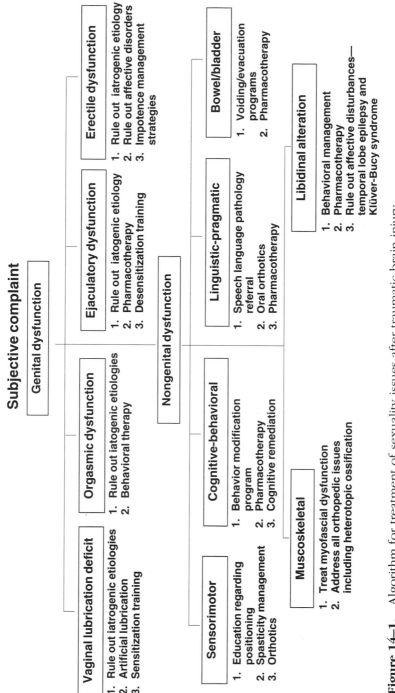

Subjective complaint

Genital dysfunction

Erectile dysfunction
1. Rule out iatrogenic etiology
2. Rule out affective disorders
3. Impotence management strategies

Ejaculatory dysfunction
1. Rule out iatrogenic etiology
2. Pharmacotherapy
3. Desensitization training

Orgasmic dysfunction
1. Rule out iatrogenic etiologies
2. Behavioral therapy

Vaginal lubrication deficit
1. Rule out iatrogenic etiologies
2. Artificial lubrication
3. Sensitization training

Nongenital dysfunction

Bowel/bladder
1. Voiding/evacuation programs
2. Pharmacotherapy

Libidinal alteration
1. Behavioral management
2. Pharmacotherapy
3. Rule out affective disturbances—temporal lobe epilepsy and Klüver-Bucy syndrome

Linguistic-pragmatic
1. Speech language pathology referral
2. Oral orthotics
3. Pharmacotherapy

Cognitive-behavioral
1. Behavior modification program
2. Pharmacotherapy
3. Cognitive remediation

Muscoskeletal
1. Treat myofascial dysfunction
2. Address all orthopedic issues including heterotopic ossification

Sensorimotor
1. Education regarding positioning
2. Spasticity management
3. Orthotics

Figure 14–1.   Algorithm for treatment of sexuality issues after traumatic brain injury.

the first 2–3 weeks). Clinically, I have had some success with serotonergic agents such as trazodone hydrochloride for suppression of libido in doses typically ranging from 3.0–5.0 mg/kg body weight. Noradrenergic agonists and/or hormonal supplementation have been used for hyposexuality, particularly in males (Blumer and Migeon 1975; Lehne 1986; McConaghy et al. 1988; Zasler and Horn 1990).

Clinicians should recall that patients with temporolimbic epilepsy may present with alterations in neuroendocrine status and sexual function. The presence of characteristic "temporal lobe personality" traits such as circumstantiality, viscosity, and obsessionalism in combination with altered sexuality, even in the absence of "clinical" seizures and/or electrographic seizures, suggests consideration for treatment with a psychoactive anticonvulsant such as carbamazepine or valproate (Gualtieri 1991). Patients with Klüver-Bucy syndrome have also shown hypersexual behaviors as part of this symptom complex that respond in a favorable fashion to treatment with psychotropic anticonvulsants such as carbamazepine (Stewart 1985).

Genital Dysfunction

Genital sexual dysfunction after TBI may take a number of potential forms. Males may present with erectile, ejaculatory, and/or orgasmic dysfunction. The present state of the art in neurological management of erectile dysfunction focuses on one of three main treatment categories: penile prostheses, intracavernosal pharmacotherapy, and external management. Enteral agents have been used, including noradrenergic agonists such as yohimbine (5.4–6.0 mg po tid) (Morales et al. 1982), as well as other drug classes such as dopamine agonists. Work is ongoing relative to the efficacy of enteral agents in this patient population. Problems with premature ejaculation should be first addressed behaviorally to assess how much of the problem is functionally based. Methods such as the "squeeze" technique, which involves application of pressure to the penile shaft just proximal to the glans penis when the male feels that he is about to ejaculate, can be taught to prolong the time until ejaculation. On occasion, medication could be considered for the male patient who complains of premature ejaculation; this could include topical anesthetics to the penile shaft (5%–10% lidocaine) or anticholinergic (imipramine 100–200 mg/day) and sympatholytic medication (phenoxybenzamine 10 mg bid to tid) administered orally. Orgasmic dysfunction is generally approached from a behavioral standpoint in both men and women. Females may complain of alterations in vaginal lubrication and/or orgasmic dysfunction. Inadequate vaginal lubrication can generally be treated with artificial lubrication using water-soluble products. Behavioral therapy, including imagery and body exploration-sensitization training, may benefit some females who have arousal or orgasmic dysfunction (Zasler 1991).

Physicians should be aware of how certain medications may produce iatrogenic sexual dysfunction. Antipsychotic medications, antihypertensives, and anticholinergic medications are some of the more common "culprits." Other drugs, including histamine, subtype 2, receptor blockers, may produce adverse effects through their anti-androgenic effect and increased central prolactin. Anticonvulsant medication such as phenytoin may decrease circulating levels of sex hormone via induction of hepatic enzyme systems, resulting in a relative secondary hypogonadism. Assessment of medications and appropriate substitutions to optimize sexual functioning is critical in the physician's role in the management of sexuality issues in this population.

Counselling Issues

There are numerous controversial issues pertaining to sexuality in this patient population that impact on medical, ethical, and legal fronts, thereby obliging us to address them. Among these issues are matters pertaining to sex education, including birth control, sexually transmitted disease, sexual abuse, sexual release, and masturbation. Other issues that may arise include decisions regarding sterilization, as well as more germane and "socially acceptable" issues such as dating, marriage, sexual preference issues, child-rearing matters, and psychosocial behavior.

Quite frequently, TBI patients will assume that they will be unable to find a compatible sexual companion because they have had a brain injury. Various recommendations can be provided to maximize community reintegration, including attending church or synagogue functions, head injury survivor meetings, local organization social gatherings, or participating in dating services for people with disabilities such as Handicapped Introductions and DateAble (Garden 1988). Professionals also can assist clients by teaching or "reteaching" the psychosocial graces that may many times be adversely affected by significant TBI, before attempting more aggressive community reentry efforts. Responsible decisions regarding sexual relations are critical for both single and married people with brain injury, and ongoing follow-up is essential to ensure that there is compliance with the recommendations, as well as sex life satisfaction.

Generally, patients who have been evaluated as competent, and having the capacity to understand and remember the ramifications of their actions, are probably capable of being sexually active in a responsible fashion. Sexually active patients, whether male or female, should be instructed in the appropriate use of condoms given the ever present fear of acquired immunodeficiency syndrome (AIDS).

For patients demonstrating poor "sexual judgment" or uncontrollable sexual behaviors, including indiscriminate masturbation or hypersexuality, the professional may need to consider either chemical or surgical sterilization. Given the variability in state laws regarding competency-capacity issues and decisions regarding sterilization, it is recommended that professionals consult legal counsel regarding each case in question.

Families and patients should be counselled regarding alternatives for sexual release, particularly for patients without active sexual partners. Masturbation should be discussed as one potential option as long as it is done in an appropriate social context. For those clients requiring external stimulation to aid in successful masturbation, sexual stimuli, for example, erotic reading materials, pictures, videotapes, and telephone sex services, can be provided. Obviously, many of the aforementioned suggestions may not be acceptable to certain people secondary to their moral and/or religious beliefs, but they should be discussed with all patients and families as appropriate.

Some health care professionals and family members have advocated, as well as condoned, the use of sexual surrogates and prostitutes in addressing the sexual frustrations of people following TBI who might otherwise never find sexual partners. Although there are differences between surrogates and prostitutes, many state laws do not make a legal distinction. In an era of high awareness regarding sexually transmitted diseases and legal liability, most professionals seem to be shying away from making use of this class of "community resources."

In my clinical experience, it is not uncommon for TBI patients who were heterosexual before their injury to turn to homosexual life-styles or at least experimentation after injury, because it may become the only way to express their sexual feelings and vent sexual needs. Professionals should counsel patient and family alike regarding dealing with alterations in sexual preference, which are more commonly a result of lack of heterosexual partners (for heterosexual patients) than a result of organically based alterations in sexual orientation due to the TBI itself (Miller et al. 1986). Appropriate counseling for heterosexuals and homosexuals alike should be available. Counselling clinicians should always inquire about the patient's sexual orientation. All patients, regardless of sexual preference, should be counselled on high-risk sexual practices.

Sexual abuse is an issue that occurs on occasion in this patient population. Although poorly documented due to a general trend toward not studying things that make us feel uncomfortable, clinicians must recognize abuse when they see it. Health care professionals are legally and morally obligated to ensure that the proper authorities are notified if a person with TBI, a family member, an attendant, or an acquaintance is engaged in sexual misconduct and/or abuse. If sexual abuse is suspected, proper measures should be taken to either remove the patient from the environment in question or remove the suspected perpetrator from the patient's immediate milieu.

Effects on Family Roles

Sexuality is a classic example of an integrative function, requiring cognitive, physical, and psychobehavioral components. A double sensitivity often exists regarding sexuality and disability (Chigier 1980), which often prevents the person with a brain injury from being seen as a sexual being. All people, whether patient, family, or treating professionals, must learn to accept the fact that sexuality issues exist for most survivors, regardless of injury severity, and must be dealt with relative to sexual function issues, sexual rights, rehabilitation interventions, and family or attendant counselling. Family issues may arise in a variety of situations, including single individuals living with parents, married people living with spouses, and parents living with children with brain injuries (Zasler and Kreutzer 1991).

Sexual problems following TBI can occur in at least three different scenarios. First, people with brain injury, classically adolescents or young adults, may be living with their parents. They commonly may be unable to maintain sexual relationships established before their injury and/or to establish new relationships after the injury. Sexual problems for these individuals include finding a suitable partner, as well as diminished their physical capabilities.

Second, some survivors are able to maintain previously established relationships. These people may be married, living with a significant other, or single and dating. Diminished frequency of intercourse and physical dysfunction may stem from emotional or physical problems.

Third, sexual problems may arise between married relatives of the injured person and may be attributable to the negative consequences of brain injury in other family members (children, siblings, or parents). The stressors associated with caring for the injured person may cause a variety of psychological reactions, including burn-out, feelings of guilt, and displacement, to name only a few, thereby resulting in spousal alienation, sexual disinterest, and potentially sexual dysfunction.

Conclusions

Professionals are only beginning to examine the neurological and functional ramifications of TBI on sexual function. Presently, there is a relative dearth of information on which clinicians can base prognostication, assessment, or treatment; however, our knowledge base is expanding slowly but surely. Better acknowledgement of the importance of sexuality and sexual function to quality of life may stimulate researchers and clinicians alike to allocate more resources to answering many of the questions that remain. The treating physician must be able to address sexuality issues effectively by relying on an approach that holistically defines problematic areas, determines what changes can realistically be made, and works toward effecting those changes and accepting what cannot be changed. In the interim, clinicians and researchers alike should remain cognizant of the importance of sexual expression relative to other areas of human function following TBI. Awareness, in and of itself, will provide an impetus for further critical examination of this important area of psychophysiological function.

References

Bauer HG: Endocrine and metabolic conditions related to pathology in the hypothalamus, a review. J Nerv Ment Dis 28:323–328, 1959

Blumer D: Changes of sexual behavior related to temporal lobe disorders in man. Journal of Sex Research 6:173–180, 1970a

Blumer D: Hypersexual episodes in temporal lobe epilepsy. Am J Psychiatry 126:1099–1106, 1970b

Blumer D, Migeon C: Hormone and hormonal agents in the treatment of aggression. J Nerv Ment Dis 160:127–137, 1975

Blumer D, Walker AE: Sexual behavior in temporal lobe epilepsy. Arch Neurol 16:31–43, 1967

Boller F, Frank E: Sexual Dysfunction in Neurological Disorders: Diagnosis, Management and Rehabilitation. New York, Raven, 1982

Bond MR: Assessment of psychosocial outcome of severe head injury. Acta Neurochir 34:57–70, 1976

Chigier E: Sexuality of physically disabled people. Clinics in Obstetrics and Gynecology 7:325–343, 1980

Cohen H, Rosen R, Goldstein L: Electroencephalographic laterality changes during human sexual orgasm. Arch Sex Behav 5:189–199, 1976

Coslett H, Heilman K: Male sexual function: impairment after right hemisphere stroke. Arch Neurol 43:1036–1039, 1986

Garden FH: Dating services for the disabled: Sexuality Update Newsletter. American Congress of Rehabilitation Medicine 1:4, 1988

Garden FH, Bontke CF, Hoffman M: Sexual functioning and marital adjustment after traumatic brain injury. Journal of Head Trauma Rehabilitation 5(2):52–59, 1990

Goutier-Smith PC: Sexual function and dysfunction. Clinical Neurobiology 1:634–642, 1986

Gualtieri CT: Neuropsychiatry and Behavioral Pharmacology. New York, Springer-Verlag, 1991

Heath RG: Pleasure response of human subjects to direct stimulation of the brain: physiologic and psychodynamic considerations, in The Role of Pleasure in Behavior. Edited by Heath RG. New York, Harper & Row, 1964, pp 219–243

Herzog A: Endocrinological aspects of epilepsy, in Neurology and Neurosurgery Update Series (5[11]). Princeton, NJ, Continuing Professional Education Center, 1984

Horn LJ, Zasler ND: Neuroanatomy and neurophysiology of sexual function. Journal of Head Trauma Rehabilitation 5(2):1–13, 1990

Kosteljanetz M, Jensen TS, Norgard B, et al: Sexual and hypothalamic dysfunction in post-concussional syndrome. Acta Neurol Scand 63:169–180, 1981

Kreutzer JS, Zasler ND: Psychosexual consequences of traumatic brain injury: methodology and preliminary findings. Brain Inj 3:177–186, 1989

Lehne GK: Brain damage and paraphilia: treatment with medroxyprogesterone acetate. Sexuality and Disability 7:145–157, 1986

Levin RJ: The physiology of sexual function in women. Clinics in Obstetrics and Gynecology 7:213–252, 1980

Lezak MD: Living with the characterologically altered brain injured patient. J Clin Psychiatry 39:592–598, 1978

MacLean P: Brain mechanisms of primal sexual functions and related behavior, in Sexual Behavior: Pharmacology and Biochemistry. Edited by Sandler M, Gessa G. New York, Raven, 1975, pp 1–11

Mauss-Clum N, Ryan M: Brain injury and the family. Journal of Neurosurgical Nursing 13:165–169, 1981

McConaghy N, Balszczynski A, Kidson W: Treatment of sex offenders with imaginal desensitization and/or medroxyprogesterone. Acta Psychiatr Scand 77:199–206, 1988

Mesulam M: Principles of Behavioral Neurology. Philadelphia, PA, FA Davis, 1985

Miller BL, Cummings JL, McIntyre H, et al: Hypersexuality or altered sexual preference following brain injury. J Neurol Neurosurg Psychiatry 49:867–873, 1986

Morales A, Surridge DHC, Marshall PG, et al: Nonhormonal pharmacological treatment of organic impotence. J Urol 128:45–47, 1982

O'Carroll RE, Woodrow J, Maroun F: Psychosexual and psychosocial sequelae of closed head injury. Brain Inj 5:303–313, 1991

Oddy M, Humphrey M: Social recovery during the first year following severe head injury. J Neurol Neurosurg Psychiatry 43:798–802, 1980

Oddy M, Humphrey M, Uttley D: Subjective impairment and social recovery after closed head injury. J Neurol Neurosurg Psychiatry 41:611–616, 1978

Padma-Nathan H: Neurologic evaluation of erectile dysfunction. Urologic Clinics of North America 15(1):77–80, 1988

Penfield W, Rasmussen T: The Cerebral Cortex of Man. New York, Macmillan, 1950

Rosenbaum M, Najenson T: Changes in life patterns and symptoms of low mood as reported by wives of severely brain-injured soldiers. J Consult Clin Psychol 44:881–888, 1976

Stewart JT: Carbamazepine treatment of a patient with Kluver-Bucy Syndrome. J Clin Psychiatry 46:496–497, 1985

Walker AE: The neurological basis of sex. Neurol India 24(1):1–13, 1976

Weddell R, Oddy M, Jenkins D: Social adjustment after rehabilitation: a two year follow-up of patients with severe head injury. Psychol Med 10:257–263, 1980

Zasler ND: Sexuality in neurologic disability: an overview. Sexuality and Disability 9(1):11–27, 1991

Zasler ND, Horn LJ: Rehabilitative management of sexual dysfunction. Journal of Head Trauma Rehabilitation 5(2):14–24, 1990

Zasler ND, Kreutzer JS: Family and sexuality after traumatic brain injury, in Impact of Head Injury on the Family System: An Overview for Professionals. Edited by Williams J, Kay T. Baltimore, MD, Paul H Brookes, 1991, pp 253–270

Chapter 15

Alcohol and Drug Disorders

Norman S. Miller, M.D.

The single greatest risk factor for traumatic brain injury (TBI) is alcohol/drug use and alcohol/drug disorder (A/DD). TBI is often an irreversible adverse consequence of the pharmacological effects and addictive use of alcohol and drugs. Of critical importance is that TBI is preventable. The prevention can include many aspects, but of primary importance is the treatment of A/DD before the onset of the TBI (Brismar et al. 1983; Brooks 1984; Field 1976; Sparadeo and Gill 1989).

The coexistence of TBI with A/DD requires concurrent treatment of both disorders. A/DD complicates the treatment of the TBI and vice versa. Acceptance of both categories of disorders as independent and interactive enhances the total treatment of the patient (Special Section 1981).

The clinicians involved in the acute and chronic management of TBI must be knowledgeable and skilled in the identification of A/DD whenever it exists in combination with TBI. If only one condition is the focus of treatment, incomplete treatment and poor prognosis are likely to result for either condition. Because the interplay between TBI and A/DD is related from onset and

471

throughout the clinical course, treatment strategies must be developed that recognize the independence of and interaction between the two categories of disorders (Freund 1985).

The treatment protocols can be implemented from the time of first contact during the acute intervention through chronic maintenance. Those who are actively involved in the treatment must be skilled in the intervention, referral, and in some cases the actual long-term management of both TBI and A/DD. Although a specialist may be employed for either category of disorder, he or she must know the ramifications of both disorders. For instance, the addiction specialist must know and work with the limitations of the alcohol or drug-addicted patient with brain injury, and at the same time the brain specialist must know the impact of both treated and untreated alcoholism and drug addiction on the patient with TBI. The two specialists, then, must work to coordinate the treatment of both disorders (Substance Abuse Task Force 1988).

Prevalence of the Problems

The incidence of intoxication or a positive blood alcohol level associated with TBI ranges from 29%–52% when total admissions to the hospital are considered, to 58% when the number of surgical admissions are considered, and to 72% when the overall number of contacts are considered. Contacts are defined as visits to the hospital, including visits to the emergency room. The high degree of association strongly suggests that alcohol and TBI are causally related. The incidence appears to be greater in males by four to one. The reported prevalence of a history of alcohol dependence (addictive drinking) ranges from 25%–68%, which suggests that the majority of those involved in TBI at any time had a serious problem with alcohol use prior to the onset of the injury (Edna 1985; Elmer and Lim 1985).

The role of drugs other than alcohol is not as well documented because often specific testing and history taking for drugs are not part of either routine clinical practice or research studies. Many hospital records do not mention the implications of drug histories where clear evidence exists. The reasons for poor documentation are complex and include poor skills in assessing the importance of drugs and alcohol and lack of knowledge that effective treatment for alcohol and drug disorders exists. Research protocols do not often include measurement of urine or blood for illicit or prescription medications that can influence the onset of TBI. The common occurrence of multiple drug and alcohol use or addiction in high-risk populations for the development of TBI, namely adolescents and young adults, makes routine assessment for alcohol and drug use mandatory in these populations when traumatic injury occurs.

The prevalence rate for alcoholism in the United States is about 15%. The long-term diagnosis of alcoholism can be made in 29% of males in the United States, and 7% of females. The mean age of onset of alcoholism is 22 years in males and 25 in females, according to the Epidemiological Catchment Area Study (Miller 1991a). The reported prevalence rate for drug addiction in the general population ranges from 9%–20%. The majority of drug-addicted individuals are addicted to alcohol, and substantial numbers of alcoholic individuals are addicted to other drugs as well. Over 90% of alcoholic individuals under the age of 30 are addicted to at least one other drug, namely cannabis, cocaine, benzodiazepines, opiates, and/or hallucinogens, in decreasing order of frequency (Miller 1991a; Schuckit 1990).

The prevalence rate for A/DD in psychiatric populations is 50%–75%, and 25%–50% in medical populations. Treatment populations of addictive disorders show consistently high rates of multiple combinations of A/DDs. The average age for males in treatment is 30–35 years, for females 25–30. The proportion of males to females in typical treatment populations is 75% to 25%, and 60% to 40% in membership surveys of Alcoholics Anonymous (Helzer and Pryzbeck 1988; Miller 1991b; Ries and Samson 1987).

Survey data provide evidence that alcohol and drugs are often involved in TBI. One hundred thousand people die annually in accidents in the United States. Fifty percent are motor vehicle accidents as the leading cause of death between the ages of 17 and

21. Of these fatal motor vehicle accidents, 50% are associated with alcohol and drugs. Seventy percent of fatal injuries are from head trauma, and two-thirds of TBIs involve motor vehicle accidents. The survival rate for people with severe TBIs has increased to 60% in the last two decades. Most are young adult males who will have long-term survival rates. Moreover, 50% of all violent deaths from any cause are alcohol or drug related (Sparadeo and Gill 1989; Sparadeo et al. 1990; Substance Abuse Task Force 1988).

A survey revealed that of 484 fatally injured drivers and pedestrians, only 32% had neither alcohol nor drug in blood samples (Sparadeo and Gill 1989). A group of studies published in 1988 (Substance Abuse Task Force 1988) showed that approximately one-third of brain injury patients have an identifiable problem and/or treatment history for chemical dependency prior to injury, and approximately 50%–70% are intoxicated at the time of injury.

The high degree of association of alcohol/drug use and addiction and TBI in young populations is clear. Despite what is known about the relationship between A/DD and TBI, there is much that is still not known. Studies of prognosis and outcome following brain injury frequently exclude individuals who are addicted to drugs and/or alcohol prior to the accidents, even though this practice produces significant and relevant distortion of the data (Sparadeo and Gill 1989; Substance Abuse Task Force 1988).

Intervention at the Acute State

The first clinical caveat is that if alcohol and/or drug addiction is implicated in TBI, it is likely to have been a problem preceding and up to the injury. Precautions for the medical and psychiatric sequelae of acute *and* chronic drug and alcohol use should be undertaken. Frequent complications include drug-drug interactions, drug overdose, increased sensitivity to medication effects, and seizures either from drug intoxication or drug/alcohol withdrawal. Other possible complications include behavior dyscontrol, hallucinations, delusions, anxiety, and depression induced by intoxication and withdrawal from drugs and alcohol, and drug seeking from the presence of an addictive disorder (Miller 1991a; Schuckit 1983) (Table 15–1).

The second clinical caveat is that the behaviors following acute intoxication and overdose are very similar to those following brain injury, such as lethargy or agitation, confusion, disorientation, respiratory depression, and others. Importantly, some intoxicated patients are discharged from the emergency room when in fact they have undiagnosed brain injuries. In a study of 167 patients (Gallagher and Browder 1968), alcohol obscured changes in consciousness, leading to misdiagnosis or delayed diagnosis of complications of brain trauma. In 21 patients, a subdural hematoma was diagnosed only at postmortem (Galbraith 1976), and others have reported similar results (Rumbaugh and Fang 1980).

For these reasons the use of pharmacological interventions acutely must take into consideration possible drug-drug interactions with known and unknown drugs, both illicit and prescription medications. Persistent history taking from the patient and family and drug screens on urine and blood are essential in identifying the influence of alcohol and drugs in the precipitation of the brain injury and possible responses of the patient to pharmacological and behavioral managements. For instance, benzodiazepines may interact with alcohol and/or other sedatives acutely to further depress consciousness. On the other hand, acute withdrawal from

---

Table 15–1.   Psychiatric sequelae from drugs and alcohol

Drug-drug interactions

Drug overdose

Increased sensitivity to medication effects

Seizures either from drug intoxication or drug or alcohol withdrawal

Behavior control

Hallucinations

Delusions

Anxiety

Depression induced by intoxication and withdrawal from drugs

Alcohol and drug seeking from the presence of an addictive disorder

---

alcohol that is not adequately treated with benzodiazepines may progress to agitation and delirium. Only the combination of clinical assessment and laboratory diagnosis will achieve the answer to these clinical dilemmas (Miller and Gold 1991).

Diagnosis of Alcohol and Drug Disorders

Once the acute stabilization is achieved, the patient and family should be further evaluated for the presence and severity of an A/DD. Alcoholism and drug addiction are diagnosable according to established criteria in DSM-IV (American Psychiatric Association 1994). Three of the seven criteria for the dependence syndrome reflect the behaviors of addiction, namely, 1) preoccupation with acquiring alcohol or drugs, 2) compulsive use of alcohol or drugs despite adverse consequences, and 3) a pattern of relapse or inability to cut down on use despite adverse consequences. Two of the seven criteria reflect development of tolerance of and dependence on alcohol and drugs. Any three of the nine criteria are required to make the diagnosis of alcohol and/or drug dependence. The loss of control over use of alcohol and drugs that is pervasive to the criteria for the dependence syndrome in DSM-IV is evident in the histories of patients with TBI. The manifest loss of control often is reflected by the circumstances surrounding and including the actual trauma that culminates in the brain injury (Table 15–2).

Alcohol dependence and drug dependence are independent diagnoses. As independent disorders, each has a characteristic course and predictable consequences. The application of exclusionary criteria for A/DD is required before establishing other psychiatric disorders using DSM-IV (Tamerin and Mendelson 1969).

There is little objective evidence that alcohol or drugs are used to "medicate" or ameliorate a mood state or an underlying or additional psychiatric disorder, including one caused by TBI. The preponderance of the studies show that alcohol and drugs cause psychiatric symptoms and worsen already-existing symptoms from psychiatric disorders, especially those associated with TBI. Al-

---

Table 15–2. Diagnostic criteria for psychoactive substance dependence

---

A maladaptive pattern of substance use, leading to clinically significant impairment or distress, as manifested by three or more of the following, occurring at any time in the same 12-month period:

1) Tolerance, as defined by either of the following:

   a) A need for markedly increased amounts of the substance to achieve intoxication or desired effect

   b) Markedly diminished effect with continued use of the same amount of the substance

2) Withdrawal, as manifested by either of the following:

   a) The characteristic withdrawal syndrome for the substance (refer to Criteria A and B of the criteria sets for Withdrawal from the specific substances)

   b) The same (or a closely related) substance taken to relieve or avoid withdrawal symptoms

3) The substance is often taken in larger amounts or over a longer period than was intended

4) There is a persistent desire or unsuccessful efforts to cut down or control substance use

5) A great deal of time is spent in activities necessary to obtain the substance (e.g., visiting multiple doctors or driving long distances), use the substance (e.g., chain smoking), or recover from its effects

6) Important social, occupational, or recreational activities are given up or reduced because of substance use

7) The substance use is continued despite knowledge of having a persistent or recurrent physical or psychological problem that is likely to have been caused or exacerbated by the substance (e.g., current cocaine use despite recognition of cocaine-induced depression, or continued drinking despite recognition that an ulcer was made worse by alcohol consumption)

Specify if:

With Physiological Dependence: evidence of tolerance or withdrawal (i.e., either Item 1 or 2 is present)

Without Physiological Dependence: no evidence of tolerance or withdrawal (i.e., neither Item 1 nor 2 is present)

Source. Reprinted from American Psychiatric Association: Diagnostic and Statistical Manual of Mental Disorders, 4th Edition. Washington, DC, American Psychiatric Association, 1994. Used with permission.

though alcoholic patients and those with drug addictions report drinking and using drugs because of anxiety and depression, objective and controlled studies fail to confirm the hypothesis that alcohol and drugs are used to improve mood and thinking. The conclusions from the studies are that continued alcohol and drug use results in an appearance and worsening of psychiatric symptoms in proportion to the amount and duration of alcohol and drug use (Mayfield and Allen 1967; Schuckit 1990; Schuckit et al. 1990).

Family history is the best predictor for the onset of alcoholism and drug addiction in a given individual. A positive family history for alcohol and drug disorders can increase the index of suspicion for the presence of an A/DD in the TBI patient. Also family members may have A/DDs that require diagnosis, intervention, and treatment. Untreated family members with addictions can have an adverse impact on the patient with A/DD and TBI that can interfere with the overall treatment (Cermak 1991; Miller et al 1990).

These findings have important treatment implications. In general, the first step in treatment of an A/DD is to discontinue the active use of alcohol and drugs. During this initial abstinence, the influence of alcohol and drugs on mood cognition and behavior, as well as the drug seeking from the addictive disorder, can be assessed. A differential diagnosis for coexisting psychiatric disorders also can be assessed longitudinally, apart from the effects of alcohol and drug intoxication and addictive use of drugs (Blankfield 1986; Miller and Mahler 1991).

Screening tests are available for alcohol disorders that can be modified for drugs by inserting drug for the word alcohol. The Brief Michigan Alcohol Screening Test (a modified version of the Michigan Alcohol Screening Test [MAST]; Selzer et al. 1975) (Table 15–3) correlates with the clinical diagnosis of alcoholism. The CAGE (Mayfield et al. 1974) (Table 15–4) is also a useful bedside screening test, which correlates well with a diagnosis of alcoholism (positive response to one question means probable alcohol dependence). The MAST and the CAGE can be self-administered and take only minutes to complete. Both correlate highly with the DSM-III-R criteria (American Psychiatric Association 1987) for substance use disorders, and they have been in use and are well-established screening instruments.

Treatment of Alcohol/Drug Withdrawal

The principles employed in the treatment of withdrawal from alcohol and drugs in addicted patients with TBI are similar to those

Table 15–3.   Brief Michigan Alcohol Screening Test (MAST)

Questions	Circle correct answer	
1. Do you feel you are a *normal* drinker? (*Normal* means that you drink *less than* or *as much as* most other people.)	Yes (0)	No (2)
2. Do friends or relatives think you are a normal drinker?	Yes (1)	No (2)
3. Have you ever attended a meeting of Alcoholics Anonymous (AA)?	Yes (5)	No (0)
4. Have you ever lost friends or girlfriends/ boyfriends because of drinking?	Yes (2)	No (0)
5. Have you ever gotten into trouble at work because of drinking?	Yes (2)	No (0)
6. Have you ever neglected your obligations, your family, or your work for two or more days in a row because of drinking?	Yes (2)	No (0)
7. Have you ever had delirium tremens (DTs) or severe shaking or heard voices or seen things that weren't there after heavy drinking?	Yes (2)	No (0)
8. Have you ever gone to anyone for help about your drinking?	Yes (5)	No (0)
9. Have you ever been in a hospital because of drinking?	Yes (5)	No (0)
10. Have you ever been arrested for drunk driving or driving after drinking?	Yes (2)	No (0)

Note. If this is used as a self-administered written instrument, the scoring system should not be shown on the form. The scores on the Brief MAST correlate well with the full MAST. A score of 6 or above could identify an alcoholic patient.
Source. Reprinted from Selzer ML, Vinokur A, van Rooijen L: "A Self-Administered Short Michigan Alcoholism Screening Test (SMAST)." *Journal of Studies on Alcohol* 36:117–126, 1975. Used with permission.

employed in patients without TBI, with some important exceptions. The identification of alcohol and drug intoxication and withdrawal follows the general principles of pharmacological dependence. The use of blood and urine toxicology is important to identify presence and levels of alcohol and drugs for assessment of intoxication and anticipation of withdrawal. The use of vital signs, particularly blood pressure, pulse, and temperature, are critical in determining the presence and severity of the withdrawal state (Miller 1991a).

The medications employed in the treatment of withdrawal in TBI patients can be similar to those employed in patients who have only drug/alcohol addiction. However, the doses should be reduced to allow for the increased sensitivity of brain injury patients to the medication/drug effect. The amount of tolerance is decreased to a wide variety of medications, particularly the sedatives used in the treatment of withdrawal and agitation. The optimal level of medications for withdrawal can be assessed in an individual on an as-needed basis (prn) according to the clinical status of the patient. The patient's behavioral and vital signs can be assigned parameters for medication treatments (Miller 1991a).

For instance, for detoxification from alcohol, a dose of benzodiazepines can be given for a systolic blood pressure greater than 150 mmHg and/or diastolic greater than 100 mmHg. For detoxification from benzodiazepines, a standing schedule can be

---

Table 15–4. CAGE

1. Have you felt you ought to *Cut* down on your drinking?
2. Have people *Annoyed* you by criticizing your drinking?
3. Have you ever felt bad or *Guilty* about your drinking?
4. Have you ever had a drink first thing in the morning to steady your nerves and get rid of a hangover? (*Eye opener*)

Scoring: Two or more positive responses suggest sufficient evidence of alcohol abuse at some point during lifetime to warrant further investigation.

Source. Mayfield D, McLeod G, Hall P: "The CAGE Questionnarire: Validation of a New Alcoholsim Screening Instrument." *American Journal of Psychiatry* 131:1121–1123. Used with permission.

designed for 2–3 weeks based on estimates of doses taken during chronic use preceding withdrawal. For alcohol withdrawal, benzodiazepines should have a shorter acting half-life (e.g., lorazepam) to avoid persistent sedation in patients with brain injury. However, for benzodiazepine withdrawal, the intermediate acting preparations (e.g., diazepam) are preferred in order to avoid sharp peaks and troughs from short-acting preparations and persistent sedation from long-acting preparations that occur during the taper (Alexander and Perry 1991; Miller and Gold 1989; Miller et al. 1988).

In general, benzodiazepines are used for alcohol withdrawal (Table 15–5), benzodiazepines or phenobarbital for sedative/hypnotic withdrawal (Table 15–6), including withdrawal from benzodiazepines (Table 15–7). For cocaine, other stimulant, and cannabis withdrawal, medications usually are not required. For opiates, either clonidine or methadone can be employed in 2-week or 4-week tapering schedules. As stated, other schemes for detoxification can be utilized, but only in lower doses for the drug sensitive TBI patient. Assessment for other drugs present is indicated through history and clinical examination (Miller 1991a).

Table 15–5.   Short- and long-acting benzodiazepines

Short-acting agents (trade names)
 Triazolam (Halcion)
 Oxazepam (Serax)
 Temazepam (Restoril)
 Lorazepam (Ativan)
 Alprazolam (Xanax)

Long-acting agents (trade names)
 Chlordiazepoxide (Libritabs and Librium)
 Diazepam (Valium)
 Halazepam (Paxipam)
 Clorazepate (Tranxene)
 Prazepam (Centrax)
 Clonazepam (Klonopin)
 Flurazepam (Dalmane)

Complications

Psychiatric Symptoms

The effects of alcohol and drugs on mood and behavior are numerous and include many psychiatric symptoms. In general, alcohol and other depressant drugs can cause depression, suicidal and homicidal thinking during intoxication, anxiety, hyperactivity, hallucinations, and/or delusions during withdrawal. Cocaine and

Table 15–6. Drug doses equivalent to 600 mg of secobarbital and 60 mg of diazepam

Drug (by class)	Dose (mg)
Benzodiazepines	
Alprazolam	6
Chlordiazepoxide	150
Clonazepam	24
Clorazepate	90
Flurazepam	90
Halazepam	240
Lorazepam	12
Oxazepam	60
Prazepam	60
Temazepam	90
Barbiturates	
Amobarbital	600
Butabarbital	600
Butalbital	600
Pentobarbital	600
Secobarbital	600
Phenobarbital	180
Glycerol	
Meprobamate	2,400
Piperidinedione	
Glutethimide	1,500
Quinazolines	
Methaqualone	1,800

Note. For patients receiving multiple drugs, each drug should be converted to its diazepam or secobarbital equivalent.

other stimulant drugs can cause anxiety, hallucinations, and delusions during intoxication, and/or depression and suicidal and homicidal thinking during withdrawal. As consequences of addictive disorders, the patient can be withdrawn, asocial, antisocial (including violent behaviors), hysterical, passive-aggressive, dependent, and/or narcissistic. Often these personality features diminish after abstinence from alcohol and drugs and specific treatment of the addictive disorder. The aim of treatment of the addictive disorder is to alter attitudes and behaviors that are detrimental to personality (Blankfield 1986; Mayfield 1979; Miller and Mahler 1991; Schuckit 1983).

Length of Stay

The length of stay in the hospital for the patient with TBI is affected by the presence of alcohol or drugs. The TBI patients who

Table 15–7. Signs and symptoms of benzodiazepine withdrawal

Symptoms of hyperexcitability	Gastrointestinal symptoms
Agitation	Abdominal pain
Anxiety	Constipation
Hyperactivity	Diarrhea
Insomnia	Nausea
	Vomiting
Neuropsychiatric symptoms	
Ataxia	**Cardiovascular symptoms**
Depersonalization	Chest pain
Depression	Flushing
Fasciculation	Palpitations
Formication	
Headache	**Genitourinary symptoms**
Hyperventilation	Incontinence
Malaise	Loss of libido
Myalgia	Urinary urgency, frequency
Paranoid delusions	
Paresthesia	
Pruritus	
Tinnitus	
Tremor	
Visual hallucinations	

are users of alcohol or drugs have a longer period of hospitalization. Sparadeo and Gill (1989) reported that patients with a negative blood alcohol level had an average length of stay less than 3 weeks, with only 9.5% staying over 3 weeks, and a maximum length of stay of 45 days. For patients with a positive blood alcohol level, twice as many patients (19.4%) stayed beyond 3 weeks, and the maximum length of stay was 102 days.

Agitation

Although the incidence of agitation is not significantly greater, the duration of agitation for patients with a positive blood alcohol level is significantly longer beyond the withdrawal effects than for nonintoxicated patients. Agitation is a serious complication for recovery from TBI in these patients because it interferes with nursing care, physical therapy, occupational therapy, speech therapy, and medical and surgical interventions. Importantly, families and staff are generally disturbed by agitated patients as well (Sparadeo and Gill 1989; Substance Abuse Task Force 1988).

Cognitive Status

Of considerable interest is that patients who were intoxicated prior to brain injury have lower global cognitive statuses at the time of discharge than do those who were not intoxicated. One could speculate that the trauma is more significant in those who are compromised by alcohol and drugs through a number of mechanisms. There is significantly and persistently reduced intellectual function in alcohol- and drug-addicted patients who use alcohol and drugs on a regular basis over time (Tarter and Edwards 1985).

Intellectual deficits appear to be in large measure reversible in those without known brain trauma, and intelligence quotients improve with abstinence as a function of time. The improvement in memory, abstraction, calculations, and other cognitive abilities occurs rapidly in the first 3–6 months and more gradually thereafter. Studies have shown improvement in intellect continuing at 2 years of abstinence, and clinical experience suggests that this continues beyond this initial period (Chelune and Parker 1981; Parsons and Leber 1981).

There is usually some loss of intellectual functioning in TBI. Brain injuries are diffuse in affecting the cortex (associated motor and sensory areas), deep white matter, and brain stem. Cognitive deficits are in attention and concentration, short-term memory, and speed of processing information. There are often significant intellectual impediments to long-term recovery from TBI (Sparadeo and Gill 1989).

Cost Effects

Studies show that a positive blood alcohol level is associated with higher costs for medical care. The longer length of stay, increased agitation, higher intensity and level of care, complications with treatment of TBI, and increased morbidity from alcohol and drug effects lead to greater expense in caring for alcohol and drug-addicted or -using patients. Early identification and treatment of alcohol and drug problems and disorders can reduce expenses and allow greater numbers of patients to be treated (Miller and Ries 1991; Sparadeo and Gill 1989; Substance Abuse Task Force 1988).

Intermediate and Long-Term Treatment

Principles

Currently, there is little integration of methods for treatment of addictive disorders in psychiatric and TBI populations. The patient with a TBI usually receives care that does not identify and treat the addictive disorders. The consequences are that the morbidity and mortality from A/DD and the interactions between A/DD and TBI often continue unabated.

Generally the most widely employed treatment for A/DD uses the 12-step approach, which considers addiction as an independent disorder. This approach includes principles of recovery derived from Alcoholics Anonymous, cognitive-behavior therapies, group and individual modalities, and long-term management of the addictive disorders in Alcoholics Anonymous or Narcotics Anonymous (Table 15–8). The results of treatment outcome studies indicate that the 12-step method is an effective form of treatment for A/DD (Harrison et al. 1991); Overall abstinence rates for 1 year were 68% in 1,663 outpatients and 60% in 8,087 inpatients in a study derived from 35 different treatment sites. The abstinence rates increased to 82% and 75% respectively with regular attendance at Alcoholics Anonymous (Hoffman and Miller 1992).

In the Harrison et al. (1991) study of 9,750 patients, motor vehicle accidents and moving traffic violations were significantly reduced in patients who received treatment for alcohol/drug addiction when rates before and after the treatment of the addictive disorder were compared. Of further interest is that the utilization of medical and psychiatric services dropped significantly and job performance improved significantly in those who received addiction treatment.

Experience in applying these treatment techniques to TBI patients is limited. Novel programs tailored to the needs of TBI patients are being used, although clinical success awaits documentation in outcome studies. Attempts are under way to integrate standard care for TBI patients with standard treatment for addictive disorders (McLaughlin and Shaffer 1985; Miller and Mahler 1991; Substance Abuse Task Force 1988; Tobis et al. 1982) (Table 15–9).

Table 15–8. Resources for treatment of addictive disorders

Alcoholics Anonymous (AA) and Narcotics Anonymous (NA) and similar groups
Support groups based on AA and NA
Individual, group, and family alcohol and drug counseling
Outpatient and inpatient alcohol and drug treatment programs
Environmental control and behavior modification
Psychopharmacology

Clinical experience suggests that patients with TBI have specific persistent problems that may interfere with participating with other patients without TBI in mainstream treatment programs. The major difference is that the effects due to pharmacological effects from alcohol and drugs are reversible, whereas those due to brain injury may not be totally reversible (Table 15–9).

It is imperative to achieve and maintain progress in addiction treatment in order to gauge any success in the treatment of the neuropsychiatric deficits from trauma. Basic principles employed generally in working clinically with brain injury individuals can be utilized in their addiction treatment as well. TBI patients require concrete and structured programs that employ techniques that reach their mental capacities. The addiction therapist must be knowledgeable in the assets and liabilities of brain injury patients and skilled in applying traditional addiction treatment specifically to their needs. On the other hand, physicians, including psychiatrists and other therapists, must be knowledgeable in the priority of alcohol/drugs in the life of addicted patients and skilled in referring and collaborating with the addiction treatment team to provide a consistent, cogent, and effective treatment plan.

Treatment Strategy and Process

The following is an example of a program that provides a therapeutic milieu for the brain injury patient to learn about and discuss his or her alcohol/drug problems.

Table 15–9. Comparative effects of brain injury and drugs and/or alcohol

Possible effects of brain injury	Effects of pharmacological agents
Poor memory	Poor memory
Impaired judgment	Impaired judgment
Fine and gross motor impairments	Fine and gross motor impairments
Poor concentration	Poor concentration
Decreased impulse control	Decreased impulse control
Impaired language skills	Impaired language skills

■ **Abstinence.**   The overall aim is for the TBI patient to achieve and maintain abstinence from alcohol and drugs. The common denominator for recovery for alcoholic or drug-addicted TBI patients is loss of control over alcohol and drugs. The focus of treatment should be on abstaining from alcohol and drugs of addiction, and what changes an individual must make in order to accomplish this goal. The process begins by admitting and optimally accepting that the use of alcohol and drugs results in adverse consequences to the individual. The success in maintaining abstinence by the addicted individual will be limited without the fundamental recognition by the therapist of the psychopathological processes in addictive use of drugs. The therapist must collaborate in the goals with the patient, and be prepared to clarify for the patient the importance of abstinence from alcohol/drugs in order to recover from addiction and TBI. At times, supportive confrontation may be necessary to dispel the denial inherent in the addictive process (Miller 1991c; Roman 1982; Vaillant 1983).

■ **Denial.**   Denial is a major feature of the psychopathology of addictive disorders. Denial is both conscious and unconscious and appears to originate from multiple sources. The denial system stems in part from the pharmacological (organic) effects of alcohol and drugs and in many ways is indistinguishable from a dementia syndrome from other causes. The pharmacological effects of alcohol and drugs include aberration in judgment, insight, planning, and motivation, functions that are subserved by the frontal lobe. The result is a poorly motivated, addicted patient with little insight and judgment in response to therapeutic intervention. The temporal lobe is also affected by alcohol and drugs such that short-term memory and the acquisition of memory for new events are impaired, resulting in faulty recall of associations between alcohol and drug use and the adverse consequences. Pharmacological disruption of the temporal lobe also leads to distortions in thinking and emotions that further augment the denial (Blanchard 1984).

The denial can be effectively confronted using the evidence of the adverse consequences from addictive use of alcohol and drugs. The associations can be made for the patient by the therapist in the concrete manner that is already employed in the approach to the TBI patient. The therapist is advised to remain in the "here and now," and concentrate on what must be done to abstain from alcohol and drugs. It is counterproductive to dwell on antecedent causes that are ultimately not directly related to the addictive use of alcohol and drugs. The addiction to alcohol/drugs is an independent and autonomous condition that is not generated by other causes. This is a crucial concept that must be incorporated into successful addiction treatment. Otherwise, distraction away from the central problem of addiction to other problems that are unrelated or secondary to the addiction will prevent the addicted patient from focusing on the addictive use of alcohol and drugs (Miller and Mahler et al. 1991; Stead and Viders 1979).

The timing and method of confrontation about deficits, including alcohol and other drug problems, should be carefully coordinated with the interdisciplinary TBI treatment team. Educational points should be presented in the most effective cognitive and sensory mode. This information is best obtained from a TBI team member knowledgeable in cognitive deficits (Kreutzer et al. 1990) (Table 15–10).

▌ **Group therapy.**   In group therapy, the primary treatment intervention is performed in a group setting where confrontation of

---

Table 15–10.   Techniques for therapy with traumatic brain injury (TBI) patients

People with TBI may digress or change course during a conversation:
1. Redirect them using appropriate cues and reinforcers.
2. Teach prevention skills to the person with TBI that can be used in more than one life setting to maximize generalization.
3. Focus on a specific prevention goal.
4. Be redundant.
5. Never assume understanding or memory from a previous session.
6. Always repeat the purpose, duration, and guidelines for each meeting.
7. Summarize previous progress and then restate where the previous meeting left off (Sparadeo et al. 1990).

---

denial and induction of acceptance of the individual's addiction are best accomplished. The group consists of peers who also have addiction(s) and brain injury and is led by professionals who are skilled in addiction therapy. The focus of the group is on the loss of control of alcohol/drug use and the attendant adverse consequences. The group members share their experience, strength, and hope with each other in a supportively confrontational atmosphere (Langley 1991; Miller and Mahler 1991).

The group has a prescribed structure and format that are facilitated by the therapist and actively employed by the patients. The patients generally speak one at a time with limited cross talk where patients "advise" other patients. The patients are encouraged to speak from their own experiences and show how these may benefit others. The identification of one patient with another is central to the therapeutic process. The identification between patients with both addiction and TBI is conducive to dissipating the destructive denial and initiating constructive therapeutic changes.

The shame, guilt, and hopelessness associated with addiction and TBI can be replaced through the mutual care and consideration of one patient toward another. There are no good studies illustrating the interactions between group members that produce the dramatic cohesion that can occur within the groups. Thus far it has been impossible to explain how patients with severe addiction and mental problems work together to produce this therapeutic milieu.

The clinical experience in this type of group process has been predominantly in addiction treatment. However, preliminary experience suggests that group therapy can be adapted to patients who also have TBI. Special techniques that are commonly used in patients with brain injury can be applied in addiction groups. Interestingly, the psychological approach to the patient with brain injury shares commonalities with that for the addiction patient. Techniques such as keeping it simple, focused, and concrete are useful in both patient populations. Being directive and supportive are also useful in patients with addiction and TBI (Sparadeo et al. 1990) (Table 15–10).

Treatment Setting

The addiction-focused groups can be adjunctive in milieus that treat TBI. The addiction groups can be combined with the other therapies as an integral part of the overall therapy of TBI patients. Because over 50% of the patients with TBI are likely to also have alcohol/drug addiction, the addiction groups can be incorporated as an essential therapeutic component for many patients in a given setting. Although it is not necessary for all members of the treatment staff to be skilled in addiction treatment, it is desirable that they have minimum knowledge regarding the nature of the illness and its impact on TBI. For instance, physicians and nurses must be able to identify drug seeking and differentiate it from other medical and psychiatric problems. In this way, addiction can be confronted and treated, and iatrogenic participation in addictive use of drugs can be minimized in the clinical care of these patients (Minkoff 1989).

All interventions should be directive in nature, short term, goal directed, and behaviorally anchored. Severe brain injuries are typically so devastating to the family system that many family members "leave the field" when they come to appreciate what has occurred. Social isolation is common for people with TBI. The family system must be assessed and reassessed because it will fluctuate markedly in the first 4 years following TBI. The clinician should accentuate positive gains using frequent social praise (Sparadeo et al. 1990).

Duration of Treatment

The duration of the addiction groups can be extended over time in a graduated fashion. The first month may have three 1-hour groups per week, on a Monday-Wednesday-Friday schedule. The remaining months may have one group per week in the setting, particularly if there is a prolonged stay. Also it is important that the patients attend meetings of Alcoholics or Narcotics Anonymous (AA, NA) either in the treatment setting or in the community. The service structure of AA offers assistance with holding meetings in institutions through the Cooperation with Professionals Committee. Also some AA and NA meetings in the community are oriented toward having patients attend on a regular basis (Chappel 1993) (see Appendices 15–1 through 15–5).

Generally, it is recommended that a patient with alcoholism and drug addiction undergo continuous treatment indefinitely. Both of these are chronic illnesses that can be characterized by a relapsing course in the untreated state. The relapse rate is highest in the first 3–6 months with up to 80% of patients returning to alcohol and drug addiction in the untreated state. With treatment intervention, the abstinence rate can be increased to 70%–80% and higher with attendance at AA or NA meetings (Hoffman and Miller 1992). Abstinence rates are unknown for addicted patients with TBI in long-term recovery.

The Hoffman and Miller (1992) treatment outcome study, as well as others in addicted non-TBI patients, further demonstrate improved cognition, emotional status, and attitudes toward self and others. The interpersonal relationships and responsibility toward self and others are improved in those alcohol- and drug-addicted patients who continue in a sustained recovery program that includes attendance at aftercare for addiction treatment and AA. Personal responsibility is the cornerstone in recovery from addictive diseases (Alcoholics Anonymous 1976).

Use of Medications in the Recovered Alcoholic or Addicted Patient With TBI

Studies do not find that standard psychiatric pharmacological and nonpharmacological treatments for depression and anxiety occurring in the setting of addiction are efficacious in reducing either the depression or the anxiety from the addiction. Antidepressants, antianxiety agents, and psychotherapy do not relieve the depression and anxiety induced by alcoholism or drug addiction or influence the overall course of the addictive use of alcohol and drugs. The same findings hold for other psychiatric disorders. Hallucinations and delusions induced by the addictive use of alcohol and drugs do not respond to conventional psychiatric pharmacological or nonpharmacological therapies, especially if the use of alcohol and drugs continues (Miller 1991a; Schuckit 1990).

Studies do confirm that specific treatment of the addictive disorders will alleviate the addictive use of alcohol and drugs and the consequent psychiatric comorbidity. A period of observation of days to weeks may be necessary to examine important causal links in the genesis of psychiatric symptoms from addictive disorders and to establish independent psychiatric disorders (Miller 1991a; Tamerin and Mendelson 1969).

Most psychotropic medications can be used to treat independent psychiatric disorders in alcohol- and drug-addicted TBI patients. Generally beyond the detoxifying period in the abstinent state, there is little evidence that the psychiatric disorders in patients with addictive disorders respond differently to most psychotropic medications. The caveat is that because of the addiction potential, alcoholic or addicted patients are more likely to overuse and lose control of virtually any medications than individuals who are not addicted, particularly those medications with already established addictive potential (Miller 1991a).

The dose of psychotropic medications should be reduced because of the increased neurosensitivity of patients with brain injury. The selection of medications can be similar to those for other psychiatric disorders, including diffuse brain damage from other causes. Miller (1991a) suggested the guiding principle of aiming for the lowest doses to reduce untoward effects while maximizing therapeutic efficacy.

The physician views medications as powerful and inherently good despite the potential for toxicity. Some psychiatrists do not view themselves as physicians or minimize their role as doctors if they do not prescribe medications for a clinical disorder. Moreover, clinicians skilled in the treatment of addictive disorders advocate that the patient who is addicted to alcohol or drugs needs a clear sensorium and access to feelings in order to make fundamental changes in attitudes and behaviors for continued abstinence. Medications may impair cognition and blunt feelings, albeit sometimes in a subtle way. A parallel illustration is the crucial point stressed by psychotherapists who advise judicious use of mood-altering chemicals that might interfere with the process of psychotherapy. This is a clinical caveat that pertains to the TBI patient as well (Miller 1991a).

During recovery, the patient with alcohol/drug addiction and TBI must take an active initiative in changing attitudes and feelings, and must abandon the long held belief that alcohol and/or drugs can "fix" or "treat" life problems and uncomfortable psychological states. Clinically acknowledged, anxiety and depression can be motivating feelings to change without which the patient has little awareness of the need to change. A commonly used expression to explain this practice among recovering individuals is "no pain, no gain." The aim of pharmacotherapy to suppress symptoms such as anxiety and depression in the recovering addicted patient must take into consideration that these symptoms may be vital to the recovery and survival of the patient with alcohol/drug addiction. Enormous misunderstanding has arisen between the physician and the patient with addiction and TBI, from a divergence in purpose and perspective toward medications and the lack of knowledge and skill in both (Miller 1991a).

The current standard of care for addictive disorders is nonpharmacological beyond the detoxification period. Several studies have shown that treatment of the addictive disorder with abstinence alone results in improvement in the psychiatric syndromes associated with alcohol and drug use/addiction. Severe depressive and anxiety syndromes induced by alcohol fulfilling criteria for major depression and anxiety disorders in DSM-III-R resolve within days to weeks following the onset of abstinence. Manic syndromes induced by cocaine resolve within hours to days, and schizophrenic syndromes with hallucinations and delusions resolve within days to weeks with abstinence as well (Mayfield and Allen 1967; Schuckit 1990).

Further studies are needed to confirm the clinical experience that psychiatric symptoms, including anxiety, depression, and personality disorders respond to the specific treatment of addiction. The cognitive-behavioral techniques used in the 12-step based treatment approach have been shown to be effective in the management of anxiety and depression associated with addiction (Miller 1991b).

Long-Term Recovery in Alcoholics Anonymous

Available data demonstrate abstinence rates of 60%–80% after 2 years from alcohol and other drugs, including cocaine, in both alcohol- and drug-addicted individuals, in treatment programs based on a 12-step approach with referrals to AA. Surveys also show recovery rates with continuous abstinence of 44% at 1 year, 83% between and 1 and 5 years, and 90% at greater than 5 years, with membership and attendance at meetings in AA (44% of alcoholic individuals in AA are also addicted to drugs) (see Appendices I and II). A recent controlled study revealed that the best treatment outcome is obtained when professional treatment and AA are combined (Keso and Salaspuro 1990). Studies are not yet available that examine the efficacy of psychiatric treatments in enhancing treatment outcome in addicted patients with psychiatric comorbidity, including TBI (Chappel 1993; Group for the Advancement of Psychiatry 1991; Schulz 1991) (see Appendices I-V).

References

Alcoholics Anonymous (AA): Alcoholics Anonymous, 3rd Edition. New York, A.A. World Services, 1976

Alexander B, Perry P: Detoxification from benzodiazepines: schedules and strategies. J Subst Abuse Treat 8:9–17, 1991

American Psychiatric Association: Diagnostic and Statistical Manual of Mental Disorders, 3rd Edition, Revised. Washington, DC, American Psychiatric Association, 1987

American Psychiatric Association: Diagnostic and Statistical Manual of Mental Disorders, 4th Edition. Washington, DC, American Psychiatric Association, 1994

Blanchard MK: Counseling Head Injured Patients. Albany, NY, New York State Head Injury Association, 1984

Blankfield A: Psychiatric symptoms in alcohol dependence: diagnostic and treatment implications. J Subst Abuse Treat 3:275–278, 1986

Brismar D, Engstrom A, Rydberg U: Head injury and intoxication: a diagnostic and therapeutic dilemma. Acta Chir Scand 149:11–14, 1983

Brooks N: Closed Head Injury. Oxford, Oxford University Press, 1984

Cermak TL: Co-addiction as a disease. Psychiatric Annals 21:266–272, 1991

Chappel J: Long term recovery in AA. Psychiatr Clin North Am 16:177–188, 1993

Chelune JC, Parker JB: Neuropsychological deficits associated with chronic alcohol abuse. Clinical Psychology Review 1:181–195, 1981

Edna T: Alcohol influence and head injury. Acta Chir Scand 148:209–212, 1985

Elmer O, Lim R: Influence of acute alcohol intoxication on the outcome of severe non-neurologic trauma. Acta Chir Scand 151:305–308, 1985

Field J: Epidemiology of Head Injury in England and Wales: With Particular Application to Rehabilitation. Leicester, England, Willsons, 1976

Freund G: Neuropathology of alcohol abuse, in Alcohol and the Brain: Chronic Effects. Edited by Tarter R, Van Thiel D. New York, Plenum, 1985, pp 3–17

Galbraith S: Misdiagnosis and delayed diagnosis in traumatic intercranial hematoma. BMJ 1:1438–1439, 1976

Gallagher JP, Browder J: Extradural hematoma experienced with 167 patients. J Neurosurg 29:1–22, 1968

Group for the Advancement of Psychiatry (GAP), Committee on Alcoholism and the Addictions: Substance abuse disorders: a psychiatric priority. Am J Psychiatry 148:1291–1300, 1991

Harrison PA, Hoffman NG, Streid SG: Drug and alcohol addiction treatment outcome, in Comprehensive Handbook of Drug and Alcohol Addiction. Edited by Miller NS. New York, Marcel Dekker, 1991, 1163–1700

Helzer JE, Pryzbeck TR: The co-occurrence of alcoholism with other psychiatric disorders in the general population and its impact in treatment. J Stud Alcohol 49:219–224, 1988

Henry K: A letter to sponsors of chemically dependent head injured persons, in Task Force on Chemical Dependency. Southborough, MA, National Head Injury Foundation, 1988, 53–57

Hoffman NG, Miller NS: Effective treatment: abstinence based programs. Psychiatric Annals 22:1–5, 1992

Keso L, Salaspuro M: Inpatient treatment of employed alcoholics: a randomized clinical trial on Hazelden-type and traditional treatment. Alcohol Clin Exp Res 14:584–589, 1990

Kreutzer J, Doherty K, Harris J, et al: Alcohol use among persons with TBI. Journal of Head Trauma Rehabilitation 5(3):9–20, 1990

Langley MJ: Preventing post-injury alcohol-related problems: a behavioral approach, in Work Worth Doing: Advances in Brain Injury Rehabilitation. Edited by McMahon BT, Shaw LR. Orlando, FL, Paul M. Deutsch, 1991

Mayfield D: Alcohol and affect: experimental studies, in Alcoholism and Affective Disorders. Edited by Goodwin DW, Erickson CK. New York, S P Medical and Scientific, 1979

Mayfield D, Allen D: Alcohol and affect: a psychopharmacological study. Am J Psychiatry 123:1346–1351, 1967

Mayfield D, McLeod G, Hall P: The CAGE questionnarire: validation of a new alcoholsim screening instrument. Am J Psychiatry 131:1121–1123

McLaughlin AM, Shaffer V: Rehabilitation or remold? family involvement in head trauma recovery. Cognitive Rehabilitation 3: 1985

Miller NS: The Pharmacology of Alcohol and Drugs of Abuse and Addiction. New York, Springer-Verlag, 1991a

Miller NS: Special problems of the alcohol and multiple-drug dependent: clinical interactions, in Clinical Textbook of Addictive Disorders. Edited by Frances RJ, Miller SJ. New York, Guilford, 1991b, pp 194–218

Miller NS: Drug and alcohol addiction as a disease, in Comprehensive Handbook of Drug and Alcohol Addiction. Edited by Miller NS. New York, Marcel Dekker, 1991c, pp 295–310

Miller NS, Gold MS: Identification and treatment of benzodiazepine abuse. Am Fam Physician 40:175–183, 1989

Miller NS, Gold MS: Alcohol. New York, Plenum, 1991

Miller NS, Mahler JC: Alcoholics Anonymous and the "AA" model for treatment. Alcoholism Treatment Quarterly 8(11):39–51, 1991

Miller NS, Rics RK: Drug and alcohol dependence and psychiatric populations: the need for diagnosis, intervention, and training. Compr Psychiatry 32:268–276, 1991

Miller NS, Gold MS, Cocores JA, et al: Alcohol dependence and its medical consequences. N Y State J Med 88:476–481, 1988

Miller NS, Gold MS, Belkin B, et al: The diagnosis of alcohol and cannabis dependence in cocaine dependents and alcohol dependence in their families. Br J Addict 84:1491–1498, 1990

Minkoff K: An integrated treatment model for dual diagnosis of psychosis and addiction. Hosp Community Psychiatry 40:1031–1036, 1989

Parsons DA, Leber WR: The relationship between cognitive dysfunction and brain damage in alcoholics: causation or epiphenomenal? Clin Exp Res 5:326–343, 1981

Ries RK, Samson H: Substance abuse among inpatient psychiatric patients. Substance Abuse 8:28–34, 1987

Roman P: Barriers to the use of constructive confrontations with employed alcoholics. J Clin Psychiatry 43:53–57, 1982

Rumbaugh CL, Fang HEH: The effects of drug abuse on the brain. Med Times 3:37–52, 1980

Schuckit MA: Alcoholism and other psychiatric disorders. Hosp Community Psychiatry 34:1022–1027, 1983

Schuckit MA: Drug and alcohol abuse: a clinical guide to diagnosis and treatment. New York, Plenum, 1990

Schuckit MA, Irwin M, Brown SA: The history of anxiety symptoms among 171 primary alcoholics. J Stud Alcohol 51:34–41, 1990

Schulz JE: Long-term treatment in recovery from drug and alcohol addiction, in Comprehensive Handbook of Drug and Alcohol Addictions. Edited by Miller NS. New York, Marcel Dekker, 1991

Selzer ML, Vinokur A, van Rooijen L: A self-administered Short Michigan Alcoholism Screening Test (SMAST). J Studi Alcohol 36:117–126, 1975

Sparadeo FR, Gill D: Focus on clinical research: effect of prior alcohol use on head injury recovery. Journal of Head Trauma Rehabilitation 4(1):75–82, 1989

Sparadeo FR, Strauss D, Barth JT: The incidence, impact, and treatment of substance abuse in head trauma rehabilitation. Journal of Head Trauma Rehabilitation 5(3):1–8, 1990

Special Section: Alcohol and health, IV: treatment and rehabilitation. Alcoh Health Res World 5(3):48–58, 1981

Stead P, Viders J: A "SHARP" approach to treating alcoholism. Social Work 24:144–149, 1979

Substance Abuse Task Force: White Paper. Washington, DC, National Head Injury Foundation, 1988

Tamerin JS, Mendelson JH: The psychodynamics of chronic inebriation. Observations of alcoholic during the process of drinking in an experimental group setting. Am J Psychiatry 125:886–899, 1969

Tarter R, Edwards K: Neuropsychology of alcoholism, in Alcohol and the Brain: Chronic Effects. Edited by Tarter R, Van Thiel D. New York, Plenum, 1985, pp 217–242

Tobis JS, Puri KB, Sheridan J: Rehabilitation of the severely brain-injured patient. Scand J Rehabil Med 14:83–88, 1982

Vaillant GE: The Natural History of Alcoholism. Cambridge, MA, Harvard University Press, 1983

Letter to Alcoholics Anonymous (AA) Sponsor of AA Member With Traumatic Brain Injury

The following is a letter to an Alcoholics Anonymous (AA) sponsor explaining the special characteristics of the alcohol- or drug-addicted individual with brain damage. A sponsor in AA (or Narcotics Anonymous [NA]) is someone who also is an alcoholic- or drug-addicted individual in recovery and assists the sponsoree in learning about the AA or NA program and "working" the steps of AA or NA.

Dear Sponsor:

As a twelve-stepper in AA or NA, you know fully well the horror chemical dependency thrusts into a person's life. Without concerted and persistent effort toward recovery, personal, family and social dimensions of life are deeply threatened and treacherously undermined. In the case of the person you are now sponsoring or are considering whether to sponsor, the addiction has been further compounded by a head injury which has, to some degree, caused damage to the brain. Because of this damage, the very physiological organ responsible for memory, language, reasoning, judgment,

Appendixes reprinted courtesy of the National Head Injury Foundation (Substance Abuse Task Force: "White Paper." Washington, DC, National Head Injury Foundation, 1988, pp. 53–59).

and behavior (among other skills and abilities) has been compromised. Consequently, problems have emerged that are a direct result of the trauma to the brain, and these problems now are inevitably overlapping and interacting with the individual's addictive nature.

At this stage in his or her recovery from the trauma, the individual with whom you are working has undoubtedly regained many of those diminished abilities. However, in all probability, there are lasting effects ("sequelae," in medical terminology) that remain and that you may now be witnessing. These residual problems may be manifested in obvious or subtle ways, and an explanation of their nature may be helpful.

The purpose of this letter is to acquaint you with some of the more common cognitive (i.e., having to do with perceiving, organizing, interpreting, and acting on information) and emotional problems that head injured people face as a direct result of brain trauma. With a good medical recovery it is not at all unusual for these individuals to appear unimpaired unless one takes a close look, and your work as a sponsor certainly will require close interaction. These comments, then, are offered in a spirit of gratitude for your help to this person who must now come to grips with himself or herself on several levels; who must now, en route to recovery from addiction, untangle a complex knot of problems including the changing pretraumatic lifestyle while dealing with the confusion and psychological pain that recently shattered cognition brings.

The human brain has specific sections that specialize in specific functions. If damage to any of these areas is severe enough, those functions—as well as higher level ones which they support—may be lastingly limited. Many of these regions of the brain interface to enable the performance of complex skills such as reading, or remembering and following through on lengthy directions. Because the brain's functioning is so dependent on the interrelationship of parts, and because any of those parts may be hurt in a trauma, many sorts of problems can result. The more prominent and frequently occurring ones, discussed in cognitive and emotional areas, are as follows:

Cognitive

Attention

This includes maintaining attention for normal periods of time, and the ability to shift attention to different areas after concentrating on one set of ideas. Also included here are difficulties screening out distractions (voices, noises, and visual things) in the environment, as well as suppressing one's own preoccupations while there is other work to be done.

Suggestions: Settle for smaller amounts of quality time rather than attempting longer amounts which may prove too fatiguing to the sponsoree. Cue him when he seems stuck in prior topics (e.g., "We're talking about now . . . ") or when he seems to have drifted away ("Tune back in now, okay . . . "). Gradually lengthen the time of expected attention and concentration as increasing abilities permit.

Memory

The most common type of deficit resulting from the brain injury is of short term memory. This appears as difficulty holding onto several pieces of information while having also to think through each item (e.g., cooking, while also staying mindful of the children's nearby play). Other common problems are in remembering to follow through on assigned tasks at specified times, and in remembering recent experiences and conversations. Fortunately, memory for pretraumatic episodes are most often unimpaired by this time in the person's medical recovery.

Suggestions: Expect the person to use journals and date books—and to review them frequently and independently—to cue himself about past and future events. If such memory aids are necessary, consider this simply another component of the program to be worked; do not shy from expecting self responsibility. If the person is overloaded by doing two or more things simultaneously, encourage him to prioritize tasks and work out a time management schedule honoring that limitation.

Language

Both ability to understand others and to express one's own ideas clearly are often affected. In both cases, a slower speed of processing language is at play. Also, delays in recalling the words needed to articulate a thought are common. When speaking, the head injured person may ramble and talk in a disorganized, circular kind of way, often failing to come to the point or himself losing it in the details of the conversation.

Suggestions: Encourage the person to ask questions and request clarification of information whenever needed to compensate for a slower rate of comprehension. For situations in which it is appropriate, encourage the head injured person also to ask speakers to slow down, to repeat points, and to explain ideas in different words. Support may be required to downplay feelings of embarrassment to do these things. As a speaker, the sponsoree may need cues to see the need for making his point more clearly, simply, or briefly; working out a system for your providing such cues that you both feel comfortable with might be useful. As a general rule, encourage him to take time to think about what he wants to say, to plan how to say it, and to be unrushed in finding the words he needs.

Reasoning and Judgment

Basic skills such as cause-effect reasoning and/or the ability to make inferences are often reduced. Thinking may be excessively concrete, giving rise to confusion and misinterpretation of others' remarks (e.g., "Come off your high horse . . ."). Similarly, problem-solving skills are often marred by impulsive decision making, difficulty in considering several solutions to problems and in envisioning potential consequences of actions. Failure to note voice or facial cues of others that convey nonverbal messages also increases the chance of inappropriate remarks. Common too are related problems in inhibiting inappropriate behavior, determining what situations require what behaviors, and reflecting on the propriety of what he has just said or done.

Suggestions: As an overall rule, do not avoid openly addressing the issues raised by the above-mentioned behaviors or misunderstandings. Apply the very same gentle but firm advice-giving anyone working in a recovery program may require. It may be helpful to point out specific incidences as example of behaviors that need to be avoided, or situations from which one can learn to "think first before saying or doing something." As you would with anyone looking to you for help, follow your good instincts to provide support in the amount, kind, and frequency that leads this particular person with this particular personality to the best levels of independence he can achieve.

Executive Functions

These refer to those abilities to initiate, organize, direct, monitor, and evaluate oneself. Self-insight is a crucial component. Owing to the very high level nature of these skills and to the vulnerability of the part of the brain responsible for their operation, they are frequently impaired in the person who has suffered a head trauma. As a result, even with other skills and abilities intact, the use of these executive functions in a directed, purposeful manner may be lacking, making the overall picture of brain operations rather like a full member, competent orchestra without a conductor to organize and lead their many mixing harmonies; or, like a ready and able work crew without a foreman to coordinate and direct their labor.

Suggestions: If impairments in executive functions are apparent in the person you sponsor, it may well become especially important for you to assume a role of guiding some of these operations within the context in which you work together. To an extent, you would do this anyway; it is a large part of sponsorship. For a head injured person, however, the need for such help may be deeper and more substantial. Your skills as a conductor, or foreman, may be particularly required. A little more firmly offered advice in decision making, for example—or better perhaps, encouragement to make one's own sound decisions with you available to monitor, affirm, give feedback, and gently correct when necessary. As noted earlier, in most cases it would be perfectly okay to talk openly about the need for your help in this regard because of the limitations imposed by the head injury. But be careful, of course, not to foster unnecessary dependence; increased well-being through healthy, clear-minded independence is always, as you know, the ultimate goal.

Emotional

There is an array of emotional problems typically related to head injury. These include irritability, poor frustration tolerance, dependence on others, insensitivity, lack of awareness of one's impact on others, and heightened emotionality. There may be tendencies toward overreaction to stressful situations, some paranoia, depression, withdrawal, or denial of problems. No single head injured person evidences all of these problems, of course, and most would show only subtle signs of some of these psychosocial difficulties. They are mentioned, however, to familiarize you with some of the emotional problems that often accompany brain trauma, and to alert you to their similarity to those characteristics of many persons with histories of alcohol and drug addiction.

Suggestions: In your sponsoring of a head injured person who may exhibit some of the above problems, the art of playing issues straight is recommended. Your sponsoree should know what problems you see impeding his progress toward greater recovery. Since his well being is the goal, your responsibility is as it would be with any other such partnership. Tactful but clear identification of problems, complete with acceptance of them as risks to continued sobriety or clean time which will necessitate work, is an appropriate attitude to adopt. Whether these sorts of problems are attributable to an addictive personality, or to the head injury, or to both, open, honest acknowledgement of the work to be done and the support needed to do it is what recovery is all about. The sponsorship concept, moreover, is a very plausible means of addressing those sorts of problems.

Please also be aware that there are three main avenues of assistance further available to you.

1. If the person with whom you work has received treatment from a rehabilitation center specializing in brain trauma, do not hesitate to contact the staff for advice. They may be aware of approaches or strategies that work well with your individual.
2. For materials on head injury and chemical dependency contact the National Head Injury Foundation (NHIF), 333 Turnpike Road, Southborough, Massachusetts 01772, (508) 485–9950.
3. Members of the NHIF's Task Force on Chemical Dependency would be happy to assist you in whatever way possible.

You are one of the main supports of the recovering chemically dependent, head injured person. You deserve great thanks. The comments in this letter are not meant to frighten or dissuade you from sponsorship, but rather to provide you with basic information with which to enhance your preparedness and diffuse any unnecessary anxieties you may feel. Trust yourself in your work; your status as a twelve-stepper well respected for your patience, intelligence, and straightforwardness. The recovering head injured person receiving your help is fortunate to have you in his corner.

Kurt Vonnegut wrote that, "Detours are dancing lessons from God." You understand chemical dependency and recovery. Confronting a major life obstacle, you have learned to dance. Your sponsorship of the head injured person with whom you are beginning involvement represents help for someone whose life has been shattered in a particularly devastating way, whose detour is indeed formidable. May your help in teaching that person to dance be gratifying, and blessed, and an occasion for joy and learning for you both.

Sincerely,
Kevin Henry, M.Ed., Task Force on Chemical Dependency
National Head Injury Foundation
333 Turnpike Road
Southborough, Massachusetts 01772

Twelve Things to Do if Your Loved One Is an Alcoholic

The following is a list of things to do if "your loved one is an alcoholic." The list may be used as a guide to families who must live and assist the patient with alcohol or drug addiction and traumatic brain injury.

1. Don't regard this as a family disgrace. Recovery from alcoholism can come about as in any other illness.
2. Don't nag, preach, or lecture to alcoholic loved one. Chances are they have already told themselves everything you can tell them. They will take just so much and shut out the rest. You may increase their need to lie or force them to make promises they cannot possibly keep.
3. Guard against the "holier-than-thou" or martyr-like attitude. It is possible to create this impression without saying a word. Alcoholics' sensitivity is such that they judges people's attitudes towards them more by small things than by spoken words.
4. Don't use the "if you loved me" appeal. Because alcoholics' drinking is compulsive and cannot be controlled by willpower, this approach only increases their guilt. It is like saying, "If you loved me, you would not have tuberculosis."
5. Avoid any threat unless you think it through carefully and definitely intend to carry it out. There may be times, of course, when a specific action is necessary to protect children. Idle threats make the alcoholic feel you don't mean what you say.
6. Alcohol may need to be removed from the house or stored in locations which are inaccessible to the injured individual.

7. Don't let alcoholic loved ones persuade you to drink with them on the grounds that it will make them drink less. It rarely does. Besides, when you condone their drinking, they put off doing something to get help.

8. Don't be jealous of the method of recovery the alcoholic chooses. The tendency is to think that love of home and family is enough incentive for seeking recovery. Frequently the motivation of regaining self-respect is more compelling for the alcoholic than resumption of family responsibilities. Or you may feel left out when the alcoholic turns to other people for help in staying sober. You wouldn't be jealous of the doctor if someone needs medical care, would you?

9. *Don't expect an immediate 100% recovery. In any illness there is a period of convalescence. There may be relapses and times of tension and resentment.*

10. Don't try to protect recovering alcoholics from drinking situations. It's one of the quickest ways to push them into a relapse. They must learn on their own to say "no" gracefully. If you warn people against serving them drinks you will stir up old feelings of resentment and inadequacy.

11. Don't do for alcoholic loved ones that which they can do for themselves or which must be done by themselves. You cannot take their medicine for them. Don't remove the problem before they can face it, solve it, or suffer the consequences.

12. *Do* offer love, support, and understanding in their sobriety.

Appendix 15–3

Original Twelve Steps of Alcoholics Anonymous

1. We admitted we were powerless over alcohol; that our lives had become unmanageable.
2. Came to believe that a Power greater than ourselves could restore us to sanity.
3. Made a decision to turn our will and our lives over to the care of God as we understood Him.
4. Made a searching and fearless moral inventory of ourselves.
5. Admitted to God, to ourselves, and to another human being the exact nature of our wrongs.
6. Were entirely ready to have God remove all these defects of character.
7. Humbly asked Him to remove our shortcomings.
8. Made a list of all persons we had harmed and became willing to make amends to them all.
9. Made direct amends to such people wherever possible, except when to do so would injure them or others.
10. Continued to take personal inventory and when we were wrong, promptly admitted it.
11. Sought through prayer and mediation to improve our conscious contact with God as we understood Him, praying only for knowledge of His will for us and the power to carry that out.
12. Having had a spiritual awakening as the result of these steps, we tried to carry this message to alcoholics and to practice these principles in all our affairs.

Appendix 15–4

Traumatic Brain Injury (TBI) Explanation of the Twelve Steps

The following are the twelve steps of Alcoholics Anonymous that have been written for the TBI patient who has cognitive and mood disturbances. These steps can be understood by those who need concrete examples for understanding and using them in the recovery program for the TBI patient.

1. Admit that if you drink and/or use drugs your life will be out of control. Admit that the use of substances after having had a TBI will make your life unmanageable.
2. You start to believe that someone can help you put your life in order. This someone could be God, an AA group, counselor, sponsor, etc.
3. You decide to get help from others or from God. You open yourself up.
4. You will make a complete list of the negative behaviors in your past and current behavior problems. You will also make a list of your positive behaviors.
5. Meet with someone you trust and discuss what you wrote in step 4.
6. Become ready to sincerely try to change your negative behaviors.
7. Ask God for the strength to be a responsible person with responsible behaviors.

Reprinted courtesy of Alcoholics Anonymous

8. Make a list of people your negative behaviors have affected. Be ready to apologize or make things right with them.

9. Contact these people. Apologize or make things right.

10. Continue to check yourself and your behaviors daily. Correct negative behaviors and improve them. If you hurt another person, apologize and make corrections.

11. Stop and think about how you are behaving several times each day. Are my behaviors positive? Am I being responsible? If not, ask for help. Reward yourself when you are able to behave in a positive and responsible fashion.

12. If you try to work these steps you will start to feel much better about yourself. Now it's your turn to help others do the same. Helping others will make you feel even better. Continue to work these steps on a daily basis.

Appendix 15–5

Original Twelve Steps of Alcoholics Anonymous for People With English as a Second Language

1. We admitted that alcohol was more powerful than ourselves. We admitted that we could not control our lives.
2. We began to believe that a Power stronger than ourselves could make our minds healthy again.
3. We decided to let God take care of our minds and our lives. We chose our own idea of who God is.
4. We made a complete list of our personality problems. We were not afraid to make this list (inventory).
5. We told God and another person about our personality problems.
6. We were completely ready to let God take away all of these personality problems.
7. We humbly asked God to remove our weaknesses.
8. We made a list of all the people we hurt in the past. We became ready to tell them we were sorry and to correct past damage.
9. We said we were sorry to the people we hurt, and we tried to correct the past damage, if possible. But we did not do this if it would hurt them or other people.
10. We continued to look at the strong and weak parts of our personality. When we were wrong, we quickly admitted it.
11. We used prayer and meditation to improve our contact with God (the idea of Him that we chose). We prayed only to know His way; and we prayed only for the power to live His way.

12. Our spirit grew because we used these twelve steps, so we tried to tell other alcoholics about the steps. And we tried to use these steps in everything we did.

Chapter 16

Seizures

Gary J. Tucker, M.D.
Vernon M. Neppe, M.D., Ph.D.

The presence of posttraumatic seizures is a major complication in the recovery of the brain injury patient. It not only brings further cognitive and behavioral changes (in addition to those caused by the brain injury itself), it also connotes a worse prognosis.

The many cognitive problems faced by the patient with traumatic brain injury (TBI), including the inability to sustain attention (Parasuraman et al. 1991) and impairments in verbal communication (Marsh and Knight 1991; Sarna 1980), handicap the social interactions of the recovering patient. Seizures in themselves, without TBI, have marked effects on cognitive functions and social performance (Matthews 1992). In addition, anticonvulsant medications can also cause cognitive changes (Farwell et al. 1990; Gillham et al. 1988; Meador et al. 1990). Aside from these cognitive effects, seizures have an enormous psychological impact on the patient's self-confidence about social interactions, because of the stigma that has always been attached to seizure disorders (Temkin 1971). The seizures, the medication effects, and the psychological effects, combined with the brain trauma, significantly complicate the rehabilitation of the brain injury patient.

Epidemiology

Several studies have examined the occurrence of seizures after TBI. Closed head injuries have a 5% incidence of posttraumatic seizures that can occur any time after brain injury. When the dura has been penetrated, 30%–50% of the patients develop posttraumatic seizures (Jennett 1975; Lishman 1987). Jennett (1975) estimated that only 1% of patients develop seizures if no seizure occurs during the first week after injury; however, if a seizure occurs during the first week, the lifetime incidence increases to 25%. In those patients who develop seizures, the long-term prognosis regarding subsequent seizures is good, that is, 50% of patients with posttraumatic seizures will no longer experience seizures 5–10 years postinjury, 25% will have good seizure control on medication, and 25% will continue to have seizures. The occurrence of seizures depends not only on the severity of the brain injury, but also on the early treatment of the injury (Temkin et al. 1990). Temkin et al. (1990) showed that patients maintained on phenytoin longer than 1 week posttrauma have more cognitive deficits and more subsequent seizures than those whose phenytoin is discontinued after the first week.

Annegers et al. (1980) provided the best available data, from a large community-based survey using the epidemiological base developed by the Mayo Clinic. They surveyed all medical records of patients with reported brain injury in Olmsted County, Minnesota, from 1935–1974, who were admitted to a hospital or an emergency room, or were seen as outpatients or on a home visit in the county. In this manner, they collected a total sample of 3,587 patients with TBI, 840 of whom were excluded either because of death within the first month or a prior history of epilepsy or TBI, or because the seizure was the result of other conditions. The remaining 2,747 patients with brain injuries were followed longitudinally for the development of posttraumatic seizures. Thus the authors avoided one of the major pitfalls in many of the studies of patients with brain injury, that is, the lack of data on those patients lost to follow-up. However, this study was not without methodological problems. The authors noted the extreme complexity in estimating the risk of seizures due to the absence, at that time, of standardized definitions of brain trauma or severity of injury. (This lack of definition is present in most of the literature before the development of the standardized rating scales for TBI.) Secondly, there is the possibility that this was an atypical sample because it was obtained from a major neurosurgical center. Thirdly, the authors noted the very poor follow-up for most patients with brain trauma. Lastly, it was often unclear whether the patient had a history of seizures prior to the injury.

In spite of these methodological concerns, this community-based study is still very valuable in presenting, to date, the most complete picture of the longitudinal course of patients with brain trauma. The patients were grouped into three categories:

1. *Mild brain trauma* (1,640 patients)—defined as those without skull fractures and without loss of consciousness, or a period of posttraumatic amnesia of less than 30 minutes.
2. *Moderate brain trauma* (912 patients)—those patients who had more than a 30-minute period of unconsciousness or posttraumatic amnesia and/or had a skull fracture.
3. *Severe brain trauma* (195 patients)—evidence of brain contusion, hematoma, or 24 hours of unconsciousness.

With this classification, Annegers et al. (1980) followed the patients over the 40-year period from 1935–1974. Seizures developed in 51 patients during the first 4 years after injury. The risk for patients with severe injury (7.1% in the first year and 11.5% within the next 5 years) was much greater than for those with moderate (0.7% in the first year and 1.6% within 5 years) or mild injury (0.1% in the first year and 1.6% within 5 years). In children with severe injury, the incidence of posttraumatic seizures was 30% compared to only 10% in adults with severe brain injury. Thus the age of the patient and the severity of the injury are crucial determinants of the subsequent development of posttraumatic seizures.

The study by Temkin et al. (1990) demonstrated that the use of anticonvulsants after TBI affected the subsequent development of seizures. Patients with severe brain trauma were treated with either phenytoin or a placebo immediately after the injury. Between drug loading and the seventh day after the trauma, 3.6% of the phenytoin group and 14.2% of the control group developed seizures. Between day eight and the end of the first year of the study, 21.5% of the phenytoin group but only 15.7% of the placebo group had seizures. At the end of the second year, the seizure rates were 27.5% for the phenytoin group and 21.1% for the control group. Both of these follow-up differences were statistically significant. The authors hypothesized that phenytoin exerts a prophylactic effect on reducing seizures during the first week after severe brain injury but may increase seizure frequency with prolonged treatment. They concluded that the drug has an early suppressive effect but not a true prophylactic one. Consequently, in view of the cognitive changes associated with phenytoin and other anticonvulsants, their continued use after the first week following the injury may be contraindicated.

Diagnosis

Electroencephalograms

A major diagnostic indicator of a seizure disorder is an abnormal electroencephalogram (EEG), generally involving paroxysms or spikes, either focal or generalized (Neppe and Tucker 1992). The presence of an epileptiform finding occurs more frequently with penetrating brain injury. It is important to emphasize, however, that a prior EEG will reveal seizure activity in only 41% of patients with symptomatic seizures (Desai et al. 1988). Consequently, this relatively low sensitivity of the EEG suggests that the presence or absence of an epileptiform spike should not be a factor in determining disability benefits for individuals with epilepsy and one should not use such abnormalities as an entry criterion for research (Desai et al. 1988). Jabbari et al. (1986) performed EEG evaluations on 515 Vietnam War victims 12–16 years after penetrating brain injury. They found that 42% of the subjects had abnormal EEGs, but only 9% demonstrated epileptiform findings. There was a significant correlation between EEG findings and the extent of brain volume loss visualized by computerized tomography. All patients with anterior temporal foci or central spike foci experienced posttraumatic seizures. Focal slowing, as would be expected, correlated significantly with localized neurological deficits such as hemiplegia and others (Jabbari et al. 1986). Salazar et al. (1985) studied 421 Vietnam veterans with penetrating brain injuries. Posttraumatic seizures developed in 53% of these patients. However, only 12% had EEG results diagnostic of a seizure disorder. The authors concluded that the EEG may not always be diagnostically helpful.

The severity of the injury increases the probability of EEG abnormality. Koufen and Hagel (1987) evaluated 100 patients with posttraumatic seizures, who also had at least one week of amnesia following brain injury, and found that 95% had focal EEG abnormalities, 70% of which were bilateral. Many of these patients had focal neurological symptoms and skull fractures as well. The EEG normalized in 48% after 2 years, but foci persisted in 22% of the patients and 30% remained diffusely abnormal. The most common abnormalities were delta rhythms (85%) and focal dysrhythmias with temporal localization (58%–82% depending upon criteria).

The majority of posttraumatic seizures are generalized; however, all types of partial seizures can also occur (Salazar et al. 1985) and, in fact, are equal in presentation to the generalized seizures. The diagnosis of seizure disorders is a clinical diagnosis because the best diagnostic test is to observe someone having a seizure. All evaluations of suspected seizure disorders should have regular EEGs, especially a sleep EEG, which is four times more likely to show an abnormality than a waking EEG (Gibbs and Gibbs 1952).

Although some researchers advocate the use of nasopharyngeal leads, these actually increase the rate of abnormal findings by 10% (Bickford 1979). A later study (Sadler and Goodwin 1989) shows that submandibular notch placement on the buccal skin surface is as effective as either nasopharyngeal or sphenoidal leads.

Prolactin levels have been shown to rise in patients with seizures and may be of some use in diagnosis (Dana-Haer and Trimble 1984). Recent studies using single photon emission tomography show about a 30%–40% chance of demonstrating a seizure focus interictally and a 70%–80% chance if the study is done ictally (Lassen and Holm 1992; Lee et al. 1988). This may prove to be a useful technique for the confirmation of seizure foci.

Pathogenesis

Although the etiology of posttraumatic seizures is not certain, the most frequently associated factor is the actual disruption of brain tissue. Almost any injury that penetrates the dura and the cortex results in a higher incidence of posttraumatic seizures. The incidence of posttraumatic epilepsy in penetrating injuries varies from 28%–50% (Salazar et al. 1985). Some seizure disorders can be treated successfully by the surgical removal of cortical scar tissue (Spencer and Katz 1990). Consequently, there may be cortical disruption, scarring, or irritability, such as the release of various endogenous neurotoxins (e.g., glutamate), which leads to the onset of posttraumatic seizures.

Heikkmen et al. (1990) noted that although the severity of injury was most predictive of the development of early seizures (within the first seven days postinjury), other specific factors were also associated with the onset of seizures, including periods of unconsciousness over 24 hours, skull fracture with dural tears, contusions, hematomas, and/or hemorrhage. The presence of subcortical atrophy or impaired local cerebral blood flow were most predictive of late onset seizures occurring in the 3–12 month period after injury (Table 16–1).

After severe brain injury, hyperexcitable neurons may produce an epileptic focus between the time of the trauma and the seizure occurrence (Kuhl et al. 1990). There is biochemical evidence from animal studies (Mori et al. 1990) that the occurrence of posttraumatic seizures may be related to a breakdown of red blood cells and hemoglobin in the cerebral cortex, leading to release of free hydroxyl radicals into the central nervous system, subsequently affecting the neuromembranes and leading to seizures. Interestingly, Weiss et al. (1982) noted a higher incidence of cerebral vascular accidents in patients with posttraumatic epilepsy. Proctor et al. (1988) used an experimental model for seizure development in closed head injury. Their research involved cats subjected to significant atmospheric fluid percussion impact (3.5 atmospheres administered to the cerebral cortex). They found that there were significant differences in seizure development related to measures of oxygenation and cytochrome A and ATP.

It is unclear why one person will develop seizures and another, with the same degree of brain trauma, will not. Weiss et al. (1982) and Salazar et al. (1985) reported that there was no genetic predisposition or a family history of seizures in those who developed seizures.

Prognosis

The area of prognosis is an extremely difficult one to tease apart in patients with posttraumatic epilepsy because the strongest correlate of the development of seizures is the severity of the brain injury. This factor constantly leaves one with the question of whether the seizures further complicate the clinical course of a patient with severe brain injury or they simply reflect the more

Table 16–1.   Risk factors for early and late seizures

Risk factors for early seizures (within the first week)	Risk factors for late seizures (after the first week)
Younger age (especially under 5 years)	Early seizures
Posttraumatic amnesia more than 24 hours	Posttraumatic amnesia more than 24 hours
Skull fracture (especially depressed)	Depressed skull fracture
Intracranial hemorrhage	Hematoma
Initial seizures	Penetrating injury
Penetrating injury	High Glasgow Coma Scale score

extensive injury. In either case, the presence of posttraumatic seizures predicts a poor prognosis. Dikmen and Reitan (1978) reported that a group of posttraumatic epilepsy patients with cortical defects on neuropsychological testing had a worse prognosis than those with posttraumatic epilepsy who showed no cortical defects. The patients with cortical deficits *and* seizures would be expected to do poorly because they are usually the most severely injured. Other studies indicate a more severe prognosis for patients with posttraumatic epilepsy. Corkin et al. (1984) showed that patients with posttraumatic epilepsy had shorter life expectancies than those with brain injuries without seizures. Walker and Blumer (1989), in a 40-year follow-up of 244 World War II veterans who had penetrating brain injuries and seizure disorders, noted that at follow-up, 101 had died (a figure much higher than one would expect in a normal population). Thus patients with posttraumatic epilepsy have an increased mortality. This observation was confirmed by Weiss et al. (1982). Interestingly, 25% of the survivors of brain injury also showed deterioration in cognitive functions and earlier signs of aging. However, of those with seizures, 75% had no seizures in the past 10 years (Walker and Blumer 1989). Walker and Blumer also pointed out that the pattern and type of injury that occurs in the military differs from civilian brain injury. Civilian brain injuries are usually in the frontal-temporal region whereas those associated with military injuries are usually penetrating and in rolandic (motor) and parietal regions and involve several cerebral lobes. Thus the mortality and neurological deficit studies may not be generalizable to civilian populations. Weiss et al. (1986), in a 15-year follow-up study of 520 veterans, noted that 95% of the patients were seizure free 3 years after the trauma. Interestingly, the presence of substance or alcohol abuse was not a factor in the cessation of seizure activity. However, Salazar et al. (1985) noted that seizures occurred up to 15 years posttrauma in a group of Vietnam veterans. Although the majority of veterans (57%) developed seizures within the first year, 15% did not develop seizures until 2 years after brain injury and 18% developed seizures within 5 years (Weiss et al. 1986).

Armstrong et al. (1990) surveyed 300 consecutive brain trauma admissions to a rehabilitation hospital and, after excluding those with penetrating brain injuries or prior histories of epilepsy, found 87 patients with posttraumatic epilepsy (37%) and 151 patients (63%) with brain trauma and no posttraumatic epilepsy. In comparing these patients, they noted that there was a greater incidence of males than females in the posttraumatic epilepsy group. Interestingly, although there were no differences between the two groups in the neurological findings in terms of skull fracture, hematomas, hemorrhages, or the Halstead-Reitan Battery results, there were marked differences in outcome in the patients who had posttraumatic epilepsy. Patients with posttraumatic epilepsy had a longer stay in the hospital, more difficulty with receptive language and intelligibility, decreased ability to perform activities of daily living, decreased motor function, and more mood and affective changes, as well as more problems with orientation, than the patients without posttraumatic epilepsy. Although all of the patients made gains from admission to discharge, the posttraumatic epilepsy group started lower and ended lower.

Table 16–2 presents a summary of these factors associated with the presence of seizures in patients with head injury. The onset of seizures in a patient with TBI is a poor prognostic sign for general recovery, although as noted, the seizures themselves are not a major complication during the recovery years. The presence of focal neurological and cognitive deficits markedly worsens the prognosis. However, it is difficult to sort out the exact contribution of the seizures to this poor prognosis because these patients usually have more severe injuries overall.

Table 16–2. Factors associated with the presence of seizures in head injury patients

Increased	Decreased
Rehabilitation hospital stays	Communicative ability
Mood and affective disorders	Motor function
Cerebrovascular accidents	Activities of daily living
	Orientation
	Life expectancy

Psychopathology

Seizure disorders are associated with increases in psychopathology (McKenna et al. 1985; Trimble 1991). The psychopathology can range from changes in personality characteristics to frank psychosis with either an episodic or a chronic course. Patients with seizure disorders, when assessed in large studies, often show statistically significant increased incidence of such personality traits as impulsiveness and irritability, emotional lability, hyposexuality, hypergraphia, viscosity, paranoia, nightmares, fluidity of thinking, chronic pain, aggression, and philosophical or religious preoccupation (Neppe and Tucker 1992). Almost every psychopathological symptom (Table 16–3) has been well noted in patients with seizure disorders (Blumer et al. 1990; Neppe and Tucker 1988a, 1988b). These characteristics also occur in patients with abnormal EEGs and probably relate to greater dysfunction of the central nervous system, rather than specifically to seizures. However, these traits can, in themselves, be an added complication to someone who already, through brain trauma, has a predisposition to such symptoms.

Perhaps most problematic to all involved in the care of these patients are the episodic affective disturbances, primarily depression, which can occur with suicidal thoughts and even suicidal attempts (Fedoroff et al. 1992). These usually occur in isolated instances, but if they increase in frequency, they can result in significant impairment. Shukla et al. (1987) analyzed 20 patients

Table 16–3. Psychopathological disorders that have been reported in seizure disorders

Mood disorders (dysphoric, euphoric, rapid cycling, and mixed)
Irritable-impulsive disorders
Schizophreniform disorders (paranoid, delusional, and hallucinatory)
Anxiety disorders (panic, phobic, and generalized)
Amnestic-confusional disorders
Somatoform disorders (pseudoseizures and pain)
Personality disorders (viscous, hyperemotional, and hypersexual)

who developed mania after brain injury and found an association with posttraumatic seizures. They emphasized that this type of mania involved irritable mood and assaultiveness, rather than euphoria. The predisposition to mania may result from posttraumatic seizures, particularly because this group had no family history of affective disorder, only 30% had any prior depressive episodes, and only 15% had prior mania.

In a similar way, the hallucinatory and psychotic experiences can occur either episodically or, in more refractory cases, be consistently and unremittingly present, forming a chronic psychotic condition. They can also occur up to 14 years after the onset of seizure. All of these conditions have been well described (McKenna et al. 1985; Neppe and Tucker, 1988a, 1988b, 1992; Trimble 1991).

There are two major groups of patients with seizure disorders. First are those who have seizures without any greater incidence of psychopathology than is found in the general population. We have called these patients the "standard" epilepsy patients and this is probably the majority of patients (McKenna et al. 1985). This contrasts with the "epilepsy plus" patients who have psychopathology. University and specialized epilepsy center populations may include a higher proportion of "epilepsy plus" patients, whereas the overwhelming majority of patients with seizures have no additional psychopathology. As a consequence of such findings, we have suggested the tiered axes for psychopathology and epilepsy to analyze all cases of psychopathology linked with seizure disturbance, including patients with brain injury. Only through such detailed analyses will we ultimately be able to tease out the exact links between psychopathology and posttraumatic epilepsy (Neppe and Tucker 1992) (Table 16–4).

Treatment of Behavioral Conditions

The basic initial treatment of the behavioral complications of seizure disorders in patients with brain trauma is the treatment of the seizures themselves. The seizures and often the psychopathology respond to traditional anticonvulsant medications (phenytoin, carbamazepine, sodium valproate, ethosuximide, primidone,

Table 16–4. Tiered axes for psychopathology and epilepsy: a two-tiered, seven-axis schema for classifying psychopathology in patients with epilepsy

Axis	Psychiatric tier
I	Psychiatric diagnosis (DSM-IV[a])
	Descriptive psychopathology diagnosis
	Severity of episode (mild, moderate, severe)
II	Personality or developmental disorder (DSM-IV)
	Personality description
III	Physical disorders (DSM-IV) (related/unrelated)
	Symptomatic etiology of psychopathology
IV	Psychosocial and environmental factors (Axis IV; DSM-IV)
V	Global assessment of functioning (current, past year, during illness, expected on recovery)
VI	Pharmacological (responsiveness, compliance, dose, levels and response, duration, dosing)
VII	Age at onset of current psychopathology (e.g., psychosis)

Axis	Epilepsy tier
I	Seizure classification
	Epilepsy syndrome
	Extent of seizure control (complete, occasional, moderate, or poor)
II	Intelligence (normal or borderline/mildly/moderately mentally retarded)
III	Time link of psychopathology and seizures (periictal, interictal, nonictal, or unclear)
IV	Electroencephalogram (localization and seizure features) and other brain tests
V	Course (deteriorating or nondeteriorating)
	Chronicity (single episode, episodic, or chronic)
VI	Pharmacological response of seizures (compliance, doses, frequency, levels, and duration)
VII	Age at onset of seizures

[a]See American Psychiatric Association 1994.

clonazepam, and phenobarbital); however, the barbiturate derivatives seem to have more cognitive and depressive effects than the
others (Brent et al. 1990; Farwell et al. 1990) (Table 16–5). Because
physicians often use anticonvulsants in a prophylactic manner in
head injury patients, one must first assure that behavioral and
cognitive problems are not due to the anticonvulsant. Consequently, in the patient without seizures, one might consider stopping the anticonvulsants if no seizures are present. This is
particularly important because studies have repeatedly shown little
benefit of prophylactic anticonvulsant treatment in preventing the
occurrence of seizures (McQueen et al. 1983; Perry et al. 1979;
Temkin et al. 1990; Young et al. 1983) in patients with brain injury.
Consequently, one should not use anticonvulsants to treat behavioral symptoms if seizures are not present. In these instances, one
should first use other psychopharmacological interventions, particularly in light of the cognitive impairments associated with anticonvulsant use (Trimble 1987).

When seizures are present with behavioral symptoms, particularly episodic symptoms of psychosis, depressive feelings, or
impulsive behavior, the first approach is to evaluate the anticonvulsants or begin anticonvulsant treatment. The behavioral symptoms seem to respond best to anticonvulsant blood levels in the
mid to upper therapeutic ranges. In our clinical experience, we
find that it is important to keep the blood levels of anticonvulsants

Table 16–5. Daily doses, effective blood levels, and serum half-lives of anticonvulsants

Anticonvulsant	Usual daily dose (mg)	Effective blood level (mg/md)	Serum half-life (hours)
Carbamazepine	200–2000	6–12	12
Clonazepam	1–10	.01–.07	18–50
Ethosuximide	1500–2000	40–100	40
Phenobarbital	60–200	10–40	96
Phenytoin	100–600	10–20	24
Primidone	250–1500	5–15	12
Valproic acid	500–3000	50–100	8

within the therapeutic window, because there can be an increased occurrence of behavioral and cognitive impairments with levels beyond the therapeutic window and even an increased risk of seizures with phenytoin at toxic levels. However, if there is no symptomatic response to anticonvulsants in the therapeutic blood level range, then medicating beyond the usual therapeutic range may be attempted to see whether the targeted behavioral symptoms decrease in frequency or occurrence. Although earlier studies have noted that carbamazepine is associated with less cognitive impairment (Dodrill and Troupin 1977; Trimble 1987), recent studies have shown that there is cognitive impairment with all anticonvulsants when used in therapeutic ranges (Dodrill and Troupin 1991; Gillham et al. 1988; Massagli 1991; Meador et al. 1990). Interestingly, the cognitive impairments noted with these anticonvulsants are in the area of attention and concentration, memory deficits, information processing, and motor speed, all of which are highly associated with brain trauma. Consequently, we can see how these medications in themselves may exacerbate certain symptoms. Therefore, if the patient worsens, one should consider a decrease in these medications, which may also improve some of the behavioral symptoms. Although most of the cognitive effects are dose dependent, they may occur in therapeutic blood level ranges. Some patients' seizures respond better to one anticonvulsant than another and if there is no response, it is useful to try changing anticonvulsants. In a similar manner, the cognitive effects may also be worse with one anticonvulsant; therefore, if the side effects are considerable, it is worth attempting a change. The drug interactions of these medications, not only with each other, but with psychotropic medications, are complex and varied (Duncan et al. 1991). As a result, frequent blood level checks are useful when anticonvulsants are combined either with each other or with other medications.

If the behavioral symptoms, particularly those of an affective or psychotic nature, do not respond to manipulation of the anticonvulsants, it is appropriate to use low doses of either neuroleptics or antidepressant medication. In our experience, these patients are extremely sensitive to medication changes, so any medication changes should be done slowly and gradually over time. Although neuroleptics and many of the antidepressant medications lower seizure thresholds, in small doses they can be extremely helpful to the behavioral symptoms of these patients.

A number of patients will respond to surgical intervention, such as scar excision or lobectomy. With surgical treatment, it has been noted that 51% of patients after 40 years had no significant seizures and 11% had focal seizures. Of those medically treated, 63% had no seizures after 40 years and only 8% had minor seizures (Walker and Blumer 1989).

As noted earlier, complicating all of this is the added emotional burden of having seizures for someone who already has a serious brain injury. The emotional impact on the patient and the family is considerable and adds significantly to the rehabilitation task. Certainly, patients with TBI and seizures can have the same emotional problems that any person with a seizure disorder has. However, the brain injury patient has specific problems that Lezak (1978) clearly defined in what has now become a classic article. She noted five broad areas where behavior may become impaired:

1. Social and interpersonal perceptiveness
2. Capacity for self-regulation and control
3. Stimulus bound behavior
4. Emotional control (e.g., apathy, irritability, and lability)
5. Inability to profit from experience

These problems are compounded by the seizure disorder because seizures have a tremendous stigma associated with them, as well as the potential to cause actual lapses in behavior and attention. These two factors combine to mandate a psychotherapeutic approach that is first psychoeducational (Helgeson et al. 1990; Whitman and Hermann 1986). The patient, and particularly the family or the caregivers, must be educated about the behavioral and cognitive effects of both TBI and seizures. The family must learn what behaviors are associated with these conditions and that the anger or apathy is not related to the patient's feelings about them but to his or her illness. They must also learn behavioral strategies to deal with these behaviors, and be counseled about how to take care of themselves and how to take time off from their caretaking responsibilities.

Conclusions

TBI is an etiologic cause of convulsive seizures. With these seizures comes the possibility of behavioral disturbances additional to the already complicated picture of the recovery from TBI. The primary treatment of these seizures is the use of anticonvulsants. Because there are many different anticonvulsants, the clinician may try many in a sequential fashion until seizure control is achieved. All of the anticonvulsants have blood levels for which therapeutic ranges have been established, so the clinician can titrate the clinical response to the dose by following the anticonvulsant blood levels. At times, if there is no response from monotherapy, two of several anticonvulsants can be tried in combined treatment, again maintaining the appropriate blood levels of both drugs. In the patient with seizures, behavioral symptoms should be treated initially with anticonvulsants, again trying to keep the blood levels in the higher therapeutic range. Of course, even without overt seizures, if the patient has the onset of clear episodic behavioral symptoms such as hallucinations, affective symptoms, and panic attacks, it may be appropriate to try anticonvulsants. If behavioral symptoms, particularly affective ones, persist, small doses of antidepressants may be tried, or if the symptoms are of a psychotic nature, neuroleptics. However, each of these patients presents a unique therapeutic problem. Because there are so few of these patients, there are almost no large scale studies of the systematic use of psychopharmacological agents in their treatment. As a result, each patient becomes a unique therapeutic challenge or experiment and one must often try many different agents or combinations of agents to achieve behavioral improvement (Neppe and Tucker 1988a, 1988b).

References

American Psychiatric Association: Diagnostic and Statistical Manual of Mental Disorders, 4th Edition. Washington, DC, American Psychiatric Association, 1994

Annegers JF, Grabow J, Groover RV, et al: Seizures after head trauma: a population study. Neurology 30:683–689, 1980

Armstrong KK, Sahgal V, Block R, et al: Rehabilitation outcomes in patients with post-traumatic epilepsy. Arch Phys Med Rehabil 71:156–160, 1990

Bickford RG: Activation Procedures and Special Electrodes in Current Practice of Clinical Electroencephalography. Edited by Kass D, Daly DD. New York, Raven, 1979

Blumer D, Neppe V, Benson DF: Diagnostic criteria for epilepsy-related mental changes. Am J Psychiatry 147:676–677, 1990

Brent DA, Crumrine PK, Varma R, et al: Phenobarbital treatment and major depressive disorder in children with epilepsy. Pediatrics 85:1086–1091, 1990

Corkin S, Sullivan EV, Carr A: Prognostic factors for life expectancy after penetrating head injury. Arch Neurol 41:975–977, 1984

Dana-Haer J, Trimble MR: Prolactin and gonadotropin changes following partial seizures in epileptic patients with and without psychopathology. Biol Psychiatry 19:329–336, 1984

Desai B, Whitman S, Bouffard DA: The role of the EEG in epilepsy of long duration. Epilepsia 29:601–606, 1988

Dikmen S, Reitan R: Neuropsychological performance in post-traumatic epilepsy. Epilepsia 19:177–183, 1978

Dodrill CB, Troupin AS: Psychometric effects of carbamazepine in epilepsy. Neurology 27:1023–1028, 1977

Dodrill CB, Troupin AS: Neuropsychological effects of carbamazepine and phenytoin: a reanalysis. Neurology 41:141–143, 1991

Duncan J, Potsalas P, Ghorvan S: Effects of discontinuation of phenytoin, carbamazepine, and valproate on concomitant antiepileptic medication. Epilepsia 32:101–115, 1991

Farwell J, Lee YJ, Hirtz DG, et al: Phenobarbital for febrile seizures: effects on intelligence and seizure recurrence. N Engl J Med 332:364–370, 1990

Fedoroff JP, Storkstein S, Forrester A, et al: Depression in patients with acute traumatic brain injury. Am J Psychiatry 149:918–923, 1992

Gibbs FA, Gibbs EL: Atlas of Electroencephalography. Cambridge, MA, Addison-Wesley, 1952

Gillham RA, Williams N, Wiedmann, et al: Concentration-effect relationships with carbamazepine and its epoxide on psychomotor and cognitive function in epileptic patients. J Neurol Neurosurg Psychiatry 51:929–933, 1988

Heikkmen ER, Routy HS, Tolonen U, et al: Development of postraumatic epilepsy. Stereotact Funct Neurosurg 54/55:25–33, 1990

Helgeson DC, Mittan R, Tan SY, et al: Sepulveda epilepsy education: the efficacy of a psychoeducational treatment program in treating medical and psychosocial aspects of epilepsy. Epilepsia 31:75–82, 1990

Jabbari B, Vengrow MI, Salazar AM, et al: Clinical and radiological correlates of EEG in the late phase of head injury: a study of 515 Vietnam veterans. Electroencephalogr Clin Neurophysiol 64:285–293, 1986

Jennett WB: Epilepsy after Non-Missile Injuries, 2nd Edition. Chicago, IL, Year Book Medical, 1975

Koufen H, Hagel KH: Systematic EEG follow-up study of traumatic psychosis. Eur Arch Psychiatry Neurol Sci 237:2–7, 1987

Kuhl DA, Boucher BA, Buhlbauer MS: Prophylaxis of post-traumatic seizures. DICP 24:277–285, 1990

Lassen NA, Holm S: Single photon emission computerized tomography (SPECT), in Clinical Brain Imaging. Edited by Mazziotta JC, Gilman S. Philadelphia, PA, FA Davis, 108–134, 1992

Lee BI, Markland ON, Wellman HN, et al: HIDPM-SPECT in patients with medically intractable complex partial seizures. Arch Neurol 45:397–402, 1988

Lezak M: Living with the characterologically altered brain injured patient. J Clin Psychiatry 39:592–598, 1978

Lishman WA: Organic Psychiatry, 2nd Edition. Oxford, Blackwell, 1987

Marsh NV, Knight R: Behavioral assessment of social competence following severe head injury. J Clin Exp Neuropsychol 13:729–740, 1991

Massagli T: Neurobehavioral effects of phenytoin, carbamazepine, and valproic acid: implications for use in traumatic brain injury. Arch Phys Med Rehabil 72:219–226, 1991

Matthews CG: The neuropsychology of epilepsy. J Clin Exp Neuropsychol 14:133–143, 1992

McKenna PJ, Kane JM, Parrish K: Psychotic syndromes in epilepsy. Am J Psychiatry 142:895–904, 1985

McQueen JK, Blackwood DNR, Harris P, et al: Low risk of late post-traumatic seizures following severe head injury. J Neurol Neurosurg Psychiatry 46:899–904, 1983

Meador KJ, Loring K, Huh BB, et al: Comparative cognitive effects of anticonvulsants. Neurology 40:391–394, 1990

Mori A, Hiromatsu M, Yoko I, et al: Biochemical pathogenesis of post-traumatic epilepsy. Pavlov J Biol Sci 25:54–62, 1990

Neppe VM, Tucker GJ: Modern perspectives on epilepsy in relation to psychiatry: classification and evaluation. Hosp Community Psychiatry 39:263–271, 1988a

Neppe VM, Tucker GJ: Modern perspectives on epilepsy in relation to psychiatry: behavioral disturbances of epilepsy. Hosp Community Psychiatry 39:389–396, 1988b

Neppe VM, Tucker GJ: Neuropsychiatric aspects of seizure disorders, in American Psychiatric Press Textbook of Neuropsychiatry. Edited by Hales R, Yudofsky S. Washington, DC, American Psychiatric Press, 1992, pp 397–425

Parasuraman R, Mutter S, Malloy R: Sustained attention following mild closed-head injury. J Clin Exp Neuropsychol 13:789–811, 1991

Perry JK, While BG, Brackett CE: A controlled prospective study of the pharmacologic prophylaxis of post-traumatic epilepsy. Neurology 29:600–601, 1979

Proctor HJ, Palladino GW, Fillipo D: Failure of autoregulation after closed head injury: an experimental model. J Trauma 28:347–352, 1988

Sadler M, Goodwin J: Multiple electrodes for detecting spikes in partial complex seizures. Can J Neurol Sci 16:326–329, 1989

Salazar AM, Jabbari B, Vance SC, et al: Epilepsy after penetrating head injury. Neurology 35:1406–1414, 1985

Sarna MT: The nature of verbal impairment after closed head injury. J Nerv Ment Dis 168:685–692, 1980

Shukla S, Cook BL, Mukherjee S, et al: Mania following head trauma. Am J Psychiatry 144:93–96, 1987

Spencer S, Katz A: Arriving at the surgical options for intractable seizures. Senior Neurology 4:422–430, 1990

Temkin O: The Falling Sickness, 2nd Edition. Baltimore, MD, Johns Hopkins University Press, 1971

Temkin N, Dikmen S, Wilensky S, et al: A randomized double-blind study of phenytoin for the prevention of post-traumatic seizures. N Engl J Med 323:497–502, 1990

Trimble MR: Anticonvulsant drugs and cognitive function: a review of the literature. Epilepsia 28 (suppl):S37–S45, 1987

Trimble MR: The psychosis of epilepsy. New York, Rover, 1991

Walker AE, Blumer D: The fate of World War II veterans with post-traumatic seizures. Arch Neurol 46:23–26, 1989

Weiss GH, Caveness WF, Eisiedei-Lechtape H, et al: Life expectancy and courses of deaths in a group of head injured veterans of World War I. Arch Neurol 39:741–743, 1982

Weiss GH, Salazar AM, Vance SC, et al: Predicting post-traumatic epilepsy in penetrating brain injury. Arch Neurol 43:771–773, 1986

Whitman S, Hermann BP: Psychopathology in epilepsy. New York, Oxford University Press, 1986

Young B, Rapp RP, Norton J, et al: Failure of prophylactically administered phenytoin to prevent late post-traumatic seizures. Neurosurgery 58:236–241, 1983

Chapter 17

The Family System: Impact, Assessment, and Intervention

Thomas Kay, Ph.D.
Marie M. Cavallo, M.A.

The Family System: Homeostasis and Involvement

The impact of traumatic brain injury (TBI) on the family system merits study for five very important reasons. First, TBI inevitably causes profound changes in every family system. Second, these changes dramatically influence the functional recovery of the person with brain injury. Third, the impact of TBI continues over the life-cycle of the family, long after the initial adjustment to disability is made. Fourth, the lives of individual family members may be profoundly affected by a brain injury in another family member. Fifth, family assessment and intervention are crucial at all stages of rehabilitation and adjustment after TBI, even when a pathological response is not present.

TBI is an event that impacts on and alters an entire family, not only the person with the injury. Families are systems with sets of relationships and roles that develop to maintain an effective balance in the day-to-day world. This homeostasis is broken at the moment one person in the family sustains a brain injury. The struggle of the family to "right itself" and reestablish a new homeostasis after TBI in one member is parallel to the process of rehabilitation and adjustment in the injured person. In the way that recovery is never complete for the individual after brain injury, the family as a unit can never return to its former "self." Assisting families in the process of reestablishing equilibrium, with new sets of roles, relationships, and goals, is the purpose of family assessment and intervention. Because of the range of physical, cognitive, and behavioral-affective changes that can result from TBI, the injured person is often more dependent on family members, and therefore more intertwined in and affected by family dynamics. Consequently, the family's relative success or failure in establishing a functional equilibrium will play a significant role in determining the relative independence of the person with brain injury, making family interventions critical to the rehabilitation process.

Although it is generally agreed among professionals that families should be involved in the rehabilitation process, family involvement is often limited to keeping families informed of treatment plans, and periodic appearances at team conferences, where families may be updated on progress and encouraged to participate in carrying out the team's care plan. This approach both lacks the active input of the family in defining the rehabilitation goals and process, and fails to appreciate the needs of the recovering family system.

Equally unfortunate is the fact that psychiatric intervention is usually the consultation of last resort: when there is a crisis that no one else can manage, when medication is required, or (especially) when someone becomes suicidal. In our opinion, this is a serious underutilization of potential psychiatric knowledge and skill in the area of family systems. The model we develop in this chapter involves not primarily tertiary psychiatric intervention in the event of crisis, but a prospective, preventive, primary intervention model, which calls for the psychodynamic and interpersonal expertise of the psychiatrist to be brought to bear in helping families cope from the moment of injury through long-term adjustment. In fact, we will be less concerned with delineating traditional psychiatric manifestations in the family, and more concerned with articulating the impact of TBI on families, how they respond, what they need, and what psychiatric interventions are appropriate along the continuum of care.

The Impact of TBI on the Family

The impact of TBI on the family can be conceptualized in three broad phases. In the acute phase, in which the primary issues are survival, medical stabilization, and minimization of permanent damage, the family coalesces and orients all of its energy toward the care of the injured person. In the rehabilitation phase, family roles are reorganized and the goal is the restoration of as much physical and cognitive functioning as possible following brain injury. In the reintegration phase, the individual recovering from the injury attempts to return as much as possible to a level of maximum engagement and productivity in the community, while the family settles into longer-term patterns and equilibrium that will allow them to resume their family life-cycle with an altered identity. The primary issues the family faces during each of these phases will be considered below in the section on Assessment and Intervention.

In the long run, however, TBI is distinguished from other catastrophic injuries in terms of impact on the family by the following facts: 1) cognitive, emotional, and behavioral sequelae, which alter the personality and capacities of the injured person, remain (Kay and Lezak 1990); 2) these deficits are permanent and the family must establish new patterns and goals to incorporate a member with brain damage; and 3) the demographics of TBI (primarily affecting young, adult males) dictate that, unlike strokes or dementing diseases affecting primarily the elderly, TBI affects families who are generally young and in the early stages of their development (Kalsbeek et al. 1980).

Research Literature on Families

The physical, emotional, psychosocial, and financial costs of TBI on the family have been documented in a number of reviews (Bond 1983; Brooks 1991; Florian et al. 1989; Livingston 1990; Romano 1989). An overview of trends since the early 1970s distinguishes an evolution of TBI family research that includes four main phases (Kay and Cavallo 1991). In *Phase I* family members were studied as "windows" on the person with the brain injury (e.g., Bond 1976; Hpay 1970; Oddy et al. 1985). These studies were useful in documenting the cognitive, affective, and personality changes after brain injury, and the persistence of symptoms over time.

In *Phase II,* studies that primarily documented the effects of brain injury on the patient also incidentally noted the impact of the injury on significant others. For example, Panting and Merry (1972) documented that 61% of wives and mothers required medication to help them cope with relatives with TBI, wives had more difficulty coping than mothers, and more than half of all relatives felt support services were inadequate. A series of studies by Oddy et al. (1978a) in London noted that increased dependence on families was associated with greater severity of injury, poorer family relationships at 1 year were associated with personality changes in the person with the brain injury (Oddy and Humphrey 1980), and personality changes were associated with greater family dependence (Weddell et al. 1980). These studies, however, did not have the family as their primary focus.

In *Phase III,* beginning in the late 1970s but peaking in the mid to late 1980s, families—or at least individual family members—became a primary focus of research. By documenting the severity of injury, presence of a range of neurobehavioral symptoms, and the reactions of family members, these studies began to identify the factors that led to distress and burden on primary caregivers. For example, Oddy et al. (1978b) found that depression in family members correlated not primarily with severity of injury (as measured by coma or posttraumatic amnesia), but with the number and extent of cognitive symptoms, as well as with the failure to return to work and social isolation of the person with the injury. This theme—that the behavioral manifestations of the injury (both neuropsychological and functional), not the neurological severity of the TBI per se, impact on family members—is a consistent one in this phase of family research.

In the 1980s Brooks and colleagues in Glasgow published a series of papers articulating the nature and causes of subjective burden of family members after TBI (see Brooks 1991 and Livingston and Brooks 1988 for reviews). A number of themes can now be considered established (summarized in Table 17–1). First, in the long run, behavioral, affective, and personality changes are most burdensome to families; physical deficits cause least burden; and cognitive deficits cause intermediate burden (Brooks and McKinlay 1983; Brooks et al. 1987; McKinlay et al. 1981).

Second, in a parallel finding, persons with brain injury and family members agree most when rating the nature and extent of physical problems, least about emotional-behavioral problems, and moderately on cognitive problems. Family members are most distressed by the changes persons with brain injury are least aware of the impulsivity, disinhibition, irritability, anger outbursts, insensitivity, and changes in personality.

Third, over the course of time, subjective family burden actually increases (Brooks et al. 1987). Subjective family burden becomes more strongly linked to personality changes (Brooks and

---

Table 17–1. Glasgow Research on Subjective Burden

1. Behavioral, affective, and personality changes cause most burden; cognitive changes intermediate; physical changes least.

2. Patients and family member agree most rating physical problems; intermediate about cognitive problems; least about emotional-behavioral problems.

3. Over time, family burden increases, becoming more linked to personality changes, and less to neurological severity.

4. No one-to-one correspondence between degree of deficits and degree of burden.

Note. For more information on subjective burden, see Brooks and McKinlay 1983; Brooks et al. 1987; Livingston 1987; McKinlay et al. 1981.

McKinlay 1983), and less strongly linked to neurological severity (McKinlay et al. 1981).

Fourth, there is no one-to-one correspondence between the degree of deficit and the degree of burden; personality characteristics of the family member appear to be a factor in how much burden that family member experiences. Although all family members experiencing high levels of burden report personality changes in the person with brain injury, it is not conversely true that whenever personality changes occur, the result is high burden on the family (Brooks and McKinlay 1983). Similarly, although low levels of burden are associated with low levels of deficit, high levels of burden may be associated with either low or high levels of deficit (Brooks et al. 1987). However, relatives who rated the patient's emotional-behavioral problems as high, also tended to have high neuroticism scores on the Eysenck Personality Scale (Eysenck and Eysenck 1975). Because this score represents a presumably durable personality trait involving maladaptive and anxiety-laden responses in stressful situations, it may be that family members with poorer ego integration experience more affective and behavioral distress from the person with the injury, and therefore feel more burden. This suggestion was reinforced by Livingston (1987), who found that the preinjury psychiatric and health history of the relative accounted for 30% of the variance in the relative's rating of subjective burden.

In summary, subjective burden of family members tends to increase, not decrease, over time; it is most related to changes in personality, emotions, and behavior, of which the person with brain injury is least aware; it is the neurobehavioral manifestations of TBI, and not the neurological severity per se, that affect family members, and the adjustment of family members plays a large role in determining the subjective burden they experience.

In *Phase IV* of the research literature, predominantly in the late 1980s, the focus shifted from individual family members to families as systems, and the impact of TBI on roles, relationships, and the family's status in society. For example, Kozloff (1987) used network analysis to document that the size of the social network of the person with the brain injury decreases, multiplex relationships increase (i.e., family members serve more and more functions, as nonrelatives drop out), and families with higher socioeconomic status are more able to maintain existing relationships. Maitz (1989) compared families with a member with TBI to a group of families who did not have a person with TBI living with them, but in which one of the members either had a sibling with TBI, or a sibling married to a person with TBI. He found, using formal measures of family functioning, that families with a member with TBI had less (and more variable) cohesiveness and more variability in conflict resolution, and showed a correlation between marital conflict and decreased cohesiveness, than those families who did not have a person with TBI living with them. Peters et al. (1990) found that good dyadic adjustment (between person with TBI and spouse) was associated with less financial strain, low spousal ratings of patient psychopathology, and less severe injuries. Life-style changes in families with TBI were documented by Jacobs (1988), who found that families tend to be primarily responsible for providing support, socialization, and assistance to persons with brain injury, with two-thirds experiencing financial adversity. Finally, the diversity of styles of family adaptation has begun to be acknowledged in recent research. Our own work at N.Y.U. Medical Center emphasizes the individuality of families, and attempts to identify subgroups of family responses to TBI (Cavallo et al. 1992).

This final phase of the research literature, the study of the family unit, depends on increasingly sophisticated and valid instruments and techniques for assessing family system functioning (see Bishop and Miller 1988, for a review of existing approaches). Most family assessment instruments are inadequately sensitive to particular issues specific to TBI. The N.Y.U. Head Injury Family Interview (HI-FI) is one attempt to systematically survey family members about the impact of TBI on the person with the injury and on the family system (Kay et al. 1988).

The HI-FI is a five-part structured interview designed for both research and clinical uses. It includes five sections (see Table 17–2) covering premorbid, accident, rehabilitation, and community resource utilization. It gathers information from both the person with the head injury and significant others, and provides a method for documenting the impact of the head injury not only on the injured person, but on other family members as well. Most questions are hierarchically organized, beginning with open-ended questions (e.g., "What changes have you noticed since the injury?"), proceeding through structured areas (e.g., "Have you no-

Table 17–2.   The New York University Head Injury Family Interview

  I. Demographic and preinjury form
     A. Demographic information
     B. Accident/medical information
     C. Preaccident history
     D. Psychiatric history
     E. Neurological history
 II. Follow-up interview
     A. Routine medical care
     B. Rehabilitation services
     C. Psychotherapy
     D. Living arrangements
     E. Legal/insurance
     F. Community service utilization
III. Significant other interview
     A. Problems and changes
     B. Problem checklist
     C. Activities of daily living
     D. Socialization and home activities
     E. Patient competency rating
 IV. Interview for person with the head injury
     A. Problems and changes
     B. Friendship and intimacy
     C. Employment status
     D. Homemaker status
     E. Educational status
     F. Problem checklist
     G. Patient competency rating
  V. Impact on the family
     A. General
     B. Questions for spouse
     C. Questions for parents
     D. Questions for adult siblings
     E. Questions for younger siblings
     F. Questions for adult children
     G. Questions for younger children

ticed any physical changes?"), and ending with focused questi
(e.g., "Do you have problems with balance?"). Many of the ma
areas of inquiry are asked both of the person with the head injury,
and a significant other. Specific sections are provided for impact
on parents, spouses, siblings, and children. The interview was
developed over nine years at the N.Y.U. Research and Training
Center on Head Trauma and Stroke, out of a need for an instrument to gather detailed clinical and codable information specific to
issues in TBI. The interview can be obtained from the authors
(Rusk Institute of Rehabilitation Medicine, 400 East 34th Street,
New York, New York 10016).

Clinical Observations

In her classic article, Lezak (1978) provided observations on what
it is like for family members living with the "characterologically
altered" person with brain injury. She described the personality
changes that have primary impact on the family: 1) an impaired
capacity for social perceptiveness, 2) stimulus-bound behavior
(i.e., a concreteness, a failure to generalize), 3) impaired capacity
for control and self-regulation, 4) emotional alterations (including
apathy, irritability, and sexual changes), and 5) an inability to profit
from experience (i.e., a tendency to repeat maladaptive patterns
and not benefit from corrective strategies). As a result, family
members may feel trapped, isolated, abandoned by outside relatives, and even abused, which often results in chronic or periodic
depression among primary caregivers. Lezak's emphasis on the
impact of *characterological* changes after brain injury (especially
involving frontal systems) anticipated the later research documenting that personality, affective, and behavioral changes in the
person with the brain injury result in the greatest family burden.

Clinical experience bears out the research and descriptive
literature cited above. Physical problems, although at times quite
severe and necessitating specific family routines or limitations, are
usually dealt with most successfully by the family in the long run,
in large part because these problems are predictable, can be
planned for, are within the awareness of the person with the brain

injury, and are visible to and acknowledged by others. Cognitive problems, such as impaired attention, concentration, and memory, are more troublesome because they are less predictable and can invade all spheres of interaction, and because their functional implications often are beyond the anticipation of the person with the brain injury. On the other hand, families often can be extremely creative in providing the external structures to minimize the impact of such deficits on everyday life. Emotional, behavioral, and personality changes, however, such as anger outbursts, self-centeredness, impulsivity, disinhibition, and social insensitivity, are extremely difficult to cope with because they can appear suddenly and unpredictably, have (even if not intended) a direct emotional impact on the recipient, are often embarrassing to others, and are extremely difficult to control. Not only do these characterological problems increase stress in internal family life, they also lead to family isolation as fewer friends visit, social outings decrease, and the immediate family bears increasing responsibility for the social network of the person with brain injury.

For example, a young father with brain stem and frontal lobe injuries after a high speed motor vehicle accident and extended coma will typically have physical, cognitive, and behavioral changes. He may learn to compensate for an ataxic gait by walking slower, using a cane on uneven surfaces, and avoiding activities requiring speed and agility. He may learn to compensate in part for severe memory deficits by keeping a detailed memory book, writing down all phone messages, keeping lists and checking things off as he does them, and posting visual cues around the house for things he needs to do. Adaptations to these physical and cognitive deficits may enable him to be a semi-productive and reliable helper at home. However, if he is behaviorally disinhibited, his outbursts of rage at his wife and children may make him difficult to be around, and unpredictable and embarrassing disparagement of guests may make it impossible to have friends over, essentially isolating the family and leading to severe emotional and interpersonal problems within it.

These generalizations tend to apply to all "families" in which two or more persons are living together. Specific variations occur, however, depending on whether the person with TBI is a parent or a child, and brain injury in the family affects spouses, parents, siblings, and children in different ways. These variable effects on family roles are considered in the following section.

Family Structure and Role Changes

The impact of TBI on various members of the family system has been documented in the literature; for example, Williams and Kay (1991) included a number of first person accounts from family members, and Lezak (1978, 1988) provided clinical commentary on various family roles.

Impact on Spouses

In many ways, the spouse, usually the wife, bears the greatest burden when the partner sustains a brain injury. An equal adult partnership has been broken, and the uninjured spouse is often thrust into the role of caregiver—both for the injured partner and for the family when there are children. The result is often financial burden, loss of support, and isolation. Younger spouses may become more dependent on their families of origin, especially if the injured partner is unable to independently carry out household responsibilities. In-law conflicts may erupt between the parents of the injured person and his or her spouse over care issues. In traditional families where the husband was the "family executive," the wife may be thrust into managing and decision-making roles for which she is not prepared. (Increasingly it is common for the wife to play this executive role.) Spouses often express the feeling of being "single parents": "My husband and I used to have two children; now I feel like I have three." Even in situations where the injury is less severe and the injured partner is able to return to some type of work, it often is far below preaccident levels, and major life-style changes are required of the family. When there are children, the spouse may be without an equal parenting partner, and in fact competition may develop between the children and the injured partner for the spouse's attention.

Especially in more severe injuries, spouses may feel married to a different person—one they no longer love or feel attracted to. Spouses face an enormous conflict between commitment and guilt if they consider leaving the relationship. This is particularly the case when the couple is young, and have either no or very young children. The spouse often realistically faces the choice of "sacrificing" his or her life to the injured partner, or leaving the relationship to develop a new family. These are difficult moral and personal choices, and the professional is best advised to help the spouse sort out the options, rather than imposing his or her own value system. In less tragic cases, enough of the personality and competence of the injured person remain on which to build a mutually satisfying commitment.

The situation in which the uninjured partner is considering divorce poses ethical and treatment dilemmas for the clinician. When the identified patient is clearly the person with TBI, it may be appropriate to find another therapist to help the partner, or the couple, deal with the divorce issues. When the identified "patient" is the family, however, it is appropriate for the clinician to work with the whole system—or the parental subsystem—to help them face these issues. Unlike many mutually agreed-upon divorces, however, divorces after TBI are often more unilaterally sought (by the uninjured partner), and the process of negotiating this transition is a combination of supporting the uninjured spouse (who is often ridden with guilt), and negotiating new support systems for the reluctant, angry, and frightened person with TBI—tasks usually more comfortably handled by two persons.

Countertransference issues often arise in working with young families with severe injuries, when the personal value system of the clinician may be at odds with the decisions of the uninjured partner. These feelings can arise in either direction: unconsciously encouraging the partner perceived as "trapped" to find a way out, or unconsciously discouraging a desperate spouse from "abandoning" the injured partner. Awareness of his or her personal feelings is crucial for the therapist, and transfer of the case is appropriate if the decisions of the uninjured partner make it impossible for the clinician to be fully supportive. Sorting out these countertransference issues, from realistically helping the partner to think through the consequences of his or her choices, is a crucial but tricky process, requiring self-searching by the therapist, and often consultation with a colleague.

Even when marriages do survive, sexuality and intimacy are often difficult. Persons with brain injury may have decreased capacity for intimacy, either heightened or lowered sexual drive, and may be impaired in their ability to perform sexually (for physiological or psychological reasons). Wives in particular may be pressed to meet the sexual demands of the injured spouse, with little satisfaction for themselves. It is not uncommon for sexual relationships to stop entirely; when the spouse chooses to stay in the marriage, he or she may seek out (with much guilt and need for support) sexual relationships outside the marriage.

Impact on Parents

When a child is injured, special burdens and pressures exist for the parents. When a young child living at home is injured, the mother usually takes on the role of primary nurturer and caregiver. This may create tension within the marital relationship, and underlying cracks or strains in the relationship may become manifest. Husbands may unconsciously compete with the injured child for the mother's limited resources. When couples are composed of persons with complementary coping styles, the stress of caring for a severely injured child may drive them to opposite extremes of reaction and threaten the relationship; for example, the father may bury himself in his work while the mother drops everything (including any attention to her husband) and devotes all her energy to the injured child. Parents may also find it difficult to apportion their time and energy to other children, or to elderly parents whom they may care for. Even when they work well together around the crisis, parents may find their lives dominated by the needs of the injured child, and may be in jeopardy of neglecting their own marital relationship (e.g., no longer spending time together separate from their children), or being cut off from adult social activities with friends.

When the injured child had been grown and out of the house, parents often are thrown back into an earlier developmental phase of caring for a dependent child, with the complication that the grown child resents and resists the dependency. This is an extremely difficult position for both parents and child, especially when the child is male, recently past adolescence, and striving for autonomy. Driving, independent living, dating, and establishing friends and intimate relationships become volatile family issues. Parents often have great difficulty accepting the permanent changes in their children, and in fact may complicate the rehabilitation process by refusing to give up unrealistic expectations ("My son *will* become a lawyer!"). Conflicts may develop between the parents over what is reasonable to expect of their adult child with brain injury.

Impact on Children

Children of parents with brain injury face special problems over which they have little control. Younger children may suddenly find that they have lost the nurturance and guidance of a formerly loving and competent parent. The injured parent may be unpredictable, irritable, or even in competition with them for the uninjured parent's attention. Older children at home usually have increased responsibilities, less attention from the other parent, and an awkward home situation into which they are uncomfortable bringing their peers. Depending on the preexisting relationship, the child may be drawn emotionally closer to, or driven farther away from and resent the injured parent. Older children may have more capacity to understand what has happened, but also more freedom to create distance. It is not uncommon for school or behavioral problems to surface in children who are depressed, angry, or guilty about their new family situation.

When an older parent incurs a brain injury, adult children who are out of the house are inevitably faced with the issue of taking on increased responsibility. Because of their own adult responsibilities, children are often limited in how much assistance they can actually contribute, with inevitable feelings of guilt. Adult children are often torn between the needs of their partners and children and those of their parents. Conflicts often develop between the caregiving adult child and his or her spouse, with resulting imbalance and conflict within the family. Interventions with spouses of adult children of parents with head injury are often the most effective way to stabilize the support system for the injured parent.

Impact on Siblings

With most attention being paid to the child with the head injury, uninjured siblings often become unrecognized "victims" of shifts in the family system after TBI. When the siblings are young and living at home with the injured child, the parents characteristically reorient all their attention and energy toward the child with the brain injury. Parents need support in finding a balance in allocating limited resources among their children. Older children at home may, like children of injured parents, have more domestic responsibilities, and perhaps also a socially awkward situation into which they are embarrassed to bring friends. Siblings of different personality styles and relationships with the injured child may also respond in very different ways, with one sibling attaching closer to the injured child, while another moves away in anger.

Older siblings who are not living at home experience stresses similar to those of adult children of injured parents. The demands of their own lives, perhaps including a spouse and children, compete against the need and desire to help their sibling. Typically one adult sibling is designated as the primary caregiver, especially if the injured sibling is unmarried and the parents are distant or too old to take on a primary caregiving role. Support from the sibling's family is essential for him or her to play an effective role.

Impact on Extended Family

The impact of TBI on extended family networks is seldom discussed. The reality is that, especially in a mobile, urban society, kinship bonds often are more tenuous than they used to be, and aunts, uncles, and cousins seldom play a significant role in the primary care of any person with brain injury. (This does not hold in cultural groups where a high value is placed on networks of extended families.) From our perspective, it is very helpful for the nuclear family, whenever possible, to involve the extended family as early as possible in learning about the injury, the recovery process, and how to normalize the new person who emerges. Nuclear families who are able to tap into the support systems of extended families, even once or twice a year for respite, have a great advantage. Families often are unable to elicit the active support of relatives, however, because extended family members who do not live with the injured person often do not understand, are less sympathetic toward the family stresses, or are simply more wary of becoming involved. It is extremely useful for professionals working with families to include extended families in family meetings, especially early on, to establish a basis for a wider support network.

Family Responses to TBI:
Stage Theories

The family's process of adjusting to TBI evolves over time; it involves becoming aware of the nature, extent, and permanence of neurobehavioral deficits, and reestablishing a new set of family roles, structure, and routines to accommodate to these changes. Successful clinical intervention with families requires the professional to be aware of where in this process of adjustment the family is; this will determine what the family is able to hear and what kind of support they need.

There are a number of useful ways to conceptualize the continuum of changes that families pass through. These are expressed as various stages, although it is clear that there is no objectively and universally true sequence. In discussing above the impact of TBI on the family, we made reference to three main stages: the acute phase, the rehabilitation phase, and the integration phase. These stages are tied to a medically defined system of rehabilitation. In the acute phase, the family is dealing with issues of survival and minimizing the extent of physical and neurological damage. The family generally is suspending normal routines and orienting all their resources toward the injured person. In the rehabilitation phase, the medically stable person enters a phase of intensive treatment aimed at restoring as high a level of functioning as possible. This is a time when high expectations for recovery predominate, and the family begins the task of receiving the injured person back into the family system, and making the necessary structural adjustments. The rehabilitation may be inpatient or outpatient, but active treatment keeps open the possibility of unlimited improvement. The integration phase is the lengthiest and most difficult, and involves integration in two senses. First, the injured person is completing formal treatment and is, as much as possible, becoming gradually reintegrated into the community—socially, vocationally, etc. Second, this is a time of reintegration for the family system. Expectations for complete recovery begin to recede as the reality of permanent neurobehavioral impairment in the injured person becomes apparent, and the family system attempts to strike a new, more permanent balance to allow its various members to proceed with their own lives. There is enormous variability during this final phase, which itself is composed of a series of stages of internal adjustment.

A number of other authors proposed stage theories of family adjustment after TBI. Rape et al. (1992) described and analyzed a number of these. These authors identified six major stages incorporated in most (but not all) of the stage theories they analyzed. (These stages are listed in Table 17–3.) Rape et al. noted that the hypothesized stages lacked empirical validation, often failed to meet the criteria for defining explanatory epigenetic stages, and contained conceptual problems (e.g., why some families adapt while others become stuck at one of the stages). They proposed integrating a family systems perspective into stage theories to solve some of these problems, and they advocated longitudinal research.

Prominent among the stage theories specific to TBI is Lezak's

(1986) six-stage model of family adjustment after TBI, which amplifies subphases in our integration phase. After the injured person returns home, the family passes through a series of perceptions, expectations, and reactions, beginning with minimizing problems and expecting full recovery, and happiness at survival (I), through bewilderment and anxiety (II), discouragement and guilt (III), depression, despair, and feeling trapped (IV); and families who will ultimately move beyond their sorrow go through two final stages of grieving (V) and reorganization-emotional disengagement (VI). Lezak emphasized that many families are unable to move beyond chronic depression and despair. In our experience, it is often 2 years or more posttrauma before family members begin the true process of mourning that will propel them to resume healthier life-cycles for the rest of the family. Even then, some families seem better adapted than others to accepting the new realities and limits, and are able to let go of old goals and hopes for complete recovery and find dignity in a new family constellation. Other families remain angry, bitter, and unaccepting, often blaming professionals for lack of recovery and constantly seeking the "right" rehabilitation program. Rape et al. (1992) provided some initial integration of systems theory and stage theory to account for these individual differences.

Kubler-Ross (1969) proposed an intrapsychic model of an individual's response to the prospect of death and dying, which is often applied to TBI, and discussed as if the family as a system, or each individual family member, were proceeding through the

---

Table 17–3. Stages of family adjustment

1. Initial shock
2. Emotional relief, denial, and unrealistic expectation
3. Acknowledgment of permanent deficits and emotional turmoil
4. Bargaining
5. Mourning or working through
6. Acceptance and restructuring

Note. Based on Rape et al. 1992.

stages of denial, anger, bargaining, depression, and acceptance. Although it is absolutely true that each family member goes through some or all of these feelings in coping with TBI, we believe that there are some problems, indeed some dangers, in applying this model too simplistically to a family's response to TBI. First, the fact that the mourned person still lives and is present interferes with the normal grieving process in and of itself. Second, the denial so often noted in families of persons with brain injury (Romano 1974) often is treated as something to be dislodged by therapists, if families do not heed therapists' prognostications early in the rehabilitation process about the permanence of deficits. The reality is that early denial—especially continuing to believe in the possibility of significant recovery—is an effective buffer against depression (Ridley 1989), may be necessary for the family to regroup, and should be respected by professionals. Third, the notion of a steady final stage of acceptance—in the sense of an emotionally uncomplicated approval of the way things are—is neither realistic nor perhaps desirable to expect. Transitions in the family's life-cycle bring episodic loss and rekindle the mourning process (see below). Most importantly, harm has been done to families in turmoil years after an injury by professionals who expect that because they are not demonstrating "acceptance" after so much time, a psychopathological process is occurring. The reality is that living with an adult with brain injury brings cycles of adjustment, disequilibrium, and reestablishment of a new balance on a periodic basis, and this recycling never ends. The Kubler-Ross stages are best seen as an individual's internal responses that are likely to be replayed numerous times over the course of the life-cycle. The family system's process of adjustment is too complex to reduce to such a set of stages.

That the grieving process following disability does not simply reach a steady state of acceptance has been recognized by a number of persons working outside the area of TBI. Olshansky (1962), for example, introduced the notion of "chronic sorrow" to describe the continued experience of sadness and ongoing adjustment that parents of mentally retarded children feel. Wikler (1981), working within the same framework, recognized that such chronic sorrow is punctuated by periods of more intense grieving at critical developmental junctures. Other formulations emphasized normal family life-cycles (Carter and McGoldrick 1980) or life "spirals"— recurrent patterns of events that cycle through family systems across generations (Combrinck-Graham 1985). These are periods of normal transition (births, graduations, new jobs, marriages, retirements) separating broader bands of life commitments (child-hood, studenthood, parenthood). Williams (1991a) applied these concepts to TBI and developed the notion of "episodic loss," in which the initial grieving process over the changed person is revisited at critical points in the family life-cycle. The son with brain injury who does not begin to date normally, does not enter college, remains unmarried through his twenties, and does not present grandchildren to his aging parents, represents a situation where the initial family adjustment to permanent disability is emotionally recreated at critical times in the family's life-cycle. Adjustment to loss is reexperienced episodically both by the injured person and by emotionally linked family members. Finally, Rolland (1987a, 1987b, 1990) developed a model that categorizes chronic illness according to its onset, course, outcome, and degree of incapacitation, describes its unfolding over time, and integrates concepts of family individuality and family life-cycles.

A Model of Assessment and Intervention

Families are thrown into crisis at the moment a person is injured. Psychiatric intervention should not be reserved for severe manage-ment problems or dysfunctional families. Family intervention should be proactive, flexible, health and prevention oriented, and responsive to the needs of families within the context of a progres-sive reestablishment of family equilibrium after brain injury.

The quality of family functioning has direct impact on the process of rehabilitation. "Dysfunctional" families may fail to join forces with the rehabilitation team, or deliver conflicting messages, or respond to behaviors in ways that undercut the team's approach, all of which results in the patient being caught between the family and treating professionals in a way that undermines the rehabilitation process. However, much of what professionals perceive as "dysfunctional" in families is the result of families being uninformed, underinvolved, and not having basic needs met, all of which may be preventable with appropriate interventions.

We propose a three-dimensional model of intervention (Table 17–4): *Where* the intervention is aimed (Concentric Circles of Intervention), *What* the intervention is (Levels of Intervention), and *When* it occurs (Stages of Intervention). Each of these dimensions itself contains three progressive levels.

Concentric Circles of Intervention

In evaluating the family of a person with brain injury, our model suggests thinking of that family as composed of three sets or units nested within each other (Figure 17–1): 1) the *individual family members,* 2) the *family as a system,* and 3) the *relationship of the family to the community.* Each of these systems must be assessed independently, and different interventions can be made at each level depending on where in the stage the family is. (The concept

Table 17–4.   A model of family assessment and intervention after traumatic brain injury

A. Concentric circles of intervention
   1. Individual family members
   2. The family as a system
   3. Relationship of family to community
B. Levels of intervention
   1. Information and education
   2. Support, problem solving, and restructuring
   3. Formal therapy
C. Stages of intervention
   1. Acute care
   2. Rehabilitation
   3. Community reintegration

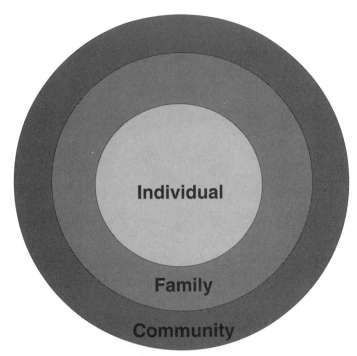

Figure 17–1. Concentric circles of intervention.

of concentric circles, as an alternative to the more traditional "unstable triad" of person, family, and society as bearing responsibility for the long-term care needs of persons with head injury, was first proposed by DeJong et al. in 1990.)

The clinician should evaluate *individual family members* in terms of their personality structure, their expectations for the injured person and the family, the individual strengths and weaknesses they bring to the family, and how they respond both to the person with the injury and to the current family situation. Individual family members may have particular attitudes, limitations, or strengths that become crucial in the rehabilitation process; for example, a mother's need for her son not to hold a menial job, a father's need to not let others make decisions for his family, or a sibling's commitment to support an injured child. Individual family members may be at risk or in crisis, or simply need support because they are shouldering a large share of the family's responsibilities. At times the most effective family intervention is a targeted intervention with an individual family member.

The *family system* must be considered as a unit above and beyond its individual members. What are the structures and roles in this family, and how have they shifted as a result of the injury? What are the patterns of relationship and communication, and how are problems solved? How cohesive is the family unit, and what is their degree of enmeshment or disengagement? How flexible is the family in responding to challenges? What specific cultural norms does the family hold that may be different from the rehabilitation team's and which will color their expectation of what is important in outcome, and how it is achieved? (See Williams and Savage 1991, for examples of cultural values applied to TBI rehabilitation.) What values does the family hold that will influence their goals and expectations? Very often the failure of the rehabilitation team to appreciate strongly held family norms, values, or needs leads to conflict and an impasse in the rehabilitation process. Assessing the family system is crucial, and often strategic interventions within the family structure are critical to enabling a family to move on and cope more effectively.

The *family's relationship to the community* also must be assessed, and often very crucial interventions need to be made not within the family system itself, but at the interface of the family and their community. The community is both the professional community of services that needs to be accessed, and the psychosocial community of friends, recreation, and extended family. The history of a family's relationships to these communities is the best predictor of how they will respond in the crisis situation of TBI. In the early stages, intervention at this level almost always involves negotiating a good working relationship between the family (often as represented by one or two key members) and the rehabilitation team. Forging a strong working alliance is crucial for successful rehabilitation. In later stages, families must learn to deal with the world of multiple, often bureaucratic community services, and if they are to overcome the natural tendency toward isolation, they must reestablish functional social and recreational opportunities.

One often overlooked community relationship in the early stages is the family's need to establish quick communication with the world of insurance and legal matters. For families with injured children, the educational world is the major community relationship. Effective family intervention pays attention not only to the internal matters of the family, but to the family's relationship to various aspects of the community as well.

Levels of Intervention

A second principle of our model is that family intervention need not equal family therapy. Effective family intervention requires that the clinician think in terms of levels of intervention that are appropriate to the situation (Muir et al. 1990; Rosenthal and Muir 1983). Our model defines three levels of intervention: 1) *information and education,* 2) *support, problem solving, and restructuring,* and 3) *formal therapy.* Figure 17–2 illustrates how these three levels of intervention—in ascending order from the most basic to the most complex—cut across the dimensions of individual, family, and community described above.

At the most basic level, families need *information and education* at all stages from coma to community. In the earliest acute phase, this is the most crucial intervention, although long-term prognostication is impossible. Families need to know what has physically happened to the person and his or her brain, what treatments are being given and why, what can be expected over the next few days and weeks, how to understand unusual behavior (e.g., confusion, agitation, and disinhibition) and how to respond to it, how to anticipate and respond to cognitive deficits (e.g., disorientation, severe memory problems, lack of language), what treatment options will need to be considered, and what their insurance and legal options are. Professionals tend to undereducate families, and avoid exposing their own uncertainty.

The timing of providing information also is crucial. In early stages of recovery, families need to sustain hope and cannot be overwhelmed with dire warnings and pessimistic projections. The seeds of long-term limitations are quietly planted early, but the skilled clinician will know when the family is ready to have them nurtured. Likewise it is unethical to steer families toward program decisions without making them aware of the full range of options. In the past 10 years, an enormous amount of informational material (of variable quality) has been developed for families, and the National Brain Injury Foundation is an excellent resource for such materials (see contact information at end of chapter). Most good rehabilitation facilities will develop specific educational programs for families to inform them about TBI in a systematic way (Klonoff and Prigatano 1987; Rosenthal and Hutchins 1991). Educational programs that include open discussions also can be an excellent indirect and nonthreatening way to enable families to face their

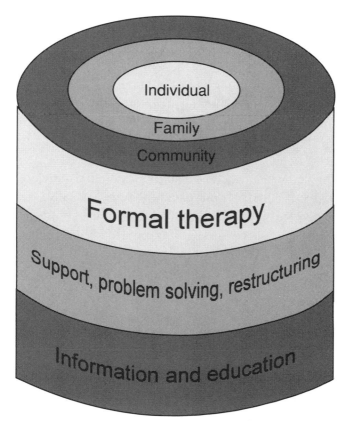

Figure 17–2. Levels of intervention.

own emotional reactions, in a way they would not if offered the more direct opportunity of group sessions run by psychologists or psychiatrists.

Support, problem solving, and restructuring can be an effective family intervention at individual, system, or community-relations levels. For example, the overwhelmed wife of a husband with a brain injury may need structure and guided problem solving in deciding how to manage a family on limited resources. A large family whose mother returns home after a brain injury may need to sit down as a group and negotiate how family responsibilities need to be reapportioned, and deal with the inevitable feelings and conflicts generated by that process. The family who feels "trapped" at home with an impulsive and aggressive teenage son may need help in finding creative ways to maintain social relationships in the community, or even how to take vacations. This level of intervention requires an active therapist who knows the realities of adjusting to brain injury and builds on the strengths and problem-solving capacities of the family and its individual members.

Formal therapy becomes appropriate when severe problems are rendering the family system, or some part of it, dysfunctional. The stress and family changes inherent in TBI may cause family members to need individual therapy (often this is a person previously seen as strong, such as a sibling or child). Individual family members who benefit from psychotherapy usually begin with issues related to brain injury, but almost always end up dealing with longer-standing personal or family of origin issues. This is what distinguishes this level of intervention from the previous two: *all* families benefit from education and problem solving; *some* family members require longer-term formal treatment because of issues outside the event of TBI. The same holds true for the family as a system. Families that were dysfunctional before the injury may require formal family therapy after the injury, with the added complication of learning to adjust their family structure. Decisions about the nature of this family therapy, and the extent to which the person with brain injury will be able to fully participate, should be based on individual circumstances and the injured person's neurobehavioral competence.

Stages of Intervention

We have broadly divided the impact of TBI on the family into three main stages: 1) *acute care,* 2) *rehabilitation,* and 3) *community reintegration,* being fully aware that the third stage is open ended and itself contains numerous subphases. This broad division, however, is useful in conceptualizing the nature of interventions that must be made during each stage. Figure 17–3 illustrates the concept that at each of these temporal stages, interventions can be conceptualized at the three levels (information and education; support, problem solving, and restructuring; formal therapy) and within the three concentric domains (individual, family, community) described above.

In *acute care* families gather their resources and organize around the injured person. This is a period of crisis intervention when education and information are crucial. Emotional support and permission to break standard family routines also are important. Later within this stage, when survival is assured, the family must quickly evaluate treatment options and insurance realities. Family intervention should be aimed at helping the family to cope effectively on numerous fronts while still in shock: practical daily realities, emotional distress, and major decision making.

Rehabilitation is defined as the intermediate stage during which formal restorative treatment, inpatient or outpatient, is the primary family focus. During this stage, there is initially relief at survival and great hope for recovery, which the therapist should support, while gradually tempering hope with cautious reality. Even when therapists realistically assess severe limits of long-term functioning, families may be angered and alienated if this message is presented prematurely or too starkly. It is much better to help families gradually *realize* (rather than be told) emerging limitations through experience. It is during this stage when major family role restructuring often takes place, and individuals may need help in adjusting to their new roles. Toward the end of the rehabilitation stage, it will begin to become apparent that even though formal treatment is ending, complete recovery has not occurred, and the family faces the prospect of living with a permanently disabled person. This is a crucial time for intervention, when the therapist begins to deal with the anxieties and fears of the family.

Community reintegration, as noted above, refers both to the person with brain injury and to the family system, as they struggle to reenter community life under drastically changed circumstances. This is when discouragement, depression, despair, and mourning begin to occur, often over the first few years after the end of rehabilitation. Family interventions usually become more needed, more intense, and longer term. The crucial turning point occurs when, after all formal rehabilitation ends, the family as a system faces the challenge of being able to reconstitute as an effective and functional system with a new balance and identity. Not all families are able to do so. In families who cannot, the life-cycle is seriously

Stages of Intervention

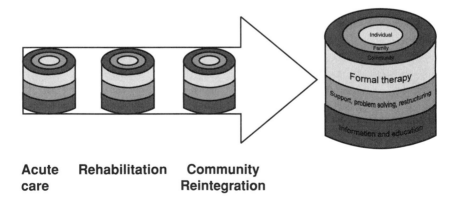

Acute   **Rehabilitation**   **Community**
care   **Reintegration**

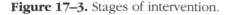

Figure 17–3. Stages of intervention.

disrupted, and individual members may be blocked from making natural life transitions in a healthy way. For example, a busy professional couple may be unable to reorganize their time and finances to care for a severely injured son who lives at home, and that role may fall to a teenage daughter. If she becomes trapped in that role, she may stay home after high school and devote herself to caring for her brother, with the result that her own development (college, career, boyfriends, marriage) may be seriously blocked. Depending on her nature, she may either become seriously depressed, or sacrifice herself for the sake of the family, to her long-term "detriment." In working with such families, clinicians must be careful to sort out what is detrimental in their eyes from what is detrimental in the eyes of different family members. The decision to intervene when the self-sacrifice is in the service of homeostasis raises difficult countertransference and ethical issues, which must be dealt with honestly both within the therapist and directly with the family. Often it is when a family member reaches a developmental transition (e.g., when the caregiving daughter's friends begin to marry) that the family becomes destabilized, and productive intervention can begin.

Even when families do make the transition, and their life-cycle resumes, transitional points can bring episodic loss and mourning (see Stage Theories, above). For example, a family may adapt quite well to a severe head injury in a young child, but when his or her peers begin Little League and he does not, when dating, high school graduation, college, and marriage do not occur as they naturally would, there is sadness for the family and a retouching of old hurts and losses. It is crucial during this period to help families build on their strength and dignity, and especially important to enable the person with the brain injury to find a productive and meaningful place in the family, with peers, and in the community.

The relationship of the family to the community is particularly important during this stage. Families need to learn to draw comfortably on the existing resources of extended family, friends, employers, churches, and other community organizations, and to resist the tendency to become isolated, ashamed and self-conscious, or shield the community from the injured person (although the conscious motive is usually the opposite). Family interventions should include a circle of support that is often wider than would initially be comfortable for the family. Family-to-family programs, self-help groups, family outreach and advocacy, and community networking, are all concepts that the savvy family therapist will utilize (Williams 1991b). Family intervention at this final stage of reintegration needs to move beyond the confines of the office into the community.

Postscripts

Family Issues in Mild TBI

A special set of dynamics apply to mild TBI, which deviates somewhat from some of the principles outlined in this chapter. Mild TBI refers to injuries with brief or no loss of consciousness, no long-term focal neurological abnormalities, usually normal computed tomography scans and magnetic resonance imaging studies, a constellation of symptoms including headache, irritability, fatigue, sleep disturbance, poor attention, concentration and memory, depression, anxiety, poor self-esteem, and general inability to function (Kay 1986). Psychological overlay accumulates with time and increases dysfunction, which usually reflects a complex interaction among organic, personality, and environmental factors. In many cases, a legitimate, if subtle, brain injury underlies and drives the dysfunction, which is layered over with maladaptive psychological reactions, many of which result from inappropriate environmental responses (Kay 1992).

Although in moderate to severe brain injury the family tends to rally around, support, and advocate for the injured person, one often sees a picture of initial concern, followed by increasing alienation, in families after mild TBI. This is the result of the injured person's apparent normalcy in the presence of his or her anxiety, depression, loss of self-esteem, and increasing dysfunction over time.

An essential part of any neuropsychiatric trea⌐ complex and difficult cases is immediate family inv⌐ Family responses and reactions to the apparent discrepan⌐ tween severity of injury and severity of symptoms can eith⌐ induce or exacerbate a dysfunctional postconcussional syndrome. The family needs information and education about the nature and consequences of concussion, and how to understand and help the patient manage his or her symptoms. Also, the alienation that exists between the injured person and the family needs to be healed. Often this involves addressing old issues, either intraper- sonal or within the family system, which are in fact contributing to the excessive level of dysfunction. It is a mistake to see the obvious emotional overlay in such cases, and dismiss the injured person as malingering or the problems as purely psychosomatic ones. The individual cannot be helped back to a level of produc- tive functioning without addressing what is usually a deteriorated family situation.

National Head Injury Foundation and Other Support Organizations

The National Head Injury Foundation (NHIF) was founded in 1980 by Marilyn Price Spivack and Martin Spivack, and a small group of families and professionals in Framingham, Massachusetts. Today it has grown into a national advocacy organization centered in Washington, DC, with affiliated chapters in most states. The NHIF encourages active participation of persons with brain injury, family members, and professionals; provides educational materials to families and professionals; organizes support groups at the local level; and acts as an advocacy organization at the state and national level for public policies and laws that support persons with brain injury and their families. At the professional level, the NHIF provides numerous opportunities for involvement through committees, task forces, and an annual national professional con- vention.

As of this writing, there is a Psychiatric Committee within NHIF charged with increasing the involvement of the professional of

Psychiatry within the field of TBI rehabilitation (as there is a Traumatic Brain Injury Task Force within the American Psychiatric Association). (NHIF, 1140 Connecticut Ave., NW, Suite 812 Washington, DC, 20036; 202-296-6443; Family Helpline: 800-444-6443.) In local areas, other support and advocacy organizations, which may not be associated with the NHIF, have also evolved.

Family Individuality and Coping

Chapters such as this one can be written only by generalizing about families. A fitting way to end is with the caveat that all families are different, and the effective clinician will respond to the conscious and unconscious needs of the individual family, and not project onto the family his or her value system of what healthy adjustment is. Precisely because the person with brain injury will be dependent on a network of significant others for his or her successful adaptation to disability, successful family intervention must proceed from within the framework of that unique family system. The rehabilitation team will not successfully impose goals, limits, or routines that are alien to the family. It is the role of the family therapist to help families meet their needs, establish a new balance and identity that works for them, and negotiate a productive alliance between the rehabilitation team and the family. This can be done only by starting—and ending—with a healthy respect for the family's individuality.

References

Bishop SD, Miller IW: Traumatic brain injury: empirical family assessment techniques. Journal of Head Trauma Rehabilitation 3:31–41, 1988

Bond MR: Assessment of psychosocial outcome of severe head injury. Acta Neurochir 34:57–70, 1976

Bond MR: Effects on the family system, in Rehabilitation of the Head Injured Adult. Edited by Rosenthal M, Griffith E, Bond M, Miller JD. Philadelphia, PA, FA Davis, 1983, pp 209–217

Brooks N: The head-injured family. J Clin Exp Neuropsychol 13:155–188, 1991

Brooks N, McKinlay W: Personality and behavioural change after severe blunt head injury—a relative's view. J Neurol Neurosurg Psychiatry 46:336–344, 1983

Brooks N, Campsie L, Symington C, et al: The effects of severe head injury upon patient and relative within several years of injury. Journal of Head Trauma Rehabilitation 2:1–13, 1987

Carter EA, McGoldrick M (eds): The Family Lifecycle: A Framework for Family Therapy. New York, Gardner, 1980

Cavallo MM, Kay T, Ezrachi O: Problems and changes after traumatic brain injury: differing perceptions between and within families. Brain Inj 6:327–335, 1992

Combrinck-Graham L: A developmental model for family systems. Fam Process 24:139–150, 1985

DeJong G, Batavia AI, Williams JW: Who is responsible for the lifelong well-being of a person with a head injury? Journal of Head Trauma Rehabilitation 5:9–22, 1990

Eysenck HJ, Eysenck SBG: Eysenck Personality Questionnaire. London, Hodder and Stoughton, 1975

Florian V, Katz S, Lahav V: Impact of traumatic brain damage on family dynamics and functioning: a review. Brain Inj 3:219–233, 1989

Hpay H: Psycho-social effects of severe head injury, in International Symposium on Head Injuries, Edinburgh and Madrid. New York, Churchill Livingstone, 1970, pp 110–119

Jacobs HE: The Los Angeles head injury survey: procedures and initial findings. Arch Phys Med Rehabil 69:425–431, 1988

Kalsbeek WD, McLauren RL, Harris BSH, et al: The National Head and Spinal Cord Injury Survey: major findings. J Neurosurg 53:S19–S31, 1980

Kay T: The Unseen Injury: Minor Head Trauma. Framingham, MA, National Head Injury Foundation, 1986

Kay T: Neuropsychological diagnosis: disentangling the multiple determinants of functional disability after mild traumatic brain injury, in Rehabilitation of Post-Concussive Disorders: Physical Medicine and Rehabilitation: State of the Art Reviews. Edited by Horn L, Zassler N. Philadelphia, PA, Hanley and Belfus, 1992, 109–127

Kay T, Cavallo MM: Evolutions: research and clinical perspectives on families, in Head Injury: A Family Matter. Edited by Williams JM, Kay T. Baltimore, MD, Paul H Brookes, 1991, pp 121–150

Kay T, Lezak M: The nature of head injury, in Traumatic Brain Injury and Vocational Rehabilitation. Edited by Corthell D. Menomonie, WI, University of Wisconsin-Stout, 1990, pp 21–65

Kay T, Cavallo MM, Ezrachi O: Administration Manual, N.Y.U. Head Injury Family Interview (Version 1.2). New York, NYU Medical Center, Research and Training Center on Head Trauma and Stroke, 1988

Klonoff P, Prigatano GP: Reactions of family members and clinical intervention after traumatic brain injury, in Community Re-Entry for Head Injured Adults. Edited by Ylvisaker M, Gobble EMR. Boston, MA, College Hill, 1987, pp 381–402

Kozloff R: Networks of social support and the outcome from severe head injury. Journal of Head Trauma Rehabilitation 2:14–23, 1987

Kubler-Ross E: On Death and Dying. New York, Macmillan, 1969

Lezak MD: Living with the characterologically altered brain injured patient. J Clin Psychiatry 39:592–598, 1978

Lezak MD: Psychological implications of traumatic brain damage for the patient's family. Rehabilitation Psychology 31:241–250, 1986

Lezak MD: Brain damage is a family affair. J Clin Exp Neuropsychol 10:111–123, 1988

Livingston MG: Head injury: the relative's response. Brain Inj 1:33–39, 1987

Livingston MG: Effects on the family system, in Rehabilitation of the Adult and Child with Traumatic Brain Injury. Edited by Rosenthal M, Griffith ER, Bond MR, et al. Philadelphia, PA, FA Davis, 1990, pp 225–235

Livingston MG, Brooks DN: The burden on families of the brain injured: a review. Journal of Head Trauma Rehabilitation 4:6–15, 1988

Maitz EA: The psychological sequelae of a severe closed head injury and their impact upon family systems. Unpublished doctoral dissertation, Temple University, 1989

McKinlay WW, Brooks DN, Bond MR, et al: The short-term outcome of severe blunt head injury as reported by relatives of the injured person. J Neurol Neurosurg Psychiatry 44:527–533, 1981

Muir CA, Rosenthal M, Diehl LN: Methods of family intervention, in Rehabilitation of the Adult and Child with Traumatic Brain Injury. Edited by Rosenthal M, Griffith ER, Bond MR, et al. Philadelphia, PA, FA Davis, 1990, pp 433–448

Oddy M, Humphrey M: Social recovery during the year following severe head injury. J Neurol Neurosurg Psychiatry 43:798–802, 1980

Oddy M, Humphrey M, Uttley D: Subjective impairment and social recovery after closed head injury. J Neurol Neurosurg Psychiatry 41:611–616, 1978a

Oddy M, Humphrey M, Uttley D: Stresses upon the relatives of head-injured patients. Br J Psychiatry 133:507–513, 1978b

Oddy M, Coughlan T, Tyerman A, et al: Social adjustment after closed head injury: a further follow-up seven years after injury. J Neurol Neurosurg Psychiatry 48:564–568, 1985

Olshansky S: Chronic sorrow: a response to having a mentally defective child. Social Casework 43:190–193, 1962

Panting A, Merry PH: The long-term rehabilitation of severe head injuries with particular reference to the need for social and medical support for the patient's family. Rehabilitation 38:33–37, 1972

Peters LC, Stambrook M, Moore AD, et al: Psychosocial sequelae of closed head injury: effects on the marital relationship. Brain Inj 4:39–47, 1990

Rape RN, Busch JP, Slavin LA: Toward a conceptualization of the family's adaptation to a member's head injury: a critique of developmental stage models. Rehabilitation Psychology 37:3–22, 1992

Ridley B: Family response in head injury: denial or hope for the future? Soc Sci Med 29:555–561, 1989

Rolland JS: Chronic illness and the life cycle: a conceptual framework. Fam Process 26:203–221, 1987a

Rolland JS: Family illness paradigms: evolution and significance. Family Systems Medicine 5:482–503, 1987b

Rolland JS: Anticipatory loss: a family systems framework. Fam Process 29:229–244, 1990

Romano MD: Family response to traumatic head injury. Scand J Rehabil Med 6:1–4, 1974

Romano MD: Family issues in head trauma, in Traumatic Brain Injury: Physical Medicine and Rehabilitation: State of the Art Reviews. Edited by Horn L, Cope DN. Philadelphia, PA, Hanley and Belfus, 1989, pp 157–168

Rosenthal M, Hutchins B: Interdisciplinary family education in head injury rehabilitation, in Head Injury: A Family Matter. Edited by Williams JM, Kay T. Baltimore, MD, Paul H Brookes, 1991, pp 273–282

Rosenthal M, Muir CA: Methods of family intervention, in Rehabilitation of the Head Injured Adult. Edited by Rosenthal M, Griffith ER, Bond MR, et al. Philadelphia, PA, FA Davis, 1983, pp 407–419

Weddell R, Oddy M, Jenkins D: Social adjustment after rehabilitation: a two-year follow-up of patients with severe head injury. Psychol Med 10:257–263, 1980

Wikler L: Chronic stresses of families of mentally retarded children. Family Relations 30:281–288, 1981

Williams JM: Family reaction to head injury, in Head Injury: A Family Matter. Edited by Williams JM, Kay T. Baltimore, MD, Paul H Brookes, 1991a, pp 81–99

Williams JM: Family support, in Head Injury: A Family Matter. Edited by Williams JM, Kay T. Baltimore, MD, Paul H Brookes, 1991b, pp 299–312

Williams JM, Kay T: Head Injury: A Family Matter. Baltimore, MD, Paul H Brookes, 1991

Williams JM, Savage RC: Family culture and child development, in Head Injury: A Family Matter. Edited by Williams JM, Kay T. Baltimore, MD, Paul H Brookes, 1991, pp 219–238

Chapter 18

Ethical and Legal Issues

Robert I. Simon, M.D.

T raumatic brain injury (TBI) patients, particularly those who manifest difficulties in judgment, mood regulation, memory, orientation, insight, and impulse control, often present complex ethical and legal problems. In addition, they are likely to have a plethora of psychiatric symptoms. In litigation, brain injuries can bring in large monetary awards, particularly if unemployability is present. In combination with current and future medical expenses, it is easy to see that compensable damages from head trauma can be substantial. Depending on functional impairment, even minor brain injuries can bring in seven-figure verdicts.

Ethical Considerations

During the first half of the twentieth century, the principle of patient autonomy was clearly recognized in the medical malpractice case, *Schloendorff v. Society of New York Hospital* (1914). Justice Cardozo firmly enunciated the principle of patient self-determination by stating that "every human being of adult years and sound mind has a right to determine what shall be done with his own body, and a surgeon who performs an operation without his patient's consent commits an assault, for which he is liable in damages" (1914, p. 126).

Since the late 1950s and early 1960s, the medical profession has moved away from an authoritarian, physician-oriented stance toward a more collaborative relationship with patients concerning their health care decisions. This is especially reflected in contemporary ethical principles (American Psychiatric Association 1989). Thus psychiatry, on ethical grounds, endorses granting competent patients the legal right to autonomy in determining their medical care. Quite apart from any legal compulsion, most psychiatrists disclose truthful and pertinent medical information to their patients in order to enhance the therapeutic alliance (Simon 1989, 1992a).

The ethical principles of beneficence, nonmaleficence, and respect for the dignity and autonomy of the patient comprise the moral-ethical foundation for the doctor-patient relationship. Accordingly, brain injury that significantly interferes with the patient's decision-making capacity requires more active intervention by the psychiatrist. For example, the psychiatrist has a legal and ethical duty to obtain consent from substitute decision makers when a patient is incapable of making an informed decision. The rights of all patients are the same—only how these rights are exercised is different (Parry and Beck 1990).

The ethics of social justice calls for the fair allocation of medical resources in accord with medical need (Ruchs 1984). Although seemingly a new development, the ethical concerns about equitable health care distribution are found in the Hippocratic Oath and in the tradition of medicine and psychiatry (Dyer 1988). For example, it would be unethical to discriminate against an individual who receives a TBI during the course of committing a felony by not providing adequate treatment and management resources.

Ethical issues arise daily for psychiatrists who treat TBI patients. Medical decision making, informed consent, resuscitation, "brain death," organ transplantation, the withholding and withdrawing of life support, and the allocation of medical resources all give rise to complex ethical and legal problems (Luce 1990). Moreover, that which is considered ethical in clinical practice today may become a legal requirement tomorrow.

I will address specific ethical issues in connection with the various clinical and legal topics discussed throughout this chapter.

Competency: The Basic Concept

Case example.

> A 47-year-old man with traumatic dementia inherits $6 million. His physician becomes concerned when the patient proposes to pay for a 90-day around-the-world trip for himself and three of his longtime friends. A psychiatric consultation is requested. The mental status evaluation reveals judgment and insight to be intact. Short-term memory is moderately disturbed. Sensorium and orientation are intact. Affective lability is present, particularly when frustration is experienced. The patient's brother requests a competency hearing and an appointment of a guardian for financial matters. After hearing testimony, the court finds that the patient has the minimal mental capacity to manage his financial matters. The court notes that decisions that seem idiosyncratic or even foolish do not necessarily denote mental incompetence.

Nearly every area of human endeavor is affected by the law and, as a fundamental condition, requires one to be mentally competent (Appendix 18–1). Essentially, *competency* is defined as "having sufficient capacity, ability . . . [or] possessing the requisite physical, mental, natural, or legal qualifications . . . " (Black 1990, p. 284). This definition is deliberately vague and ambiguous because competency is a broad concept encompassing many different legal issues and contexts. As a result, its definition, requirements, and application can vary widely depending on the circumstances in which it is measured (e.g., health care decisions, executing a will, or confessing to a crime).

As noted in the case example, *competency* refers to some *minimal* mental, cognitive, or behavioral ability, trait, or capability required to perform a particular legally recognized act or to assume some legal role. The term *incapacity,* which is often interchanged with incompetency, refers to an individual's functional inability to understand or to form an intention with regard to some act, as determined by a health care provider (Mishkin 1989). In TBI patients, fluctuations in mental capacity are common, particularly in the days and even months following injury.

The legal designation of *incompetent* is applied to an individual who fails one of the mental tests of capacity and is therefore considered *by law* not mentally capable of performing a particular act or assuming a particular role. The adjudication of incompetence by a court is subject or issue specific. For example, the fact that a TBI patient is adjudicated incompetent to execute a will does not automatically render that patient incompetent to do other things, such as consenting to treatment, testifying as a witness, marrying, driving, or making a legally binding contract. Generally, the law will recognize only those decisions or choices that have been made by a competent individual. The law seeks to protect incompetent individuals from the harmful effects of their acts. People over the age of majority, which is now 18, are presumed to be competent (*Meek v. City of Loveland* 1929; The Legal Status of Adolescents 1980, published in 1981). This presumption, however, is rebuttable by evidence of an individual's incapacity (*Scaria v. St. Paul Fire & Marine Ins Co* 1975). For the TBI patient, perception, short- and long-term memory, judgment, language comprehension, verbal fluency, and reality orientation are mental functions that a court will scrutinize regarding capacity and competency.

The issue of competency, whether in a civil or criminal context, is commonly raised when the person is a minor or is mentally disabled. In many situations, minors are not considered legally competent and therefore require the consent of a parent or designated guardian. There are exceptions to this general rule, however, such as minors who are considered emancipated (Smith 1986), mature (*Gulf S I R Co v. Sullivan* 1928), or competent to consent in some cases of medical need (*Planned Parenthood v. Danforth* 1976) or emergency (*Jehovah's Witnesses v. King County Hospital* 1967, published in 1968).

The mentally disabled, which often include TBI patients, present more complex problems in evaluating competency. Lack of capacity or competency *cannot* be presumed either from treatment for mental disorders (*Wilson v. Lehman* 1964) or from institutionalization of such persons (*Rennie v. Klein* 1978). Mental disability or disorder does *not,* in and of itself, render a person incompetent or incompetent in all areas of functioning. Nor do idiosyncratic or foolish decisions, by themselves, denote mental incompetence. Making foolish decisions is part of the human condition. Instead, scrutiny should be given to determine whether there are specific functional incapacities that render a person incapable of making a particular kind of decision or performing a particular type of task.

Respect for individual autonomy (*Schloendorff v. New York Hospital* 1914) demands that individuals be allowed to make decisions of which they are capable, even if they are seriously mentally ill, developmentally arrested, or organically impaired. As a rule, a patient with a TBI that produces mental incapacity generally must be judicially declared incompetent before that patient's exercise of his or her legal rights can be abridged. The person's current or past history of physical and mental illness is but one factor to be weighed in determining whether a particular test of competency is met.

Health Care Decision Making

Informed Consent

Case example.

A 56-year-old man with a traumatic amnestic syndrome develops a major depression. In order to obtain informed consent for treatment, the psychiatrist describes the risks and benefits of antidepressant medications to the patient. The psychiatrist quickly realizes that the patient lacks the mental capacity to retain this information long enough to consider it. In frustration and embarrassment, the patient consents to take any medication. The psychiatrist obtains the proxy consent of the patient's wife after explaining the diagnosis, risks and benefits of treatment, alternative treatments with their risks and benefits, and the prognosis with and without treatment. Proxy consent by next of kin is permitted by statute in the state where the patient lives.

Because patients with TBI frequently demonstrate impaired mental capacity, obtaining a valid informed consent to proposed diagnostic procedures and treatments can be both challenging and frustrating. The capacity to consent, particularly following brain injury, may be present one moment and gone the next. Lucid intervals may permit the obtaining of competent consent for health care decisions.

The need to obtain competent, informed consent is not negated simply because it appears that the patient is in need of medical intervention or would likely benefit from it. Instead, clinicians must assure themselves that the patient or an appropriate substitute decision maker has given a competent consent before proceeding with treatment. In the case example, the psychiatrist realized that the patient was giving an incompetent consent to treatment and obtained proxy consent. When patients agree to treatment, their competency to assent is often not questioned. An increasing number of states require a judicial determination of incompetence and the court's substituted consent prior to the administration of neuroleptic treatment to a patient who is deemed by a health care provider to lack the functional mental capacity (Simon 1992a).

Under the doctrine of informed consent, health care providers have a legal duty to abide by the treatment decisions made by competent patients unless a compelling state interest exists. The term *informed consent* is a legal principle in medical jurisprudence, which holds that a physician must disclose to a patient sufficient information to enable the patient to make an informed decision about a proposed treatment or procedure (Black 1990, p. 779). In order for a patient's consent to be considered informed, it must adequately address three essential elements: competency, information, and voluntariness. In general, the patient must be given enough information to make a truly knowledgeable decision and that decision (consent) must be made voluntarily by a person who is legally competent. Each of these elements must be met or any consent given will not be considered informed and legally valid (Table 18–1).

The law recognizes several circumscribed exceptions to the requirement of informed consent (Rozovsky 1984). The most notable is the "emergency exception," which states that consent is implied in circumstances in which the patient is unable to give consent (e.g., unconsciousness) and has an acute, life-threatening crisis that requires immediate medical attention. The TBI patient often is initially brought for emergency care. Because the patient may be unconscious or manifest significant impairment in consciousness, treatment may be initiated under implied emergency consent. Another common clinical situation in which this exception might arise is in the treatment of the violent TBI patient. For instance, patients diagnosed with frontal lobe or temporal lobe damage are known to have sudden, violent outbursts that usually require immediate intervention in order to prevent serious injury to the patient or nearby third parties (Devinsky and Bear 1984).

Only a *competent* person is legally recognized as able to give informed consent. Competent patients must not be treated against their objections. This is particularly important for health care providers working with patients who sometimes are of questionable competence due to brain injury. Obtaining valid informed consent from these patients can be intimidating because of their vacillating and unpredictable mental state (Carlson 1977).

From a legal perspective, the term *competency* is narrowly defined in terms of *cognitive* capacity. There are no established criteria for determining a patient's competence. A very basic level of decision-making capacity exists when the patient is able to understand

---

Table 18–1.   Informed consent: reasonable information to be disclosed

Although there exists no consistently accepted set of information to be disclosed for any given medical or psychiatric situation, as a rule of thumb, five areas of information are generally provided:

1. Diagnosis—description of the condition or problem
2. Treatment—nature and purpose of proposed treatment
3. Consequences—risks and benefits of the proposed treatment
4. Alternatives—viable alternatives to the proposed treatment including risks and benefits
5. Prognosis—projected outcome with and without treatment

Source. Reprinted from Simon RI: *Clinical Psychiatry and the Law,* 2nd Edition. Washington, DC, American Psychiatric Press, 1992, p. 128. Used with permission.

the particular treatment choice proposed, make a treatment choice, and communicate that decision (Table 18–2).

The problem with this standard of decision-making capacity is that it obtains a simple consent from the patient rather than an informed consent because alternative treatment choices are not provided. A review of case law and scholarly literature on this issue reveals four general standards for determining incompetency in decision making (Appelbaum et al. 1987). In order of levels of mental capacity required, these standards include 1) communication of choice, 2) understanding of information provided, 3) appreciation of one's situation and the risks and benefits of options available, and 4) rational decision making. Psychiatrists generally feel most comfortable with a rational decision-making standard in determining incompetency. Most courts prefer the first two standards. An informed consent reflecting the patient's autonomy and personal needs and values occurs when rational decision making is applied to the risks and benefits of appropriate treatment options provided to the patient by the clinician. When the patient seems competent, a decision that appears irrational is not, by itself, a basis for a determination of incompetence (Benesch 1989). Persons who are fully competent may make foolish decisions. Legal advice may be needed if the competency issue cannot be resolved by additional medical and psychiatric consultation.

The psychiatrist planning to treat a TBI patient suspected of having neuropsychiatric deficits should conduct a thorough and systematic assessment of cognitive functioning. The sole objective of such an evaluation should be the determination of the TBI patient's ability to meet the minimal requirements for consent. At the very least, a mental status assessment of the patient's language, memory, judgment, insight, affect, orientation, and attention span

---

Table 18–2.   Minimal health care decision-making capacity

Understand the particular treatment being offered

Make a discernible decision regarding the treatment that has been offered

Communicate the decision verbally or nonverbally

---

should be performed (Folstein et al. 1975). Certain TBI patients may be cognitively intact but manifest such severe affective lability that they are rendered mentally incompetent.

Except in an emergency, an authorized representative or appointed guardian must make health care decisions on behalf of patients with TBI who lack health care decision-making capacity (*Aponte v. United States* 1984; *Frasier v. Department of Health and Human Resources* 1986). Table 18–3 lists a number of consent options that may be available for such patients, depending on the jurisdiction.

Incompetent Patients

In what was hoped to be the "final word" on this very difficult and personal question of patient autonomy, the United States Supreme Court ruled in *Cruzan v. Director, Missouri Department of Health* (1990) that the state of Missouri could refuse to remove a food and water tube surgically implanted in the stomach of Nancy Cruzan without clear and convincing evidence of her wishes. She had been

---

Table 18–3. Common consent options for patients lacking the mental capacity for health care decisions

---

Proxy consent of next of kin

Adjudication of incompetence; appointment of a guardian

Institutional administrators or committees

Treatment review panels

Substituted consent of the court

Advance directives (living will, durable power of attorney, and health care proxy)

Statutory surrogates (spouse or court-appointed guardian)[a]

---

[a]Because of the frequent absence of advance directives, statutory surrogate laws have been enacted in some states. These laws authorize certain persons, such as a spouse or court-appointed guardian, to make health care decisions when the patient has not stated his or her wishes in writing. At least 14 states currently have enacted statutory surrogate laws (American Medical News 1991).

Source. Reprinted from Simon RI: *Clinical Psychiatry and the Law,* 2nd Edition. Washington, DC, American Psychiatric Press, 1992, p. 109. Used with permission.

in a persistent vegetative state for seven years. In other words, without clear and convincing evidence of a patient's decision to have life-sustaining measures withheld in a particular circumstance, the state has the right to maintain that individual's life, even against the family's wishes.

Although this decision seems to leave unanswered more questions than it answers, the Court's decision does buttress the position of "right to refuse" treatment advocates in the following three significant ways:

1. The Court seemed to give constitutional status to a competent person's right to refuse treatment. Furthermore, if individuals appoint relatives or friends to make decisions about medical treatment should they become incompetent, states "may well be constitutionally required" to defer to the wishes of such "surrogate decision makers."
2. The Court did not distinguish between artificially administered food and water and other life-sustaining measures, such as respirators. This distinction has been a hotly contested sticking point in some previous, lower court decisions.
3. An incompetent person who makes his or her wishes known in advance, such as through a living will, may have a constitutional right to halt life-sustaining intervention, depending on the proof of those wishes.

The *Cruzan* decision is important for clinicians who treat severely or terminally impaired TBI patients because it requires that they seek clear and competent instructions regarding foreseeable treatment decisions. This information is best provided in the form of a living will, durable power of attorney agreement, or health care proxy. However, any written document that clearly and convincingly sets forth the patient's wishes would serve the same purpose. Although physicians have historically feared civil or criminal liability for stopping life-sustaining treatment, liability may now arise from overtreating critically or terminally ill patients (Weir and Gostin 1990).

Do-Not-Resuscitate Orders (DNR)

Case example.

A 42-year-old woman with TBI has a cardiac arrest and is resuscitated. A psychiatric consult determines that the patient retains sufficient mental capacity to make health care decisions. The patient instructs her physician not to resuscitate her if another cardiac arrest occurs. The family disagrees. They want the patient to be resuscitated because they feel the DNR decision is based on impaired judgment caused by the brain injury. Nevertheless, the primary physician determines that the patient is competent when she makes the request. The physician writes the DNR order.

Cardiopulmonary resuscitation (CPR) is a medical life-saving technology. To be effective it must be applied immediately, leaving no time to think about the consequences of reviving a patient. Ordinarily, patients requiring CPR have not thought about or expressed a preference for or against its use.

In the critically ill TBI patient, the psychiatrist and the substitute medical decision maker have time to consider whether CPR should be offered based on the patient's earlier expressed wishes. The ethical principle of patient autonomy justifies the position that the patient or substitute decision maker should make the final decision regarding the use of CPR. However, some patients and families who are not offered CPR may feel helpless and abandoned. Psychiatrists must remain mindful of this reaction to properly assist the patient and family. As illustrated in the case example, the patient's direction concerning DNR should be followed if made competently. Malpractice liability for not offering or providing futile care is unlikely and the psychiatrist is exposed to greater liability exposure if such care is provided (March and Staver 1991). Schwartz (1987) noted that two key principles have emerged concerning DNR decisions:

1. In accordance with the ethical principle of autonomy and with the legal doctrine of informed consent, DNR decisions should be reached consensually by the attending physician and the patient or substitute decision maker.

2. DNR orders should be written and the reasoning for the DNR order documented in the chart.

Hospital CPR policies make DNR decisions discretionary (Luce 1990). However, psychiatrists should be familiar with the specific hospital policy whenever a DNR order is written. Medicolegal-ethical principles have been promulgated concerning CPR and emergency cardiac care (American Medical Association 1991, 1992).

Advance Directives

The use of advance directives such as a living will, health care proxy, or a durable medical power of attorney is recommended in order to avoid ethical and legal complications associated with requests to withhold life-sustaining treatment measures (Simon 1992a; Solnick 1985). The Patient Self-Determination Act, which took effect on 1 December 1991, requires hospitals, nursing homes, hospices, managed care organizations, and home health care agencies to advise patients or family members of their right to accept or refuse medical care and to execute an advance directive (LaPuma et al. 1991). These advance directives provide a method for individuals, while competent, to choose proxy health care decision makers in the event of future incompetency. A living will can be contained as a subsection of a durable power of attorney agreement. In the ordinary power of attorney created for the management of business and financial matters, the power of attorney generally becomes null and void if the person creating it becomes incompetent.

Federal law does not specify the right to formulate advance directives; therefore, state law applies. Recently, state legislators have recognized that individuals may want to indicate who should make important health care decisions in case they become incapacitated and unable to act in their own behalf. All 50 states and the District of Columbia permit individuals to create a *durable* power of attorney (i.e., one that endures even if the competence of the creator does not) (*Cruzan v. Director, Missouri Department of Health* 1990, n 3). A number of states and the District of Columbia have durable power of attorney statutes expressly authorizing the appointment of proxies for making health care decisions (*Cruzan v. Director, Missouri Department of Health* 1990, n 2).

Generally, durable power of attorney has been construed to empower an agent to make health care decisions. Such a document is much broader and more flexible than a living will, which covers only the period of a diagnosed terminal illness, specifying only that no "extraordinary treatments" may be utilized that would prolong the act of dying (Mishkin 1985). In order to rectify the sometimes uncertain status of the durable power of attorney as applied to health care decisions, a number of states have passed or are considering health care proxy laws. The health care proxy is a legal instrument akin to the durable power of attorney but specifically created for health care decision making (see Appendix 18–2). Currently, efforts are underway to tailor the living will into a psychiatric living will as an alternative to involuntary treatment. The legal sufficiency of such a document remains untested (Cody 1991). Despite the growing use of advance directives, there is increasing evidence that physician values rather than patient values are more critical in end-of-life decisions (Orentlicher 1992).

In a durable power of attorney or health care proxy, general or specific directions are set forth about how future decisions should be made in the event one becomes unable to make these decisions. The determination of a patient's competence, however, is not specified in most durable power of attorney and health care proxy statutes. Because this is a medical or psychiatric question, the examination by two physicians who confirm the patient's ability to understand the nature and consequences of the proposed treatment or procedure, the ability to make a choice, and the ability to communicate that choice is usually minimally sufficient. This information, like all significant medical observations, should be clearly documented in the patient's file.

Because of the frequent absence of advance directives, statutory surrogate laws have been enacted in some states. These laws authorize certain persons, such as a spouse or court-appointed guardian, to make health care decisions when the patient has not stated his or her wishes in writing. At least 14 states currently have enacted statutory surrogate laws (American Medical News 1991).

The application of advance directives to neuropsychiatric patients presents some difficulties. The classic example arises when a currently asymptomatic TBI patient, with organic personality syndrome and occasional bouts of severe affective instability, draws up a durable power of attorney agreement or health care proxy directing that, "If I become mentally unstable again, administer medications even if I strenuously object or resist." This has been described as the "Ulysses Contract" (T. Gutheil, personal communication, September 1985). In Greek mythology, Ulysses was bound to the mast of his ship so he could hear the beautiful, although lethal, sirens' song. All the other sailors covered their ears. When he heard the irresistible song of the sirens, Ulysses tried to struggle loose to go to them. When that failed, he demanded to be untied. Similarly, when mood instability recurs, the TBI patient may strenuously object to treatment.

Because durable power of attorney agreements or health care proxies can be easily revoked, the treating psychiatrist or institution has no choice but to honor the patient's refusal, even if there is reasonable evidence that the patient is incompetent. Legal consultation also should be considered at this point. If the patient is grossly disordered and is an immediate danger to self and others, the physician or hospital is on firmer ground medically and legally to temporarily override the patient's treatment refusal. Otherwise, it is generally better to seek a court order for treatment than to risk legal entanglement with the patient by attempting to enforce the original terms of the advance directive. Typically, unless there are compelling medical reasons to do otherwise, courts will generally honor the patient's original treatment directions given while competent.

Guardianship

A guardianship is a method of substitute decision making for individuals who have been judicially determined as unable to act for themselves (Brakel et al. 1985). Historically, the state or sovereign possessed the power and authority to safeguard the estates of incompetent persons (Regan 1972).

This traditional role still reflects the purpose of guardianship today. In some states, there are separate provisions for the appointment of a "guardian of one's person" (e.g., health care decision making) and for a "guardian of one's estate" (e.g., authority to make contracts to sell one's property) (Sale et al. 1982, p. 461). This latter guardian is frequently referred to as a conservator, although this designation is not used uniformly throughout the United States. A further distinction, also found in some jurisdictions, is *general (plenary)* versus *specific* guardianship (Sale et al. 1982, p. 462). As the name implies, the latter guardian is restricted to exercising decisions about a particular subject area. For instance, the specific guardian may be authorized to make decisions about major or emergency medical procedures and the disabled person retains the freedom to make decisions about all other medical matters. General guardians, in contrast, have total control over the disabled individual's person, estate, or both (Sale et al. 1982, pp. 461–462).

Guardianship arrangements, which are increasingly utilized for patients who demonstrate dementia, particularly acquired immunodeficiency syndrome (AIDS)-related dementia and Alzheimer's disease, can also be of use for TBI patients (Overman and Stoudemire 1988). Under the Anglo-American system of law, an individual is presumed to be competent unless adjudicated incompetent. Thus incompetence is a legal determination made by a court of law based on evidence, provided by health care providers and others, that the individual's functional mental capacity is significantly impaired. Laws governing competency in many states are based on the Uniform Guardianship and Protective Proceeding Act or the Uniform Probate Code (Mishkin 1989). Drafted by legal scholars and practicing attorneys, Uniform Acts serve as models whose purpose is to achieve uniformity among the state laws by enactment of model laws.

General incompetency is defined by the Uniform Guardianship and Protective Proceeding Act as

> Impaired by reason of mental illness, mental deficiency, physical illness or disability, advanced age, chronic use of drugs, chronic intoxication, or other cause (except minority) to the extent of lacking sufficient understanding or capacity to make or communicate reasonable decisions.

A significant number of TBI patients meet the above definition. Generally, the appointment of a guardian is limited to situations in which the individual's decision-making capacity is so impaired that he or she is unable to care for personal safety or provide such necessities as food, shelter, clothing and medical care, likely resulting in physical injury or illness (*In re Boyer* 1981). The standard of proof required for a judicial determination of incompetency is *clear and convincing evidence*. Although the law does not assign percentages to proof, clear and convincing evidence is in the range of 75 percent certainty (Simon 1992b).

States vary concerning the extent of their reliance on psychiatric assessments. Nonmedical personnel such as social workers, psychologists, family members, friends, colleagues, and even the individual who is the subject of the proceeding may testify.

Substituted Judgment

Psychiatrists often find that the time required to obtain an adjudication of incompetence is unduly burdensome and frequently interferes with the provision of quality treatment on a timely basis. Moreover, families often are reluctant to face the formal court proceedings necessary in order to declare their family member incompetent, particularly when sensitive family matters are disclosed. A common solution to both of these problems is to seek the legally authorized proxy consent of a spouse or relative serving as guardian, when the refusing TBI patient is believed to be incompetent. Proxy consent, however, is not available in every state (Simon 1992a).

There are clear advantages associated with having the family serve as decision maker (Perr 1984). First, use of responsible family members as surrogate decision makers maintains the integrity of the family unit and relies on the sources that are most likely to know the patient's wishes. Second, it is more efficient and less costly than adjudication. However, there are some disadvantages. Proxy decision making requires synthesizing the diverse values, beliefs, practices, and prior statements of the patient for a given specific circumstance (Emanuel and Emanuel 1992). As one judge characterized the problem, any proxy decision making in the absence of specific directions is "at best only an optimistic approximation" (*In re Jobes* 1987). Ambivalent feelings, conflicts within the family and with the patient, and conflicting economic interest may make certain family members suspect as guardians (Gutheil and Appelbaum 1980). Also relatives may be unavailable or unwilling to become involved.

The President's Commission for the Study of Ethical Problems in Medicine and Biomedical and Behavioral Research (1982) recommended that the relatives of incompetent patients be selected as proxy decision makers for the following reasons:

1. The family is generally most concerned about the good of the patient.
2. The family will also usually be most knowledgeable about the patient's goals, preferences, and values.
3. The family deserves recognition as an important social unit to be treated, within limits, as a single decision maker in matters that intimately affect its members.

A number of states permit proxy decision making by statute, mainly through their informed consent statute (Solnick 1985). Some state statutes specify that another person may authorize consent on behalf of the incompetent patient; others mention specific relatives. Unless proxy consent by a relative is provided by statute or by case law authority in the state where the psychiatrist practices, it is not recommended that the good faith consent of next of kin be relied on in treating a TBI patient believed to be incompetent (Klein et al. 1983). The legally appropriate procedure is to seek judicial recognition of the family member as the substitute decision maker.

Some TBI patients treated in an emergency may be expected to recover competency during lucid intervals or within a few days. As soon as the patient is able to competently consent to further treatment, such consent should be obtained directly from the patient. For the patient who continues to lack mental capacity for health care decisions, an increasing number of states provide administrative procedures authorized by statute that permit involuntary treatment of the incompetent and refusing mentally ill patients who do not meet current standards for involuntary civil commitment (Hassenfeld and Grumet 1984; Zito et al. 1984). In most jurisdictions, a durable power of attorney agreement permits the next of kin to consent through durable power of attorney statutes (Solnick 1985). In some instances, however, this procedure may not meet judicial challenge. To avoid this problem, a number of states have created health care proxies specifically for advance health care decision making.

Criminal Proceedings

Among criminal defendants, a history of severe brain injury frequently is present. The possibility of TBI must be thoroughly investigated in criminal defendants. For example, Lewis et al. (1986) studied 15 death row inmates who were chosen for examination because of imminent execution rather than evidence of neuropathology. In each case, evidence of severe brain injury and neurological impairment was found.

The causal connection between brain damage and violence, however, remains frustratingly obscure. Violent behavior spans a wide spectrum, from a normal response to a threatening situation to violence emanating directly from an organic brain disorder such as Klüver-Bucy syndrome, hypothalamic tumors, or temporal lobe epilepsy (Strub and Black 1988). Moreover, violent behavior is the result of the interaction between a specific individual and situation. Brain damage or mental illness may or may not play a significant role in this equation. Psychiatrists must acknowledge limitations in their expertise concerning the possible connection between brain damage and violence.

Criminal Intent (*Mens Rea*)

Under the common law, the basic elements of a crime are 1) the mental state or level of intent to commit the act (known as the *mens rea* or "guilty mind"), 2) the act itself or conduct associated with committing the crime (known as *actus reus* or "guilty act"), and 3) a concurrence in time between the guilty act and the guilty mental state (*Bethea v. United States* 1977). To convict a person of a particular crime, the state must prove beyond a reasonable doubt that the defendant committed the criminal act with the requisite intent. All three elements are necessary in order to satisfy the threshold requirements for the imposition of criminal sanctions.

The question of intent is a particularly vexing problem for the courts. For example, everyone would agree that killing another person is deplorable conduct. But should the accidental death of a child in a car accident, the heat-of-passion shooting by a husband of his wife's lover, and the cold blooded murder of a bank teller by a robber all result in the same punishment? The determination of the defendant's intent, or *mens rea,* at the time of the offense is the law's "equalizer" and trigger mechanism for deciding criminal culpability and the appropriate division of retribution. For instance, a person who deliberately plans to commit a crime is more culpable than the person who accidentally commits one.

There are two classes of intent used to categorize *mens rea:* specific and general. Specific intent refers to the *mens rea* in those crimes in which a *further intention is present* beyond that which is identified with the physical act associated with an offense. For instance, the courts will frequently state that the intent necessary for first degree murder includes a "specific intent to kill" or a person might commit an assault "with the intent to rape" (Melton et al. 1987). Unlike general criminal intent, specific criminal intent cannot be presumed from the unlawful criminal act but must be proven independently.

General criminal intent is more elusive. General criminal intent may be presumed from commission of the criminal act. It usually is used by the law to explain criminal liability where a defendant was merely conscious or should have been conscious of his or her physical actions at the time of the offense (Melton et al. 1987). For example, proof that the owner of a boat sold it without first paying off the loan creates a presumption that the owner intended to defraud the lender. In order to deal with the vagueness of these two standards, many states have enacted their own definitions of intent.

Persons with certain mental handicaps or impairments, such as the TBI patient, represent a challenge for prosecutors, defense counsel, and judges in determining what, if any, retribution is justifiable. Mental impairment often raises serious questions about the intent to commit a crime and the appreciation of its consequences.

In addition to *mens rea,* a defendant's mental status can play a deciding role in whether he or she will be ordered to stand trial to face the criminal charges (*Dusky v. United States* 1960), be acquitted of the alleged crime (M'Naughten's Case 1943), be sent to prison, be hospitalized (Mental Aberration and Post Conviction Sanctions 1981), or in some extreme cases, be sentenced to death (*Ford v. Wainwright* 1986). Before any defendant can be criminally prosecuted, the court must be satisfied that the accused is competent to stand trial, that is, he or she understands the charges and is capable of rationally assisting counsel with the defense.

Competency To Stand Trial

In every situation in which competency is a question, the law seeks to reiterate a common theme: that only the acts of a rational individual are to be given recognition by society (*Neely v. United States* 1945). In doing so, the law attempts to reaffirm the integrity of the individual and of society in general.

The legal standard for assessing pretrial competency was established by the United States Supreme Court in *Dusky v. United States* (1960). Throughout involvement with the trial process, the defendant must have "sufficient present ability to consult with his lawyer with a reasonable degree of rational understanding—and whether he has a rational as well as factual understanding of the proceedings against him" (*Dusky v. United States* 1960).

Typically, the impairment that raises the question of the defendant's competence will be associated with a mental disease or defect. A person may be held to be incompetent to stand trial even if there is no mental disease or defect as defined by DSM-IV (American Psychiatric Association 1994). Although the majority of impairments implicated in competency examinations are functional, rather than organic (Reich and Wels 1985), various forms of neuro-psychiatric impairments will typically raise questions about a defendant's competency to stand trial. For example, in *Wilson v. United States* (1968), the defendant had no memory regarding the time of the alleged robbery because of permanent retrograde amnesia. This amnesia was caused by injuries he sustained in an automobile accident that occurred as he was being pursued by the police after the offense. Of the various criteria the court established in determining the defendant's competence to stand trial, the following are directly relevant to the issue of neuropsychiatric impairment:

1. The extent to which the amnesia affected the defendant's ability to consult with and assist his lawyer, and
2. The extent to which the amnesia affected the defendant's ability to testify in his own behalf.

Amnesia by itself is insufficient to support a finding of incompetency to stand trial or not guilty by reason of insanity (Rubinsky and Brandt 1986). Significant impairment of cognitive and communicative abilities, however, is likely to affect the decision regarding a defendant's competency. Nevertheless, it is the actual functional mental capability to meet the minimal standard of trial competency and not the severity of the deficits that will determine whether an individual is cognitively capable of being tried.

Numerous commentators have sought to identify clinical guides that could be used in assessing the general standards established in *Dusky*. One such attempt is the "Competency to Stand Trial Instrument" ("CSTI") designed by the Laboratory of Community Psychiatry (McGarry 1973). The CSTI involves the consideration of 13 functions "related to what is required of a defendant in criminal proceedings in order that he may adequately cope with and protect himself in such proceedings."

The purpose of the CSTI is to standardize, objectify, and qualify relevant criteria for the determination of an individual's competency to stand trial. The presentation of these functions is written so the CSTI can be useful and acceptable to both the legal and the medical professions.

The following are the recommended 13 functions to be assessed:

- Ability to appraise the legal defenses available
- Level of unmanageable behavior
- Quality of relating to attorney
- Ability to plan legal strategy
- Ability to appraise the roles of various participants in the courtroom proceedings
- Understanding of court procedure
- Appreciation of the charges
- Appreciation of the range and nature of possible penalties
- Ability to appraise the likely outcome
- Capacity to disclose to attorney available pertinent facts surrounding the offense
- Capacity to challenge prosecution witnesses realistically
- Capacity to testify relevantly
- Manifestation of self-serving versus self-defeating motivation

The degree of a defendant's impairment in one particular function, however, does not automatically render him or her incompetent. For example, the fact that the defendant is manifesting certain deficits due to damage to the parietal lobe does not necessarily mean that he or she lacks the requisite cognitive ability to aid in the defense at trial (Tranel 1992). The ultimate determination of incompetency is solely for the court to decide (*United States v. David* 1975). Moreover, the impairment must be considered in the context of the particular case or proceeding. Mental impairment may render an individual incompetent to stand trial in a complicated tax fraud case but not incompetent for a misdemeanor trial.

Psychiatrists and psychologists who testify as expert witnesses regarding the effect of TBI on a defendant's competency to stand trial will be most effective if their findings are framed according to the degree to which the defendant is cognitively capable of meeting the standards enunciated in *Dusky*. Use of instruments such as the CSTI to pragmatically illustrate actual functional conformity to competency standards is especially useful.

Insanity Defense

In American jurisprudence, one of the most controversial issues is the insanity defense. Defendants with TBI who are found competent to stand trial may seek acquittal on the basis that they were not criminally responsible for their actions due to insanity at the time the offense was committed.

The vast majority of criminals commit crimes for a variety of reasons, but the law presumes that all of them do so rationally and of their own free will. As a result, the law concludes that they are deserving of some form of punishment. Some offenders, however, are so mentally disturbed in their thinking and behavior that they are thought to be incapable of acting rationally. Under these circumstances, civilized societies have deemed it unjust to punish a "crazy" or insane person (Blackstone 1769). This is in part due to fundamental principles of fairness and morality. Additionally, the punishment of a person who cannot rationally appreciate the consequences of his or her actions thwarts the two major tenets of punishment—retribution and deterrence. Although the insanity defense is rarely used, a successful insanity defense is even rarer.

A generally accepted, precise definition of legal insanity does not exist. Over the years, tests of insanity have been subject to much controversy, modification, and refinement (Brakel et al. 1985, p. 707). The development of the insanity defense standard in the United States has had four basic elements (Table 18–4). The existence of a mental disorder has remained a consistent core of the insanity defense whereas the other elements have varied over time (Brakel et al. 1985, p. 709). Thus there is variability in the insanity defense standard in the United States, depending on which state or jurisdiction has control over the defendant raising the defense.

Following the acquittal by reason of insanity of John Hinckley, Jr., on charges of attempting to assassinate President Reagan and murder others, an outraged public demanded changes in the insanity defense. Federal and state legislation to accomplish that result ensued. Between 1978 and 1985, approximately 75% of all states made some sort of substantive change in their insanity defense (Perlin 1989). A number of states continued to adhere to the American Law Institute insanity defense standard or a version of it. The American Law Institute provides

> A person is not responsible for criminal conduct if at the time of such conduct as a result of mental disease or defect he lacks substantial capacity either to appreciate the criminality [wrongfulness] of his conduct or to conform his conduct to the requirements of law.
>
> As used in this Article, the terms *mental disease* or *mental defect* do not include an abnormality manifested only by repeated criminal or otherwise anti-social conduct (Model Penal Code 4.01 [1962], 10 U.L.A. 490-91 [1974]).

This standard contains both a cognitive and a volitional prong. The cognitive prong derives from the M'Naughten rule, pronounced in England in 1843, exculpating the defendant who does not know the nature and quality of the alleged act or does not know the act was wrong. The volitional prong is a vestige of the irresistible impulse rule, which states that the defendant who is overcome by an irresistible impulse that leads to an alleged act is not responsible for that act. It is on the volitional prong that experts disagree the most in individual criminal cases.

In contrast, defendants tried in a federal court are governed by the insanity defense standard enunciated in the Comprehensive Crime Control Act of 1984 (Pub. L. No. 98-473, 98 Stat 1837). The Comprehensive Crime Control Act provides that insanity is an affirmative defense to all federal crimes in which, at the time of the offense, "the defendant, as a result of a severe mental disease or defect, was unable to appreciate the nature and quality or the wrongfulness of his acts. Mental disease or defect does not otherwise constitute a defense" (Id 402, 98 Stat at 2057). This codification

Table 18–4. Basic elements of insanity defense

Presence of a mental disorder

Presence of a defect of reason

A lack of knowledge of the nature or wrongfulness of the act

An incapacity to refrain from the act

eliminates the volitional or irresistible impulse portion of the insanity defense. That is, it does not allow an insanity defense based on a defendant's inability to conform his or her conduct to the requirements of the law. The defense is now limited to only those defendants who are unable to appreciate the wrongfulness of their acts (i.e., the *cognitive portion* of the defense).

Case example.

A 29-year-old woman sustains a TBI in an automobile accident. She is subsequently diagnosed as having an organic personality syndrome secondary to frontal lobe damage. The patient is taking carbamazepine to control severe affective lability and poor impulse control. During an argument with her boyfriend, she impulsively pulls out a loaded gun from a drawer and kills him. She is charged with second-degree murder. She pleads not guilty by reason of insanity. Experts on both sides agree on the diagnosis. The defense forensic psychiatric expert testifies that the defendant was unable to form any intent to commit murder. Although she knew what was happening, it was like a bystander watching a murder take place. Rather, the shooting was a momentary impulsive act arising from her TBI. The prosecution expert testifies that the defendant has little cognitive impairment. Furthermore, she kept a loaded gun readily available, despite the knowledge of her own poor impulse control. At the moment of the murder, the defendant knew that she was killing her boyfriend. Because the case is heard in federal court, the insanity defense standard enunciated in the Comprehensive Crime Control Act of 1984 is applied. The court finds the defendant guilty of second-degree murder because she was "able to appreciate the nature and quality or the wrongness of her act."

The case example illustrates that the threshold issue in making an insanity determination is not the existence of a mental disease or defect per se, but the lack of substantial mental capacity because of it. Therefore, the lack of capacity due to other causes besides TBI may be sufficient. For instance, mental retardation may represent an adequate basis for the insanity defense under certain circumstances.

Diminished Capacity

It is possible for a person to have the required *mens rea* and yet still not be found criminally responsible. For instance, a defendant's actions may be considered so bizarre that a jury finds the defendant criminally insane and therefore not legally responsible. Yet the defendant's knowledge of the criminal act (e.g., committing a murder) was relatively intact. Accordingly, the law recognizes that there are "shades" of mental impairment that obviously can affect *mens rea* but not necessarily to the extent of completely nullifying it. In recognition of this fact, the concept of "diminished capacity" was developed (Melton et al. 1987).

Diminished capacity permits the defendant to introduce medical and psychological evidence that relates directly to the *mens rea* for the alleged crime, without the necessity of pleading insanity (Melton et al. 1987). For example, in a case of assault with the intent to kill, psychiatric testimony would be permitted to address whether the offender acted with the purpose of committing homicide. When a defendant's *mens rea* for the criminal charge is nullified by psychiatric evidence, the defendant is acquitted only of that charge (Melton et al. 1987). In the above example, the prosecutor may still try to convict the defendant of an offense requiring a lesser *mens rea*, such as manslaughter. TBI patients who commit criminal acts may be eligible for a diminished capacity defense.

The diminished capacity concept has been gradually losing ground largely due to the unevenness of its application by the courts (Brakel et al. 1985, p. 711). In California, where it originated, the use of diminished capacity has been abolished by state statute largely in response to a public outcry against the court's ruling in the notorious "Twinkie defense" of Dan White (Cal Penal Code 28[b] [West 1981]), who was charged with killing the mayor of San Francisco and a county supervisor. Dan White was found guilty by a jury of voluntary manslaughter rather than first degree murder. A diminished capacity defense was used based on testimony that mental distress was aggravated by chemical imbalances caused by the ingestion of large quantities of refined sugar (*People v. White,* 117 Cal App 3d 270, 172 Cal Rptr 612 [1981]).

Guilty But Mentally Ill

In a number of states, an alternative verdict of guilty but mentally ill (GBMI) has been established. Under GBMI statutes, if the defendant pleads not guilty by reason of insanity, this alternative verdict is available to the jury (Slovenko 1982). Under an insanity plea, the verdict may be

- Not guilty
- Not guilty by reason of insanity
- Guilty but mentally ill
- Guilty

The problem with GBMI is that it is an alternative verdict without a difference from finding the defendant plain guilty. The court must still impose a sentence on the convicted person. Although the convicted person will receive psychiatric treatment if necessary, this treatment provision is also available to any other prisoner. Moreover, the frequent unavailability of appropriate psychiatric treatment for prisoners adds an additional element of spuriousness to the GBMI verdict.

Exculpatory and Mitigating Disorders

Psychotic disorders of differing etiology form the most common basis for an insanity defense. But in addition to the major psychiatric and organic brain disorders, a number of other conditions may provide a foundation for an insanity or diminished capacity defense.

▪ **Automatisms.** For conviction of a crime, not only must there be a criminal state of mind (*mens rea*) but also the commission of a prohibited act (*actus reus*). The physical movement necessary to satisfy the *actus reus* requirement must be conscious and volitional. In addition to statutory and common law in many jurisdictions, Section 2.01(2) of the Model Penal Code (1962) specifically excludes from the *actus reus* the following:

(a) a reflex or convulsion; (b) a bodily movement during unconsciousness or sleep; (c) conduct during hypnosis or resulting from
hypnotic suggestion; [and] (d) a bodily movement that otherwise
is not the product of the effort or determination of the actor. . . .

A defense claiming that the commission of a crime was an
involuntary act usually is referred to as an automatism defense.

The classic, although rare, example is the person who commits
an offense while "sleepwalking." Courts have held that such an
individual does not have conscious control of his or her physical
actions and therefore acts involuntarily (*Fain v. Commonwealth*
1879; *H.M. Advocate v. Fraser* 1878). A conscious, reflexive action
carried out under stressful circumstances may qualify for an automatism defense. For example, a driver who is being attacked in his car
by a bee loses control in attempting to swat the insect. The car
strikes a pedestrian who is killed. An automatism defense may exist
to a charge of vehicular homicide. Other situations, relevant to
psychiatry in which the defense might be used, arise when a crime
is committed during a state of altered consciousness caused by a
concussion following a head injury, involuntary ingestion of drugs
or alcohol, hypoxia, metabolic disorders such as hypoglycemia, or
epileptic seizures (Low et al. 1982).

There are, however, limitations to the automatism defense.
Most notably, some courts hold that if the person asserting the
automatism defense was aware of the condition prior to the offense
and failed to take reasonable steps to prevent the criminal occurrence, then the defense is not available. For example, if a defendant
with a known history of uncontrolled epileptic seizures loses control of a car during a seizure and kills someone, that defendant will
not be permitted to assert the defense of automatism.

■ **Intoxication.**   Ordinarily, intoxication is not a defense to a
criminal charge. Because intoxication, unlike mental illness, mental
retardation, and most neuropsychiatric conditions, is usually the
product of a person's own actions, the law is naturally cautious
about viewing it as a complete defense or mitigating factor. Most
states view voluntary alcoholism as relevant to the issue of whether

the defendant possessed the *mens rea* necessary to commit a specific crime or whether there was premeditation in a crime of murder. Generally, however, the mere fact that the defendant was voluntarily intoxicated will not justify a finding of automatism or insanity. A distinct difference does arise when, because of chronic, heavy use of alcohol, the defendant demonstrates an alcohol-induced organic mental disorder, such as alcohol hallucinosis, withdrawal delirium, amnestic disorder, or dementia associated with alcoholism. If competent psychiatric evidence is presented that an alcohol-related neuropsychiatric disorder caused significant cognitive or volitional impairment, a defense of insanity or diminished capacity could be upheld.

❙ **Temporal lobe seizures.**   Another "mental state" defense occasionally raised by defendants regarding assault-related crimes is that the assaultive behavior was involuntarily precipitated by abnormal electrical patterns in the brain. This condition is frequently diagnosed as temporal lobe epilepsy (Devinsky and Bear 1984). Episodic dyscontrol syndrome (Elliot 1978; Monroe 1978) has also been advanced as a neuropsychiatric condition causing involuntary aggression. Studies have hypothesized that there are "centers of aggression" in the temporal lobe or limbic system—primarily the amygdala. This hypothesis has promoted the idea that sustained aggressive behavior by these persons may be primarily the product of an uncontrollable, randomly occurring, abnormal brain dysrhythmia. Hence the legal argument is raised that these individuals should not be held accountable for their actions. Despite its simplicity and occasional success in the courts, there is little empirically significant data to support this theory at this time (Blumer 1984).

❙ **Metabolic disorders.**   Defenses based on metabolic disorders have also been tried. The so-called Twinkie defense was used as part of a successful diminished capacity defense of Dan White in the murders of San Francisco Mayor George Mosconi and Supervisor Harvey Milk. This defense was based on the theory that the ingestion of large amounts of sugar contributed to a state of temporary insanity (*People v. White* 1981). The forensic psychiatric report stated that the defendant had been "filling himself up with Twinkies and Coca-Cola" (Blinder 1981–1982, p. 16). After specifying a number of factors that contributed to the murders, the forensic examiner concluded with the following opinion concerning Dan White's ingestion of certain food:

> Finally, there is much evidence to suggest recently recognized physiological aberrations consequent to consumption of noxious edibles by susceptibles. There are cases in the literature challenged with large quantities of refined sugar. Furthermore, there are studies of cerebral allergic reactions to the chemicals in highly processed foods; some studies have documented a marked reduction in violent and antisocial behavior in "career criminals" upon the elimination of these substances from their diet, as well as the production of rage reactions in susceptible individuals when challenged by the offending food substances. For these reasons, I would suggest a repeat electroencephalogram preceded by a glucose-tolerance test, as well as a clinical challenge of Mr. White's mental functions with known food antigens, in a controlled setting. (Blinder 1981–1982, pp. 21–22)

Hypoglycemic states also may be associated with significant psychiatric impairment (Kaplan and Sadock 1989). The brain is dependent on a steady supply of glucose through the blood stream. When the glucose level drops significantly, the brain has no backup energy source to compensate. When this occurs, metabolism naturally slows down and cerebral function is impaired. Because the cerebral cortex and parts of the cerebellum metabolize glucose at the highest rate, they are the first to show impairment when there is an energy depletion (Wilson et al. 1991). When a substantial depletion occurs, a wide variety of responses may occur, including episodic and repetitive dyscontrol, temporary amnesia, depression, and hostility with spontaneous recovery (quick recovery following the consumption of appropriate nutrients). The degree of mental abnormality associated with hypoglycemic states varies from mild to severe according to the blood glucose level. It is the degree of disturbance, not the mere presence of an etiologic metabolic component, that determines a mental state defense. This principle also applies to mental dysfunctions produced by disorders originating in the hepatic, renal, adrenal, and neuroendocrine systems (premenstrual syndrome) (Parry and Berga 1991).

Civil Litigation

Expert Testimony

The ensuing civil litigation in brain injury cases generally requires the evaluation and testimony of psychiatrists as well as neurologists, psychologists, neuropsychologists, and other mental health professionals. Psychiatrists can become involved in litigation as witnesses in one of two ways: as treaters or as forensic experts. An increasing number of psychiatrists are practicing the subspecialty of *forensic psychiatry,* which is defined as

> a subspecialty of psychiatry in which scientific and clinical expertise is applied to legal issues in legal contexts embracing civil, criminal, correctional or legislative matters. (American Academy of Psychiatry and the Law 1987, p. 1)

The Treating Clinician

Psychiatrists who venture into the legal arena must be aware of the fundamentally different roles that exist between a treating psychiatrist and the forensic psychiatric expert. Treatment and expert roles do not mix. For example, unlike the orthopedist who possesses objective data such as the X ray of a broken limb to demonstrate orthopedic damages in court, the treating psychiatrist must rely heavily on the subjective reporting of the patient. In the treatment context, psychiatrists are interested primarily in the patient's perception of his or her difficulties, not necessarily the objective reality. As a consequence, many treating psychiatrists do not speak to third parties or check pertinent records to gain additional information about patients or to corroborate their statements. The law, however, is interested only in that which can reasonably be established by facts. Uncorroborated, subjective patient data is frequently attacked in court as speculative, self-serving, and unreliable. The treating psychiatrist usually is not well equipped to counter these charges.

Credibility issues also abound. The treating psychiatrist is, and must be, a total ally of the patient. This bias toward the patient is a proper treatment stance that fosters the therapeutic alliance. Furthermore, to be an effective therapist, the psychiatrist should "like" the patient reasonably well. No practitioner can treat a patient for very long whom he or she fundamentally dislikes. Moreover, the psychiatrist looks for mental disorders to treat. This again is an appropriate bias for the treating psychiatrist.

When testifying in court, a treating psychiatrist must possess credibility. Opposing counsel will take every opportunity to portray the treating psychiatrist as a subjective mouthpiece for the patient-litigant—which may or may not be true. Also court testimony by the treating psychiatrist may compel the disclosure of information that may not be legally privileged, but nonetheless is viewed as intimate and confidential by the patient. This disclosure by the previously trusted therapist is bound to cause psychological damage to the therapeutic relationship (Strasburger 1987). In addition, psychiatrists must be careful to inform patients about the consequences of releasing treatment information, particularly in legal matters. Section 4, Annotation 2 of the Principles of Medical Ethics with Annotations Especially Applicable to Psychiatry (American Psychiatric Association 1989) states

> The continuing duty of the psychiatrist to protect the patient includes fully apprising him/her of the connotations of waiving the privilege of privacy. This may become an issue when the patient is being investigated by a government agency, is applying for a position, or is involved in legal action. (p. 6)

Finally, when the treating psychiatrist testifies concerning the patient's need for further treatment, a conflict of interest is readily apparent. In making such treatment prognostications, the psychiatrist stands to benefit economically from the recommendation of further treatment. Although this may not be the intention of the psychiatrist at all, opposing counsel is sure to point out that the psychiatrist has a financial interest in the case.

The American Academy of Psychiatry and the Law (1987), in its ethics statement, advises that

> A treating psychiatrist should generally avoid agreeing to be an expert witness or to perform an evaluation of his patient for legal purposes because a forensic evaluation usually requires that other people be interviewed and testimony may adversely affect the therapeutic relationship. (p. 4)

The treating psychiatrist should attempt to remain solely in a treatment role. If it becomes necessary to testify on behalf of the patient, the treating psychiatrist should testify only as a fact witness, not as an expert witness. As a fact witness, the psychiatrist will be asked to describe the number and length of visits, diagnosis, and treatment. Generally, no opinion evidence will be requested concerning causation of the injury or extent of damages. In some jurisdictions, however, the court may convert a fact witness into an expert at the time of trial. Psychiatrists must remain ever mindful of the many double agent roles that can develop when mixing psychiatry and litigation (Simon 1992a).

The Forensic Expert

The forensic expert, on the other hand, is usually free from these encumbrances. During forensic evaluation, no doctor-patient relationship is created with a treatment bias toward the patient. The expert can review a variety of records and speak to a number of people who know the litigant. Furthermore, the forensic expert, because of a clear appreciation of the litigation context and the absence of treatment bias, is not easily distracted from considering exaggeration or malingering. Finally, the forensic psychiatrist is not placed in a conflict of interest position of recommending treatment from which he or she would personally benefit. The forensic expert, however, is frequently viewed by opposing counsel as a "hired gun."

Particularly in evaluating the TBI patient, both the treating psychiatrist and the expert psychiatric witness will need to coordinate their efforts with other medical and nonmedical professionals. Obtaining additional information from others who are also assisting the patient creates both good treatment and credible testimony.

The Forensic Psychiatric Evaluation of the TBI Claimant

The forensic psychiatric evaluation of the TBI *claimant* differs in a number of significant ways from the traditional psychiatric evaluation of the TBI *patient*. In the litigation context, the distinction between the role of treating psychiatrist and that of forensic evaluator must be firmly maintained. Problems invariably arise for the clinician when these roles are confused. The psychiatrist who enters the legal arena must understand that equities usually exist on both sides of a case; otherwise it would probably not have been brought to litigation in the first place. The fact that opposing experts disagree does not necessarily mean that one side or the other is wrong. The opinions of opposing experts should be carefully considered.

Team Approach

The comprehensive forensic psychiatric evaluation requires cooperation with a number of other practitioners and specialists. Usually, the forensic psychiatrist who is evaluating the TBI claimant will require the input of a neurologist, a psychologist, and an internist or general practitioner. Depending on the complexities of the case, a number of other disciplines may need to be consulted. The forensic evaluator also must consider the findings of other examinations performed at the request of opposing counsel. The burgeoning number of ever more complicated brain studies currently available make consultation with a qualified neurologist virtually a necessity in cases involving claims of brain injury.

No Doctor-Patient Relationship

The psychiatrist should inform the claimant at the time of the examination that no doctor-patient relationship will be formed. That is, the psychiatrist will not treat the claimant in any fashion. The psychiatrist should explain that he or she has been retained (name the specific party) to perform an independent psychiatric examination. The sole purpose of the examination is to provide information to the party retaining the psychiatrist.

No Confidentiality

The claimant must be informed that, unlike the usual doctor-patient relationship, confidentiality surrounding the forensic evaluation may not exist. Once the retaining attorney decides to disclose the findings of the evaluation in litigation, the information will be available to both sides and will likely become a public record.

Standard Diagnostic Schema

The diagnostic evaluation of TBI claimants should be made according to the multiaxial classification system contained in DSM-IV. All five axes should be employed. Axis I permits the clinician to consider the major clinical psychiatric syndromes, either single or multiple. It is not unusual for the TBI claimant to have concurrent Axis I diagnoses. For example, the presence of alcohol or drug abuse may have directly contributed to the brain injury. Concurrent Axis I disorders may have preexisted or been exacerbated by the brain injury.

Axis II forces the clinician to consider personality disorders that are often overlooked or ignored in the forensic evaluation of a claimant. The occurrence of significant brain injuries is high among the violent criminal population where a higher incidence of antisocial personality disorders exists (Lewis et al. 1986; Petursson and Gudjonsson 1981).

On Axis III, the relationship of medical disorders and their treatments to the patient's clinical presentation on Axis I must be carefully evaluated. TBI claimants may have a number of injuries requiring extensive pharmacotherapy that may further complicate the clinical picture. Moreover, a host of medical disorders may present or have associated symptoms of cerebral dysfunction. Prior brain injuries or preexisting central nervous system disorders must be considered. For example, young adults who have a history of learning disabilities or attention-deficit disorder are likely to develop serious incapacity when they sustain a TBI.

Axis IV permits the evaluation of psychosocial and environmental problems occurring within the year preceding the current evaluation, which may have contributed to the development of a new mental disorder, recurrence of a prior mental disorder or have become a focus of treatment. Posttraumatic stress disorder is an exception to the 1-year rule. The search for multiple psychosocial stressors must be carefully conducted. It is the rare claimant who has only one psychosocial stressor impacting on his or her life. A brain injury often occurs in the context of other preexisting psychosocial stressors, such as sustained interpersonal difficulties, financial problems, occupational distress, or other personal losses.

Finally, functional impairment should be assessed on Axis V according to the DSM-IV Global Assessment of Functioning Scale in combination with other standard methods of evaluation of psychiatric impairment discussed below.

Collateral Sources of Information

In the treatment situation, the psychiatrist relies almost exclusively on the subjective reporting of the patient. The patient is presumed to be candid and without conscious hidden agendas. In litigation, however, the claimant must naturally be expected to favor his or her own legal case. The possibility of malingering must always be kept in mind (Table 18–5). Malingering is not limited to the fabrication of symptoms. More often, malingering is manifested by the exaggeration of symptoms. Thus the psychiatrist must consider a broad array of information.

Usually, during the course of legal discovery by both parties to the suit, a great deal of information is developed. The forensic examiner should request that the retaining lawyer provide all relevant information. Proceeding to court with incomplete information will likely be exposed by opposing counsel, undercutting the psychiatrist's testimony and irreparably damaging the claimant's case. The forensic psychiatrist should review all data carefully before coming to a conclusion. The collateral source information list in Table 18–6, although not exhaustive, indicates major areas for inquiry.

Mental Status Examination

In evaluating the mental status of the claimant, the psychiatrist must conduct a thorough and reliable mental status examination. Usually, it is better to conduct the examination in divided sessions over the course of two days because of, among other things, possible fluctuations in the mental status of the TBI claimant. The practice of performing a perfunctory mental status examination or relying solely on the assessment of the neuropsychologist is unwarranted. Neuropsychological assessment can be a very valuable adjunct to the neuropsychiatric assessment of the TBI claimant (Becker and Kay 1986). Nevertheless, the psychiatrist will have little basis for critically reviewing the neuropsychological findings unless he or she can perform a competent mental status examination. Moreover, the mental status assessment is an integral part of the psychiatric

Table 18–5. Increased index of suspicion for malingering

Litigation context (financial compensation, evading criminal prosecution)

Marked discrepancy between clinical findings and subjective complaints

Lack of cooperation with evaluation and treatment

Antisocial personality traits or disorder

Overdramatization of complaints

History of recurrent accidents or injuries

Evidence of self-induced injuries

Vaguely defined symptoms

Poor work history

Unable to work but retains capacity for pleasurable activities examination that cannot be delegated to others. The mental status examination as described by Strub and Black (1988) provides a scored, comprehensive, reliable format for mental status evaluation.

The role of neuropsychological testing must be critically evaluated in each case. Neuropsychological tests are not totally objective. The qualifications and experience of the neuropsychologist are critical variables. Tests of behavior in neuropsychological testing are subject to the control of the person performing the task. Thus the consideration of motivation is critical. Also low test scores may be caused by factors other than brain damage (see Table 18–7). For example, the impact of somatic therapies and psychopathology as confounding factors in neuropsychological testing has been noted recently (Cullum et al. 1991; Finlayson and Bird 1991). Doctors, not tests, make diagnoses. A neuropsychological test score, by itself, cannot point to a specific cause of the litigant's injury. In litigation, causation is a matter for the finder of fact to determine.

A base rate occurrence of neuropsychological deficits typically exists in the normal population. If impairments are noted without evaluation of the claimant's prior history and level of neuropsychological functioning, overinterpretation of the test data is likely. The critical review of school and work records to determine

---

Table 18–6.   Collateral information sources

Other physicians and health care providers (reports, direct discussions)
Hospital records
Family
Other third parties
Military records
School records
Police records
Witness information
Work records
Work products—letters, work projects
Legal discovery—depositions, legal documents
Prior medical and psychiatric records
Prior psychological and neuropsychological evaluations

---

the prior level of intellectual functioning is important in establishing baseline performance. Neuropsychological impairments observed among a normal population increase with the age of the population. Lower IQ score and slower responses are also associated with normal aging.

Brain Injury Mimics

A number of psychiatric disorders may mimic TBI. Some of the more common TBI mimics include conversion, factitious, somatization, and depressive disorders presenting with symptoms of neurological and cerebral dysfunction. Conversion disorder symptoms classically mimic neurological disease. Dissociative symptoms may present with amnesia or atypical memory loss. Depressive pseudodementia is a commonly recognized clinical disorder in the elderly. Posttraumatic stress disorder manifesting symptoms of difficulty in concentration and psychogenic amnesia may also mimic brain injury. Similarly, anxiety disorders may be associated with memory complaints secondary to the inability to concentrate. On the other hand, TBI may produce anxiety and depression, so these may occur together with TBI.

To complicate matters, TBI litigants may be receiving psychoactive substances, either for their symptoms of brain injury or for concurrent psychiatric and medical disorders or both. Neuroleptics,

---

Table 18–7.   Major factors affecting neuropsychological test findings

Original endowment
Environment (e.g., education, occupation, and life experiences)
Motivation (effort)
Physical health
Psychological distress
Psychiatric disorders (e.g., affective and somatoform disorders)
Medications (e.g., anticonvulsants and psychotropics)
Qualifications and experience of neuropsychologist
Errors in scoring
Errors in interpretation

---

antidepressants, lithium, and particularly benzodiazepines can produce side effects that mimic neurological and brain disorders. Psychoactive substances may produce serious memory difficulties, either directly on brain chemistry or indirectly through sedation. Unfortunately, it is common for practitioners to prescribe two or more drugs simultaneously, particularly when the claimant appears refractory to treatment during the course of litigation. As a result, medications may interact to produce a host of side effects that involve the central nervous system. Psychoactive drug abuse is distressingly common in these cases, especially when the TBI litigant complains of persistent pain. Narcotics and barbiturates, especially in combination with nonnarcotic pain medications, are commonly abused.

Comorbidity and drug effects also must be considered when evaluating the results of neuropsychological test assessments. Questionable results will be obtained in the neuropsychological testing if the effects of concurrent psychiatric disorders and medications are not considered.

Disability Determinations

In addition to the psychiatric diagnosis, an assessment of functional impairment and disability must be made. In litigation, it is the degree of functional impairment, not the psychiatric diagnosis per se, that determines the amount of the monetary damage award. The psychiatrist also must understand the difference between impairment and disability. An impaired individual may not necessarily be disabled. Psychiatric impairment is considered disabling only when a psychiatric disorder limits a person's capacity to meet the demands of living. The American Medical Association's Guides to the Evaluation of Permanent Impairment gives the example of the impact of the loss of the fifth finger on the left hand to illustrate this point (American Medical Association 1993, pp. 1–2). For a bank president, the occupational impact will likely be negligible. The concert pianist, however, will probably be totally disabled.

Similarly, a TBI patient may have moderate impairment but only mild disability in social or occupational functioning due to the development of compensatory coping mechanisms. On the other hand, practically every psychiatric clinician has seen the TBI patient who has little or no actual impairment but nevertheless is seriously disabled. This latter situation is particularly common in the litigation context. For claimants presenting such a picture, the psychiatrist should pay particular attention to the possible presence of concurrent Axis IV psychosocial and environmental problems, comorbidity, polypharmacy, and the effect of litigation on the clinical presentation of the TBI claimant.

Standard impairment assessment methods should be used in combination with the DSM-IV Axis V global assessment of functioning. The credible psychiatric assessment of functional impairment will avoid strictly subjective, idiosyncratic, ex cathedra pronouncements about the claimant's impairment and the need for future treatment. Instead, whenever possible, the TBI claimant's functional impairment and future treatment needs should be evaluated according to the American Medical Association's Guide to the Evaluation of Permanent Impairment (American Medical Association 1993, pp. 227–233). The guide closely follows the Social Security Administration's guidelines for the assessment of disability. Assessment of permanent impairment should not be made until maximum medical improvement has been achieved.

Conclusions

The ethical and legal issues surrounding the treatment and management of the TBI patient are challenging and complex. The legally informed psychiatrist is in a stronger position to provide good clinical care to the TBI patient within the burgeoning regulation of psychiatry by the courts and through governmental legislation. Moreover, psychiatrists will be increasingly required to testify in court concerning TBI patients. Familiarity and comfort with the role of fact or expert witness will facilitate competent psychiatric testimony.

References

American Academy of Psychiatry and the Law: Ethical Guidelines for the Practice of Forensic Psychiatry. Baltimore, MD, American Academy of Psychiatry and the Law, Adopted May 1987 (Revised October 1989 and 1991)

American Medical Association: Guidelines for the appropriate use of do-not-resuscitate orders (Council on Ethical and Judicial Affairs). JAMA 265:1868–1871, 1991

American Medical Association: Guidelines on cardiopulmonary resuscitation and emergency cardiac care, part VIII: ethical considerations in resuscitation. JAMA 268:2282–2288, 1992

American Medical Association: Guides to the Evaluation of Permanent Impairment, 4th Edition. Chicago, IL, American Medical Association, 1993, pp 1–2, 291–302

American Medical News, April 8, 1991, p 14

American Psychiatric Association: Opinions of the Ethics Committee on the Principles of Medical Ethics with Annotations Especially Applicable to Psychiatry. Washington, DC, American Psychiatric Press, 1989

American Psychiatric Association: Diagnostic and Statistical Manual of Mental Disorders, 4th Edition. Washington, DC, American Psychiatric Association, 1994

Aponte v United States, 582 FSupp 555, 566–69 (D PR 1984)

Appelbaum PS, Lidz CW, Meisel A: Informed Consent: Legal Theory and Clinical Practice. New York, Oxford University Press, 1987, p 84

Becker B, Kay GC: Neuropsychological consultation in psychiatric practice. Psychiatr Clin North Am 9:255–265, 1986

Benesch K: Legal issues in determining competence to make treatment decisions, in Legal Implications of Hospital Policies and Practices. Edited by Miller RD. San Francisco, CA, Jossey-Bass, 1989, pp 97–105

Bethea v United States, 365 A2d 64, (DC 1976) cert denied, 433 US 911 (1977)

Bisbing SB: Competency and Capacity in Legal Medicine, 2nd Edition. St. Louis, MO, Mosby Year Book, 1991

Black HC: Black's Law Dictionary, 6th Edition. St Paul, MN, West Publishing, 1990, p 284

Blackstone W: Commentaries vol. 4, 24–25 (1769); Coke E: Third Institute 6 (1680)

Blinder M: My examination of Dan White. American Journal of Forensic Psychiatry 2:12–22, 1981–1982

Blumer D: Psychiatric Aspects of Epilepsy. Washington, DC, American Psychiatric Press, 1984

Brakel SJ, Parry J, Weiner BA: The Mentally Disabled and the Law, 3rd Edition. Chicago, IL, American Bar Foundation, 1985, p 370

Carlson RJ: Frontal lobe lesions masquerading as psychiatric disturbances. Canadian Psychiatric Association Journal 22:315–318, 1977

Cody P: Psychiatric "living will" gaining popularity as alternative to involuntary commitment. Psychiatric News, November 15, 1991, pp 9, 21

Cruzan v Director, Missouri Department of Health, 110 S Ct 284 (1990)

Cullum CM, Heaton RK, Grant I: Psychogenic factors influencing neuropsychological performance: Somatoform disorders, factitious disorders and malingering, in Forensic Neuropsychology: Legal and Scientific Bases. Edited by Doerr HO, Carlin AS. New York, Guilford, 1991, pp 141–171

Devinsky P, Bear DM: Varieties of aggressive behavior in patients with temporal lobe epilepsy. Am J Psychiatry 141:651–655, 1984

Dusky v United States, 362 U.S. 402 (1960)

Dyer AR: Ethics and Psychiatry: Toward Professional Definition. Washington, DC, American Psychiatric Press, 1988

Elliot FA: Neurological aspects of antisocial behavior, in The Psychopath. Edited by Reid WH. New York, Brunner/Mazel, 1978

Emanuel EJ, Emanuel LL: Proxy decision making for incompetent patients—an ethical and empirical analysis. JAMA 267:2067–2071, 1992

Fain v Commonwealth, 78 Ky 183 (1879)

Finlayson MAJ, Bird DR: Psychopathology and neuropsychological deficit, in Forensic Neuropsychology: Legal and Scientific Bases. Edited by Doerr HO, Carlin AS. New York, Guilford, 1991

Folstein MF, Folstein SE, McHugh PR: "Mini-Mental State": a practical method of grading the cognitive state of patients for the clinician. J Psychiatr Res 12:189–198, 1975

Ford v Wainwright, 477 US 399 (1986); Note, The Eighth Amendment and the Execution of the Presently Incompetent, 32 Stan L Rev:765 (1980)

Frasier v Department of Health and Human Resources, 500 So2d 858, 864 (La Ct App 1986)

Gulf S I R Co v Sullivan, 155 Miss 1, 119 So 501 (1928)

Gutheil TG, Appelbaum PS: Substituted judgment and the physician's ethical dilemma: with special reference to the problem of the psychiatric patient. J Clin Psychiatry 41:303–305, 1980

Hassenfeld IN, Grumet B: A study of the right to refuse treatment. Bull Am Acad Psychiatry Law 12:65–74, 1984

H.M. Advocate v Fraser, 4 Couper 70 (1878)

In re Boyer, 636 P2d 1085 1089 (Utah 1981)

In re Jobes, 108 NJ 394 (1987)

Jehovah's Witnesses v King County Hospital, 278 FSupp 488 (WD Wash 1967), affd, 390 US 598 (1968)

Kaplan HI, Sadock BJ: Comprehensive Textbook of Psychiatry, 5th Edition, Vol 2. Baltimore, MD, Williams & Wilkins, 1989, pp 1219–1220

Klein J, Onek J, Macbeth J: Seminar on Law in the Practice of Psychiatry. Washington, DC, Klein & Farr, 1983, p 28

LaPuma J, Orentlicher D, Moss RJ: Advance directives on admission: clinical implications and analysis of the Patient Self-Determination Act of 1990. JAMA 266:402–405, 1991

Lewis DO, Pincus JH, Feldman M, et al: Psychiatric, neurological and psychoeducational characteristics of 15 death row inmates in the United States. Am J Psychiatry 143:838–845, 1986

Low P, Jeffries J, Bonnie R: Criminal Law: Cases and Materials. Mineola, NY, The Foundation Press, 1982, pp 152–154

Luce JM: Ethical principles in critical care. JAMA 263:696–700, 1990

March FH, Staver A: Physician authority for unilateral DNR orders. J Leg Med 12:115–165, 1991

McGarry AL: Competency to Stand Trial and Mental Illness, a monograph sponsored by the Center for Studies of Crime and Delinquency, National Institute of Mental Health, DHEW Pub. No. (HSM) 73-9105, Rockville, MD, 1973

Meek v City of Loveland, 85 Colo 346, 276 P 30 (1929)

Melton GB, Petrila J, Poythress NG, et al: Psychological evaluation for the courts. New York, Guilford, 1987, p 128

Mental Aberration and Post Conviction Sanctions, 15 Suffolk UL Rev:1219 (1981); State v Hehman, 110 Ariz 459, 520 P2d 507 (1974); Commonwealth v Robinson, 494 Pa 372, 431 A2d 901 (1981)

Mishkin B: Decisions in Hospice. Arlington, VA, The National Hospice Organization, 1985

Mishkin B: Determining the capacity for making health care decisions, in Issues in Geriatric Psychiatry (Advances in Psychosomatic Medicine Series, Vol 19). Edited by Billig N, Rabins PV. Basel, Karger, 1989, pp 151–166

M'Naughten's Case, 10 Cl. F. 200, 8 Eng. Rep. 718 (H.L. 1943); United States v. Brawner, 471 F2d 969 (DC Cir 1972)

Monroe RR: Brain Dysfunction in Aggressive Criminals. Lexington, MA, Lexington Books, 1978

Neely v United States, 150 F2d 977 (DC Cir), cert denied 326 US 768 (1945)

Orentlicher D: The illusion of patient choice in end-of-life decisions. JAMA 267:2101–2104, 1992

Overman W, Stoudemire A: Guidelines for legal and financial counseling of Alzheimer's disease patients and their families. Am J Psychiatry 145:1495–1500, 1988

Parry JW, Beck JC: Revisiting the civil commitment/involuntary treatment stalemate using limited guardianship, substituted judgment and different due process considerations: A work in progress. Medical and Physical Disability Law Reporter 14:102–114, 1990

Parry BL, Berga SL: Neuroendocrine correlates of behavior during the menstrual cycle, in Psychiatry, Vol 3. Edited by Cavenar JO. Philadelphia, PA, JB Lippincott, 1991, pp 1–22

People v White, 117 Cal App 3d 270, 172 Cal Rptr 612 (1981)

Perlin MJ: Mental Disability Law: Civil and Criminal, Vol 3. Charlottesville, NC, Michie, 1989, p 404

Perr IN: The clinical considerations of medication refusal. Legal Aspects of Psychiatric Practice 1:5–8, 1984

Petursson H, Gudjonsson GH: Psychiatric aspects of homicide. Acta Psychiatr Scand 64:363–372, 1981

Planned Parenthood v Danforth, 428 US 52, 74 (1976) (abortion); Ill Ann Stat ch. 91 1/2, para 3-501(a) (Smith-Hurd Supp 1990) (mental health counseling)

President's Commission for the Study of Ethical Problems in Medicine and Biomedical and Behavioral Research: Making Health Care Decisions, Vol 1. (A report on the ethical and legal implications of informed consent in the patient-practitioner relationship.) Washington, DC, Superintendent of Documents, October 1982

Regan M: Protective services for the elderly: commitment, guardianship, and alternatives. William & Mary Law Review 13:569, 570–573, 1972

Reich J, Wels J: Psychiatric diagnosis and competency to stand trial. Compr Psychiatry 26:421–432, 1985

Rennie v Klein, 462 FSupp 1131 (DNJ 1978), modified, 653 F2d 836 (3d cir 1981), vacated, 458 US 1119 (1982), on remand, 720 F2d 266 (3d Cir 1983)

Rozovsky FA: Consent to Treatment: A Practical Guide. Boston, MA, Little, Brown, 1984, pp 87–122

Rubinsky EW, Brandt J: Amnesia and criminal law: a clinical overview. Behavioral Sciences and the Law 4:27–46, 1986

Ruchs VR: The "rationing" of medical care. N Engl J Med 311:1572–1573, 1984

Sale B, Powell DM, Van Duizend R: Disabled Persons and the Law: State Legislative Issues, 1982

Scaria v St. Paul Fire & Marine Ins Co, 68 Wis2d 1, 227 NW2d 647 (1975)

Schloendorff v Society of New York Hospital, 211 NY 125, 105 NE 92 (1914), overruled, Bing v Thunig, 2 NY2d 656, 143 NE2d 3, 163 NYS2d 3 (1957)

Schwartz HR: Do not resuscitate orders: The impact of guidelines on clinical practice, in Geriatric Psychiatry and the Law. Edited by Rosner R, Schwartz HR. New York, Plenum, 1987, p 91

Simon RI: Beyond the doctrine of informed consent—a clinician's perspective. Journal for the Expert Witness, The Trial Attorney, The Trial Judge 4(Fall):23–25, 1989

Simon RI: Clinical Psychiatry and the Law, 2nd Edition. Washington, DC, American Psychiatric Press, 1992a

Simon RI: Clinical Psychiatry and the Law, 2nd Edition. Washington, DC, American Psychiatric Press, 1992b; citing, Addington v Texas, 441 US 418 (1979)

Slovenko R: Commentaries on psychiatry and the law: "Guilty but Mentally Ill." J Psychiatry Law 10:541–555, 1982

Smith JT: Medical Malpractice: Psychiatric Care. Colorado Springs, CO, Shephards McGraw-Hill, 1986, pp 178–179

Solnick PB: Proxy consent for incompetent nonterminally ill adult patients. J Leg Med 6:1–49, 1985

Strasburger LH: "Crudely, without any finesse": the defendant hears his psychiatric evaluation. Bull Am Acad Psychiatry Law 15:229–233, 1987

Strub RL, Black FW: Neurobehavioral Disorders: A Clinical Approach. Philadelphia, PA, FA Davis, 1988

The Legal Status of Adolescents 1980, U.S. Department of Health & Human Services, 41 (1981)

Tranel D: Functional neuroanatomy: neuropsychological correlates of cortical and subcortical damage, in American Psychiatric Press Textbook of Neuropsychiatry, 2nd Edition. Edited by Hales RE, Yudofsky SC. Washington, DC, American Psychiatric Press, 1992, pp 70–75

Uniform Guardianship and Protective Proceeding Act (UGPPA) 5–101

United States v David, 511 F2d 355 (DC Cir 1975)

Weir RF, Gostin L: Decisions to abate life-sustaining treatment for nonautonomous patients: ethical standards and legal liability for physicians after Cruzan. JAMA 264:1846–1853, 1990

Wilson v Lehman, 379 SW2d 478, 479 (Ky 1964)

Wilson v United States, 391 F2d 460, 463 (DC Cir 1968)

Wilson JD, Braunwald E, Isselbacher KJ: Harrison's Principles of Internal Medicine, 12th Edition, Vol 2. New York, McGraw-Hill, 1991, p 1759

Zito JM, Lentz SL, Routt WW, et al: The treatment review panel: a solution to treatment refusal? Bull Am Acad Psychiatry Law 12:349–358, 1984

_____ *Appendix 18–1* _____

Some Areas of Law in Which Competency Is an Issue

Civil law
Act in public or professional capacity
Authorize disclosure of medical records
Consent to treatment
Contract
Guardianship—care for one's self and property
Make a will
Obtain a driver's license
Receive benefits
Retain private counsel
Sue or be sued
Testify in court
Vote

Criminal law
Assume responsibility for a criminal act
Be executed
Consent to sexual intercourse
Entertain premeditation or "specific intent" of a crime
Make a confession
Make a plea
Provide testimony in court
Stand trial
To be sentenced
Waive the insanity defense
Waive the right to counsel

Family law
  Adopt
  Divorce
  Marry
  Terminate parental relations with a child

Adapted from Bisbing SB: *Competency and Capacity in Legal Medicine,* 2nd Edition. St. Louis, MO, Mosby Year Book, 1991.

Appendix 18–2

Living Will Declaration, Health Care Proxy, and Durable Power of Attorney Forms

Living Will Declaration

INSTRUCTIONS: Consult this column for help and guidance.

To My Family, Doctors, and All Those Concerned with My Care

This declaration sets forth your directions regarding medical treatment.

I, _____ , being of sound mind, make this statement as a directive to be followed if I become unable to participate in decisions regarding my medical care.

If I should be in an incurable or irreversible mental or physical condition with no reasonable expectation of recovery, I direct my attending physician to withhold or withdraw treatment that merely prolongs my dying. I further direct that treatment be limited to measures to keep me comfortable and to relieve pain.

You have the right to refuse treatment you do not want, and you may request the care you do want.

These directions express my legal right to refuse treatment. Therefore I expect my family, doctors, and everyone concerned with my care to regard themselves as legally and morally bound to act in accord with my wishes, and in so doing to be free of any legal liability for having followed my directions.

You may list specific treatment you do <u>not</u> want. For example:

I especially do not want: _____

_____

_____

Cardiac resuscitation Mechanical respiration Artificial feeding/fluids by tubes

_____

_____

Otherwise, your general statement, top right, will stand for your wishes.

_____

_____

_____

You may want to add instructions for care you <u>do</u> want—for example, pain medication; or that you prefer to die at home if possible.

Other instructions/comments: _____

_____

_____

_____

_____

If you want, you can name someone to see that your wishes are carried out, but you do not have to do this.

Proxy designation clause: Should I become unable to communicate my instructions as stated above, I designate the following person to act in my behalf:

Name _____

Address _____

If the person I have named above is unable to act in my behalf, I authorize the following person to do so:

Name _____

Address _____

Sign and date here in the presence of two adult witnesses, who should also sign.

Signed _____

Date _____

Witness _____

Witness _____

Keep the signed original with your personal papers at home. Give signed copies to your doctors, to your family, and to your proxy.

Reprinted by permission of the Society for the Right to Die, 250 West 57th Street, New York, NY 10107.

Durable Power of Attorney for Health Care

Information About This Document

This is an important legal document. Before signing this document it is vital for you to know and understand these facts:

- This document gives the person you name as your agent the power to make health care decisions for you if you cannot make decisions for yourself.
- Even after you have signed this document, you have the right to make health care decisions for yourself so long as you are able to do so. In addition, even after you have signed the document, no treatment may be given to you or stopped over your objection.
- You may state in this document any types of treatment that you do not desire and those that you want to make sure you receive.
- You have the right to revoke (take away) the authority of your agent by notifying your agent or your health care provider orally or in writing of this desire.
- If there is anything in this document that you do not understand, you should ask for an explanation.

You will be given a copy of this document after you have signed it, and a copy will be sent to each person you name as your agent or alternative agent.

Durable Power of Attorney for Health Care

I, _____

hereby appoint

_____	_____
Name	**Home address**
_____	_____
Home telephone number	**Work telephone number**

as my agent to make health care decisions for me if and when I am unable to make my own health care decisions. This gives my agent the power to consent to giving, withholding, or stopping any health care, treatment, service, or diagnostic procedure. My agent also has the authority to talk with health care personnel, get information, and sign forms necessary to carry out those decisions.

If the person named as my agent is not available or is unable to act as my agent, then I appoint the following person(s) to serve in the order listed below:

_____   _____
Name   **Home address**

_____   _____
Home telephone number

_____   _____
Work telephone number

By this document I intend to create a power of attorney for health care that shall take effect upon my incapacity to make my own health care decisions and shall continue during that incapacity.

My agent shall make health care decisions as I direct below or as I make known to him or her in some other way.

(a) STATEMENT OF DESIRES CONCERNING LIFE-PROLONGING CARE, TREATMENT SERVICES, AND PROCEDURES;

_____

_____

_____

_____

(b) SPECIAL PROVISIONS AND LIMITATIONS:

_____

_____

_____

BY SIGNING HERE I INDICATE THAT I UNDERSTAND THE
PURPOSE AND EFFECT OF THIS DOCUMENT.

I sign my name to this form on   **(Date)**

at:

[address]

(You sign here)

WITNESSES

I declare that the person who signed or acknowledged this document is personally known to me, that he/she signed or acknowledged this durable power of attorney in my presence, and that he/she appears to be of sound mind and under no duress, fraud, or undue influence. I am not the person appointed as agent by this document, nor am I the patient's health care provider or an employee of the patient's health care provider.

First Witness

Signature:

Home address:

Print name:

Date:

Second Witness

Signature:

Home address:

Print name:

Date

AT LEAST ONE OF THE ABOVE WITNESSES MUST ALSO
SIGN THE FOLLOWING DECLARATION.

I further declare that I am not related to the patient by blood,
marriage, or adoption, and, to the best of my knowledge, I am not
entitled to any part of his/her estate under a will now existing or by
operation of law.

Signature: _____

Signature: _____

Health Care Proxy

(1) I, _____ hereby

appoint _____
        (Name, home address, and telephone number)

as my health care agent to make any and all health care
decisions for me, except to the extent that I state otherwise.
This proxy shall take effect when and if I become unable to
make my own health care decisions.

(2) Optional instructions: I direct my agent to make health care
decisions in accord with my wishes and limitations as stated
below, or as he or she otherwise knows. [Attach additional
pages if necessary.]

_____

_____

[Unless your agent knows your wishes about artificial nutrition
and hydration (feeding tubes), your agent will not be allowed to
make decisions about artificial nutrition and hydration. See instructions below for samples of language you could use.]

(3) Name of substitute or fill-in agent if the person I appoint above is unable, unwilling, or unavailable to act as my health care agent.

_____

(Name, home address, and telephone number)

_____

(4) Unless I revoke it, this proxy shall remain in effect indefinitely, or until the date or conditions stated below. This proxy shall expire [specific date or conditions, if desired]:

_____

(5) Signature _____

Address _____

Date _____

Statement by Witnesses (must be 18 or older)

I declare that the person who signed this document is personally known to me and appears to be of sound mind and acting of his or her own free will. He or she signed (or asked another to sign for him or her) this document in my presence.

Witness 1 _____

Address _____

Witness 2 _____

Address _____

About the Health Care Proxy

This is an important legal form. Before signing this form, you should understand the following facts:

1. This form gives the person you choose as your agent the authority to make all health care decisions for you, except to the extent you say otherwise in this form. "Health care" means any treatment, service, or procedure to diagnose or treat your physical or mental condition.
2. Unless you say otherwise, your agent will be allowed to make all health care decisions for you, including decisions to remove or provide life-sustaining treatment.
3. Unless your agent knows your wishes about artificial nutrition and hydration (nourishment and water provided by a feeding tube), he or she will not be allowed to refuse or consent to those measures for you.
4. Your agent will start making decisions for you when doctors decide you are not able to make health care decisions for yourself.

You may write on this form any information about treatment that you do not desire and/or those treatments that you want to make sure you receive. Your agent must follow your instructions (oral and written) when making decisions for you.

If you want to give your agent written instructions, do so right on the form. For example, you could say:

> *If I become terminally ill, I do/don't want to receive the following treatments: . . .*
> *If I am in a coma or unconscious, with no hope of recovery, then I do/don't want . . .*
> *If I have brain damage or a brain disease that makes me unable to recognize people or speak and there is no hope that my condition will improve, I do/don't want . . .*
> *I have discussed with my agent my wishes about _____ and I want my agent to make all decisions about these measures.*

Examples of medical treatments about which you may wish to give your agent special instructions are listed below. This is not a complete list of the treatments about which you may leave instructions.

- Artificial respiration
- Artificial nutrition and hydration (nourishment and water provided by feeding tube)
- Cardiopulmonary resuscitation (CPR)
- Antipsychotic medication
- Electroconvulsive therapy
- Antibiotics
- Psychosurgery
- Dialysis
- Transplantation
- Blood transfusions
- Abortion
- Sterilization

Talk about choosing an agent with your family and/or close friends. You should discuss this form with a doctor or another health care professional, such as a nurse or social worker, before you sign it to make sure that you understand the types of decisions that may be made for you. You may also wish to give your doctor a signed copy. **You do not need a lawyer to fill out this form.**

You can choose any adult (over 18), including a family member, or close friend, to be your agent. If you select a doctor as your agent, he or she may have to choose between acting as your agent or as your attending doctor; a physician cannot do both at the same time. Also, if you are a patient or resident of a hospital, nursing home, or mental hygiene facility, there are special restrictions about naming someone who works for that facility as your agent. You should ask staff at the facility to explain those restrictions.

You should tell the person you choose that he or she will be your health care agent. You should discuss your health care wishes and this form with your agent. Be sure to give him or her a signed copy. Your agent cannot be sued for health care decisions made in good faith.

Even after you have signed this form, you have the right to

make health care decisions for yourself as long as you are able to do so, and treatment cannot be given to you or stopped if you object. You can cancel the control given to your agent by telling him or her or your health care provider orally or in writing.

Filling Out the Proxy Form

Item (1)	Write your name and the name, home address, and telephone number of the person you are selecting as your agent.
Item (2)	If you have special instructions for your agent, you should write them here. Also, if you wish to limit your agent's authority in any way, you should say so here. If you do not state any limitations, your agent will be allowed to make all health care decisions that you could have made, including the decision to consent to or refuse life-sustaining treatment.
Item (3)	You may write the name, home address, and telephone number of an alternate agent.
Item (4)	This form will remain valid indefinitely unless you set an expiration date or condition for its expiration. This section is optional and should be filled in only if you want the health care proxy to expire.
Item (5)	You must date and sign the proxy. If you are unable to sign yourself, you may direct someone else to sign in your presence. Be sure to include your address.

Two witnesses at least 18 years of age must sign your proxy. The person who is appointed agent or alternate agent cannot sign as a witness.

From Simon RI: *Clinical Psychiatry and the Law,* 2nd Edition. Washington, DC, American Psychiatric Press, 1992, pp. 606–610, 614–617. Used with permission.

Treatment of Traumatic Brain Injury

Chapter 19

Psychopharmacology

Jonathan M. Silver, M.D.
Stuart C. Yudofsky, M.D.

Many useful therapeutic approaches are available for the large number of people who have experienced brain injury. As has been found with treatment of psychiatric disorders such as depression, panic disorder, and obsessive-compulsive disorder, a combination of therapeutic interventions administered simultaneously provides more effective treatment than using a single modality (Frank et al. 1990; Hogarty et al. 1986; Mitchell et al. 1990; Weisman et al. 1979). Individual, cognitive, behavioral, and family therapy, as well as environmental manipulation, all may affect symptoms and the patient's ability to cope with them (see Chapters 17 and 20–22). For many patients, the appropriate use of medications can be beneficial in the treatment of neuropsychiatric symptoms. In this chapter, we review the psychopharmacologic treatment of these symptoms when they occur after traumatic brain injury (TBI).

_____
Portions of this chapter were previously published in Silver JM, Hales RE, Yudofsky SC: "Neuropsychiatric Aspects of Traumatic Brain Injury," in *The American Psychiatric Press Textbook of Neuropsychiatry,* 2nd Edition. Edited by Yudofsky SC, Hales RE. Washington, DC, American Psychiatric Press, 1992, pp. 363–395. Used with permission.

Table 19–1.   Psychiatric side effects of neurological drugs

Symptom	Medications	Comments
Depression	Amantadine	Common at usual doses.
	Anticonvulsants	Usually at higher blood levels.
	Corticosteroids, ACTH	More common with high doses; may occur on withdrawal.
	Benzodiazepines	Depression may also decrease in anxious, depressed patients.
	Barbiturates	Common side effect.
	Narcotics	
	L-Dopa	Greater risk with prolonged use.
	Antihypertensives	Has been reported with many preparations.
	Propranolol	Can occur at usual doses.
	Vinblastine	Rare.
	Asparaginase	Common side effect with higher doses.
	Cimetidine	
	Oral contraceptives	In as many as 15% of all cases.
	Ibuprofen	Rare.
	Metoclopramide	Usual doses.
Mania	Baclofen	Usually appears after sudden withdrawal.
	Bromocriptine	Symptoms may continue after drug is withdrawn.
	Captopril	Symptoms may continue after drug is withdrawn.
	Corticosteroids, ACTH	Usually at higher doses.
	Dextromethorphan	
	L-Dopa	More frequent in elderly patients; risk increases with prolonged use.
	Antidepressants	In bipolar and some patients with chronic depression.
	Digitalis	In bipolar patients with higher doses.
	Cyclobenzaprine	Reported in one patient.
Hallucinations	Amantadine	Rare; more common in elderly patients.
	Anticonvulsants	Visual and auditory.
	Antihistamines	Especially with higher doses.
	Anticholinergics	Usually with delirium.
	Corticosteroids, ACTH	See above.[a]
	Digitalis	Usually at higher blood levels.
	Indomethacin	Especially in elderly patients.
	Methysergide	Occasional.
	Propranolol	At usual or increased doses.
	Methylphenidate	More likely in children.
	L-Dopa	See above.[a]
	Ketamine	Common.
	Cimetidine	Usually in higher doses and in elderly patients.

Table 19–1.   Psychiatric side effects of neurological drugs *(continued)*

Symptom	Medications	Comments
Nightmares	Antidepressants	When entire dose is taken at night.
	Amantadine	Especially in elderly patients.
	Baclofen	Usually after sudden withdrawal.
	Ketamine	Also produces hallucinations, crying, changes in body image, and delirium.
	L-Dopa	Often after dosage increase.
	Pentazocine	During treatment.
	Propranolol	See above.[a]
	Digitalis	See above.[a]
Paranoia	Asparaginase	May be common.
	Bromocriptine	Not dose related.
	Corticosteroids, ACTH	See above.[a]
	Amphetamines	Even at low doses.
	Indomethacin	Especially in elderly patients.
	Propranolol	At any dose.
	Sulindac	Reported in a few patients.
Aggression	Bromocriptine	Not dose related; may persist.
	Tranquilizers and hypnotics	A release phenomenon.
	L-Dopa	See above.[a]
	Phenelzine	May be separate from mania.
	Digitalis	See above.[a]
	Carbamazepine	In children and adolescents.

Note. ACTH = adrenocorticotropic hormone.
[a]Same comments apply as for previous reactions on this drug.
Source. Reprinted from Dubovsky SL: "Psychopharmacological Treatment in Neuropsychiatry," in *The American Psychiatric Press Textbook of Nueropsychiatry,* 2nd Edition. Washington, DC, American Psychiatric Press, 1991, pp. 694–695. Used with permission.

Evaluation

It is critical to conduct a thorough assessment of the patient before any intervention is initiated. For purposes of discussion, we assume that a complete psychiatric, developmental, and neurological history has been obtained, as presented in Chapter 3. Two issues require particular attention in the evaluation of the potential use of medication. First, the presenting complaints must be carefully assessed, defined, and operationalized, including the use of objective rating scales, such as the Overt Aggression Scale (Silver and

Yudofsky 1991) (see Chapter 10) or the Neurobehavioral Rating Scale (Levin et al. 1987) (see Chapter 3), which are invaluable in following symptoms throughout treatment. Second, the current treatment must be reevaluated. Although consultation may be requested to decide whether medication would be helpful, it is often the case that 1) other treatment modalities have not been properly applied, 2) there has been misdiagnosis of the problem, or 3) there has been poor communication among treating professionals. On occasion, a potentially effective medication has not been beneficial because it has been prescribed in a dose that is too low or for a period of time that is too brief. In other instances, the most appropriate pharmacological recommendation is that no medication is required and that other therapeutic modalities need to be reassessed.

In reviewing the patient's current medication regimen, two key issues should be addressed: 1) the indications for all drugs prescribed and whether they are still necessary and 2) the potential side effects of these medications. Patients who have had severe brain trauma may be receiving many medications that result in psychiatric symptoms such as depression, mania, hallucinations, insomnia, nightmares, cognitive impairments, restlessness, paranoia, or aggression (Table 19–1). For example, many patients with TBI have been prescribed anticonvulsant drugs (ACDs), and may still be receiving them at the time of the consultation. The first question is why the ACD was prescribed initially, because it is important, as discussed in Chapter 16, to ascertain whether it has been given for the treatment of active seizures or for prophylaxis. Because ACDs do not appear efficacious in preventing the appearance of seizures in a patient with TBI who has never had a seizure (Temkin et al. 1990), the latter use should be reconsidered. Regarding the side effects of specific ACDs, phenytoin and phenobarbital have the greatest potential to produce adverse effects on cognition and mood (Corbett et al. 1985; Gallassi et al. 1988). Treatment with more than one anticonvulsant has been implicated in increased adverse neuropsychiatric reactions (Reynolds and Trimble 1985). Phenytoin has been demonstrated to have negative effects on cognition when given to patients with TBI (Dikmen et al. 1991). Wroblewski et al. (1989) substituted carbamazepine for phenytoin, phenobarbital, or primidone in 21 patients with TBI who were being treated for previous seizures or who were believed to be at high risk for the development of seizures. Only one patient experienced an increase of seizures with drug substitution.

General Principles of Pharmacological Treatment of Psychiatric Syndromes Associated With TBI

There have been few controlled clinical trials to assess the effects of medication in patients with brain injury. Therefore, the decision regarding which medication (if any) to prescribe is based on 1) current knowledge of the efficacy of these medications in other psychiatric disorders, 2) side effect profiles of the medications, 3) the increased sensitivity to side effects shown by patients with brain injury, 4) analogies from the brain injury symptoms to the recognized psychiatric syndromes (i.e., amotivational syndrome after TBI may be analogous to the deficit syndrome in schizophrenia), and 5) hypotheses regarding how the neurochemical changes after TBI may affect the proposed mechanisms of action of psychotropic medications.

There are several general guidelines that should be followed in the pharmacological treatment of the psychiatric syndromes that occur after TBI. They are

1. Start low; go slow.
2. Therapeutic trial of all medications.
3. Continuous reassessment of clinical condition.
4. Monitor drug-drug interactions.
5. Augment partial response.

Patients with brain injury of any type are far more sensitive to the side effects of medications than are patients who do not have brain injury. Doses of psychotropic medications must be raised and lowered in small increments over protracted periods of time, although patients ultimately may require the same doses and serum levels that are therapeutically effective for patients without brain injury (Silver et al. 1990a, 1990b, 1991, 1992).

When medications are prescribed, it is important that they are given in a manner to enhance the probability of benefit and to reduce the possibility of adverse reactions. Medications should be initiated at dosages that are lower than those usually administered to patients without brain injury. Dose increments should be made gradually, to minimize side effects and enable the clinician to observe adverse consequences. However, it is also critical that the medications be given sufficient time to work. Thus when a decision is made to administer a medication, the patient must receive an adequate therapeutic trial of that medication in terms of dosage and duration of treatment.

Because of frequent changes in the clinical status of patients after TBI, continuous reassessment is necessary to determine whether the medication is required. For depression, the standard guidelines for the treatment of major depression should be used, including continuation of medication for a minimum of 6 months after remission of symptoms. For other psychiatric conditions, however, the guidelines are less clear. For example, agitation that occurs during the early phases of recovery from TBI may last days, weeks, or months. The periods of underarousal and unresponsiveness may have similar variability of symptom duration. In general, if the patient has responded favorably to medication treatment, the clinician must use sound judgment and apply risk benefit determinations to each specific case in deciding whether and exactly when to taper and attempt to discontinue the medication following TBI. Continuous reassessment is necessary because there may have been spontaneous remission, in which case the medication can be permanently discontinued, or a carryover effect of the medication may occur (i.e., its effects may persist after the duration of treatment), in which case a reinstatement of the medication may not be required.

When a new medication is initiated in combination with medications previously prescribed, the clinician must monitor drug-drug interactions that may occur. These interactions may be based on pharmacokinetics that result in increased half-lives and serum levels of medications such as anticonvulsants or in changes in pharmacodynamics such as increased sedative effects when several sedating medications are administered simultaneously.

If a patient does not respond favorably to the initial medication prescribed, several alternatives are available. If there has been no response, changing to a medication with a different mechanism of action is usually indicated, as is done routinely in the treatment of depressed patients without brain injury. If there has been a partial response to the initial medication, the clinician may add another medication with consideration of the mechanisms of action, the side effect profiles, and the potential interactions of each drug.

Neurotransmitter Changes After TBI

There have been several studies of neurochemical changes subsequent to TBI (Silver et al. 1991, 1992). These studies have shown that neurotransmitter systems including norepinephrine, serotonin, dopamine, and acetylcholine are dramatically affected by TBI. Two studies found markedly elevated plasma norepinephrine levels after acute head injury (Clifton et al. 1981; Hamill et al. 1987). Elevated plasma levels of norepinephrine were correlated with more severe injury and poorer clinical outcome. The results of four studies of serotonin activity after TBI are inconsistent. Vecht et al. (1975) found that lumbar cerebrospinal fluid (CSF) 5-hydroxyindoleacetic acid (5-HIAA) was below normal in conscious patients and normal in patients who were unconscious. Bareggi et al. (1975) found normal lumbar 5-HIAA levels in patients after severe TBI, whereas ventricular CSF 5-HIAA levels were elevated in patients within days of severe TBI (Porta et al. 1975). Van Woerkom et al. (1977) investigated patients with frontotemporal contusions and those with diffuse contusions. They documented decreased levels of 5-HIAA in patients with frontotemporal contusions, but increased 5-HIAA levels in those with more diffuse contusions. Two investigators (Bareggi et al. 1975; Vecht et al. 1975) found a decrease in lumbar CSF homovanillic acid (HVA) levels, whereas Porta et al. (1975) demonstrated elevated ventricular CSF HVA levels after severe TBI. Elevated serum dopamine may be related to the severity of the injury and to poor outcome (Hamill et al. 1987). Patients with TBI had elevated acetylcholine levels in fluid obtained from intraventricular catheters or lumbar puncture (Grossman et al. 1975).

Specific lesions may deplete norepinephrine and serotonin by interrupting the nerve tracts of these pathways (Morrison et al. 1979). The norepinephrine nerve tracts course from the brain stem anteriorly to curve around the hypothalamus, the basal ganglia, and the frontal cortex. Similarly, the serotonin system has projections to the frontal cortex. Diffuse axonal injury or contusions can affect both of these systems. Secondary neurotoxicity that is caused by excitotoxins and lipid peroxidation may further damage the neuronal systems that mediate norepinephrine and serotonin.

Pharmacological Treatment of Specific Psychiatric Syndromes

In the following section, we review the major psychiatric syndromes following TBI that may respond to medications. We also present guidelines for the use of psychotropic medications to treat these syndromes, as well as review their significant side effects (Silver et al. 1992). Information about the use of psychopharmacologic agents in patients without brain injury can be found in Dubovsky (1992) and Silver et al. (in press).

Affective Illness

■ **Depression: usage guidelines and side effects of antidepressants.** Affective disorders subsequent to brain damage are common and usually highly detrimental to a patient's rehabilitation and socialization (Silver et al. 1990b, 1991). However, the literature is sparse regarding the effects of antidepressant agents and/or electroconvulsive therapy (ECT) in the treatment of patients with brain damage in general and TBI in particular (Silver et al. 1990b, 1991; Zwil et al. 1992). Saran (1985) conducted a crossover study of phenelzine and amitriptyline administered at therapeutic doses to patients with "minor brain injury." No response to medication was observed. Although the patients were reported to be the "melancholic" subtype, they did not have significant weight loss or difficulty sleeping, which are symptoms associated with melancholia; therefore, the diagnostic categorization of these patients must be questioned. Varney et al. (1987) found that 82% of 51 patients with major depressive disorder and TBI who received treatment with either tricyclic antidepressants (TCAs) or carbamazepine reported at least moderate relief of depressive symptoms. Cassidy (1989) conducted an open trial using fluoxetine for 8 patients with severe TBI and associated depression. He found that 2 had marked improvement and 3 had moderate improvement. Interestingly, half the patients experienced sedative side effects, and 3 out of 8 patients reported an increase in anxiety. Bessette and Peterson (1992) reported the case of a 41-year-old woman who experienced an episode of major depression after a minor brain injury and responded favorably to treatment with fluoxetine 20 mg/day.

The choice of an antidepressant depends predominantly on the desired side effect profile (Table 19–2). Usually, antidepressants with the fewest sedative, hypotensive, and anticholinergic side effects are preferred. Fluoxetine (Prozac) (starting at 5–10 mg/day) and sertraline (Zoloft) (starting at 25 mg/day) are specific serotonin reuptake inhibitors without anticholinergic effects. Fluoxetine can be initiated at a low dosage by using the elixir formulation. Because fluoxetine and its metabolites have a half-life of several weeks, 20-mg capsules can be prescribed on an every-other-day basis for equivalence to a 10-mg/day dosing schedule. Occasionally, patients with brain injury and depression may become sedated during treatment with fluoxetine, whereas others become restless and experience insomnia. If a TCA is chosen, we suggest nortriptyline (initial doses of 10-mg/day) or desipramine (initial doses of 10 mg tid), and careful monitoring to achieve plasma levels in the therapeutic range for the parent compound and its major metabolites (i.e., nortriptyline levels 50–100 ng/ml;

Table 19–2. Selected antidepressant drugs, dosages, and side effects

Drugs (by class)	Trade name	Usual daily maximum oral dose (mg)	Side effects	
			Sedative	Anticholinergic
Teritary amine tricyclics				
Imipramine	Tofranil Tofranil PM SK-Pramine Janimine	300	++	+++
Amitriptyline	Elavil Endep	300	+++	+++
Doxepin	Adapin Sinequan	300	+++	+++
Trimipramine	Surmontil	200	+++	+++
Secondary amine tricyclics				
Desipramine	Norpramin Pertofrane	300	+/−	+
Nortriptyline	Aventyl Pamelor	150	+	++
Protriptyline	Vivactyl	60	0	+++
Tetracyclic				
Maprotiline	Ludiomil	200	+++	++
Dibenzoxazepine				
Amoxapine	Asendin	400	+	++
Triazolopyridine				
Trazodone	Desyrel	600	+++	0
Selective serotonin reuptake inhibitors				
Fluoxetine	Prozac	60	0	0
Sertraline	Zoloft	150	0	0
Paroxetine	Paxil	60	0	0
Unicyclic				
Bupropion	Wellbutrin	450	0	0

Note. 0 = none; + = mild; ++ moderate; +++ = severe/significant; +/− = questionable.
Source. Adapted from Silver et al. (in press). Used with permission.

desipramine levels greater than 125 ng/ml) (Task Force on the Use of Laboratory Tests in Psychiatry 1985). If the patient becomes sedated, confused, or severely hypotensive, the dosage should be reduced.

ECT remains a highly effective and underutilized modality for the treatment of depression in general, and in the case of depression following acute TBI, it can be used effectively (Ruedrich et al. 1983). We recommend using treatment with the lowest possible energy levels that will generate a seizure of adequate duration (greater than 20 seconds), using pulsatile currents, increased spacing of treatments (2–5 days between treatments), and fewer treatments in an entire course (four to six). If there is preexisting memory impairment, nondominant unilateral ECT should be used.

The most common and disabling side effects of antidepressants in patients with TBI are the anticholinergic effects. Additionally, the lowering of the seizure threshold by antidepressants can result in seizures. Several antidepressants (e.g., doxepin, amitriptyline, trimipramine, imipramine, maprotiline, and trazodone) are highly sedating, resulting in significant problems of arousal in the TBI patient (Table 19–2).

Many psychotropic medications have *anticholinergic effects*, especially the older TCAs. These medications may impair attention, concentration, and memory, especially in patients with brain lesions. For example, patients with Parkinson's disease have shown increased confusion when treated with anticholinergic medications (De Smet et al. 1982; Dubois et al. 1990). The antidepressants amitriptyline, trimipramine, doxepin, and protriptyline have high affinities for the muscarinic receptors, and thus are highly anticholinergic and should be prescribed only after careful consideration of alternative medications. Fluoxetine, paroxetine, sertraline, trazodone, and bupropion all have minimal or no anticholinergic action.

The available evidence suggests that all antidepressants may be associated with a greater frequency of *seizures* in patients with brain injury. In particular, the antidepressants maprotiline and bupropion have been associated with a higher incidence of seizures (Davidson 1989; Pinder et al. 1977). Wroblewski et al. (1990)

reviewed the records of 68 patients with TBI who received antidepressant treatment for at least 3 months. The frequency of seizures was compared for the 3 months before treatment, during treatment, and after treatment. Seizures occurred among 6 patients during the baseline period, 16 during antidepressant treatment, and 4 after treatment was discontinued. Fourteen patients (20%) had seizures shortly after the initiation of treatment. For 12 of these patients, no seizures occurred after treatment was discontinued. Importantly, 7 of these patients were receiving anticonvulsant medication before and during antidepressant treatment. The occurrence of seizures was related to greater severity of brain injury. However, Zimmer et al. (1992) treated 17 patients with neurological disorders (e.g., TBI, stroke, and degenerative disease) with bupropion at an average dosage of 200 mg/day. No seizures occurred in this group of patients. Also Ojemann et al. (1987) found that seizure control does not appear to worsen if psychotropic medication is introduced cautiously and if the patient is on an effective anticonvulsant regimen. We conclude that although antidepressants can be used safely and effectively in patients with severe TBI, they should be prescribed only with extreme caution and continuous monitoring.

There are several important *drug interactions* that may occur among antidepressants and other drugs commonly prescribed for neurological conditions (Dubovsky 1992). Many antiparkinsonian drugs and neuroleptics have anticholinergic effects that are additive to those of the antidepressants. Antidepressant levels are likely to be decreased—often below therapeutic range—by the anticonvulsants phenytoin, carbamazepine, and phenobarbital. Similarly, antidepressants such as fluoxetine may raise the plasma levels of the anticonvulsants phenytoin (Jalil 1992), valproic acid (Sovner and Davis 1991), and carbamazepine (Grimsley et al. 1991). Therefore, neurological drugs that require therapeutic blood level monitoring should have more frequent monitoring when antidepressants are administered. Although they are highly efficacious drugs, monoamine oxidase inhibitors (MAOIs) should be less frequently prescribed for the treatment of depression in patients who are taking certain other drugs that affect the central nervous system. For example, interactions with stimulants, such as dextro-amphetamine, and L-dopa may result in lethal hypertensive reactions. (For a review of the safe use of MAOIs, see Silver et al., in press).

■ **Mania.** Manic episodes that occur after TBI have been successfully treated with lithium carbonate, carbamazepine (Stewart and Nemsath 1988), valproic acid (Pope et al. 1988), clonidine (Bakchine et al. 1989), and ECT (Clark and Davison 1987). Because of the increased incidence of side effects when lithium is prescribed for patients with brain lesions, we limit the use of lithium in patients with TBI to those with mania or recurrent depressive illness that preceded their brain damage. Further, to minimize lithium-related side effects, we begin with low doses (300 mg/day) and assess the response to low therapeutic blood levels (e.g., 0.2–0.5 mEq/L).

Lithium has been reported to aggravate confusion in patients with brain damage (Schiff et al. 1982), as well as to induce nausea, tremor, ataxia, and lethargy in this population. In addition, lithium may lower seizure threshold (Massey and Folger 1984). Hornstein and Seliger (1989) reported a patient with preexisting bipolar disorder who experienced a recurrence of mania after closed head injury. This patient's mania, before injury, was controlled with lithium carbonate without side effects. However, subsequent to brain injury, dysfunctions of attention and concentration emerged that reversed when the lithium dosage was lowered.

For patients with mania subsequent to TBI, carbamazepine should be initiated at a dosage of 200 mg bid and adjusted to obtain plasma levels of 8–12 µg/ml.

As for patients without histories of TBI, the clinician should be aware of the potential risks associated with carbamazepine treatment, particularly bone marrow suppression (including aplastic anemia) and hepatotoxicity. Complete blood counts and liver function tests should be regularly monitored (Silver et al. 1994). Hematologic monitoring (complete blood count and platelet count) should be obtained every 2 weeks for the first 2 months of treatment, and every 3 months thereafter. Liver function monitoring (serum glutamic-oxaloacetic transaminase [SGOT], serum glu-tamic-pyruvic transaminase [SGPT], lactate dehydrogenase [LDH], and alkaline phosphatase) should be obtained every month for the first 2 months of treatment, and every 3 months thereafter.

The most common signs of neurotoxicity include lethargy, confusion, drowsiness, weakness, ataxia, nystagmus, and in-creased seizures. Pleak et al. (1988) described the development of mania, irritability, and aggression with carbamazepine treatment; however, in our own experience, this reaction is unusual. Brain damage increases the susceptibility to neurotoxicity induced by combination therapy with carbamazepine and lithium (Parmelee and O'Shanick 1988).

Valproic acid is begun at a dosage of 200 mg bid and gradually increased to obtain plasma levels of 50–100 µg/ml. Tremor and weight gain are common side effects. Hepatotoxicity is rare, and usually occurs in children who are treated with multiple anticon-vulsants (Dreifuss et al. 1987). We have seen one case of increased aggressive behavior in a patient treated with high plasma levels of carbamazepine and valproic acid; the aggressive behavior sub-sided when the doses of both medications were lowered.

∎ **Lability of mood and affect.** Antidepressants may be used to treat the labile mood that frequently occurs in the presence of neurological disease. However, it appears that the control of lability of mood and affect may differ from that of depression, and the mechanism of action of antidepressants in treating mood lability in patients with brain injury may differ from that in the treatment of patients with "uncomplicated" depression (Lauterbach and Schweri 1991; Panzer and Mellow 1992; Schiffer et al. 1985; Seliger et al. 1992; Sloan et al. 1992). Ross and Rush (1981) reported the case of a 38-year-old woman who had TBI with loss of consciousness extending 2–3 weeks after the accident. The authors examined the patient 2 years later and found her to be irritable, with pathological laughing and crying, weight gain, and pervasive feelings of sadness and helplessness. Cerebral tomogra-phy revealed bilateral prefrontal atrophy. Nonetheless, the patient exhibited a "remarkable improvement in her behavior, with total resolution of her dysphoria," after treatment with nortriptyline 100 mg/day. Schiffer et al. (1985) conducted a double-blind crossover study with amitriptyline and placebo in 12 patients with pathological laughing and weeping secondary to multiple sclerosis. Eight patients experienced a dramatic improvement after treatment with amitriptyline at a maximum dose of 75 mg/day.

There have been several reports of the beneficial effects of fluoxetine for "emotional incontinence" secondary to several neurological disorders (Panzer and Mellow 1992; Seliger et al. 1992; Sloan et al. 1992). In general, these investigators began treatment with 20 mg/day of fluoxetine, and patients often exhibited response within 5 days. The authors have had similar success with fluoxetine raised to higher doses (40–80 mg/day) and with sertraline, starting at 25 mg/day and increasing gradually to 100 mg/day. Other antidepressants, such as nortriptyline, can also be effective for emotional lability. We emphasize that for many patients it may be necessary to administer these medications at standard antidepressant dosages to obtain full therapeutic effects, although response may occur for others within days of initiating treatment at relatively low doses.

Cognitive Function and Arousal

Stimulants, such as dextroamphetamine and methylphenidate, and dopamine agonists, such as amantadine and bromocriptine, may be beneficial in treating patients with apathy and impaired concentration, to increase arousal and diminish fatigue (Table 19–3).

Table 19–3.   Medications to treat impairment of cognition and arousal

Drug	Initial dose	Maximum dose
Dextroamphetamine	2.5 mg bid	60 mg/day
Methylphenidate	5 mg bid	60 mg/day
Amantadine	50 mg bid	400 mg/day
Bromocriptine	2.5 mg/day	90 mg/day
Sinemet (L-dopa/carbidopa)	10/100 tid	25/250 qid

These medications all act on the catecholaminergic system, but in different ways. Dextroamphetamine blocks the reuptake of norepinephrine and, in higher doses, blocks the reuptake of dopamine. Methylphenidate has a similar mechanism of action. Amantadine acts both presynaptically and postsynaptically at the dopamine receptor and may increase cholinergic and gabaminergic activity. Bromocriptine is a dopamine, subtype 1, receptor antagonist and a dopamine, subtype 2, receptor agonist. It appears to be a dopamine agonist at mid-range doses (Berg et al. 1987). Assessment of improvement in attention and arousal may be difficult (Whyte 1992), and further work needs to be conducted in this area to determine whether these medications affect outcome. Therefore, careful objective assessment, with appropriate neuropsychological tests, may be helpful in determining response to treatment.

■ **Stimulants.**   Evans et al. (1987) reported that impairments in verbal memory and learning, attention, and behavior were alleviated with either dextroamphetamine (0.2 mg/kg body weight bid) or methylphenidate (0.3 mg/kg body weight bid) in a 24-year-old man with severe TBI. Other reports have also indicated that these medications may be beneficial (Lipper and Tuchman 1976; Weinstein and Wells 1981). Weinberg et al. (1987) treated a 33-year-old man who had a subdural hematoma after a seizure. He was in coma for 3 weeks and became abulic and aphonic several months later. After treatment with methylphenidate in dosages increasing to 60 mg/day, he "became fully alert and performed certain automatic movements and occasional automatic speech expressions" (p. 58). This patient was also transiently treated with physostigmine with variable results. In the authors' opinion, methylphenidate resulted in persisting benefit, even after the drug was discontinued. Gualtieri and Evans (1988) studied 15 patients with TBI who were currently functioning at a Rancho Los Amigos Scale (see Table 3–3, Chapter 3, this volume) level of 7 or 8. They received methylphenidate in a double-blind, placebo-controlled crossover study. Patients received 2-week treatment with either placebo, methylphenidate 0.15 mg/kg body weight bid, or methylphenidate 0.30 mg/kg body weight bid. Of the 15 patients treated,

14 improved on active medication, with increased scores on ratings of mood and performance. Gualtieri and Evans observed that this acute response was not sustained over time. Methylphenidate should be initiated at 5 mg bid and dextroamphetamine at 2.5 mg bid. The maximum dosage of each medication is 60 mg/day bid or tid.

▮ **Dopamine agonists.** Lal et al. (1988) reported on the use of L-dopa/carbidopa (Sinemet) in the treatment of 12 patients with brain injury (including anoxic damage). With treatment, patients exhibited 1) improved alertness and concentration; 2) decreased fatigue, hypomania, and sialorrhea; and 3) improved memory, mobility, posture, and speech. Dosage administered was 10/100 mg to 25/250 mg qid. Eames (1989) suggested that bromocriptine may be useful in treating cognitive initiation problems of brain injury patients who are at least 1 year subsequent to injury. He recommended starting at 2.5 mg/day and treatment for at least 2 months at the highest dose tolerated (up to 100 mg/day). Other investigators found that patients with nonfluent aphasia (Gupta and Mlcoch 1992), akinetic mutism (Echiverri et al. 1988), and apathy (Catsman-Berrevoets and Harskamp 1988) improved after treatment with bromocriptine. Parks et al. (1992) suggested that bromocriptine exerts specific effects on the frontal lobe, thus increasing goal-directed behaviors.

Amantadine may be beneficial in the treatment of anergia, abulia, mutism, and anhedonia subsequent to brain injury (Chandler et al. 1988; Gualtieri et al. 1989). These authors also reported that improvement may occur in impulsivity and emotional lability. Initial dosages should be 50 mg bid, and increased every week by 100 mg/day to a maximum dosage of 400 mg/day.

▮ **Side effects.** Adverse reactions to medications for impaired concentration and arousal are related most often to increases in dopamine activity. Dextroamphetamine and methylphenidate may lead to paranoia, dysphoria, agitation, and irritability. Because depression often occurs on discontinuation, stimulants should be discontinued using a slow regimen. Interestingly, there may be a role for stimulants to increase neuronal recovery subsequent to brain injury (Crisostomo et al. 1988). Side effects of bromocriptine include sedation, nausea, psychosis, headaches, and delirium. Amantadine may cause confusion, hallucinations, edema, and hypotension; these reactions occur more often in elderly patients than in younger patients.

Some clinicians have been concerned that stimulant medications may lower seizure threshold in patients with TBI who are at increased risk for posttraumatic seizures. Recently, Wroblewski et al. (1992) reviewed their experience with methylphenidate in 30 patients with severe brain injury and seizures and examined changes in seizure frequency after initiation of methylphenidate. The seizure frequency was monitored for 3 months before treatment with methylphenidate, 3 months during treatment, and 3 months after treatment was discontinued. They found that whereas only 4 patients experienced more seizures during methylphenidate treatment, 26 had either fewer or the same number of seizures during treatment.

Wroblewski et al. (1992) concluded that there was no significant risk in lowering seizure threshold with methylphenidate treatment in this high-risk group. Although many patients in this study were treated concomitantly with anticonvulsant medications that may have conferred some protection against the development of seizures, this does not explain why 13 patients had fewer seizures when treated with methylphenidate.

In a double-blind placebo-controlled study of the effects of methylphenidate (0.3 mg/kg body weight bid) in 10 children with well-controlled seizures and attention-deficit disorder, no seizures occurred during the 4 weeks of treatment with either active drug or placebo (Feldman et al. 1989). Dextroamphetamine has been used adjunctively in the treatment of refractory seizures (Livingston and Pauli 1975), and bromocriptine may also have some anticonvulsant properties (Rothman et al. 1990). Amantadine may lower seizure threshold (Gualtieri et al. 1989); we also have observed several patients who had not experienced seizures for months before the administration of amantadine, but did have a seizure weeks after it was prescribed.

Psychosis

■ **Antipsychotic and neuroleptic medications.** The psychotic ideation resulting from TBI is generally responsive to treatment with antipsychotic medications. However, side effects such as hypotension, sedation, and confusion are common. Also patients with brain injury are particularly subject to dystonias, akathisias, and other parkinsonian side effects—even when relatively low doses of antipsychotic medications are prescribed (Wolf et al. 1989). Antipsychotic medications have also been reported to impede neuronal recovery after brain injury (Feeney et al. 1982). Therefore, we advise that antipsychotics should be used sparingly during the acute phases of recovery after the injury. When clinically essential, haloperidol (Haldol) 0.5 mg bid, or fluphenazine (Prolixin) 0.5 mg bid may be used as initial treatment. Therapeutic effect may not be evident for 3 weeks after treatment at each dosage. In general, we recommend a low-dose neuroleptic strategy for all patients with neuropsychiatric disorders (Silver and Yudofsky 1988). Table 19–4 summarizes the antipsychotic medications available and their usual dosages. Clozapine is a novel and effective antipsychotic medication that does not produce extrapyramidal side effects (EPS). Although its use in patients with neuropsychiatric disorders has yet to be investigated fully, its side effect profile poses many potential disadvantages (discussed below). It is highly anticholinergic, produces significant sedation and hypotension, lowers seizure threshold profoundly, and is associated with a 1% risk of agranulocytosis that requires lifetime weekly monitoring of blood counts. Psychopharmacologic options for the treatment of posttraumatic psychosis are summarized in Table 19–5. (This topic is discussed further in Chapter 8.)

■ **Side effects: EPS and seizures.** Table 19–6 summarizes the most disabling side effects that occur when neuroleptics are prescribed to patients with TBI. In general, the low-potency antipsychotic medications such as thioridazine, mesoridazine, and chlorpromazine are sedating, have greater anticholinergic properties, and cause greater orthostatic hypotension. High-potency neu-

Table 19–4. Selected antipsychotic drugs and dosages

Drugs (by class)	Trade name	Dose equivalent to 100 mg chlorpromazine	Usual maintenance oral dose (mg)[a]
Phenothiazines			
Aliphatic			
Chlorpromazine hydrochloride	Thorazine	100	200–600
Piperidine	Mellaril	90–104	200–600
Thoridazine hydrochloride			
Mesoridazine besylate	Serentil	50–62	150–200
Piperazine	Stelazine	2.4–3.2	5–10
Trifluoperazine			
Fluphenazine hydrochloride	Prolixin Permitil	1.1–1.3	2.5–10
decanoate enanthate	Prolixin	0.61	10 mg/day oral fluphenazine = 12.5–25 mg/ 2 weeks fluphenazine decanoate
Perphenazine	Trilafon	8.9–9.6	16–24
Thiozanthenes			
Thiothixene	Navane	3.4–5.4	6–30
Chlorprothixene	Taractan	36–52	75–200
Butyrophenones			
Haloperidol	Haldol	1.1–2.1	2–12
Haloperidol decanoate			10 mg/day oral haloperidol = 100–200 mg/ 4 weeks haloperidol decanoate
Dibenzoxazepine			
Loxapine	Moban	10	20–60
Indole derivatives			
Molindone hydrochloride	Moban Lidone	5.1–6.9	15–60
Pimozide	Orap	2	2–10
Dibenzodiazepine			
Clozapine	Clozaril	50	200–900

[a]Dose ranges required for patients varies. Adjustment in doses may be required depending on the patient's clinical status and responsiveness to medication.
Source. Adapted from Silver et al. (in press).

roleptics such as haloperidol and fluphenazine result in greater EPS (see below). The medium potency antipsychotic drugs such as trifluoperazine and thiothixene are intermediate in their side effect profiles.

With the exception of clozapine, all antipsychotic drugs block postsynaptic dopamine receptors and may result in a number of EPS, including acute dystonic reactions, parkinsonian syndrome, akathisia, akinesia, tardive dyskinesia, and the neuroleptic malig-

Table 19–5. Psychopharmacological treatment of posttraumatic psychosis

Agent	Indications	Special clinical considerations
Any specific neuroleptic	History of good response for a particular patient in a similar episode	Evaluate for EPS and TD before and during treatment
Standard neuroleptic	Schizophrenia-like target symptoms (hallucinations, delusions, and thought disorder)	Evaluate for EPS and TD before and during treatment
Pimozide	Monosymptomatic delusional disorder	Electrocardiographic abnormalities
Clozapine	Schizophrenia-like psychosis with poor response or intolerable side effects with standard neuroleptics	Lowers seizure threshold; lifelong risk of agranulocytosis
Anticonvulsants (carbamazepine and valproic acid)	Seizure disorder, manic episode or prominent mood swings, aggression, poor response to neuroleptics	Bone marrow suppression (carbamazepine) Hepatotoxicity (valproic acid and carbamazepine)
Clonazepam	Manic symptoms; alternative to anticonvulsants for psychosis with epilepsy	Tolerance and dependence
Lithium	Manic syndrome; possible bipolar or schizoaffective disorder	Neurotoxicity or confusion
Beta-blockers	Chronic aggression or violent behavior	May not affect psychosis

Note. EPS = extrapyramidal side effects; TD = tardive dyskinesia.
Source. See Table 8–7 (Chapter 8, this volume).

nant syndrome (Silver et al., in press). These effects may also occur with antiemetic drugs, such as metoclopramide and prochlorperazine. Consistent with their greater sensitivity to medications affecting the CNS, patients with brain injury are more sensitive to the development of EPS (Rosebush and Stewart 1989; Vincent et al. 1986; Wolf et al. 1989; Yassa et al. 1984a, 1984b). Acute dystonic reactions are disturbing and frightening and most often occur within hours or days of the initiation of antipsychotic therapy. The most common feature of this syndrome includes uncontrollable tightening of the face and neck and spasm and distortions of the patient's facial musculature and/or back (opisthotonos). These reactions are terrifying to the patient who has no prior experience with this condition or no prior knowledge of this side effect. In patients with brain injury who may already have loss of neuromuscular function, these reactions may intensify their fear of taking medications. Intravenous or intramuscular administration of anticholinergic drugs provides rapid treatment of acute dystonia.

The parkinsonian syndrome (or pseudoparkinsonism) has many of the classic features of idiopathic Parkinson's disease: diminished range of facial expression (masked facies), cogwheel rigidity, slowed movements (bradykinesia), drooling, small handwriting (micrographia), and "pillrolling" tremor. The onset of this side effect is gradual and may not appear for weeks to months

---

Table 19–6.   Side effects of neuroleptics

Oversedation

Hypotension (falls)

Confusion

Neuroleptic malignant syndrome

Parkinsonian side effects

Akathisia

Dystonia

Tardive dyskinesia

Source. Reprinted from Yudofsky SC, Silver JM, Hales RE: "Pharmacologic Management of Aggression in the Elderly." *Journal of Clinical Psychiatry* 51 (Suppl. 10):22–28, 1990. Copyright 1990, Physicians Postgraduate Press. Used with permission.

after neuroleptics have been administered. These symptoms are treated with anticholinergic drugs, which include trihexyphenidyl, benztropine mesylate, and diphenhydramine. Amantadine is also effective, and has the advantage of not possessing anticholinergic effects that can produce confusion.

Akathisia is an extrapyramidal disorder consisting of a highly unpleasant restlessness and the inability to sit still. It is a common reaction and most often occurs within days to weeks after the initiation of antipsychotic drugs. Unfortunately, akathisia is frequently mistaken for an exacerbation of psychotic symptoms, anxiety, and/or depression, thus obviating the corrective clinical actions (e.g., discontinuation of the antipsychotic medication or a trial of propranolol) that will ameliorate the condition.

Akinesia, another extrapyramidal side effect of antipsychotic medication, is characterized by apathy, diminished spontaneity of speech and movement, and difficulty in initiation. Akinesia may appear after several weeks of therapy and may be mistaken as depression. Anticholinergic drugs are effective treatments.

Tardive dyskinesia is a dangerous and disabling side effect of antipsychotic medication that is characterized by involuntary movements of the face, trunk, or extremities. The diagnostic features of tardive dyskinesia are listed in Table 19–7. The treatment of any patient with antipsychotic medication requires an evaluation for abnormal movements before treatment has begun, and every 6 months thereafter. A procedure for examining a patient for tardive dyskinesia can be found in Table 19–8. Although the most common form of "tardive disorder" is the dyskinetic variety, other types have been observed, including tardive akathisia, tardive dystonia, and tardive tics. Prevention is the most important aspect of the treatment of tardive dyskinesia, because this disorder can be irreversible. A 50% reduction in dyskinetic movement is documented in most patients by 18 months after discontinuation of antipsychotic agents (Glazer et al. 1984).

Neuroleptic malignant syndrome is a potentially life-threatening disorder that may emerge after the use of any antipsychotic agent. The patient with neuroleptic malignant syndrome becomes severely rigid and occasionally catatonic. There is fever, elevated white blood cell count, tachycardia, abnormal blood pressure fluctuations, tachypnea, and diaphoresis. Although medications such as bromocriptine and dantrolene sodium have been suggested to treat neuroleptic malignant syndrome, the most important therapeutic interventions are discontinuation of antipsychotic medications, treatment of any underlying infections, and symptomatic treatment of fever and hypertension (Rosebush et al. 1991).

Many psychotropic medications affect seizure threshold (Silver and Yudofsky 1988). This can be of concern because of the frequent problem of posttraumatic seizures after TBI. Among all the first-generation antipsychotic drugs, molindone and fluphenazine have consistently demonstrated the lowest potential for lowering the seizure threshold (Oliver et al. 1982; Silver et al., in press). Clozapine treatment is associated with a significant dose-

---

Table 19–7.   Clinical features of tardive dyskinesia

The following abnormal movements may be seen in tardive dyskinesia:

Facial and oral movements

  a. Muscles of facial expression: involuntary movement of forehead, eyebrows, periorbital area, and/or cheeks; involuntary frowning, blinking, smiling, and/or grimacing.

  b. Lips and perioral area; involuntary puckering, pouting, and/or smacking.

  c. Jaw: involuntary biting, clenching, chewing, mouth opening, and/or lateral movements.

  d. Tongue: involuntary protrusion, tremor, and/or choreoathetoid movements (rolling, wormlike movement without displacement from the mouth).

Extremity movements

  a. Involuntary movement of upper arms, writs, hands, and/or fingers: choreic movements (rapid, objectively purposeless, irregular, and/or spontaneous), athetoid movements (slow, irregular, complex, and/or serpentine), tremor (repetitive, regular, and/or rhythmic).

  b. Involuntary movement of lower legs, knees, ankles, and/or toes: lateral knee movement, foot tapping, foot squirming, and/or inversion and eversion of foot.

Trunk movements

  Involuntary movement of neck, shoulders, and/or hips: rocking, twisting, squirming, and/or pelvic gyrations.

Source. Adapted from National Institue of Mental Health 1976.

related incidence of seizures (ranging from 1% to 2% of patients who receive doses below 300 mg/day, and 5% of patients who receive 600–900 mg/day) (Lieberman et al. 1989), and thus must be prescribed for patients with TBI only with extreme caution and when clearly indicated for the relief of psychotic symptoms.

Table 19–8. Examination procedure for tardive dyskinesia

Either before or after completing the examination procedure, unobstrusively observe the patient at rest (e.g., in waiting room). The chair to be used in this examination should be a hard, firm one without arms.

Examination procedure

1. Ask patient whether there is anything in his or her mouth (e.g., gum or candy) and if there is, to remove it.
2. Ask patient about the current condition of his or her teeth. Ask patient if he or she wears dentures. Do teeth or dentures bother patient now?
3. Ask patient whether he or she notices any movements in mouth, face, hands,or feet. If yes, ask to describe and to what extent they currently bother patient or interfere with his or her activities.
4. Have patient sit in chair with hands on knees, legs slightly apart, and feet flat on floor. (Look at entire body for movements while patient is in this position.)
5. Ask patient to sit with hands hanging unsupported. If male, between legs, if female and wearing a dress, hanging over knees. (Observe hands and other body areas.)
6. Ask patient to open mouth. (Observe tongue at rest within mouth.) Do this twice.
7. Ask patient to protrude tongue. (Observe abnormalities of tongue movement.) Do this twice.
8. Ask patient to tap thumb, with each finger, as rapidly as possible for 10 to 15 seconds; separately with right and then with left hand. (Observe facial and leg movements.)
9. Flex and extend patient's left and right arms (one at a time). (Note any rigidity.)
10. Ask patient to stand up. (Observe in profile. Observe all body areas again, hips included.)
11. Ask patient to extend both arms outstretched in front with palms down. (Observe trunk, legs, and mouth.)
12. Have patient walk a few paces, turn, and walk back to chair. (Observe hands and gait.) Do this twice.

Source. Adapted from National Institue of Mental Health 1976.

Anxiety Disorders and Posttraumatic Stress Disorder

Because of the side effects and danger of dependence associated with benzodiazepine use, we generally prefer to treat complaints of anxiety in brain injury patients with supportive psychotherapy and social interventions. TBI is very highly associated with alcoholism and drug dependency (see Chapter 15), which further increases our caution in prescribing benzodiazepines for these patients. However, when the symptoms are so severe that they require pharmacological intervention, treatment with benzodiazepines or buspirone should be considered. Side effects of benzodiazepines include sedation and memory impairment, which often affect the cognitive performance of patients with brain injury.

Buspirone, a serotonin 5-HT_1 agonist, has less deleterious effect on cognitive functioning in patients with TBI than do benzodiazepines, and the former is not associated with dependency. Buspirone's therapeutic effects occur after a latency of several weeks. Gualtieri (1991a, 1991b) found that four out of seven patients with "postconcussion syndrome" experienced "decreased anxiety, depression, irritability, somatic preoccupation, inattention, and distractibility" after treatment with buspirone. Side effects from buspirone are dizziness, lightheadedness, and paradoxically increased anxiety.

Patients with brain injury also may develop other anxiety disorders, such as panic disorder, obsessive compulsive disorder, posttraumatic stress disorder (PTSD), and phobias. Medications, particularly antidepressants, are often indicated for these conditions, with the caveat that brain injury patients are highly susceptible to antidepressant side effects. The most important step in the treatment of the patient with PTSD is the careful assessment and diagnosis of comorbid DSM-IV Axis I or II conditions (American Psychiatric Association 1994). When no pervasive comorbid condition is diagnosed, antidepressant medications should be the initial pharmacological treatment. The positive symptoms of PTSD, including reexperiencing of the event and increased arousal, often improve with medication. The negative symptoms of avoidance and withdrawal usually respond poorly to pharmacotherapy. Depending on the response to this initial treatment, several therapeutic strategies are suggested. Figure 19–1 summarizes our approach to the pharmacological treatment of PTSD (Silver et al. 1990c).

Benzodiazepines may produce sedation and impair memory and motoric function, in addition to other side effects of their use in patients with brain injury (Table 19–9).

In some instances, sedation may be the desired effect of benzodiazepines, but usually this side effect impairs the patient's psychosocial functioning. Problems with balance, ataxia, and coordination that occur subsequent to brain injury are likely to be exacerbated by benzodiazepines. These drugs can produce amnesia (Angus and Romney 1984; Lucki et al. 1986; Roth et al. 1980) and will worsen preexisting memory difficulties.

Walburga et al. (1992) examined the effects of anxiolytic medications (buspirone and diazepam) on driving performance of outpatients with generalized anxiety disorder who had no neurological impairment. Each week, the subjects were tested for driving ability by a 100-kilometer on-the-road driving test. Among the patients who received diazepam, two subjects could not complete the test during the first 2 weeks of treatment, and the entire group showed significantly impaired performance in the first, second, and third weeks. No impairment was detected in the subjects who received buspirone. These subjects did not have any cognitive impairments before the study, and did not have a previous history

Table 19–9.   Side effects of benzodiazepines

Oversedation

Motor disturbances (poor coordination)

Mood disturbances

Memory impairment, confusion

Dependency, overdoses, withdrawal syndromes

Paradoxical violence

Source.   Reprinted from Yudofsky SC, Silver JM, Hales RE: "Pharmacologic Management of Aggression in the Elderly." *Journal of Clinical Psychiatry 51* (Suppl. 10):22–28, 1990. Copyright 1990, Physicians Postgraduate Press. Used with permission.

of drug or alcohol abuse. We recommend careful monitoring of the driving of all patients who receive psychotropic drugs—especially those who take benzodiazepines.

Sleep

Sleep patterns of patients with brain damage are often disordered, with impaired rapid-eye-movement (REM) recovery and multiple nocturnal awakenings (Prigatano et al. 1982). Hypersomnia that occurs after severe penetrating head injury most often resolves within the first year after injury, whereas insomnia that occurs in patients with long periods of coma and diffuse injury has a more chronic course (Askenasy et al. 1989). Barbiturates and long-acting

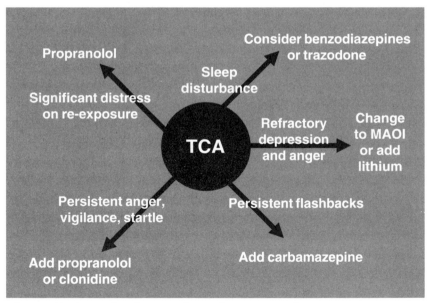

Figure 19–1. Psychopharmacological treatment of posttraumatic stress disorder. TCA = tricyclic antidepressant; MAOI = monoamine oxidase inhibitor.
Source. Reprinted from Silver JM, Sandberg DP, Hales RE: "New Approaches in the Pharmacotherapy of Posttraumatic Stress Disorder." *Journal of Clinical Psychiatry* 51 (Suppl. 10):33–38, 1990c. Copyright 1990, Physicians Postgraduate Press. Used with permission.

benzodiazepines should be prescribed for sedation with great caution, if at all. These drugs interfere with REM and stage 4 sleep patterns, and may contribute to persistent insomnia (Buysse and Reynolds 1990). Clinicians should warn patients of the dangers of using over-the-counter preparations for sleeping and for colds because of the prominent anticholinergic side effects of these agents.

Trazodone, a sedating antidepressant medication that is devoid of anticholinergic side effects, may be used for nighttime sedation. A dose of 50 mg should be administered initially; if ineffective, doses up to 150 mg may be prescribed. Nonpharmacological approaches should be considered, including minimizing daytime naps, maintaining regular sleep onset times, and engaging in regular physical activity during the day.

Aggression and Agitation

Table 19–10 summarizes our recommendations for the use of various classes of medication in the treatment of chronic aggressive disorders associated with TBI. Acute aggression may be treated by using the sedative properties of neuroleptics or benzodiazepines. In treating aggression, the clinician, where possible, should diagnose and treat underlying disorders and use, where possible, antiaggressive agents specific for those disorders. When there is partial response after a therapeutic trial with a specific medication, adjunctive treatment should be instituted with a medication possessing a different mechanism of action. For example, a patient with partial response to beta-blockers may have more complete improvement with the addition of an anticonvulsant. (This area is discussed in detail in Chapter 10.)

Concerns Regarding Pharmacotherapy

There has been a bias held by patients, families, and often treatment centers against the use of medications for the treatment of neuropsychiatric disorders in patients with brain injury. These issues are important, because the psychiatrist is often faced with resistance from patients, families, and staff about the use of medications. The bias against the use of psychiatric medications may have several sources, including the stigma associated with mental illness and psychiatry, and the patient's previous suboptimal experience with psychotropic medications. Stigma may relate to the view that psychiatric symptoms are signs of weakness, indolence, or even moral decline. We have suggested that the neuropsychiatric paradigm that uses a "medical model" reduces the misleading demarcation between "brain" and "mind," and emphasizes neurobiological effects (without negating emotional and psychological factors) as our strongest weapon against stigma

Table 19–10. Psychopharmacological treatment of chronic aggression

Agent	Indications	Special clinical considerations
Antipsychotics	Psychotic symptoms	Oversedation and multiple side effects
Benzodiazepines	Anxiety symptoms	Paradoxical rage
Anticonvulsants		
Carbamazepine (CBZ)	Seizure disorder	Bone marrow suppression
Valproic acid (VPA)		(CBZ) and hepatoxicity (CBZ and VPA)
Lithium	Manic excitement or bipolar disorder	Neurotoxicity and confusion
Buspirone	Persistent, underlying anxiety and/or depression	Delayed onset of action
Propranolol (and other beta-blockers)	Chronic or recurrent aggression	Latency of 4–6 weeks
Antidepressants	Depression or mood lability with irritability	May need usual clinical doses

Source. Reprinted from Yudofsky SC, Silver JM, Hales RE: "Pharmacologic Management of Aggression in the Elderly." *Journal of Clinical Psychiatry* 51 (Suppl. 10):22–28, 1990. Copyright 1990, Physicians Postgraduate Press. Used with permission.

(Yudofsky and Hales 1989). It is helpful to tell patients that their symptoms may be due to alterations in neurotransmitter function, which may be treated with centrally active medications.

Unfortunately, for patients with TBI, a common experience with the use of psychotropic medications indeed has often been a negative one. Neuroleptics are widely misused as a general "tranquilizer" to sedate patients agitated after TBI, with resulting impairment in alertness, cognition, and initiation, and the production, over time, of severe EPS. For example, we evaluated in consultation one patient who had been treated with low-dose fluphenazine to control agitated behavior. One month later, the staff and family complained that she was "underaroused." On our examination, the patient had severe cogwheel rigidity that had not been diagnosed previously. One hour after administration of benztropine 1 mg, she was "active" again.

Another fear about medication is that it will interfere with a "natural healing process" that occurs after TBI. Evidence obtained from animal models suggests that certain drugs may interfere with recovery following neuronal injury. Feeney et al. (1982) studied the effect of D-amphetamine on recovery from hemiplegia after ablation of the sensorimotor cortex in rats. They found that D-amphetamine accelerated the rate of recovery, and that this effect was blocked by haloperidol. In addition, haloperidol, when administered alone, resulted in delayed recovery. Importantly, recovery was affected only when the animal was allowed to move during drug administration. This implies that haloperidol delays a process during active rehabilitation, rather than interfering with spontaneous recovery. In another model, Hovda et al. (1985) found that haloperidol blocked the positive effect of D-amphetamine on recovery of depth perception after visual cortex injury. It has been suggested that the mechanism of action of haloperidol in delaying recovery is through effects as an α-adrenergic antagonist (Sutton et al. 1987). Clonidine, an α_2-adrenergic agonist, and prazosin, an α_1-adrenergic antagonist reinstates deficits after sensorimotor cortex ablation (Sutton and Feeney 1987), an effect not seen with propranolol (Boyeson and Feeney 1984). Other studies have demonstrated that clonidine has deleterious effects on recovery (Feeney and Westerberg 1990; Goldstein and Davis 1990). It should be noted that these experimental methods in animals do not produce the same neuropathological findings as contusions or diffuse axonal injury in humans, and, therefore, may not apply to many patients with TBI. These results also suggest that patients must be in active rehabilitation during drug administration for these effects to occur.

In animal studies involving the neurotransmitter γ-aminobutyric acid (GABA), increase in GABA function has been associated with greater neuromotor deficits and poorer recovery (Boyeson 1991). Increased production of GABA associated with benzodiazepine administration may result in greater glutamate neurotoxicity (Simantov 1990). Diazepam has been found to block recovery of sensory deficits after rat neocortex ablation (Schallert et al. 1986).

The studies cited above relating psychotropic use to impaired neuronal recovery after laboratory-induced brain injury have all used animal models. There have been no carefully controlled clinical trials of this important relationship in humans. Interestingly, when the medical records of recovering stroke patients were reviewed, the use of antihypertensive medications or haloperidol was associated with poorer recovery (Porch et al. 1985). Goldstein and Davis (1990) found that when patients who had had ischemic strokes were administered phenytoin, benzodiazepines, dopamine receptor antagonists, clonidine, or prazosin, they showed poorer sensorimotor function and lower activities of daily living than stroke patients who did not receive those drugs.

Conclusions

Ideally, it would be desirable if psychosis, depression, anxiety, aggression, and agitation could be controlled without medications. However, these states are associated with great pain and disability and if not treated may even endanger the patient and others. In many cases, behavioral treatment and cognitive rehabilitation cannot be effective until psychopharmacologic interventions are initiated. In other psychiatric conditions such as major depression, there is evidence that delay of effective treatment may result in refractoriness of the condition. Post (1992) reported that recurrent affective disorder becomes more difficult to treat the longer the condition persists. Thus there are theoretical reasons for prompt initiation of pharmacological treatment of psychiatric syndromes in patients with TBI.

Brain injury invariably leads to emotional damage in the patient. In this chapter, we have reviewed the role of medication in the treatment of the most frequently occurring psychiatric symptomatologies that are associated with TBI. When appropriately administered, medications may significantly alleviate these symptoms and improve rehabilitation efforts.

References

American Psychiatric Association: Diagnostic and Statistical Manual of Mental Disorders, 4th Edition. Washington, DC, American Psychiatric Association, 1994

Angus WR, Romney DM: The effect of diazepam on patients' memory. J Clin Psychopharmacol 4:203–206, 1984

Askenasy JJM, Winkler I, Grushkiewicz J, et al: The natural history of sleep disturbances in severe missile head injury. Journal of Neurological Rehabilitation 3:93–96, 1989

Bakchine S, Lacomblez L, Benoit N, et al: Manic-like state after bilateral orbitofrontal and right temporoparietal injury: efficacy of clonidine. Neurology 39:777–781, 1989

Bareggi SR, Porta M, Selenati A, et al: Homovanillic acid and 5-hydroxyindoleacetic acid in the CSF of patients after a severe head injury, I: lumbar CSF concentration in chronic brain post-traumatic syndromes. Eur Neurol 13:528–544, 1975

Berg MJ, Ebert B, Willis DK, et al: Parkinsonism—drug treatment, part I. Drug Intell Clin Pharmacy 13:10–21, 1987

Bessette RF, Peterson LG: Fluoxetine and organic mood syndrome. Psychosomatics 33:224–225, 1992

Boyeson MG: Neurochemical alterations after brain injury: clinical implications for pharmacologic rehabilitation. Neurorehabilitation February:33–43, 1991

Boyeson MG, Feeney DM: The role of norepinephrine in recovery from brain injury. Soc Neuroci Abstr 10:68, 1984

Buysse DJ, Reynolds III CF: Insomnia, in Handbook of Sleep Disorders. Edited by Thorpy MJ. New York, Marcel Dekker, 1990, pp 373–434

Cassidy JW: Fluoxetine: a new serotonergically active antidepressant. Journal of Head Trauma Rehabilitation 4:67–69, 1989

Catsman-Berrevoets CE, Harskamp FV: Compulsive pre-sleep behavior and apathy due to bilateral thalamic stroke: response to bromocriptine. Neurology 38:647–649, 1988

Chandler MC, Barnhill JL, Gualtieri CT: Amantadine for the agitated head-injury patient. Brain Inj 2:309–311, 1988

Clark AF, Davison K: Mania following head injury: a report of two cases and a review of the literature. Br J Psychiatry 150:841–844, 1987

Clifton GL, Ziegler MG, Grossman RG: Circulating catecholamines and sympathetic activity after head injury. Neurosurgery 8:10–14, 1981

Corbett JA, Trimble MR, Nichol TC: Behavioral and cognitive impairments in children with epilepsy: the long-term effects of anticonvulsant therapy. Journal of the American Academy of Child Psychiatry 24:17–23, 1985

Crisostomo EA, Duncan PW, Propst M, et al: Evidence that amphetamine with physical therapy promotes recovery of motor function in stroke patients. Ann Neurol 23:94–97, 1988

Davidson J: Seizures and bupropion: a review. J Clin Psychiatry 50:256–261, 1989

De Smet Y, Ruberg M, Serdaru M, et al: Confusion, dementia, and anticholinergics in Parkinson's disease. J Neurol Neurosurg Psychiatry 45:1161–1164, 1982

Dikmen SS, Temkin NR, Miller B, et al: Neurobehavioral effects of phenytoin prophylaxis of posttraumatic seizures. JAMA 265:1271–1277, 1991

Dreifuss FE, Santilli N, Langer DH, et al: Valproic acid hepatic fatalities: a retrospective review. Neurology 37:379–385, 1987

Dubois B, Pillon B, Lhermitte F, et al: Cholinergic deficiency and frontal dysfunction in Parkinson's disease. Ann Neurol 28:117–121, 1990

Dubovsky SL: Psychopharmacological treatment in neuropsychiatry, in The American Psychiatric Press Textbook of Neuropsychiatry, 2nd Edition. Edited by Yudofsky SC, Hales RE. Washington, DC, American Psychiatric Press, 1992, pp 663–701

Eames P: The use of Sinemet and bromocriptine. Brain Inj 3:319–320, 1989

Echiverri HC, Tatum WO, Merens TA, et al: Akinetic mutism: pharmacologic probe of the dopaminergic mesencephalo-frontal activating system. Pediatr Neurol 4:228–230, 1988

Evans RW, Gualtieri CT, Patterson D: Treatment of chronic closed head injury with psychostimulant drugs: a controlled case study and an appropriate evaluation procedure. J Nerv Ment Dis 175:106–110, 1987

Feeney DM, Gonzalez A, Law WA: Amphetamine, haloperidol, and experience interact to affect rate of recovery after motor cortex injury. Science 217:855–857, 1982

Feeney DM, Westerberg VS: Norepinephrine and brain damage: alpha noradrenergic pharmacology alters functional recovery after cortical trauma. Can J Psychol 44:233–252, 1990

Feldman H, Crumrine P, Handen BL, et al: Methylphenidate in children with seizures and attention-deficit disorder. Am J Dis Child 143:1081–1086, 1989

Frank E, Kupfer DJ, Perel JM, et al: Three-year outcomes for maintenance therapies in recurrent depression. Arch Gen Psychiatry 47:1093–1099, 1990

Gallassi R, Morreale A, Lorusso S, et al: Carbamazepine and phenytoin: comparison of cognitive effects in epileptic patients during monotherapy and withdrawal. Arch Neurol 45:892–894, 1988

Glazer WM, Moore DC, Schooler NR, et al: Tardive dyskinesia: a discontinuation study. Arch Gen Psychiatry 41:623–627, 1984

Goldstein LB, Davis JN: Clonidine impairs recovery of beam-walking after a sensorimotor cortex lesion in the rat. Brain Res 508:305–309, 1990

Grimsley SR, Jann MW, Carter JG, et al: Increased carbamazepine plasma concentration after fluoxetine coadministration. Clin Pharmacol Ther 50:10–15, 1991

Grossman R, Beyer C, Kelly P, et al: Acetylcholine and related enzymes in human ventricular and subarachnoid fluids following brain injury. Proceedings of the 5th Annual Meeting for Neuroscience 76:3:506, 1975

Gualtieri CT: Buspirone for the behavior problems of patients with organic brain disorders. J Clin Psychopharmacol 11:280–281, 1991a

Gualtieri CT: Buspirone: neuropsychiatric effects. Journal of Head Trauma Rehabilitation 6:90–92, 1991b

Gualtieri CT, Evans RW: Stimulant treatment for the neurobehavioural sequelae of traumatic brain injury. Brain Inj 2:273–290, 1988

Gualtieri CT, Chandler M, Coons TB, et al: Amantadine: a new clinical profile for traumatic brain injury. Clin Neuropharmacol 12:258–270, 1989

Gupta SR, Mlcoch AG: Bromocriptine treatment of nonfluent aphasia. Arch Phys Med Rehabil 73:373–376, 1992

Hamill RW, Woolf PD, McDonald JV, et al: Catecholamines predict outcome in traumatic brain injury. Ann Neurol 21:438–443, 1987

Hogarty GE, Anderson CM, Reiss DJ, et al: Family psychoeducation, social skills training, and maintenance chemotherapy in the aftercare treatment of schizophrenia, II: two-year effects of a controlled study on relapse and adjustment. Arch Gen Psychiatry 43:633–642, 1986

Hornstein A, Seliger G: Cognitive side effects of lithium in closed head injury (letter). J Neuropsychiatry Clin Neurosci 1:446–447, 1989

Hovda DA, Sutton RL, Feeney DM: Haloperidol blocks amphetamine-induced recovery of binocular depth perception after bilateral visual cortex ablation in cat. Proc West Phramacol Soc 28:209–211, 1985

Jalil P: Toxic reaction following the combined administration of fluoxetine and phenytoin: two case reports. J Neurol Neurosurg Psychiatry 55:414–415, 1992

Lal S, Merbitz CP, Grip JC: Modification of function in head-injured patients with Sinemet. Brain Inj 2:225–233, 1988

Lauterbach EC, Schweri MM: Amelioration of pseudobulbar affect by fluoxetine: possible alteration of dopamine-related pathophysiology by a selective serotonin reuptake inhibitor. J Clin Psychopharmacol 11:392–393, 1991

Levin HS, High WM, Goethe KE, et al: The Neurobehavioral Rating Scale: assessment of the behavioral sequelae of head injury by the clinician. J Neurol Neurosurg Psychiatry 50:183–193, 1987

Lieberman JA, Kane JM, Johns CA: Clozapine: guidelines for clinical management. J Clin Psychiatry 50:329–338, 1989

Lipper S, Tuchman MM: Treatment of chronic post-traumatic organic brain syndrome with dextroamphetamine: first reported case. J Nerv Ment Dis 162:266–371, 1976

Livingston S, Pauli LL: Dextroamphetamine for epilepsy. JAMA 233:278–279, 1975

Lucki I, Rickels K, Geller AM: Chronic use of benzodiazepines and psychomotor and cognitive test performance. Psychopharmacology 88:426–433, 1986

Massey EW, Folger WN: Seizures activated by therapeutic levels of lithium carbonate. South Med J 77:1173–1175, 1984

Mitchell JE, Pyle RL, Eckert ED, et al: A comparison study of antidepressants and structured intensive group psychotherapy in the treatment of bulimia nervosa. Arch Gen Psychiatry 47:149–157, 1990

Morrison JH, Molliver ME, Grzanna R: Noradrenergic innervation of cerebral cortex: widespread effects of local cortical lesions. Science 205:313–316, 1979

National Institue of Mental Health: Abnormal Involuntary Movement Scale, in EDCEU Assessment Manual. Edited by Guy W. Rockville, MD, U.S. Department of Health, Education, and Welfare, 1976

Ojemann LM, Baugh-Bookman C, Dudley DL: Effect of psychotropic medications on seizure control in patients with epilepsy. Neurology 37:1525–1527, 1987

Oliver AP, Luchins DJ, Wyatt RJ: Neuroleptic-induced seizures: an in vitro technique for assessing relative risk. Arch Gen Psychiatry 39:206–209, 1982

Panzer MJ, Mellow AM: Antidepressant treatment of pathologic laughing or crying in elderly stroke patients. J Geriatr Psychiatry Neurol 4:195–199, 1992

Parks RW, Crockett DJ, Manji HK, et al: Assessment of bromocriptine intervention for the treatment of frontal lobe syndrome: a case study. J Neuropsychiatry Clin Neurosci 4:109–110, 1992

Parmelee DX, O'Shanick GJ: Carbamazepine-lithium toxicity in brain-damaged adolescents. Brain Inj 2:305–308, 1988

Pinder RM, Brogden RN, Speight TM, et al: Maprotiline: a review of its pharmacological properties and therapeutic efficacy in mental states. Drugs 13:321–352, 1977

Pleak RR, Birmaher B, Gavrilescu A, et al: Mania and neuropsychiatric excitation following carbamazepine. J Am Acad Child Adolesc Psychiatry 27:500–503, 1988

Pope Jr. HG, McElroy SL, Satlin A, et al: Head injury, bipolar disorder, and response to valproate. Compr Psychiatry 29:34–38, 1988

Porch B, Wyckes J, Feeney DM: Haloperidol, thiazides and some antihypertensives slow recovery from aphasia (abstract). Society for Neuroscience Abstracts 11:52, 1985

Porta M, Bareggi SR, Collice M, et al: Homovanillic acid and 5-hydroxyindoleacetic acid in the CSF of patients after a severe head injury, II: ventricular CSF concentrations in acute brain post-traumatic syndromes. Eur Neurol 13:545–554, 1975

Post RM: Transduction of psychosocial stress into the neurobiology of recurrent affective disorders. Am J Psychiatry 149:999–1010, 1992

Prigatano GP, Stahl ML, Orr WC, et al: Sleep and dreaming disturbances in closed head injury patients. J Neurol Neurosurg Psychaitry 45:78–80, 1982

Reynolds EH, Trimble MR: Adverse neuropsychiatric effects of anticonvulsant drugs. Drugs 29:570–581, 1985

Rosebush P, Stewart T: A prospective analysis of 23 episodes of neuroleptic malignant syndrome. Am J Psychiatry 146:717–725, 1989

Rosebush PI, Stewart T, Mazurek MF: The treatment of neuroleptic malignant syndrome: are dantrolene and bromocriptine useful adjuncts to supportive care? Br J Psychiatry 159:709–712, 1991

Ross ED, Rush J: Diagnosis and neuroanatomical correlates of depression in brain-damaged patients. Arch Gen Psychiatry 38:1344–1354, 1981

Roth T, Hartse KM, Saab PG, et al: The effects of flurazepam, lorazepam, and triazolam on sleep and memory. Psychopharmacology 70:231–237, 1980

Rothman KJ, Funch DP, Dreyr NA: Bromocriptine and puerperal seizures. Epidemiology 1:232–238, 1990

Ruedrich I, Chu CC, Moore SI: ECT for major depression in a patient with acute brain trauma. Am J Psychiatry 140:928–929, 1983

Saran AS: Depression after minor closed head injury: role of dexamethasone suppression test and antidepressants. J Clin Psychiatry 46:335–338, 1985

Schallert T, Hernandez TD, Barth TM: Recovery of function after brain damage: severe and chronic disruption by diazepam. Brain Res 379:104–111, 1986

Schiff HB, Sabin TD, Geller A, et al: Lithium in aggressive behavior. Am J Psychiatry 139:1346–1348, 1982

Schiffer RB, Herndon RM, Rudick RA: Treatment of pathologic laughing and weeping with amitriptyline. N Engl J Med 312:1480–1482, 1985

Seliger GM, Hornstein A, Flax J, et al: Fluoxetine improves emotional incontinence. Brain Inj 6:267–270, 1992

Silver JM, Yudofsky SC: Psychopharmacology and electroconvulsive therapy, in American Psychiatric Press Textbook of Psychiatry. Edited by Talbott JA, Hales RE, Yudofsky SC. Washington, DC, American Psychiatric Press, 1988, pp 767–853

Silver JM, Yudofsky SC: The Overt Aggression Scale: Overview and clinical guidelines. J Neuropsychiatry Clin Neurosci 3 (suppl):S22–S29, 1991

Silver JM, Hales RE, Yudofsky SC: Psychiatric consultation to neurology, in American Psychiatric Press Review of Psychiatry, Vol 9. Edited by Tasman A, Goldfinger SM, Kaufmann CA. Washington, DC, American Psychiatric Press, 1990a, pp 433–465

Silver JM, Hales RE, Yudofsky SC: Psychopharmacology of depression in neurologic disorders. J Clin Psychiatry 51 (suppl 1):33–39, 1990b

Silver JM, Sandberg DP, Hales RE: New approaches in the pharmacotherapy of posttraumatic stress disorder. J Clin Psychiatry 51 (suppl 10):33–38, 1990c

Silver JM, Yudofsky SC, Hales RE: Depression in traumatic brain injury. Neuropsychiatry, Neuropsychology, and Behavioral Neurology 4:12–23, 1991

Silver JM, Hales RE, Yudofsky SC: Neuropsychiatric aspects of traumatic brain injury, in American Psychiatric Press Textbook of Neuropsychiatry, 2nd Edition. Edited by Yudofsky SC, Hales RE. Washington, DC, American Psychiatric Press, 1992, pp 363–395

Silver JM, Yudofsky SC, Hurowitz GI: Psychopharmacology and electroconvulsive therapy, in American Psychiatric Press Textbook of Psychiatry, 2nd Edition. Edited by Hales RE, Yudofsky SL, Talbott JA. Washington, DC, American Psychiatric Press, (in press)

Simantov R: Gamma-aminobutyric acid (GABA) enhances glutamate cytotoxicity in a cerebellar cell line. Brain Res Bull 24:711–715, 1990

Sloan RL, Brown KW, Pentland B: Fluoxetine as a treatment for emotional lability after brain injury. Brain Inj 6:315–319, 1992

Sovner R, Davis JM: A potential drug interaction between fluoxetine and valproic acid (letter). J Clin Psychopharmacol 11:389, 1991

Stewart JT, Nemsath RH: Bipolar illness following traumatic brain injury: treatment with lithium and carbamazepine. J Clin Psychiatry 49:74–75, 1988

Sutton RL, Feeney DM: Yohimbine accelerates recovery and clonidine and prazosin reinstate deficits after recovery in rats with sensorimotor cortex ablation (abstract). Society for Neuroscience Abstracts 13:913, 1987

Sutton RL, Weaver MS, Feeney DM: Drug-induced modifications of behavioral recovery following cortical trauma. Journal of Head Trauma Rehabilitation 2:50–58, 1987

Task Force on the Use of Laboratory Tests in Psychiatry: Tricyclic antidepressants: blood level measurements and clinical outcome (APA Task Force Report). Am J Psychiatry 142:155–162, 1985

Temkin NR, Dikmen SS, Wilensky AJ, et al: A randomized, double-blind study of phenytoin for the prevention of post-traumatic seizures. N Engl J Med 323:497–502, 1990

Van Woerkom TCAM, Teelken AW, Minderhoud JM: Difference in neurotransmitter metabolism in frontotemporal-lobe contusion and diffuse cerebral contusion. Lancet 1:812–813, 1977

Varney NR, Martzke JS, Roberts RJ: Major depression in patients with closed head injury. Neuropsychology 1:7–9, 1987

Vecht CJ, Van Woerkom TCAM, Teelken AW, et al: Homovanillic acid and 5-hydroxyindoleacetic acid cerebrospinal fluid levels. Arch Neurol 32:792–797, 1975

Vincent FM, Zimmerman JE, Van Haren J: Neuroleptic malignant syndrome complicating closed head injury. Neurosurgery 18:190–193, 1986

Walburga van Laar M, Volkeerts ER, van Willigenburg APP: Therapeutic effects and effects on actual driving performance of chronically administered buspirone and diazepam in anxious outpatients. J Clin Psychopharmacol 12:86–95, 1992

Weinberg RM, Auerbach SH, Moore S: Pharmacologic treatment of cognitive deficits: a case study. Brain Inj 1:57–59, 1987

Weinstein GS, Wells CE: Case studies in neuropsychiatry: post-traumatic psychiatric dysfunction—diagnosis and treatment. J Clin Psychiatry 42:120–122, 1981

Weisman MM, Prusoff BA, DiMascio A, et al: The efficacy of drugs and psychotherapy in the treatment of acute depressive episodes. Am J Psychiatry 36:1450–1456, 1979

Wolf B, Grohmann R, Schmidt LG, et al: Psychiatric admissions due to adverse drug reactions. Compr Psychiatry 30:534–545, 1989

Wroblewski BA, Glenn MB, Whyte J, et al: Carbamazepine replacement of phenytoin, phenobarbital and primidone in a rehabilitation setting: effects on seizure control. Brain Inj 3:149–156, 1989

Wroblewski BA, McColgan K, Smith K, et al: The incidence of seizures during tricyclic antidepressant drug treatment in a brain-injured population. J Clin Psychopharmacol 10:124–128, 1990

Wroblewski BA, Leary JM, Phelan AM, et al: Methylphenidate and seizure frequency in brain-injured patients with seizure disorders. J Clin Psychiatry 53:86–89, 1992

Yassa R, Nair V, Schwartz G: Tardive dyskinesia and the primary psychiatric diagnosis. Psychosomatics 25:135–138, 1984a

Yassa R, Nair V, Schwartz G: Tardive dyskinesia: a two-year follow-up study. Psychosomatics 25:852–855, 1984b

Yudofsky SC, Hales RE: The reemergence of neuropsychiatry: definition and direction. J Neuropsychiatry Clin Neurosci 1:1–6, 1989

Yudofsky SC, Silver JM, Hales RE: Pharmacologic management of aggression in the elderly. J Clin Psychiatry 51 (suppl 10):22–28, 1990

Whyte J: Neurologic disorders of attention and arousal: assessment and treatment. Arch Phys Med Rehabil 73:1094–1103, 1992

Zimmer B, Garber HJ, Price TRP, et al: Bupropion use in patients at risk for seizures. Proceedings of the New Research American Psychiatric Association 145th Annual Meeting, Washington, DC, May 1992, pp 2–7

Zwil AS, McAllister TW, Price TRP: Safety and efficacy of ECT in depressed patients with organic brain disease: review of a clinical experience. Convulsive Therapy 8:103–109, 1992

Chapter 20

Individual Psychotherapy

Irwin W. Pollack, M.D.

U ntil quite recently, psychiatrists as individuals and psychiatry as a whole demonstrated little interest in working with people who had experienced significant brain trauma. They, like most of their colleagues in neurology and neurosurgery, believed that after a brief postinjury period, during which time a limited spontaneous recovery occurred, no further improvement could be brought about by any type of therapeutic intervention. Most often about six months after the injury, families were told, "What you see is what you'll have." The role for psychiatrists, when there was one at all, was limited to prescribing medication to control fear and agitation in the early postinjury phase and treating depression and paranoia in the long-term recovery phase. Usually, the psychiatrist functioned as a consultant and not as a key member of the treatment team.

Undeterred by the skepticism of many physicians, psychologists were reporting success in modifying postinjury maladaptive behaviors through the use of behavioral techniques, and social workers were finding that by modifying certain environmental conditions, they too could improve long-term outcomes. Despite growing evidence that the behavior of a person with brain injury could be changed by therapeutic techniques, many psychiatrists still failed to see a role in the rehabilitation process for the more traditional approaches to psychotherapy. Certainly, people with significant brain damage did not fit the usual image of an "appropriate candidate" for psychotherapy.

The traditional approach to treatment is based on the assumption that the primary source of a person's emotional problems resides within that person and not in the outside world. Provided that a person possesses certain abilities, it is assumed that he or she has the potential to function more effectively and to gain greater satisfaction from life, a potential that can be actualized through the therapeutic process. A list of those requisite abilities includes the capacity for abstract thinking, a degree of self-awareness and the ability to self-monitor, the ability to tolerate frustration and anxiety, memory intact enough to recall significant information both within and across therapy sessions, and the ability to transfer what is learned in the treatment environment to other life situations. These abilities are rarely found in a population of people with significant brain injury (Bennett 1989; Ludwig 1980; Miller 1991). Rather, far more commonly, these individuals may be impulsive, emotionally labile, and only minimally able to tolerate anxiety and frustration. They may be unable to assume an abstract attitude and may have a limited ability to profit from experience. They may not self-monitor effectively and as a result they may fail to recognize the existence of significant problems even when they are quite obvious to others (Conboy et al. 1986; Eames 1988; Goldstein 1952; Prigatano 1987). When one now contrasts this list of deficits with the aforementioned list of abilities that are assumed to be necessary for a successful psychotherapeutic experience, the reasons for the continuing doubts become quite obvious.

Psychotherapy and the Psychotherapies

Although the various schools of psychotherapy tend to emphasize their uniqueness, they share key characteristics. Perhaps in its simplest form *psychotherapy* can be defined as "the treatment of emotional and personality problems and disorders by psychological means. The most important therapeutic factor common to all types of psychotherapy is the therapist-patient relationship" (Kolb and Brodie 1982, p. 746). The major forms of psychotherapy are distinguished by theoretical emphasis. This in turn, in large part, determines the goals of therapy, the techniques used, and the roles played by therapist and patient. Ludwig (1980) divided psychotherapy into four major types: 1) cognitive therapies subdivided into insight-oriented therapies and rational therapies, 2) behavior therapies, 3) experiential therapies, and 4) environmental manipulative or supportive therapies. These types agree in most aspects with those proposed by Kolb and Brodie (1982). For the most part, only the behavioral and supportive therapies have been considered appropriate vehicles for treating people with brain injury.

But the life experiences of brain injury patients are not so different from those of their neighbors to justify limiting their treatment options on an a priori basis. After their accidents, brain injury patients, like their neighbors, may struggle with unresolved internalized conflicts; operate from irrational assumptions about themselves and their world; demonstrate anxiety, depression, phobias and obsessions; feel alienated and devoid of feeling; and be confronted by environmental circumstances that threaten to overwhelm them. All these conditions are known to respond to psychotherapeutic intervention. Within limits, the fact that a person has sustained a traumatic brain injury (TBI) should not change this assessment. The problem is not that TBI patients do not respond to psychotherapy, but rather that every aspect of their being, of their sense of self, has been affected in ways that cannot be managed successfully by any single form of psychotherapy.

TBI and Loss of Sense of Self

Every TBI, even if it is termed *mild*, causes some disturbance of the patient's sense of self. The extent of this disruption can range from feelings of differentness or estrangement to a total disconnection from the person's past identity. Although brain injury patients may be unaware of the reasons for these changes, they usually are quite aware that something profoundly disturbing has occurred.

In the short term, the impairing effects of brain injury stem from the person's physical and cognitive deficits, but the longer term effects, those that are most disabling, are the result of personality changes and behavioral dyscontrol. Although physical, language, and cognitive difficulties almost invariably decline in frequency and severity over time, emotional difficulties, depression, and social isolation increase. Loneliness is both the most common and the most distressing of the long-term effects of brain injury (Fordyce 1983; Weddell et al. 1980).

The Psychotherapeutic Process

The primary goal of psychotherapy in the treatment of brain injury patients, then, is the same as that of the other therapeutic modalities involved in the rehabilitation process: to enable the injured person to reestablish, or in the case of more minor brain injury, to reconfirm the sense of self (Banja 1988; Condeluci and Gretz-Lasky 1987).

To accomplish this, the downhill course leading to social isolation and loneliness must be stopped and then reversed, but all too often the physical, cognitive, and emotional residuals of the brain injury and their social consequences compromise the patient's ability to regain the initiative without professional assistance. This is no less the case for many people with minor brain injuries who, over time, have become too bewildered and demoralized to put their lives back together without help.

The Starting Point

To enable brain injury patients to breach the walls of their isolation and begin once again to relate to other people effectively, therapists and their patients must find areas of shared meaning (Stuewe-Portnoff 1988). The therapist and the patient must come to share an understanding of the nature of the problem as it is experienced by the patient (Cicerone 1989; Pollack 1989; Prigatano 1989). Prigatano (1989) expressed the view that therapists working with TBI patients need symbols, concepts, or analogies that adequately represent, for both the therapist and the patient, what it is like to have a damaged brain. These concepts provide a base from which a series of other shared experiences can evolve, eventually culminating in the reestablishment of the injured person's sense of self. In most cases, initially it is the therapist who must provide a model for what has happened as a result of the injury.

If the patient is competent enough to understand, he or she should be reassured that it is the brain injury, not a neurotic or psychotic process, that is causing these disturbances. As much as possible, specific complaints should be taken up and their relationship to the injury should be explained in nontechnical language. The patient should be told that although the final outcome of his or her injuries is not wholly predictable, some improvement in physical and cognitive abilities is to be expected and the degree of this improvement often can be enhanced through rehabilitation activities. The patient should be forewarned that his or her efforts will be of the greatest importance, because therapy of whatever kind will not be fruitful without this active participation, and that even under the best of circumstances, positive changes will be slow in coming, so great patience will be required. The patient should be discouraged from returning to his or her regular routine prematurely, that is, before relevant abilities have progressed to the point at which success can be reasonably expected, in order to avoid failing unnecessarily and becoming demoralized.

In the case of very impaired people, the explanation of the effects of brain injury should be brief, concrete, and directed specifically at clarifying the most significant of the patient's complaints.

On occasion, it is the injured person, usually one who has sustained minor brain trauma, who provides the model. One young patient described her postinjury experience in this way:

> It's like being in a place where all the major well-marked highways are intact but where occasional side roads and bridges have been knocked out. Because of this when I leave the highway, I never can be sure whether I will be able to reach my destination or, if I am blocked, whether I will be able to find another path or even whether I will be able to find my way back to the highway.

This analogy, which incorporates experiences common to many people, provided an initial point of meaningful contact between therapist and patient. At times, a single successful transaction such as this can be a major turning point early in the patient's rehabilitation.

The Importance of an Historical Perspective

Although the importance of obtaining an adequate history is emphasized in all areas of medical practice, in therapeutic work with brain injury patients it is the sine qua non. Not only must therapists acquire in-depth information about the circumstances surrounding the injury, the person's preinjury personality, and postinjury symptoms, abilities, and behaviors, but the therapist must also know about that person's preinjury level of physical and social development, interests and values, school and work experiences, cultural background, friendships and family relationships, as they existed both before and after the brain injury (Cicerone 1989; Ellis, 1989; Prigatano 1989). Events surrounding the injury can have far reaching experiential and symbolic significance for the patient, and the disinhibition that frequently follows as a consequence of brain injury can result in the reemergence of previously resolved psychological issues perhaps dating back to childhood (Bennett 1989; Silver et al. 1992). These factors all contribute to a patient's vulnerabilities and predispositions, so it is important to distinguish symptoms that are associated with one or another of these factors from those associated with the brain injury itself, because these distinctions will affect the therapeutic approach (Prigatano 1989).

Patient Changeability:
The Need for Therapist Flexibility

To paraphrase Heraclitus, for the psychiatrist, in the early stages of his or her attempts to understand the patient's postinjury behaviors, the only unchanging characteristic is change itself. As noted by Gardner (1976),

> I have never seen a brain damaged individual, with the possible exception of those either completely demented or virtually recovered, who did not display sizable variations in performance from day to day, if not across hours or minutes . . . no skill seems to be completely destroyed or wholly intact; rather, each seems to be in a partial state of disrepair, and, depending upon such factors as the surrounding conditions, the extent of fatigue, the events of the preceding minutes, motivation at the given moment, the degree of alertness or attentiveness, the patient may succeed strikingly or fail dismally on a given set of tasks. This variability is all important because it precludes a ready foolproof description of the patient—as most consulting physicians soon learn, one must speak of the patient at-a-given-moment-in-time, or in particular circumstances, rather than as a fixed set of mechanized routines always performing at the same level. (p. 431)

Not only their behaviors but the entire beings of brain injury patients are in a state of flux. Most are rather young when they are injured, in their adolescence or early adulthood, and still in the process of evolving both physically and psychosocially (Lewis and Rosenberg 1990). Additionally, over time, they usually show a progressive improvement in their physical and cognitive capacities, thereby enhancing their ability to analyze and comprehend the significance of their subjective experiences (Stein 1988). Successful psychotherapeutic work with people who have experienced a TBI usually requires the therapist to utilize several different approaches to treatment. It is most common for a therapist to begin the treatment process with an approach that is almost entirely under his or her control: history taking and educational activities related to the effects of brain injury directed to both the patient and the family, and preliminary environmental manipulation such as reports to insurance carriers, recommendations relating to work or school assignments, consultation with other members of the rehabilitation team, and others.

After arriving at a mutual understanding of what has happened to the patient as a result of the brain injury, therapeutic efforts should focus on selected concrete problems. Preferably these issues should be raised by the client and pursued even if they are not considered to be important by the therapist. The patient should be assisted in attaining a clear picture of the problem as it affects both the patient and the family. At first, therapeutic efforts should be focused on the here and now even when it is clear that the patient's preinjury personality is playing a significant role. Therapist and patient together should determine how best to modify ineffectual responses, although at times, direct suggestions and advice will be necessary. On occasion a second approach to treatment may be required, for example, adding behavioral or family therapy. In addition, environmental manipulation may be indicated and for this reason the family, employer, and/or friends will need to be brought into the therapeutic situation.

The psychiatrist should emphasize the patient's remaining assets and help the patient see how these can be used to manage present problems. Success should be rewarded with acknowledgement and praise, failure with acknowledgement and support. Emphasis should be placed on what the patient can learn from each experience, and the therapist must recognize that, for the most part, it is the process that is therapeutic, not the patient's insights.

As the therapeutic relationship develops and the patient makes additional gains in cognitive abilities, the approach to therapy should gradually shift to one that places greater demands on the patient (e.g., rational or insight-oriented therapy). However, as noted above, because of the patient's extreme changeability, the psychiatrist may need to shift the approach from treatment session to treatment session or even within a single treatment session.

Because truly empathic relationships between therapists and TBI patients may be impossible to achieve, psychodynamic interpretations should be made tentatively. On the other hand, decisiveness is most appropriate when offering guidance. Cicerone (1989) suggests that interpretations should be used to make explicit connections that the patient has been unable to make.

The need for therapist flexibility is clear, because no single therapeutic approach will suffice. The psychiatrist must be prepared to shift tactics as dictated by the patient's change in state and/or by the behaviors present at the moment; only through these measures will the ensuing transactions between therapist and patient be effective in promoting further recovery.

The course of recovery from even a mild brain injury is slow and uneven, whereas the impact on the life of the injured person and his or her family and friends is devastating. Because loss of morale and increased anxiety and depression are continuing threats to the patient's successful rehabilitation, the psychotherapist must make every effort to instill hope in the patient and the family without making insubstantial predictions of a successful rehabilitation outcome (Prigatano 1986). Moreover, implicit in all contacts with even moderately impaired brain injury patients is a quality of uncertainty that tends to engender a level of anxiety in anyone (family, friends) who desires or needs to maintain a close relationship with them. A therapist can allay this anxiety most effectively through the sharing of information about the nature of the brain injury, the problems that can be expected, and the progress that the injured person is making in his or her therapy. The therapeutic tactics described in the preceding sections are summarized in Table 20–1.

Mild Brain Injury

Recent animal and human studies strongly suggest that there is a continuum of neurological damage and functional impairment from mild to severe brain injury (Eisenberg and Levin 1989; Genarelli 1981; Rutherford 1989). Although they are more subtle, at times becoming obvious only on neuropsychological testing, the cognitive impairments that result from minor brain injuries are

Table 20–1. The psychotherapeutic process—suggested tactics

Tactic	Description
Gain a historical perspective.	Obtain information from family, friends, employers, and teachers concerning preinjury growth and development, health, education, occupation, personality, interests, values, goals, impediments.
Find areas of shared meaning.	Determine what having a brain injury means to the patient, how he or she perceives its effects. At first, the psychiatrist may have to take the initiative, explaining the mechanism of traumatic brain injury in simple terms and relating the patient's difficulties to the injury, and describing the problems, events, and so on, that can be expected in the future.
Encourage the patient to take the lead.	Concentrate on the concrete "real life" difficulties that the injury has caused the patient. Early in treatment, focus on the "here and now," avoid discussing the past (it requires good memory, and it is over), avoid discussing the future (it requires the ability to abstract, and at this point is beyond comprehension).
Help the patient develop simple coping strategies.	For example, keep a notebook, follow a sequence of predetermined steps, rest before becoming too fatigued, request that a confusing message be repeated slowly and in simpler terms, set up priorities for a series of necessary tasks.
Manipulate aspects of the environment to enable the patient to function more effectively	For example, organize household equipment, utensils, dishes, and so on, in a systematic fashion, label drawers and closets, have patient use an alarm or calendar watch.
Mobilize assistance.	Mobilize the assistance of family members, employers, teachers, and friends to help keep the social and work demands as noncomplex and as manageable as possible.
Build on the patient's assets.	Build on the patient's remaining assets, avoid focusing on the residual deficits. Do not make every task seem like a test.
Recognize that the patient's world may differ from that of the psychiatrist.	Interpret the meaning of behavior with caution. Provide guidance to improve inappropriate behavior with authority.

Table 20–1. The psychotherapeutic process—suggested tactics (*continued*)

Tactic	Description
Maintain flexibility.	Many patients are adolescents or young adults in various stages of development; some improvement in physical condition and cognitive function can be expected over time; the patient's abilities and emotional state can vary from moment to moment depending on preceding events, the character of the task, the degree of alertness and motivation, and the environmental conditions.
The approach to therapy should change as the patient changes.	This should happen both within and across treatment sessions. Ideally, the treatment approach should move gradually from one that is concerned primarily with the management of concrete, here and now, practical problems to one that places greater demands on the patient to consider psycho-dynamic issues.
Instill hope.	Instill hope in the patient and family without expressing unwarranted optimism.

essentially the same as many of those that are seen after major brain trauma. Commonly, these impairments include decrements in attention, concentration, short-term memory, and rapid and/or complex mental processing (Conboy et al. 1986; Rimel et al. 1981). For some individuals, the overall impact of these seemingly low-level deficits can be devastating, in large part because the quality of their combined effect is difficult to define and almost impossible to communicate effectively. As a result, the person with a mild brain injury often is seen as overreacting and neurotic. In such circumstances the individual, feeling misunderstood, maligned, and without support can become confused, frightened, and angry.

Lezak, calling on her extensive experience in evaluating and treating patients with mild brain injuries, described a triad of subtle sequelae: perplexity, distractibility, and fatigue (Lezak 1978, 1989). Perplexity is reflected in the individual's distrust of his or her own abilities and in the validity of his or her thought processes. In interpersonal situations, perplexity is expressed as confusion, uncertainty, and self-doubt (Piotrowski 1937). Distractibility results when an individual cannot screen out unwanted or irrelevant stimulation. Because of its subtlety, it is quite common for the patient not to recognize that this problem exists. He or she is aware only of a discomfort when interacting in groups of people, and an intolerance of noise and random activity.

Unusual fatigability is found routinely following any brain injury. The patient tires more easily probably because formerly automatic activities and functions now require concentrated and sustained effort.

These subtle consequences of minor head injury, which are difficult to recognize and even more difficult to comprehend, can engender secondary feelings of confusion, anxiety, anger, and depression in both the brain injury patient and members of the family. These painful emotions tend to cause the person with a minor brain injury to overestimate the degree of cognitive and physical impairments. Unlike many patients with profound brain injuries, who do not complain, tending rather to deny the seriousness of their deficits, patients who have experienced a minor brain injury frequently complain of their symptoms, and mourn the loss of their former competencies.

Although some subtle impairments may be life-long, most people who have experienced minor brain injuries are able to resume the key aspects of their lives within a period of 3 to 6 months. Symptoms that persist beyond 6 months usually are fueled by an interplay of the neurological damage, the patient's premorbid personality traits, and his or her psychological response to the trauma (Levin et al. 1989). Lishman (1973) reported that psychological difficulties are more likely to follow minor brain injuries when the premorbid personality was characterized by insecurity and feelings of inadequacy.

Case example.

Ms. D, a 40-year-old married bank officer, was seen for neuropsychiatric evaluation 3 years after she had been involved in a minor automobile accident. At the time, she experienced a very brief loss of consciousness, perhaps 1 or 2 minutes in duration. A neurological evaluation done in the local hospital emergency room was essentially within normal limits and Ms. D was discharged to her home after being advised to return if any one of a prescribed list of symptoms should appear. Over the next several months, Ms. D began to notice difficulties in a number of areas of function that tended to reduce her effectiveness both at home and at work. She noticed that her short-term memory and her ability to concentrate had deteriorated and she described having problems finding the appropriate words to express her thoughts. She frequently became distracted during business discussions and often felt so fatigued when she arrived home in the evening that she was unable to meet her family obligations.

Over the next 3 years, Ms. D was evaluated by a number of physicians whom she saw either at her own initiative or at the request of her insurance company. The various consultants, most of whom were neurologists or psychiatrists, agreed on two points; first, there was no evidence of residual neurological damage, and second, Ms. D appeared to be overreacting to ordinary life stresses. In Ms. D's opinion, she had received neither understanding nor relief from her numerous contacts with members of the medical profession. As time passed, Ms. D became increasingly confused and overwhelmed by her continuing problems. Her work at the bank slipped badly and her position there was in jeopardy. At home, the quality of her interaction with her husband and children deteriorated so far that she was afraid that her husband was about to leave her.

During our initial meeting, Ms. D described the impact of her brain injury in the following manner. "Since my injury I feel that there is not enough of me to cope. . . . Everywhere I look I have a sense of 'not me.' It seems like I've been fractured internally [pointing to her head]. I have panic attacks! Something is terribly wrong!"

After completing the remainder of the evaluation, Ms. D was assured that her complaints were those that typically follow a mild brain injury. A simplified explanation of what occurs in the brain when the head is forcefully impacted upon was presented to her and some strategies that could help her to manage her workload more effectively were suggested.

When Ms. D returned 1 week later for her second visit, she reported that the strategies had worked and that she was feeling less anxious and confused and that she felt more in control than she had at any time since her accident. Obviously, this was not the end of Ms. D's problems but an alliance had been forged that would support her further recovery.

In every case of minor brain injury, the best treatment is prevention; prevention of the secondary emotional responses that are most disabling. Patients and families should be warned that the after effects of even a mild brain injury take time to clear. To prevent unnecessary and demoralizing failures during the early recovery period, the patient's activities should be limited, the immediate environment should be structured and predictable, and the demands on his or her time and effort should be minimal.

Both patient and family should be made aware of the nature of the problems that frequently follow a mild brain injury, and a simple explanation of the pathophysiology involved should be presented. Strategies to reduce stress and increase coping ability should be developed cooperatively with the participation of the patient, the patient's family, and when indicated the patient's employer or teachers (Conboy et al. 1986). Frequently, these preventive measures are sufficient to assure an uneventful recovery. When the expected progress fails to occur, more formal psychotherapeutic intervention is indicated.

Special Therapeutic Problems

Transference and Countertransference Issues

Any significant threat to the integrity of a person's sense of self, whether caused by brain injury, abnormal brain chemistry, or some catastrophic environmental or human event, precipitates anxiety. In an effort to alleviate this anxiety, the brain injury patient, who has a compromised ability to adapt, may attempt to modify or structure elements in the surrounding physical environment in order to increase its orderliness, and therefore its predictability, thus reducing the probability that unexpected and/or un-manageable demands will arise.

For the same reason, that is, to reduce anxiety, interpersonal transactions may be managed, manipulated, interpreted, and evaluated in terms of the level of emotional stress that they provoke or alleviate. Under these circumstances, rather than reflecting the true character and motives of the other person or people involved in these transactions, evaluation of that person(s) behavior will be based, almost entirely, on the level of comfort that is experienced by the brain injury patient at that moment. Under these circumstances, it should be expected that the injured person's specific attitudes and responses will stem, in most part, from earlier interpersonal experiences, that is, transference phenomena, rather than from the present circumstances. Because people who have survived a significant brain injury frequently have limited self-awareness and impaired self-monitoring abilities, potentially orienting and corrective interpersonal experiences may not be attended to or may be misinterpreted and discounted.

Psychotherapists who work with brain injury patients must be alert to the fact that countertransference forces, both positive and negative, lie just below the surface of every encounter (Goldstein 1952). Such forces can lead a therapist to underestimate the severity of the patient's disabilities and overestimate the degree of recovery that reasonably can be expected following treatment. As a result, a therapist may encourage a patient to incorporate impossible personal goals and adopt social values that are in conflict with those of the community to which the patient eventually must return, thereby setting the stage for the patient's eventual failure.

Although it is common for the positive changes that result from *any* psychotherapeutic process to be slow in forthcoming, an unusual level of patience is required of the psychotherapist in the treatment of brain injury patients, because of their memory problems, inflexibility, and impaired comprehension.

Not infrequently, a patient appears to comprehend the relevance of a therapeutic exchange, but because of frontal cortex damage, still fails to initiate an appropriate action, or indeed any action at all. Because the patient initially appeared to understand that there was a need to act and had repeatedly expressed his or her good intentions, inactivity and/or other "inappropriate" behaviors may be interpreted as a lack of motivation or even as an act of rebelliousness and sabotage. When the patient does not meet the therapist's expectations, feelings of frustration and anger emerge and the quality of the therapeutic alliance begins to deteriorate. When the therapist gradually becomes aware of the wish to abandon the patient, feelings of guilt become the only glue that for a short period prevents the relationship from fracturing.

At the same time, the patient, as might be expected, is feeling hurt and confused. If his or her expressions of pain and anger fail to communicate to the psychiatrist the depth of despair, and no improvement in the quality of the relationship is forthcoming, the patient's angry feelings can change to hate. Hate directed toward the therapist can serve as evidence for the patient that some sort of relationship continues to exist, which thereby defends the patient against the possibility that he or she actually is alone (Gan 1983).

Unless the therapist can clarify what has been transpiring and can begin to redirect the process, the alliance inevitably will dissolve. To avoid this unfortunate state of affairs, the psychiatrist, from the very first, must work to moderate the transference-countertransference effects. Positive aspects of the transference relationship may be nurtured, but the boundaries between patient and therapist must be kept well defined. The negative aspects of both transference and countertransference reactions must be confronted and tested against reality in order to preserve the therapeutic alliance.

Denial

Perhaps the most striking of the many phenomena associated with brain injury is the capacity of many seriously impaired people to deny the existence of their impairments. In almost every case, several interacting factors contribute to the patient's distorted view of his or her abilities and limitations.

First, it is widely recognized that denial can be the direct result of brain injury. In this instance denial is characterized by a lack of awareness or recognition of the presence and/or the significance of functional impairments. This phenomenon, termed *anosognosia* by Babinski (1914), is reported most frequently in stroke patients who appear to be unaware of their hemiplegia and/or hemianopsia. Denial also is found in patients with cortical blindness and people with amnestic conditions (Heilman et al. 1985; McGlynn and Schacter 1989).

People who have experienced a TBI frequently deny their memory deficits and the changes in their personalities that are usually associated with frontal lobe injury (Bond 1984). In fact, brain injury patients frequently exhibit some awareness of their physical and intellectual deficits while at the same time denying the existence of the changes in temperament that are described by relatives and friends (Cicerone 1989; Fahy et al. 1967; Thomsen 1974). It is important to recognize that organically mediated denial is not motivated and serves no known defensive purpose for the injured person. On the other hand, so-called psychological denial is known to occur in the absence of brain injury. This kind of denial is mobilized either consciously or unconsciously in an effort to allay anxiety and/or other unpleasant affects that can arise when an individual's integrity is threatened (Beisser 1979; Cicerone 1989; Rosen 1986; Weinstein and Kahn 1955). It is probable that motivated unawareness (psychological denial) always plays some role in a person's effort to cope with the effects of brain injury.

Although at times denial may disrupt the treatment process, several investigators have pointed out that frequently there are discrepancies between what patients say and what they do. Despite verbally denying the significance of their deficits, many patients continue to participate appropriately in prescribed treatment activities (Fordyce 1983; Tyerman and Humphrey 1984).

To make appropriate inferences that will help to explain a brain injury patient's responses in therapy, it is important for the therapist to distinguish between the neurogenic and psychogenic aspects of the patient's denial, to discriminate between those components which the patient is unable to change from those which he or she is unwilling to change.

The management of denial is one of the most difficult problems confronting a psychiatrist working with brain injury patients. As a rule, direct confrontation of the patient's denial is ineffective and may impact negatively on the therapeutic relationship. Beisser (1979) advised that "if the physician takes an adversary stance to the patient's view, there is a risk either of the patient's compliance at the risk of his or her own integrity or opposition in the service of maintaining his or her integrity" (p. 1029).

Perhaps the most effective intervention in a situation where denial is hampering the patient's progress in therapy is the structuring of an environment that supports reality in a consistent but nonthreatening manner (Cicerone 1989; Rosen 1986).

When denial is not an immediate impediment to the patient's progress, therapy should concentrate on enabling the patient to recognize and strengthen his or her preserved assets. When the patient's sense of competence increases and self-esteem improves, the need for the protection afforded by denial will be reduced, and perhaps eventually may even be eliminated. Beisser (1979) further stated that "if the integrity of the person is respected, the person is more likely to move toward those aspects of reality which will serve his or her needs" (p. 1029).

Catastrophic Conditions

A person who has had a significant brain injury tends to limit both the range of his or her activities and the physical and social situations in which these activities are carried out, in order to keep them manageable. If for any reason, the patient's efforts to keep the elements of his or her world contained are not successful, and a task must be confronted that is beyond his or her present capabilities, a catastrophic condition occurs (Goldstein 1952; Miller 1991; Prigatano 1988).

The catastrophic condition was described by Goldstein (1952) in this way:

> When the patient is unable to fulfill a task set before him . . . the overt behaviors [that result] appear very much the same as [they do in] a person in a state of anxiety. . . . In the catastrophic

condition, the patient not only is incapable of performing a task which exceeds his impaired capacity but he also fails for a longer or shorter period in performances which he is able to carry out in the ordered state. (p. 255)

By a process of selective modification of behaviors and routines, brain injury patients may be able to eliminate, or at least to decrease, the number of catastrophic episodes that they experience. For example, when they are threatened with the possibility of being overwhelmed, they may withdraw in order to reduce the number and intensity of stimuli impacting on them, may show a lack of interest or involvement in the task at hand, may deny its relevance to their situation, may question the competence and/or motives of the therapist, and may ridicule other patients who have willingly worked on the same task. Usually a brain injury patient's defensive maneuvers are confined to words and avoidance behaviors, but these can escalate to physical assault if other tactics fail to reduce the stress.

Therefore, as a first priority, psychotherapists working with this exceedingly vulnerable group of patients must strive to avoid precipitating a catastrophic condition. In particular, open-ended, anxiety-provoking comments and questions must be avoided. New concepts should be introduced gradually and in as simple a form as possible, so they can be processed effectively. It is most important to avoid presenting each new task as though it constitutes another test of the injured person's abilities. If the onset of a catastrophic condition appears to be imminent, active manipulation of one or more aspects of the therapeutic situation many avert a crisis. For example, the psychiatrist can rephrase a question or a comment and/or give additional information in order to further clarify and simplify the patient's task. Or the patient can be presented with several possible solutions or alternative strategies that would permit the given task to be pursued more effectively. At times, it can be useful for the psychiatrist to acknowledge to the patient that explanations may have been unclear or expectations may have been unreasonably high for that point in the recovery process. Obviously, the therapist should not assume responsibility for the patient's growing anxiety unless he or she actually believes this to be case. Ultimately, the best way to manage the catastrophic condition is to prevent it in the first place, because patients have few assets to assist them in reestablishing their equilibrium once it has been disturbed.

Guilt, Shame, and Punishment

It is not uncommon for a person who survives significant brain trauma to experience distressing feelings of guilt and shame. If that person was the driver of a vehicle involved in a collision and especially if he or she was drinking beforehand, the occurrence of these feelings would be quite understandable. If a passenger in the vehicle was seriously injured or killed as a result of that collision, these feelings certainly would be appropriate. Often, however, even when an injury is caused by a series of unavoidable events, intense feelings of guilt and shame add their weight to the brain injury patient's already heavy burden.

Robert Murphy, an anthropologist who was profoundly physically impaired as the result of a spinal cord tumor, wrote about guilt, shame, and punishment as they are experienced by seriously disabled people. What he has to say applies as well to those who have had a significant TBI (Murphy 1987):

> The usual formula is that a wrongful act leads to a guilty conscience; if the guilt becomes publicly known, then shame must be added to the sequence, followed by punishment. . . . A fascinating aspect of disability is that it dramatically and completely reverses the progression, while preserving every step. The sequence of the person damaged in body goes from punishment (the impairments) to shame, to guilt and finally to the crime. This is not a real crime but a self-delusion that lurks in our fears and fantasies; in the never articulated question, "What did I do to deserve this?" (p. 93)

This pressing question deserves a meaningful answer, one that is possible for the patient to find through the process of psychotherapy.

Stigmatization and Marginality:
Society's Response to Disability

The classical model of psychotherapy starts with the assumption that the patient's problems arise from early life experiences and that, within limits, the character of the current outside world has limited impact on the patient's potential for recovery. This certainly is not the case for people who have been disabled by a TBI. They do not have a benign or even neutral physical and social environment with which to contend during their struggle toward recovery.

In its effects, TBI, at one and the same time, is a condition of the injured person's body and an aspect of his or her social identity. The process is set in motion by a physical insult but is given definition and meaning by society (Murphy 1987; Thomsen 1984; Weddell et al. 1980). In fact, "very often, social relations between [brain injury patients] and their noninjured peers are tense, awkward and problematic" (Murphy 1987, p. 86).

In our society, brain injury is a condition that is deeply discrediting and stigmatizing (Goffman 1963). "By definition, the person with stigma is not quite human [and] on this assumption all varieties of discrimination are practiced through which the [injured] person's life choices are effectively reduced" (Murphy 1987, p. 6). Survivors of brain injuries may be treated as incompetent, stupid, or crazy. Frequently they are held responsible for their situations, for example, "he drove too fast; she wasn't paying attention to the road conditions; he should have known that it is dangerous to drink and drive." In fact, many brain injury patients exist in a kind of marginal state: neither in society nor fully out of it, not sick nor entirely well—a fact that is reflected in the confusion over how they should be categorized: patient, client, survivor? Governmental agencies do not agree about whether brain injury patients come under guidelines for the physically impaired, the mentally ill, or the developmentally disabled. School officials, needing to categorize the group for educational purposes, do not agree on whether to label them neurologically impaired, emotionally impaired, learning disabled, or a combination of all three. For these agencies, brain injury does not exist as a distinct category, and as a result people with TBI often get lost in the bureaucratic shuffle.

People who cannot be categorized neatly and therefore whose behaviors are not predictable tend to provoke anxiety in others (Murphy 1987; Murphy et al. 1988). Both of these qualities—not being easily categorized and being unpredictable—cause people with brain injury to be frequently demeaned or ignored. This is an inescapable fact of life for a person with brain injury and its significance must not be excluded from the psychotherapeutic process.

Loneliness

Almost every person who survives a TBI, including many whose injuries are characterized as "mild," will experience periods of significant loneliness. This is not the sort of loneliness that is brought on by the break-up of a marriage, by the absence of friends, or by the unavailability of rewarding social activities, although certainly these situations occur with dismaying frequency following brain injury. Rather, the condition of loneliness to be considered here has a far more profound impact on the injured person and on those close by. It has been described as "an unhappy compound of having lost one's points of reference, of suffering the fate of individual and collective discontinuity, and of living through, or dying from, a crisis of identity to the point of alienation from oneself" (Binswanger 1942).

Following a TBI, impaired cognitive function and alterations in emotional responsivity can interfere with the person's ability to interact empathically with others. As a result, the injured person begins to experience the world in ways that are significantly different from those of other people.

With the continued loss of meaningful interpersonal relationships, the individual begins to lose faith in the validity of his or her sense of self. In fact, the condition of intense loneliness is tantamount to a suspension in the very fashioning of identity (Becker 1962).

In an understandable effort to maintain consistency in their world as well as control over it, lonely people, brain injury survivors included, attempt to construct plausible explanations for their unhappy lives. In these efforts there is a tendency to develop inaccurate or distorted standards for social relations that are impossible for others to meet in a consistent fashion (Peplau et al. 1982). Then, in order to explain the reasons for the recurring disappointments, while denying the possible sources in themselves, lonely individuals evaluate the motives of others negatively, and from this, paranoid thinking can follow.

Psychiatrists working with TBI survivors who have become socially isolated should keep in mind that a sense of profound loneliness cannot be communicated verbally. Fromm-Reichmann (1959) related that "unlike other non-communicable emotional experiences, it cannot even be shared empathetically perhaps because the other person's empathetic abilities are obstructed by the anxiety arousing quality of its emanations" (p. 5). Lonely people and especially those who have had a brain injury can communicate and be communicated with only in the most concrete terms; therefore, at least in its earliest phase, psychotherapy should emphasize behavior rather than words.

Because person-to-person contacts are imbued with meaning by virtue of the transactions between them, the most direct means of gathering understanding is to say or do something that affects the other person. Ideally, the patient's responses to the psychiatrist's overtures will enable the therapist to begin to comprehend the quality of the patient's dilemma (Stuewe-Portnoff 1988).

Meaningful communication with a lonely brain injury patient is not possible at all until some degree of that patient's isolation is breached. This may be accomplished by the psychiatrist's mere presence in the room without making demands, expecting nothing more than to be eventually accepted as a person who is there. To progress from that point, because the sense of profound loneliness is so difficult for the patient to communicate, it may be necessary for the psychiatrist to take the initiative and open the discussion about it (Fromm-Reichmann 1959).

The special therapeutic problems and the suggested therapist responses that were discussed in the preceding sections are summarized in Table 20–2.

Some Further Suggestions for Effective Psychotherapy and Concluding Comments

∎ **The psychiatrist must be responsive.** An effective therapeutic relationship is one in which the patient's words and actions elicit appropriate and overt responses. There is no place for therapeutic passivity, open-ended questions, or nondirective comments in the treatment of individuals who have experienced significant brain injuries; nor is there room for intrusiveness or authoritarianism. Psychiatrists must be careful not to force their values and life goals upon patients who, threatened as they are with further disruption of their identities, are quite vulnerable and therefore more likely to accept the therapist's values no matter how inappropriate they may be (Pollack, in press).

∎ **The patient must be permitted to lead the way.** Whenever possible, the therapeutic endeavor should be guided by the present concerns of the patient, by what he or she believes is relevant or can accept as relevant, not by what the therapist thinks will be of greater significance for the patient at some future date. For most people, whether they have brain injury or not, the ability to sustain attention is limited when they feel forced to attend to tasks against their present intentions in order to secure some future goal (Lichtenberg and Norton 1970). In the words of one of my own patients, "I hate it when I hear, 'It's for your own good!'" In treating brain injury patients, psychotherapists are limited in their ability to "tune in" fully to or empathize deeply with their patients, because they experience the world differently from their patients. For these reasons, therapists must follow the leads of their patients; only in this way can they come to understand the world in which their patients exist.

The need to follow the patient's lead applies also to practical

Table 20–2. Special therapeutic problems: management issues

Condition	Description	Therapist response
Transference and countertransference reactions	Transference: loss or threat to sense of self, limited adaptability, intolerance of anxiety; all promote the rapid development of intense transference relationships, both positive and negative in nature. Countertransference: therapists' overidentification, overoptimism, impatience, inflexibility, and lack of awareness of the cognitive and emotional effects of brain injury stimulate countertransference reactions. Patients' slow progress, apparent lack of involvement and motivation, changeability, and emotional dyscontrol also contribute.	Be aware of the probability of some disruptive transference and countertransference reactions; negative transference reactions in the patient and all countertransference reactions in the psychiatrist must be confronted and resolved without delay; positive transference reactions may be supported, but the boundaries between psychiatrist and patient must be kept well defined.
Denial	Determined by several interacting factors, including the direct effect of the injury, feelings of shame and/or guilt, family attitudes, the unconscious defenses against threats to the person's integrity (psychological denial).	Emphasize preserved intellectual and psychological assets to improve self-esteem; structure environment in ways that support reality; direct confrontation rarely succeeds, because it further threatens the person's integrity (sense of self).

Table 20–2. Special therapeutic problems: management issues (*continued*)

Condition	Description	Therapist response
Catastrophic condition	Intense anxiety occurs when patients are confronted by situations that are beyond their capacities. Patients respond with withdrawal and other self-defensive measures, including reduced involvement in therapy; increased denial, verbal and, at times, physical aggression.	Prevention is the best therapy; avoid open-ended, anxiety-provoking comments and questions; introduce new tasks or concepts gradually and in as simple a form as possible; if a catastrophic condition is imminent, provide additional information and structure; further simplify the task or discontinue the activity.
Guilt and shame	Common responses after traumatic brain injuries even when patients are entirely without responsibility for the event.	Consider the question "Why did this happen to me?" only after a stable therapeutic alliance has developed. Early reassurances are not helpful and may disturb the developing relationship.
Stigmatization and marginality	Brain injury patients are neither sick nor well, neither in society nor entirely out; their postinjury behaviors are difficult to understand and to categorize; their responses may appear to be unpredictable, causing anxiety and even fear in others who then tend to discredit and devaluate the source of their discomfort.	Patients must be helped to deal with the realities of an often "hostile" world.

| Loneliness | Most common long-term residual of traumatic brain injuries; patients have impaired abilities to respond to others empathically. Subsequent losses of meaningful relationships contribute to the further disruption of their already-disturbed sense of self; failed attempts to comprehend what has happened to their relationships, and their impaired self-monitoring abilities lead to negative evaluations of the motives of other people and subsequently to paranoia. | Recognize that the sense of profound loneliness is difficult to communicate; a consistent supportive approach and a patient nondemanding attitude can help to breach the isolation. Provide practical concrete assistance, avoid dealing with abstract concepts. |

issues such as the frequency and duration of therapy sessions and the length of the total psychotherapeutic endeavor. For example, many patients cannot attend effectively for more than 15 or 20 minutes. As the information that they must process increases, they become more and more confused and fatigued. In these circumstances, at best, patients absorb very little, and at worst, they may be threatened with the onset of a catastrophic condition. Usually, with improvement in their cognitive abilities, patients are able to work productively for longer periods. However, the psychiatrist must be aware of the possibility that simplification or shifting topics, or even termination of a treatment session, may be necessary according to the moment-to-moment evaluation of the patient's ability to cope.

The frequency of therapy sessions should be determined not only by the psychiatrist's appraisal of the emergent nature of the patient's problems, but also by an evaluation of the patient's new learning ability. A patient with significant short-term memory difficulties may initially have to be scheduled on a daily basis in order to ensure carry-over from treatment session to treatment session.

The length of the total therapeutic endeavor, in large part, depends on the patient's goals. Indeed, a significant part of the treatment involves helping the patient to set appropriate goals, goals that are fashioned after the patient has become aware of both strengths and liabilities and has accepted and incorporated a new sense of self.

∎ **The importance of group experiences.** Every treatment program for brain injury patients must include both formal and informal group experiences in addition to psychotherapy because "the real world" that they hope to reengage is composed of groups—large groups, small groups, quartets, triads, and pairs. In "the real world" no one functions in isolation; there are always others present if only in one's memory and imagination (Pollack 1989).

People who have experienced significant brain injuries process information slowly and have difficulty attending to more than one thing at a time, consequently high levels of anxiety can be generated when they engage in group activities. To avoid the onset of a catastrophic condition, the injured person may withdraw from the group or, if that is not possible, may express distress in an immoderate fashion. Controlled and graduated group experiences can assist brain injury patients in expressing their feelings appropriately and communicating their ideas effectively.

▮ **Family members must be involved in the treatment process.** In every case, the impact of brain injury is "infectious" and affects not only the patient but also the patient's family, disrupting its integrity, disturbing the interrelatedness of its members, and tending to isolate them from each other, as well as from the community at large (Brooks 1991; Lezak 1986; Thomsen 1984).

Frequently, family members are confronted by old needs, long thought to be outgrown, and new demands that they can neither comprehend nor fulfill. In this situation, family members may feel guilty and responsible for events over which they have little control. They may then direct their anger inwardly and become self-punitive and depressed, or may direct their feelings or frustration outwardly, seeking others in the family, including the one with brain injury, to blame for their pain (Mwaria 1990).

Because the support of the family is crucial for the successful rehabilitation of the patient, each member of the therapeutic team must work to encourage ongoing healthy family interactions, not only in reference to the impaired family member, but also with respect to each other and to the community.

▮ **Reasonable risk taking should be encouraged.** Finally, therapists must be prepared to encourage reasonable risk taking by their patients. For this to happen, therapists must be prepared to allow and accept failure by their patients and by themselves because the road that brain injury patients must travel to reestablish an acceptable sense of self is uncertain and therefore cannot be risk free. Without the possibility of failure, a person can never achieve true independence and the right to make choices in his or her own behalf (Banja 1988; Dybwad 1964).

References

Babinski MJ: Contribution to the study of mental disturbance in organic cerebral hemiplegia (anosognosia). Revue Neurologique 12:845–848, 1914

Banja JD: Independence and rehabilitation: a philosophic perspective. Arch Phys Med Rehabil 69:381–382, 1988

Becker E: The Birth and Death of Meaning. New York, Macmillan, 1962

Beisser AR: Denial and affirmation in illness and health. Am J Psychiatry 136:1026–1030, 1979

Bennett TL: Individual psychotherapy and minor head injury. Cognitive Rehabilitation 7:10–16, 1989

Binswanger L: Grundformen und Erkenntnis Menschlichen Daseins. Zurich, Niehaus, 1942

Bond M: The psychiatry of closed head injury, in Closed Head Injury. Edited by Brooks N. Oxford, Oxford University Press, 1984, pp 148–178

Brooks DN: The head injured family. J Clin Exp Neuropsychol 13:155–188, 1991

Cicerone KD: Psychotherapeutic interventions with traumatically brain injured patients. Rehabilitation Psychology 34:105–114, 1989

Conboy TJ, Barth J, Boll TJ: Treatment and rehabilitation of mild and moderate head trauma. Rehabilitation Psychology 31:203–215, 1986

Condeluci A, Gretz-Lasky S: Social role valorization: A model for community re-entry. Journal of Head Trauma Rehabilitation 2:49–56, 1987

Dybwad G: Challenges in Mental Retardation. New York, Columbia University Press, 1964

Eames P: Behavior disorders after severe head injury: their nature and causes and strategies for management. Journal of Head Trauma Rehabilitation 3:1–6, 1988

Eisenberg HM, Levin HS: Computed tomography and magnetic resonance imaging in mild to moderate head injury, in Mild Head Injuries. Edited by Levin HS, Eisenberg HM, Benton AL. New York, Oxford University Press, 1989, pp 217–228

Ellis DW: Neuropsychotherapy, in Neuropsychological Treatment After Brain Injury. Edited by Ellis DW, Christensen AL. Boston, MA, Kluwer Academic, 1989, pp 241–269

Fahy TJ, Irving MH, Millac P: Severe head injuries: a six-year follow-up. Lancet 2:475–479, 1967

Fordyce WE: Denial of disability in spinal cord injury: a behavioral perspective. Paper presented at the 91st Annual Convention of the American Psychological Association, Anaheim, CA, 1983

Fromm-Reichmann F: Loneliness. Psychiatry 22:1–15, 1959

Gan JS: Hate in the rehabilitation setting. Arch Phys Med Rehabil 64:176–179, 1983

Gardner H: The Shattered Mind: The Person After Brain Damage. New York, Knopf, 1976

Genarelli TA: Cerebral concussion and diffuse brain injuries, in Head Injury. Edited by Cooper PR. Baltimore, MD, Williams & Wilkins, 1981, pp 83–97

Goffman E: Stigma. Englewood Cliffs, NJ, Prentice-Hall, 1963

Goldstein K: The effect of brain damage on the personality. Psychiatry 15:245–260, 1952

Heilman KM, Watson RT, Valenstein E: Neglect and related disorders, in Clinical Neuropsychology, 2nd Edition. Edited by Heilman KM, Valenstein E. New York, Oxford University Press, 1985, pp 243–284

Kolb LC, Brodie HK: Modern Clinical Psychiatry, 10th Edition. Philadelphia, PA, WB Saunders, 1982

Levin HS, Eisenberg HM, Benton AL (eds): Mild Head Injuries. New York, Oxford University Press, 1989

Lewis L, Rosenberg S: Psychoanalytic psychotherapy with brain-injured adult psychiatric patients. J Nerv Ment Dis 178:69–77, 1990

Lezak MD: Subtle sequelae of brain damage: perplexity, distractibility and fatigue. Am J Phys Med 57:9–15, 1978

Lezak MD: Psychological implications of traumatic brain damage for the patient's family. Rehabilitation Psychology 31:241–250, 1986

Lezak MD: The walking wounded of head injury: when subtle deficits can be disabling. Trends in Rehabilitation 3:4–9, 1989

Lichtenberg P, Norton DG: Cognitive and Mental Development in the First Five Years of Life: A Review of the Recent Literature. Rockville, MD, National Institutes of Mental Health, 1970

Lishman WA: The psychiatric sequelae of head injury: a review. Psychol Med 3:304–318, 1973

Ludwig AM: Principles of Clinical Psychiatry. New York, The Free Press, 1980, pp 424–425

McGlynn SM, Schacter DL: Unawareness of deficits in neuropsychological syndromes. J Clin Exp Neuropsychol 11:143–205, 1989

Miller L: Psychotherapy of the brain-injured patient: principles and practices. Cognitive Rehabilitation 9:24–30, 1991

Murphy RF: The Body Silent. New York, Henry Holt, 1987, pp 6, 85–110

Murphy RF, Scheer J, Murphy Y, et al: Physical disability and social liminality: a study in the rituals of adversity. Soc Sci Med 26:235–242, 1988

Mwaria CB: The concept of self in the context of crisis: a study of families of the severely brain injured. Soc Sci Med 30:889–893, 1990

Peplau LA, Miceli M, Morasch B: Loneliness and self-evaluation, in Loneliness: A Source Book of Current Theory, Research, and Therapy. Edited by Peplau LA, Perlman D. New York, Wiley, 1982, pp 135–151

Piotrowski Z: The Rorschach ink blot method in organic disturbances of the central nervous system. J Nerv Ment Dis 86:525–537, 1937

Pollack IW: Traumatic brain injury and the rehabilitation process: a psychiatric perspective, in Neuropsychological Treatment After Brain Injury. Edited by Ellis DW, Christensen AL. Boston, MA, Kluwer Academic, 1989, pp 105–125

Pollack IW: Reestablishing an acceptable sense of self: a guiding principle for brain injury rehabilitation, in Educational Programming for Children and Young Adults With Acquired Brain Injuries. Edited by Savage RC, Wolcott GF. Boston, MA, College Hill (in press)

Prigatano GP: Neuropsychological Rehabilitation After Brain Injury. Baltimore, MD, Johns Hopkins University Press, 1986

Prigatano GP: Neuropsychological deficits, personality variables and outcome, in Community Re-Entry for Head Injured Adults. Edited by Ylvisaker M, Gobble ER. Boston, MA, College Hill, 1987, pp 1–23

Prigatano GP: Emotion and motivation in recovery and adaptation after brain damage, in Brain Injury and Recovery. Edited by Finger S, Levere TE, Almi CR, et al. New York, Plenum, 1988, pp 335–350

Prigatano GP: Work, love and play after brain injury. Bull Menninger Clin 53:414–431, 1989

Rimel RW, Giordani B, Barth JT, et al: Disability caused by minor head injury. Neurosurgery 9:221–228, 1981

Rosen M: Denial and the head trauma client: a developmental formulation and treatment plan. Cognitive Rehabilitation 4:20–22, 1986

Rutherford W: Post concussional symptoms, in Mild Head Injuries. Edited by Levin HS, Eisenberg HM, Benton AL. New York, Oxford University Press, 1989, pp 217–228

Silver JM, Hales RE, Yudofsky SC: Neuropsychiatric aspects of traumatic brain injury, in American Psychiatric Press Textbook of Neuropsychiatry, 2nd Edition. Edited by Yudofsky SC, Hales RE. Washington, DC, American Psychiatric Press, 1992, pp 363–395

Stein DG: In pursuit of new strategies for understanding recovery from brain damage: problems and perspectives, in Clinical Neuropsychology and Brain Function. Edited by Boll T, Bryant B. Washington, DC, American Psychological Association, 1988, pp 9–55

Stuewe-Portnoff G: Loneliness: lost in the landscape of meaning. J Psychol 122:545–555, 1988

Thomsen IV: The patient with severe head injury and his family. Scand J Rehabil Med 6:180–183, 1974

Thomsen IV: Late outcome of very severe head trauma: 10–15 year second follow-up. J Neurol Neurosurg Psychiatry 47:260–268, 1984

Tyerman A, Humphrey M: Changes in self-concept following severe head injury. Int J Rehabil Res 7:11–23, 1984

Weddell R, Oddy M, Jenkins D: Social adjustment after rehabilitation: a two-year follow-up of patients with severe head injury. Psychol Med 10:257–263, 1980

Weinstein EA, Kahn RL: Denial of Illness. Springfield, IL, Charles C Thomas, 1955

Chapter 21

Cognitive Rehabilitation

Jack Rattok, Ph.D.
Barbara P. Ross, Ph.D.

Traumatic brain injury (TBI) is distinguished by characteristics not readily demonstrable in a majority of other medical problems. The effects of these injuries encompass physical, emotional, and cognitive sequelae that must all be addressed in the treatment of patients with head injuries (H. S. Levin et al. 1982). Most medical interventions are directed toward a primary malfunction of the organism that may have secondary consequences. In TBI, because there is by definition injury to the brain, the physical, emotional, and cognitive systems of the patient are all affected on a primary level. For example, depression may result in secondary cognitive deficits but when depression is alleviated, in the absence of dementia, intellectual functioning will return to its previous level without any specific cognitive remediation. In cases of brain injury, however, resolving the emotional difficulty will not alleviate the cognitive problems and vice versa.

Traditionally, the population availing themselves of comprehensive therapeutic services for TBI consisted of those who experienced brain injury as a result of motor vehicle accidents or work-related incidents. Currently, a wider population of patients with nondevelopmental neurological impairment (e.g., stroke and anoxic brain injury subsequent to cardiac arrest) has also been shown to benefit from these services. In this chapter, we describe the nature of the cognitive deficits in patients with TBI from the standpoint of how these patients function. We will delineate the treatment of these deficits, and discuss the contributions of psychiatrists and other professionals to the treatment process.

History of Rehabilitation of Head Injury

The early history of rehabilitation in TBI demonstrates that little was done to address the cognitive deficits of patients. It was known that, after damage, there is only limited regeneration of the central nervous system and the belief was held that cognitive functions lost due to brain injury could not be repaired. Indeed, from the end of the previous century until the early 1970s, there were only a few scientists who attempted to address treatment issues of cognitive malfunction. Their work was carried on in an individual and isolated manner and did not lead to comprehensive treatment efforts or ongoing services (Boake 1989).

During the early 1970s, scientists at Rusk Institute of Rehabilitation Medicine in New York City began to conduct systematic research to document the particular functional cognitive deficits of various stroke patients, with the goal of developing treatment programs. Their research led to the conclusion that attempts to remediate the cognitive deficits of these patients could enhance their ability to function (Diller et al. 1974). However, at that time the American rehabilitation system was not yet ready to implement these findings.

At approximately the same time, as a result of massive shelling activity between Israel and Egypt in the early 1970s, the Israeli Army had several hundred young men who had experienced traumatic brain injuries. Although the Israeli rehabilitation system attempted to maximize the recovery of their soldiers using known physical medicine and rehabilitation procedures, these veterans continued to exhibit serious and persistent cognitive and emotional difficulties that prevented them from resuming mainstream life. Consequently, in 1975, the Israeli Veterans Administration, together with Rusk Institute and Tel Aviv University, began the first modern postacute clinical research rehabilitation program for TBI. This program was not built on theories of brain recuperation, but rather was based on the notion of functional training in deficits of five cognitive domains (Table 21–1) derived from the research done at Rusk Institute in the early 1970s. One of the conclusions drawn following this pilot clinical program was that the social and emotional sequelae of TBI need to be addressed in tandem with the cognitive training of these patients (Ben-Yishay et al. 1978).

The success of the Israeli program led to the establishment of the first clinical research rehabilitation program for TBI in the United States. It was started at Rusk Institute in 1978 and led to the development of other programs (Boake 1989). At the present time, several hundred programs exist in the United States providing comprehensive postacute rehabilitation for brain injury patients. In these programs cognitive rehabilitation is considered a crucial part of the clinical service (Mazmanian et al. 1991).

Theories of Recovery From Brain Injury

In practice, it has been shown that certain types of cognitive exercises improve the functionality of the TBI patient (Weinberg et

Table 21–1.   Five cognitive domains of training

Attention and concentration
Fine motor coordination
Constructional praxis
Verbal information processing
Visual information processing

al. 1979). Scientists have looked for possible explanations of this phenomenon. There are presently two major views held of how cognitive recovery occurs (Meir et al. 1987). The first holds that recovery is a natural phenomenon and with amelioration of the transient trauma, brain functions recuperate as the trauma abates and then reach whatever level of functioning is inherently possible, postinjury. This explanation would deem cognitive rehabilitation unnecessary, because improvement would occur due to spontaneous recovery. The second view of the mechanism of action of cognitive treatment is that recovery takes place as a result of the brain's ability to compensate for an injury and transfer functioning from damaged cells to other cells, with the help of therapeutic stimulation via physical and cognitive exercises. For example, a patient who has a lesion in the Broca's area of the brain will experience difficulties with verbal information processing. Typically, during the initial recovery period the patient will not be able to utilize verbal information. According to the first view of recovery as a natural phenomenon, as the trauma abates, the patient will spontaneously recover some degree of verbal capability according to the amount of undamaged tissue remaining. The second view holds that early intervention will aid the brain in transferring function from the damaged area to other areas and will result in a more optimal return of verbal functions.

It should be noted that rehabilitation programs providing treatment and follow-up are relatively new phenomena. In the past, patients were discharged from acute care, and little further information was available to assess long-term results (Jacobs 1987). Therefore, the first notion has been more readily accepted in the medical field because it stemmed from extensive research and follow-up done in the acute and early stages of coma while spontaneous recovery was taking place.

The early rehabilitation programs, in both Israel and the United States, treated only those patients who were at least 1 year posttrauma (average 3 years posttrauma) and therefore well past the initial stages of recovery. The successful outcome of these programs is not consistent with the notion of spontaneous recovery leading to maximum cognitive functioning. Although the two

explanations mentioned above are not mutually exclusive, research outcomes are more explanatory of the second theory that,
with retraining, the brain has the capacity to compensate for lost
functions. It appears that once the cognitive system is relatively
stable, the processes that take place and augment the recovery are
therefore better explained in terms of compensation (Cope 1985).

Whatever the various theoretical explanations, they address
the physiology of the brain and do not lend themselves to any
practical interventions. Therefore, cognitive rehabilitation employs
a functional method, which does not deal with repairing the
physiology of the brain, but utilizes means of reorganizing and
retraining the cognitive system (Meir et al. 1987).

Definition of Cognitive Rehabilitation

For rehabilitation purposes, cognition is the capacity of a person
(via the CNS) to perceive stimuli in the immediate environment,
analyze and compare these stimuli to information stored in memory, organize this information, and make decisions about the
appropriate response to the environment (Adamovich 1991). Any
interruption in this chain of events will result in impairment of
cognitive-intellectual functioning. Cognitive rehabilitation is the
process of introducing remedial exercises to improve impaired
mental functions. The results of cognitive rehabilitation can be
explained either as improvement of function through restoration of
damaged areas in the brain, or as improvement of function by
compensation (the transfer, to undamaged areas, of mental functions impaired as a result of injury to the brain). To date, there is
not sufficient precise technology to measure the contribution of
one or the other.

Cognitive rehabilitation can be divided into two general levels,
the functional and the generic. The functional is the level on which
we train activities that are necessary to the orderly execution of
practical functions such as how to dress or how to prepare a meal.

On the second level we train generic cognitive skills such as the abilities to pay attention, remember, and solve problems.

Direct Delivery of Service

Cognitive rehabilitation services are provided by professionals from a variety of disciplines (Table 21–2). Occupational therapists train the cognitive aspects necessary for activities of daily living and functioning in the community. Typical training routines involve teaching the sequencing and execution of morning routines and organizing and practicing activities such as shopping, cooking, and commuting. Occupational therapists utilize kitchens, bathrooms, supermarkets, and others. The training consists of in vivo practice of activities. For example, the occupational therapist may ask the patient to prepare a dinner, which may involve the planning of a menu, actual shopping, and then preparation of a meal. At each step the occupational therapist will observe the patient's performance and provide training as necessary.

Speech therapists concentrate on improving both the assimilation, retention, comprehension and production of language, and the efficient processing of verbal information, as well as on

Table 21–2. Providers of cognitive rehabilitation

Providers	Service
Direct providers	
Occupational therapists	Functional (ADL) training
Speech therapists	Speech and communication
Neuropsychologists	Generic cognitive training
Cognitive technicians	Computer exercises
Indirect providers	
Neuropsychiatrists	Management for behavioral problems
Neurologists	General medical management
Neuro-ophthalmologists	Visual management

Note. ADL = activities of daily living.

teaching effective communication skills. If a patient is aphasic and unable to talk, a speech therapist may use computerized biofeedback instruments to stimulate speech. The speech therapist uses pictures and objects to facilitate object recognition and naming, and educational materials to retrain and improve academic skills.

Neuropsychologists are concerned primarily with improving generic brain functions such as attention, memory, and visual information processing. The neuropsychologist may use computerized exercises to improve reaction time and other components of basic attention. The patient is presented with story and picture materials, and asked to memorize the information and recall it. The patient is trained to use techniques for recalling information, thus improving memory.

Cognitive technicians represent a more novel delivery of service. They are individuals trained in the implementation of specific exercises (mainly using the computer) and their work is a technical follow-up and reinforcement of the rehabilitation techniques handled by the other disciplines mentioned above. For example, a patient who is unable to write legibly because of motor problems can be trained by a cognitive technician to use a computer.

Indirect Delivery of Service

Individuals who experience TBI often display various syndromes that can prevent cognitive rehabilitation from taking place. These syndromes require the intervention of a variety of medical specialists (Table 21–2).

A review of 300 cases treated by us and our colleagues over a 4-year period shows that 35% of patients are unaware of the nature of their cognitive difficulties and refuse, in varying degrees, to cooperate with therapeutic procedures. This phenomenon seems to stem from a combination of the genuine incapacity, in TBI, of a defective cognitive system to reflect upon and analyze its own situation, and the individual's use of the mechanism of psychological denial. Lack of motivation to participate in cognitive rehabilitation can additionally be attributed to a high level of anxiety, depression, fatigue, and lack of impulse control. To give an example, a patient who entered a cognitive rehabilitation program exhibited such intense anxiety about his situation, that verbal perseverations about what would become of him overwhelmed him and prevented him from assimilating any exercises. He would sit in front of a computer rocking back and forth exclaiming, "What is going to happen to me?" TBI patients can display an array of behaviors ranging from total withdrawal, to unenthusiastic cooperation, to agitation and/or aggressive behavior during treatment.

In the majority of these cases, a neuropsychiatric consultation is necessary in order to manage behavior with the aid of medication. This type of intervention should proceed in a judicious manner, because the majority of psychiatric medications are known to have side effects that may result in a reduction in cognitive abilities. With any reduction in cognition, TBI patients tend to be even less cooperative. In such cases it is important to maintain ongoing consultation between the neuropsychiatrist and the therapist providing cognitive rehabilitation, in order to maintain an optimal level of functioning for the patient (Silver et al. 1992).

Patients with TBI who are judged medically stable may still experience ongoing neurological episodes that affect the cognitive system, such as seizure activity. It is not uncommon to see a patient who has made substantial gains in cognitive functioning lose much of this gain following a neurological episode. In such cases, ongoing consultation and follow-up with a neurologist is necessary to ensure successful cognitive rehabilitation (Kingston 1985). Often, individuals with TBI experience difficulties with their visual systems. Because a large part of cognitive rehabilitation depends upon presenting material in the visual mode, in cases where the patient's visual system is impaired, a neuro-ophthalmology consult is necessary. For example, attention to visual detail cannot be learned by a patient who has double vision.

Through the early 1990s, none of the disciplines mentioned above, whether direct or indirect providers of service, are incorporating the treatment of TBI as a subspeciality of training in graduate curriculums. Knowledge and expertise in the field are developing as a result of on-the-job training, specialized journals dealing with head injury rehabilitation (see Appendix 21–1), and periodic workshops given on the treatment of TBI, which are listed in these journals. Experience is the sole yardstick for judging professional competence. TBI programs attached to mainstream medical facilities, with a proven record of experience, are the best choice for treatment. The National Head Injury Foundation issues an annual directory of TBI centers.

Cognitive Deficits Following TBI

TBI can impair several levels of the cognitive system (Table 21–3). The primary level involves the actual locus of injury. Localization of brain function has been well documented (Milner 1971). When injury occurs to a specific area of the brain, the cognitive function associated with this area will be impaired, for example, damage to the Broca's area of the brain results in difficulty with the organization and production of speech. Specific cognitive deficits on this level have been extensively documented in the literature (Meir et al. 1987) and are ameliorated in part by spontaneous recovery, and in part through treatment during the acute stage.

The secondary level of the cognitive system involves impairment of general cognitive functions not necessarily associated with

Table 21–3. Levels of cognitive impairment following traumatic brain injury

Deficits in specific modalities	Deficits in global processing
Motor	Arousal (attention)
Sensation	Inefficiency (slow processing)
Vision	Modulation (flexibility)
Audition	Assimilation (memory)
Language	Organization (executive skills)

localization of injury (Binder and Rattok 1988). These are the global processes of cognitive functioning identified in Table 21–3.

Attention

Trauma to the brain almost always eventuates in declined arousal, resulting in impairment of the attentional system. These deficits can range from inability to concentrate and perceive a simple stimulus, to difficulty in maintaining attention for more than several minutes, to problems in selective attention (Posner and Rafal 1987). Patients with TBI who experience difficulties with basic attention do not perceive environmental cues and are therefore unable to act upon the environment in a meaningful manner. Inability to maintain attention over more than a short time span, even if basic attention is adequate, can result in difficulties with both perceiving information and acting upon it within a reasonable span of time (Mack 1986). Problems in selective attention, even if basic attention and span of attention are both functional, will lead to difficulty in interaction with the environment when several stimuli are presented at the same time. For example, an individual with TBI may be able to conduct a meaningful conversation with one other person, yet be unable to maintain the thread of conversation, comprehend, and interact appropriately when several people are engaged.

Inefficiency

An important phenomenon is the general slowing of the cognitive system in patients with TBI (Tromp and Mulder 1991). Although in some cases most of the components of the system may be operating normally, the interactions necessary to create smooth execution of a task are slowed to the point of inefficiency (Rattok 1986). For example, when a patient with TBI who is so affected attempts to drive a car, his or her processing of cues will be too slow for an adequate reaction under normal traffic conditions. An example of a more subtle deficit is that of a physician who, after experiencing a mild TBI, maintains all the knowledge and cognitive skills necessary for his or her work, yet discovers that a patient examination that usually takes 20 minutes to perform now takes 50 minutes, with the result that he or she is unable to continue practicing in the chosen specialty.

Memory

Deficits in memory comprise the most pervasive cognitive problem after TBI (Benton 1979). Functional memory problems can appear in the form of retrograde amnesia, wherein the person forgets information stored in his or her cognitive system before the trauma, and/or anterograde amnesia, wherein the person has difficulty retrieving information and events assimilated after the trauma (often referred to as short-term memory problems). Retrograde amnesia can be inferred to result from injury to the permanent memory mechanisms of the brain. A patient with retrograde amnesia was a mechanical engineer before his injury. Although his memory for all current activities is within the normal range, he has forgotten most of the information necessary to the practice of his profession and is unable to resume his preinjury vocation. Anterograde amnesia seems to be more a result of the inability of the brain to absorb and process information. In this case, storage either does not occur, or takes place in such a manner that information cannot be adequately retrieved. The inability to absorb, process, and store information in memory can create deficits in verbal memory, visual memory, or both, depending on whether verbal and/or visual systems are affected. A patient who was an accountant remembered all the rules and regulations pertaining to accounting procedures. However, he could not remember current information given to him over the telephone by a client, could not remember discussions, and therefore was not able to retain enough information to continue working as an accountant.

Modulation

Modulation involves the ability to perceive situations from differing perspectives, to see similarities in disparate situations, and to be able to discover multifaceted solutions (abstract thinking). Once this cognitive process occurs, it is important that an individual be able to adapt his or her behavior accordingly (Lezak 1989). Often after TBI, an individual who maintains his or her basic intellectual functioning cannot see more than one aspect of a problem and will offer only a narrow solution, because of an inability to flexibly entertain a range of possibilities (concrete behavior). The inability to use cognitive information to modulate behavior frequently results in interpersonal conflict between the patient and the environment. For example, a young man who has sustained a brain injury may spend his evenings harassing family members to switch off lights and appliances, regardless of their needs at the time, because he wants to save household money by conserving electricity.

Organization

The appropriate organization of our behavior depends upon executive skills. The capacities of the brain to integrate multichannel complex information from various modalities, and to act upon this information in an efficient and purposeful manner, constitute the executive skills (Kay and Silver 1989). The brain must be capable of first, correctly perceiving the environment, and second, flexibly and efficiently analyzing it to derive the most adaptive and adequate solutions. All systems must then be organized to take into account social factors, personal factors, time and place factors, and the environment's reactions to our decisions and actions. These capabilities are the executive skills of cognition and they embody the highest level of cognitive organization and functioning. To give an example, a patient who had been the foreman of a large auto mechanic repair shop prior to his TBI was still capable of performing as an auto mechanic but could no longer function as a foreman, which involved planning and directing the work of others.

Both modulation and organization are skills that do not have a specific locus, but instead represent overall brain function. These skills are impacted by both cognitive malfunction and the typical behavioral difficulties accompanying TBI, such as impulsivity, anxiety, and depression. Unfortunately, they are the first skills to be lost in almost every case of TBI (Rattok 1985).

Treatment

Population

The seminal research on cognitive rehabilitation was done in the early 1970s with stroke patients. The rationale for the choice of this population was that the site of damage could be accurately documented. Therefore, it was possible to design controlled studies. A brief pilot study was carried out with stroke patients (Diller and Weinberg 1977). During the first 10 years of actual treatment, however, due to funding considerations, the population consisted mainly of young adults who had acquired TBI as a result of motor vehicle accidents. With the widening availability of specialized clinical services, treatment was broadened to include other populations who experienced the same types of cognitive difficulties because of nondevelopmental neurological impairments. These included traumatic brain injuries caused by open and closed head injury, Cardiovascular aneurysm (stroke and others), brain diseases such as meningitis, encephalitis and others, anoxia, radiation therapy, and postoperative impairments.

Types of Service

Services are usually provided in acute rehabilitation hospital settings, postacute residential transitional programs, day programs, or 1-hour individual treatment sessions (Cope 1985).

Acute rehabilitation services are provided through the department of Physical Medicine and Rehabilitation. Treatment is provided under the medical model and is appropriate for TBI patients who are not medically stable and/or are physically impaired to the degree that they are not independent in basic activities of daily living (e.g., they are incontinent, have severe difficulties in mobility or communication, or are unable to feed themselves). The patient is under the care of the psychiatrist and the daily program includes medical treatment, as well as intensive physical therapy, occupational therapy, and speech therapy oriented mainly toward the physical disability.

The next level of care is usually a postacute residential transitional program. Some programs are part of a medical center, others are separate treatment centers, but all treat only TBI. These programs are suitable for patients who are medically stable, but upon discharge from acute rehabilitation may still experience symptoms such as cognitive confusion, behavioral problems, and dependency, to the extent that activities of daily living cannot be discharged in the home environment. The treatment provided in these programs incorporates the elements of acute rehabilitation but extends treatment into more advanced levels of patient functionality and emphasizes cognitive rehabilitation. The key to success in such a program lies in the provision of integrated comprehensive care (see Table 21–4). Day programs for brain injury patients may be attached to medical centers or may function as independent facilities. Day programs are similar to transitional residential programs, but the patient's symptoms are less severe and he or she is able to live in a home environment. (For an example of a typical day in a transitional day program, see Table 21–5.)

Table 21–4.   Comprehensive care

Medical coordination

Physical therapy

Occupational therapy

Speech therapy

Cognitive training

Individual and family counseling

Social follow-up

Vocational aspects

Table 21–5.   A day in a transitional residential program[a]

Time	Activity
7 A.M. to 8 A.M.	Morning routines
8 A.M. to 9 A.M.	Breakfast
9 A.M. to 10 A.M.	Community meeting
10 A.M. to 11 A.M.	Orientation I and II
11 A.M. to 12 P.M.	Communication/life skills[b]
12 P.M. to 1 P.M.	Lunch
1 P.M. to 2 P.M.	Cognitive remediation
2 P.M. to 3 P.M.	Counseling/prevocational[b]
3 P.M. to 4 P.M.	Physical therapy
4 P.M. to 5 P.M.	Evening community meeting
5 P.M. to 6 P.M.	Homework
6 P.M. to 7 P.M.	Dinner

[a]Day program follows the same routine as residential program from 10 A.M. to 4 P.M.
[b]Provided on alternate days.

One-hour individual cognitive treatment sessions are recommended toward the end of the rehabilitation process. At this time the patient should be ready for his or her return to some activities in mainstream life. This therapy concentrates on addressing specific areas of deficit identified in the home, school, or work environment, and usually entails one or two treatment sessions per week.

Decisions concerning the type of program needed for an individual TBI patient are complex and require specialized training. It is now common practice for those involved in discharge planning at medical facilities to request that treatment centers for TBI send their specialists to evaluate patients and judge their suitability for each type of program. This service is usually provided free of charge by treatment centers within the geographical area.

It should be noted that when TBI is acquired from motor vehicle accidents or work-related accidents, cognitive rehabilitation is a service recognized by insurance providers. However, because it is a relatively new form of treatment, cognitive rehabilitation remains in a "gray area" for most health insurance providers, including Medicare and Medicaid. Insurance eligibility in these situations is a complicated issue, and providers of postacute brain injury rehabilitation can be contacted to provide help in these matters.

Treatment of Attention Disorder

Currently, treatment of basic attention is accomplished primarily with the aid of computers. The exercises are based upon improving reaction time to simple stimuli and then gradually introducing more and more complex stimuli. The computer measures the time that it takes to react to a correct stimulus such as the onset of a light, appearance of pictures, or simple words. Reaction time is an indicator of the capacity to pay attention. Normal reaction time to a simple stimulus is 250 milliseconds (msec). Patients with TBI who are impaired in basic attention may register a reaction time of 400 msec or more before training. In most circumstances, a few weeks of training can bring the individual with TBI to within normal ranges on tests of attention. The improvement occurs with continuous practice and the use of positive reinforcement that motivates the person to speed his or her performance (Rattok et al. 1982).

The second level of attention extends the capacity to pay attention for longer and longer periods of time, and is based on principles similar to those described above. However, the presentation of stimuli is more varied and the task has more intellectual demand (e.g., visual tracking or a response repetition to a continuous series of auditory stimuli). These tasks are presented in serial manner and are stretched over longer time spans.

The third level of attention involves the capacity to attend to stimuli coming from various simultaneous sources, for example, maintaining a conversation with several people. Training at this level is done in small structured group situations. Four to seven individuals with TBI sit together and are given simple verbal material within the level of their comprehension (e.g., a brief newspaper article) to read and then to explain to one another. There then follows verbal interaction with comments about the presented material. The emphasis of this exercise is on the capacity to attend to information coming from several sources, rather than on the quality of presentation.

Improving attentional function is crucial for advanced cognitive training. Ability to maintain an adequate level of attention is a precursor for any further cognitive functioning. Research (Ben-Yishay et al. 1987) shows that in some cases training of attention by itself can increase IQ scores significantly, because patients who are deficient in basic attention cannot attend to the test proceedings and will thus score very low regardless of their true intellectual capacities.

Efficiency

Boosting the efficiency of the cognitive system is not solely dependent upon any single cognitive exercise per se. Rather, it is embedded in the overall structure of the cognitive rehabilitation program. Patients with TBI are given feedback in the form of a quantified assessment of their progress on each and every task, utilizing summary scores and charts (Rattok et al. 1981). This method of constant reinforcement cuts across all domains of cognitive training. Programs are highly structured and organized in a workman-like manner. The patient has a weekly schedule of activities and aside from lunch and free time, only acute medical necessity is an excuse for nonparticipation.

Memory

Assimilation of information is enhanced by training in various aspects of memory and by the teaching of compensatory techniques. Basic memory training is provided using computer exercises that repetitively present simple sequential information. The successful completion of each step in the sequence is dependent on information retained from the previous step. Memory is augmented in this process, because a solution cannot be reached unless previous steps are retained (Wilson 1987).

Patients are taught how to use diaries, log books, and pocket computerized calendars to record events, activities, and schedules. In cases where a patient forgets, he or she is asked to look in the log, rather than request the information from someone else. These log books serve the patient as a memory aid and tool, but more importantly, the continual writing down of information ensures processing by the cognitive system and therefore helps to enhance memory (Deaton 1991).

Each morning, the program starts with a special orientation group in which clients discuss, with the aid of their logs, the events of the previous day and what is going to take place today. Such activity reinforces the day-to-day sense of continuity so dramatically disturbed by memory problems. In addition, it ensures that clients are paying attention to the general plan of daily events, thus supporting adequate storage of information in memory for later retrieval (Deaton 1991).

Modulation

The cognitive precursors of modulation include the capacity for verbal and visual abstractions. Cognitive training to improve abstraction utilizes both computer and paper and pencil exercises. Verbal abstractions are trained using exercises that involve verbal categorization, verbal analogies, and verbal inferences from information presented. For example, "In what way are an apple and an orange alike?" or, "Dog is to cat as car is to . . . 1) chair, 2) boat, 3) house?" Visual abstraction is trained using pictorial information that requires the patient to perceive similarities and differences and reach a correct solution (Figure 21–1).

Training in flexibility of thought, and its application to actual behavior, is done in structured group situations. Patients are presented with hypothetical real-life situations that can be viewed from different perspectives and have various possible solutions. The patients must discuss the situation and offer solutions to the problem (Ross et al. 1982).

Organization

Organizational (executive) skills are improved using special structured groups in which the patients are presented with specific topics and asked to discuss them and offer opinions and solutions. Because the ability to use executive skills represents the highest level of cognitive functioning, these skills are usually addressed toward the end of the cognitive rehabilitation program (Rattok and Ross 1986). In conjunction with this final period of cognitive training, preparation is begun for various vocational solutions to be implemented upon discharge. The topic of vocation is therefore a useful one for discussion in the groups designed to strengthen organizational skills (Rattok et al. 1983).

At this stage, patients are given individual projects to execute independently. For example, a construction supervisor was asked to plan a relatively complicated building project, and a judge was asked to evaluate and write an opinion on a case. These projects are designed to occupy great amounts of an individual's time both in the program and after hours. The patient is given a deadline for submission of the work and is responsible for pacing the time allotted for the plan and its completion.

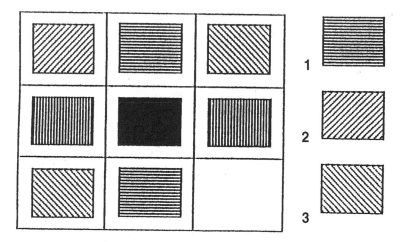

Figure 21–1. Visual abstraction training instrument. Patient is required to perceive similarities and differences and reach a correct solution.

Efficacy

Although the use of cognitive training as a central tool in the rehabilitation of TBI began in the 1970s, only a few hundred people worldwide had been treated by the mid 1980s. Early approaches were experimental and functional in nature and did not provide outcome data on specific cognitive domains (Gordon 1987). To measure the efficacy of cognitive retraining, a neuropsychological battery was administered to each patient. During the training procedures, we pretested on the specific task within a domain (e.g., information processing—visual scanning, verbal categorization), and provided training in a controlled environment (one treatment modality at a time). We posttested on the specific task to measure improvement and then readministered the entire neuropsychological battery to demonstrate generalization of that specific task to others in the same domain and to overall cognitive functioning. In addition, we administered a scale to measure changes in activities of daily living and general quality of life.

Unfortunately, for the few researchers who attempted to follow this design, results have been equivocal (Niemann et al. 1990), because the neuropsychological batteries currently in use are not sensitive enough to detect small changes in specific cognitive domains. Under a properly controlled experimental research design, cognitive rehabilitation would have to be provided as the sole form of intervention being conducted at the time. Due to the emotional and physical difficulties we encounter in patients with TBI, it is impossible to provide cognitive retraining in isolation from other forms of treatment. As of the early 1990s, the efficacy of cognitive retraining is inferred from outcome results of comprehensive programs in which cognitive retraining is a part of the treatment (usually 25% to 40% of the treatment hours). The measures used to assess these results are rating scales of general functioning and vocational outcome measures (Ruff and Camenzuli 1991).

The proof of efficacy of outcome in cognitive retraining lies in overall improvement of everyday life activities, social life, and work-related situations. Many researchers cite lack of generalization as the prime problem of cognitive remediation (Gordon 1987). Some clinicians believe that eventually they will discover a specific training procedure that will generalize better than others. However, there is skepticism regarding whether it is possible to achieve generalization from any specific cognitive domain to overall cognitive functioning, because the capacity for cognitive generalization is itself damaged in the majority of TBI patients (Ruff et al. 1989).

Use of the Computer in Cognitive Retraining

In the early stages of cognitive retraining, it became evident that some aspects of training, such as exercises in attention and visual information processing, required electronic devices to deliver the training stimuli and measure reaction time. Other types of retraining, such as verbal information processing, could be done using paper and pencil exercises.

In the mid 1970s, when cognitive rehabilitation began, personal computers were not yet available. Some researchers devised and built their own special electronic instruments for use in cognitive retraining. When personal computers became widely available in the mid 1980s, it became evident that they 1) could replace these costly and commercially unavailable electronic devices and 2) had important applicability as a more accurate and efficient tool than paper and pencil tasks. Objections that "the computer will replace the clinician" in the decision-making process were soon dispelled. Professionals began to use the computer and came to accept it as an elaborate tool, rather than an intellectual entity.

Today, the computer is widely used in cognitive rehabilitation (W. Levin 1991). However, we should be reminded that it is not a magical therapeutic panacea and can be easily misused. Leaving a patient to work alone at the computer as a method of cognitive treatment does not provide cognitive enhancement. Without the structure, motivation, and constant feedback provided by a trained therapist, computerized cognitive exercises are virtually useless. Some of the scientific journals mentioned in Appendix 21–1 include sections about practical issues related to computerized cognitive rehabilitation. They often include evaluations and recommendations of hardware and software.

Provision of cognitive therapy solely through use of the computer will rarely generalize to overall intellectual functioning. Training on the computer entails the use of discrete cognitive capacities that do not represent the entire array of cognitive functions. In addition to computerized cognitive exercises, the use of individual and group methods mentioned earlier in this chapter are necessary to ensure improvement of overall functioning.

Length of Treatment

Decisions about time of discharge from acute rehabilitation following TBI are based on criteria concerning the patient's medical status. Discharge from postacute residential programs usually follows an evaluation of the patient's ability to return to his or her home environment based on cognitive alertness, functioning of activities of daily living, and appropriate behaviors. Decisions regarding length of time in a day program or one-hour treatment sessions are more complicated, because these programs are heavily weighted toward cognitive rehabilitation. This form of intervention is more a learning process than a medical treatment, and although rate of improvement declines slowly over time, a patient can continue to benefit for many years.

Three major research programs attempted to resolve the issue of length of treatment by providing 6 months of cognitive rehabilitation followed by 6 months of vocational follow-up (Ezrachi 1983; Prigatano 1984; Scherzer 1986). Patients in these programs were mildly to moderately impaired and suitable for a day program. Results showed that patients completing these two phases were either able to return to some form of work or deemed unemployable. Employment was defined in broad terms: gainfully employed, sheltered workshop, school, or homemaking (Ezrachi et al. 1991).

For practical purposes, when programs are not financed by research funds, it is impossible to engage patients and their insurance carriers for a predefined period of 6 to 12 months in a day program. Through the early 1990s there has been no research that provides a breakdown of discrete cognitive deficits and norms for length of treatment or scientific definitions of plateau. Therefore, common practice is to establish functional goals at the beginning of treatment and reevaluate these goals on a monthly basis. In most cases of TBI, treatment will be terminated due to insurance limitations, employer requirements, and/or personal considerations, rather than the patient's inability to benefit from further treatment.

In the other forms of treatment mentioned above, the individual with TBI generally receives 1 to 5 hours per day of treatment 5 days per week. An average period of cognitive training lasts 6 months and the patient receives between 200 and 300 hours of cognitive rehabilitation.

Conclusions

Cognitive rehabilitation is central to any treatment program designed for the traumatically brain injured individual. Although specific cognitive exercises have their own unique place as training tools, when used in isolation, they are of doubtful value in aiding a traumatically brain injured person to attain true functionality. However, when utilized as part of a comprehensive interdisciplinary program of rehabilitation for TBI, they can be crucial and efficacious components of treatment.

Such an interdisciplinary program for treatment of TBI must include the cognitive, social, behavioral, and medical aspects of treatment. The psychiatrist has an important role to play in stabilizing the emotional condition of the patient. Such stabilization is a primary necessity, because without it, the individual with TBI is unable to attend to, participate in, and benefit from the rehabilitation process.

References

Adamovich BL: Cognition, language, attention, and information processing following closed head injury, in Cognitive Rehabilitation for Persons With Traumatic Brain Injury: A Functional Approach. Edited by Kreutzer JS, Wehman PH. Baltimore, MD, Paul H Brookes, 1991, pp 75–86

Ben-Yishay Y, Ben-Nachum Z, Cohen A, et al: Digest of a two-year comprehensive clinical rehabilitation research program for outpatient head injured Israeli veterans, in Working Approaches to Remediation of Cognitive Deficits in Brain Damaged Persons (Rehabilitation Monograph). Edited by Ben-Yishay Y. New York, NYU Medical Center, Institute of Rehabilitation Medicine, 1978, pp 1–61

Ben-Yishay Y, Piasetsky EB, Rattok J: A systematic method for ameliorating disorders in basic attention, in Neuropsychological Rehabilitation. Edited by Meir MJ, Diller L, Benton AL. London, Churchill Livingstone, 1987, pp 165–181

Benton AL: Behavioral consequences of closed head injury, in Central Nervous System Trauma Research Status Report. Edited by Odom GL. Washington, DC, National Institute of Neurological, Communicative Disorders and Stroke, 1979, pp 220–231

Binder LM, Rattok J: Assessment of the postconcussive syndrome after mild head trauma, in Assessment of the Behavioral Consequences of Head Trauma. Edited by Lezak MD. New York, Alan R Liss, 1988, pp 37–48

Boake C: A history of cognitive rehabilitation of head-injured patients, 1915–1980. Journal of Head Trauma Rehabilitation 4:1–8, 1989

Cope ND: Traumatic closed head injury: Status of rehabilitation treatment. Seminars in Neurology 3:212–220, 1985

Deaton AV: Group intervention for cognitive rehabilitation, increasing the challenges, in Cognitive Rehabilitation for Persons With Traumatic Brain Injury: A Functional Approach. Edited by Kreutzer JS, Wehman PH. Baltimore, MD, Paul H Brookes, 1991, pp 191–200

Diller L, Weinberg J: Hemi-inattention in rehabilitation: the evolution of a rational remediation program, in Advances in Neurology. Edited by Weinstein E, Friedland R. New York, Raven, 1977, pp 63–82

Diller L, Ben-Yishay Y, Weinberg J, et al: Studies in Cognition and Rehabilitation in Hemiplegia (Rehabilitation Monograph). New York, NYU Medical Center, Institute of Rehabilitation Medicine, 1974

Ezrachi O, Ben-Yishay Y, Rattok J, et al: Rehabilitation of gocnitive and perceptual defects in people with traumatic brain damage: a five-year clinical research study, in Working Approaches to Remedication of Cognitive Deficits in Brain Damaged Persons (Rehabilitation Monograph). Edited by Ben-Yishay Y. New York, NYU Medical Center, Institute of Rehabilitation Medicine, 1983, pp 53–78

Ezrachi O, Ben-Yishay Y, Kay T, et al: Predicting employment in traumatic brain injury following neuropsychological rehabilitation. Journal of Head Trauma Rehabilitation 6:71–84, 1991

Gordon WA: Methodological considerations in cognitive remediation, in Neuropsychological Rehabilitation. Edited by Meir MJ, Diller L, Benton AL. London, Churchill Livingstone, 1987, pp 111–131

Jacobs HE: The Los Angeles Head Injury Survey: project rationale and design implications. The Journal of Head Trauma Rehabilitation 2:37–50, 1987

Kay T, Silver SM: Closed head trauma assessment for rehabilitation, in Assessment of the Behavioral Consequences of Head Trauma. Edited by Lezak MD. New York, Alan R Liss, 1989, pp 145–170

Kingston WJ: Treatable neurologic complications encountered during rehabilitation of head-injured adult. Seminars in Neurology 3:260–264, 1985

Levin HS, Benton AL, Grossman RG: Neurobehavioral Consequences of Closed Head Injury. New York, Oxford University Press, 1982

Levin W: Computer applications in cognitive rehabilitation, in Cognitive Rehabilitation For Persons With Traumatic Brain Injury: A Functional Approach. Edited by Kreutzer JS, Wehman PH. Baltimore, MD, Paul H Brookes, 1991, pp 163–179

Lezak MD: Assessment of psychosocial dysfunctions resulting from head trauma, in Assessment of the Behavioral Consequences of Head Trauma. Edited by Lezak MD. New York, Alan R Liss, 1989, pp 113–143

Mack JL: Clinical assessment of disorders of attention and memory. Journal of Head Trauma Rehabilitation 3:22–33, 1986

Mazmanian PE, Martin KO, Kreutzer JS: Professional development and educational program planning in cognitive rehabilitation, in Cognitive Rehabilitation for Persons With Traumatic Brain Injury: A Functional Approach. Edited by Kreutzer JS, Wehman PH. Baltimore, MD, Paul H Brookes, 1991, pp 35–51

Meir MJ, Strauman S, Thompson WG: Individual differences in neuropsychological recovery: an overview, in Neuropsychological Rehabilitation. Edited by Meir MJ, Diller L, Benton AL. London, Churchill Livingstone, 1987, pp 71–110

Milner B: Interhemispheric differences in the localization of psychological processes in man. Br Med Bull 27:272–275, 1971

Niemann H, Ruff R, Baser C: Computer-assisted attention retraining in head-injured individuals: a control efficacy study of an outpatient program. J Consult Clin Psychol 58:811–817, 1990

Posner MI, Rafal RD: Cognitive theories of attention and the rehabilitation of attentional deficits, in Neuropsychological Rehabilitation. Edited by Meir MJ, Diller L, Benton AL. London, Churchill Livingstone, 1987, pp 182–201

Prigatano GP, Fordyce DJ, Zeimer HK, et al: Neuropsychological rehabilitation after closed head injury. J Neurol Neurosurg Psychiatry 478:505–513, 1984

Rattok J: The nature of cognitive deficits following traumatic head injury. J Clin Exp Neuropsychol 7:613, 1985

Rattok J: Intellectual Efficiency Following Mild Head Injury. Baltimore, MD, American Academy of Physical Medicine and Rehabilitation, 1986

Rattok J, Ross B: Cognitive remediation post traumatic head injury. J Clin Exp Neuropsychol 8:143, 1986

Rattok J, Ben-Yishay Y, Thomas JL, et al: A remedial module for systematic training of traumatic head injured patients in the area of visual information processing, in Working Approaches to Remediation of Cognitive Deficits in Brain Damaged Persons (Rehabilitation Monograph). Edited by Ben-Yishay Y. New York, NYU Medical Center, Institute of Rehabilitation Medicine, 1981, pp 43–67

Rattok J, Ben-Yishay Y, Ross B, et al: A diagnostic remedial system for basic attentional disorders in head trauma patients undergoing rehabilitation, in Working Approaches to Remediation of Cognitive Deficits in Brain Damaged Persons (Rehabilitation Monograph). Edited by Ben-Yishay Y. New York, NYU Medical Center, Institute of Rehabilitation Medicine, 1982, pp 177–187

Rattok J, Ross B, Silver S, et al: Understanding the world of work: a small-group exercise for head trauma patients in rehabilitation, in Working Approaches to Remediation of Cognitive Deficits in Brain Damaged Persons (Rehabilitation Monograph). Edited by Ben-Yishay Y. New York, NYU Medical Center, Institute of Rehabilitation Medicine, 1983, pp 92–112

Ross B, Ben-Yishay Y, Lakin P, et al: Using a "therapeutic community" to modify the behavior of head trauma patients, in head trauma patients undergoing rehabilitation, in Working Approaches to Remediation of Cognitive Deficits in Brain Damaged Persons (Rehabilitation Monograph). Edited by Ben-Yishay Y. New York, NYU Medical Center, Institute of Rehabilitation Medicine, 1982, pp 57–91

Ruff RM, Cameznuli LF: Research challenges for behavioral rehabilitation searching for solutions, in Cognitive Rehabilitation for Persons With Traumatic Brain Injury: A Functional Approach. Edited by Kreutzer JS, Wehman PH. Baltimore, MD, Paul H Brookes, 1991, pp 23–34

Ruff RM, Baser CA, Johnson JW, et al: Neuropsychological rehabilitation: an experimental study with head-injured patients. Journal of Head Trauma Rehabilitation 4:20–36, 1989

Scherzer BP: Rehabilitation following severe head trauma: results of a three-year program. Arch Phys Med Rehabil 67:366–374, 1986

Silver JM, Hales RE, Yudofsky SC: Neuropsychiatric aspects of traumatic brain injury, in The American Psychiatric Press Textbook of Neuropsychiatry, 2nd Edition. Edited by Yudofsky SC, Hales RE. Washington, DC, American Psychiatric Press, 1992, pp 363–395

Tromp E, Mulder T: Slowness of information processing after traumatic head injury. J Clin Exp Neuropsychol 13:821–830, 1991

Weinberg J, Diller L, Gordon WA, et al: Visual scanning training effect on reading related tasks in acquired right brain damage. Arch Phys Med Rehabil 58:479–496, 1979

Wilson BA: Rehabilitation of Memory. New York, Guilford, 1987

Appendix 21–1

Specialized Sources of Information on Head Injury Rehabilitation

Information concerning the services for patients with head injuries in all regions of the United States is available from the National Head Injury Foundation (NHIF). The NHIF is a nonprofit organization based in Washington, DC, that provides free information for patients and professionals.

National Head Injury Foundation
1140 Connecticut Avenue, N.W.
Washington, D.C. 20036
1-800-444-NHIF

Most mainstream professional journals published by the American Medical Association and the American Psychiatric Association contain more and more research articles about head injury. The following publications specialize in issues of head injury:

Brain Injury
A bimonthly journal published by

Taylor & Francis, Ltd.
1900 Frost Road
Bristol, Pennsylvania 19007

NeuroRehabilitation: An Interdisciplinary Journal
A quarterly journal published by

Andover Medical
80 Montvale Avenue
Stoneham, Massachusetts 02180

The Journal of Head Trauma Rehabilitation
A quarterly journal published by

Aspen Publishers, Inc.
16792 Oakmont Avenue
Gaithersburg, Maryland 20877
1-800-638-8437

The Journal of Neuropsychiatry and Clinical Neurosciences
A quarterly journal published by

American Psychiatric Press, Inc.
1400 K Street, N.W.
Washington, D.C. 20005
1-800-368-5777

Chapter 22

Behavioral Treatment

Patrick W. Corrigan, Psy.D.
Marjory R. Jakus, B.A.

In addition to the various neuropathological, cognitive, personality, and mood changes that follow traumatic brain injury (TBI), severe and acute insult to the central nervous system typically results in discrete behavioral problems that often wreak major disruption on patients' quality of life. Some of these problems spontaneously remit as the immediate impact of the injury subsides. Other behavioral problems diminish as alternate treatment modalities (e.g., neurosurgery and psychopharmacology) are effective in remediating the pronounced cognitive and physical sequelae of TBI. However, many problems do not ameliorate easily and thereby require use of strategic behavioral interventions. In this chapter, we outline the form of these behavioral problems and appropriate intervention strategies.

Typically, severe behavioral problems of TBI patients are not the purview of private practitioners during one-to-one, weekly consultation. Rather, these patients are referred to behavioral and cognitive rehabilitation *programs* in which patients' idiosyncratic problems are addressed vis-à-vis the programmatic framework of treatment strategies and staffing patterns. Rehabilitation programs frequently fail because staff members implementing component strategies are not faithful to the intent or application of these strategies. Methods that enhance staff fidelity to behavioral treatments can avert this pitfall, and we review these methods in this chapter as well.

Behavior therapy has developed a lexicon of its own such that many terms may sound foreign to the uninitiated practitioner. Dictionaries of behavioral techniques have been developed to address this problem (Bellack and Hersen 1985). Terms used frequently in this chapter are defined in Table 22–1 as a guide for the uninitiated reader.

Behavioral Problems of TBI

Although anatomical, physiological, psychophysiological, and cognitive consequences of TBI have been well documented, few studies have examined the behavioral and psychosocial correlates of head injury in great depth. This is ironic given that several investigations have shown that the greatest postinjury deficits occur in the psychosocial domains (Adams et al. 1985; Klonoff et al. 1986; Tellier et al. 1990; Thomsen 1984). Nevertheless, clinical methods from behavior therapy suggest strategies that can be utilized to understand behavioral difficulties.

Behavioral problems characteristically have been represented dichotomously, either as a significant decrease in the frequency of appropriate target behaviors or as an increase in inappropriate behaviors. Using this distinction, the range of behavioral deficits that a TBI patient might show is outlined in Table 22–2. Patients with large prosocial and self-care skill deficits, as well as pronounced antisocial behaviors, experience a more tortuous route to recovery, including longer stays in the hospital.

Behavioral Assessment

Careful assessment of the frequency of behavioral deficits and excesses is the sine qua non of behavior therapy (Barlow and Hersen 1984; Cone and Hawkins 1977). In some ways, behavioral

---

Table 22–1. Terms frequently used in behavior treatment

ABA single-case design: An experimental design involving a single subject, in which no treatment is applied to the target behavior in the A phase (or baseline period), treatment is implemented to increase or decrease the rate of the target behavior in the B phase (or treatment condition), and treatment for the target behavior is then withdrawn in the A phase. An increase or decrease in the rate of the target behavior when comparing A to B is assumed to reflect the efficacy of treatment. Also known as a reversal design.

Assertiveness training: A method for addressing a skill deficit based on social learning theory in which various prosocial behaviors that help patients meet their needs are acquired. Examples include saying no, making a complaint, and expressing appreciation.

Baseline period: In an experimental design, the rate of the target behavior prior to the application of treatments.

Behavioral assessment: A description of the frequency, duration, and conditions related to a target behavior.

Classical conditioning: A learning principle, in which a neutral stimulus (the conditioned stimulus or CS) is repeatedly paired with an unconditioned stimulus (or UCS) that always elicits an unconditioned response (UCR). After repeated pairings, the CS will elicit a conditioned response similar in form to the UCR. Also known as respondent conditioning.

Cognitions: The numerous components of mental operations and their products.

Contingency contract: An operant conditioning strategy designed to increase or decrease the performance of a target behavior by rewarding or punishing that behavior.

Deficit: A lack of or a loss of behavioral skills, of which the patient may not be aware.

Fixed-interval schedule: A reinforcer is applied to the target behavior after a specific period of time.

Fixed-ratio schedule: A reinforcer is applied to the target behavior following a specific number of responses.

Negative reinforcement: An operant conditioning strategy in which the withdrawal of a stimulus results in an increase in the frequency of the target behavior.

Operant conditioning: A learning principle in which the frequency of a behavior in a specific situation covaries with the rewards and punishers experienced in that situation. Also known as instrumental conditioning.

Overcorrection: An intervention that combines time-out from reinforcement with a requirement that patients restore a situation they may have messed up in anger.

Table 22–1. Terms frequently used in behavior treatment *(continued)*

Positive punishment: An operant conditioning strategy in which the rate of a target behavior is reduced by presenting an aversive stimulus (e.g., shock, hitting, yelling) immediately after the behavior.

Positive reinforcement: An operant conditioning intervention in which the presentation of a desired commodity or activity increases the frequency of the target behavior.

Single-case design: An illustration of the frequency, duration, and conditions related to the target behavior of the subject. Most frequently indicated by the ABA single case design.

Response cost: An operant conditioning strategy in which the rate of a response is reduced by withdrawing a reinforcing consequence (e.g., no dessert if you don't eat your vegetables).

Self-monitoring: The systematic charting, displaying, or recording of a patient's target behavior by the patient.

Social learning theory: A learning theory principle in which individuals acquire new behaviors by modeling the reinforced behavior of others. Also known as vicarious conditioning.

Target behavior: A specific response to be changed, modified, or treated through the application of behavioral strategies.

Time-out from reinforcement: An operant conditioning procedure in which the patient is removed from a rewarding environment in an effort to decrease the rate of the target behavior.

Token economy: A behavioral program frequently used in hospital settings in which patients are rewarded with tokens that can be exchanged for commodities and activities in a token store.

Transfer of training: A behavior method used to increase the rate of the target behavior across settings other than the environment where the response was learned.

Variable interval and ratio schedules: An intermittent contingency schedule in which a reinforcer is applied irregularly.

---

assessment is relatively adiagnostic—uninterested in the original causes of a problem—and instead exerts more effort on the description of behaviors and the conditions currently maintaining them. Hence, mental health professionals working with TBI patients might ignore the location of the brain lesion that has caused aggressive outbursts, instead trying to describe the environmental antecedents and consequences of the behavior. This does not mean that psychophysiological and neurochemical tests are irrelevant to building behavioral plans. Biologically based information may serve as a useful adjunct to describing patients' social and self-care deficits.

Behavioral assessment tracks the frequency of specific behaviors over time. "Single case research" is the culmination of behavioral frequency monitoring with the ABA as the prototypic single case design (Barlow and Hersen 1984). Examples of ABA designs are included in Figure 22–1. During A or baseline, the frequency in which a targeted behavior occurs with no treatment is recorded. When focusing on diminished prosocial behaviors (like poor conversation skills) that resulted from TBI, the behavioral assessor would expect the base rate of targets to be relatively low. Conversely, the rate of an inappropriate behavior such as interpersonal aggression would be relatively high.

The subsequent B phase represents the frequency of the targeted behavior after implementing treatment. Treatments may include skill-training programs or reinforcement contracts. Treatments that are expected to increase the rate of prosocial, self-care, or coping behavior should show an elevation in frequency when comparing A to B. Treatments that decrease the rate of maladaptive or antisocial behavior will demonstrate a frequency deflation. Significant change between A and B may possibly result from subtle concurrent effects in the environment unrelated to the treatment. For example, perhaps a patient's decreased aggression from A to B was caused by a change in roommates rather than the skill-training program he or she attended. To rule out this confound, clinicians withdraw the treatment and return to baseline in the second A phase. Conclusions about treatment efficacy are supported if the target behavior returns to baseline when the treatment is stopped.

Lack of Awareness of Behavioral Problems

As an observation-based strategy, behavioral assessment may be especially appropriate for many TBI patients who lack awareness

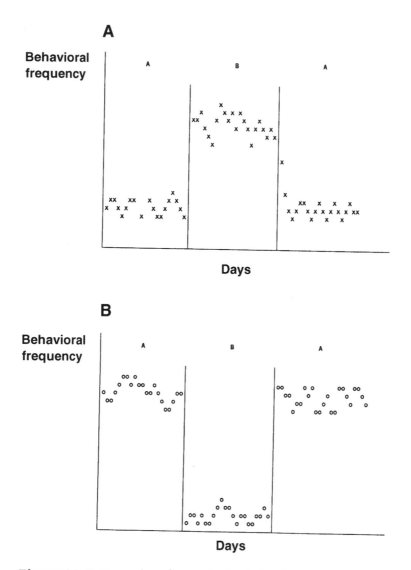

Figure 22–1. Examples of quantitative behavior assessment using single case designs. *Panel A:* The number of minutes per day of conversation with staff or peers is low at baseline, increases markedly after introduction of a token economy, and then decreases when the treatment is withdrawn. *Panel B:* An inappropriate behavior is targeted using a contingency contract. Note how it decreases from an unsatisfactory high level at baseline to a more manageable lower level after treatment is begun.

of their behavioral deficits. Research has shown that self-reports reflecting the social competence of patients with brain disease or injury are significantly disparate from more accurate reports provided by family members or treatment staff (Prigatano and Altman 1990; Sunderland et al. 1983, 1984). In fact, deficit unawareness is a problem shown by 40% of patients after severe TBI (Oddy et al. 1985). The cause of this deficit is unclear. Findings from two investigations suggested that neglect of deficits is related to extent and severity of injury (Levin et al. 1982; Prigatano and Altman 1990). However, Weinstein and Kahn (1955) found no relationship between deficit awareness and degree of brain insult; they concluded that premorbid emotional and motivational factors may account for this deficit. Perhaps some patients learn that denial of illness will be rewarded by their peers; for example, family members may be more supportive when the patient ignores his or her

Table 22–2.　Behavior deficits commonly seen in traumatic brain injury patients

Aggressive behaviors[a]	**Interpersonal skills**
Biting	Poor basic conversation skills
Harming self	Poor assertion skills
Spitting	Inability to complete tasks in a timely manner
Swearing	Lethargic and disinterested
Yelling .	Unmotivated
Hitting or kicking others	**Coping skills**
Scratching	Refusing medications
Self-care skills	Poor response to stressors
Diminished sleeping	Unable to problem solve
Doesn't feed self	**Cognitive-related skills**
Diminished eating	Poor attention and concentration
Doesn't clean clothes	Pool memory and learning
Doesn't wash	Poor social comprehension
Doesn't make bed	Diminished reading and writing skills
Doesn't brush teeth	
Doesn't keep area clean	
Doesn't comb hair	

[a]Note that in behavioral treatment, aggressive behaviors are decreased; for the skills contained in the remainder of this table, improvement of the deficit consists of increasing the targeted behaviors.

injury and reports, "I will be back to my old self soon."

Research has suggested a reciprocal relationship between problem unawareness and treatment outcome (McGlynn 1990). Patients demonstrating this syndrome show diminished motivation and interest in treatment (Prigatano and Fordyce 1986), are less likely to comply with behavioral prescriptions (Cicerone and Tupper 1986), and frequently set unrealistic therapy goals (Ben-Yishay et al. 1985). To diminish problems related to treatment compliance, Fordyce (Fordyce and Roueche 1986; Prigatano and Fordyce 1986) tested an awareness-training program that targets patients' appreciation of the consequences of their injury. Awareness training includes 1) education regarding the impact of TBI, 2) patient self-monitoring of behaviors that staff believe have been affected by the injury, and 3) videotaped feedback of targeted inappropriate behaviors. Results of an evaluation of awareness training showed that about half of a sample of TBI patients who were misperceiving their level of deficits significantly improved awareness after participating in the training program (Fordyce and Roueche 1986).

Behavior therapy may be especially well suited to treat unawareness of symptoms. In reviewing the literature on whether awareness is a prerequisite for learning, Bandura (1971) concluded that frequency of some behaviors may be increased or decreased without the subject's being fully aware of the targeted behavior or reinforcing consequences. For example, Sasmor (1966) was able to increase the frequency of imperceptible muscular responses (detected by the examiner with electronic amplification) through contingent reward. Hence, even if patients with brain damage do not accept their social deficits, improved interpersonal functioning can be facilitated by involving the patient in a strong contingency management program.

Models of Behavioral Rehabilitation

Several models of behavioral rehabilitation have been developed to treat patients with neuropsychiatric disorders; these are summarized in Table 22–3. Most of these models have not been tested in terms of treatment outcome per se. Rather, they serve as heuristic guidelines for the development and future evaluation of rehabilitation programs.

The Integrative Model

The *integrative* model situated behavioral rehabilitation within a synergy of relatively disparate professional perspectives that define the TBI patients' problems: the neurologist's definition of the insult in terms of neuroanatomical foci and physiological sequelae, the neuropsychologist's perspective on test description of the behavioral and cognitive deficits associated with the injury, and the behaviorist's treatment plans targeting the profile of behavioral problems (Diller and Gordon 1981). This view developed out of the professional consensus regarding the need for blending what had previously been the independent domains of each profession (Horton and Miller 1984; Horton and Sautter 1986; Horton and Wedding 1984). The optimal behavioral plans are those that include insights into the localization of the brain injury and the cognitive and emotional sequelae of the localized insult.

Table 22–3. Conceptual models of behavioral rehabilitation for the traumatic brain injury patient

Model	Strengths
Integrative (Diller and Gordon 1981)	Combines strategies of neuropsychological assessment, neurological lab tests, and behavior intervention
Evaluative (Glasgow et al. 1977; Lewinsohn et al. 1977)	Uses neuropsychological data to develop and evaluate behavioral treatment plans
Recovery (Gazzaniga 1974)	Defines impact of behavioral rehabilitation in terms of neurological models of recovery
Two-Phase Developmental (Passler 1987)	Combines strategies used for developmentally delayed patients with behavior modification
Process (Corrigan et al. 1990)	Bases interventions in terms of processes that might cause behavioral deficits and excesses

The Evaluative Model

Lewinsohn and colleagues developed a similar model of behavioral rehabilitation (Glasgow et al. 1977; Lewinsohn et al. 1977). According to the *evaluative* model, the information from neuropsychological assessment was used as a template for developing behavioral plans. Subsequent evaluations then served as feedback information to help determine successes and failures of the behavioral plan vis-à-vis this template and to titrate individual strategies accordingly. The behavioral plan and evaluative feedback loop began in a well-controlled laboratory setting and was transferred to the "real world" as limitations to the generalizability of treatment strategies were worked out.

Recovery Model

Gazzaniga (1974, 1978) believed that behavioral strategies augmented remaining neural and cognitive processes that led to the individual's recovery; his view was based on anatomical and physiological evidence regarding the natural *recovery* process after injury. Hence, behavioral strategies served as prosthetics, which the TBI patient might adopt to perform everyday interpersonal and self-care skills. For example, in the same way that patients without a leg were able to walk with the assistance of artificial limbs and crutches, people who have difficulty resolving interpersonal conflicts were able to reconcile these difficulties using a behavioral aide such as, for example, the steps of problem solving (D'Zurilla 1986).

The Two-Phase Developmental Model

Passler (1987) likened the behavioral deficits of many TBI patients to the problems of developmentally delayed individuals. Hence, he proposed a two-phase *developmental* rehabilitation program with the first phase focusing on the developmental limitations of TBI patients using the Kaufman Developmental Scale (KDS: Kaufman 1975). A developmental stimulation program based on the KDS outlined a series of graded tasks that were progressively more demanding of developmental abilities. For example, tasks for an initial developmental profile for gross motor activity included jumping off the ground in place, jumping from a one-foot level, balancing on one foot for one second, and broad jumping. Similarly, fine motor tasks might include copying a circle, tracing a line, drawing a cross by imitation, drawing a six-part human figure, and exhibiting motor control with dots. As patients mastered these tasks, the frustrations commensurate with developmental limitations were diminished and TBI patients were more receptive to the second phase, typical behavioral interventions.

The Process Model

Unlike the other models that yielded behavioral strategies in terms of the descriptive paradigms of neurology and neuropsychology, the *process* model defined behavioral strategies by the more generic, dynamic, and interlocking processes that accounted for the original formation and/or subsequent maintenance of behavioral problems. This model was first developed to explain behavioral rehabilitation for severely mentally ill populations (Corrigan et al. 1988, 1990), but was easily adaptable to the disabilities of TBI patients. As outlined in Figure 22–2, it includes four component processes:

❚ **Acquisition.** Severely mentally ill patients may lack interpersonal or self-care skills because they did not acquire these behaviors during their tumultuous premorbid adolescence. Rather than never having acquired the skills, TBI patients may have lost prosocial skills previously in their repertoire as a result of brain damage. Skill-training strategies help patients in both groups to (re)acquire necessary skills. In addition, TBI patients may learn symptom management skills and other behavioral prosthetics (e.g., stress management and problem-solving skills) that will help them to manage life stressors associated with wide-ranging disabilities.

❚ **Performance.** Several factors impede reinforcing conditions that provide patients' with an incentive to use their limited prosocial skills. For example, TBI patients may be relatively insensitive to many of the normal social reinforcers that maintain interpersonal skills. Moreover, friends and family members may be unwilling to provide sufficient reinforcers for what they consider insignificant behavior. Incentive strategies such as contingency management and token economies facilitate skill performance.

▮ **Generalization.** Even if TBI patients learn a range of skills and perform them in the training milieu, these skills frequently do not generalize outside of the treatment setting. Transfer-training skills (e.g., homework, in vivo practice, and training the family) foster situational and response generalization.

▮ **Cognition.** The cognitive deficits common to brain injury diminish the other component processes. For example, memory

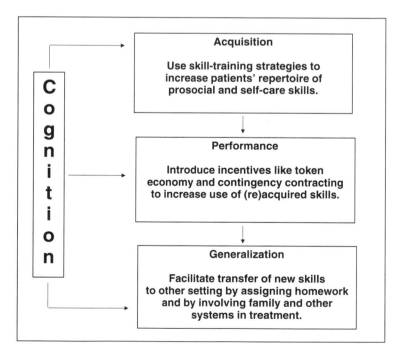

Figure 22–2. Components of the process model of behavioral rehabilitation.

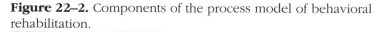

deficits that hamper learning may impair skill acquisition. Patients with attentional deficits may neglect reinforcers meant to govern the performance of certain behaviors. Furthermore, lack of sensitivity to the way in which real-world situations are similar to the training environment may hamper generalization. Cognitive rehabilitation strategies help TBI patients overcome problems such as these; these strategies are reviewed in Chapter 21. We discuss points relevant to this model throughout the remainder of the chapter.

The process model is useful for rehabilitation of TBI patients because treatment strategies are clearly wedded to the specific, deficient process in question, that is, to the phenomena that brought about the behavioral excess and deficit and to the phenomena that maintain these disabilities. When combined with the neuropsychiatrist's and neuropsychologist's perspectives, the process model yields a potent programmatic approach to the treatment of the behavioral excesses and deficits of TBI patients. We outline below the manner in which a behavioral rehabilitation program for TBI patients is organized utilizing the three components of the process model.

Acquisition

Skill-training methods, developed and tested extensively for treatment of severely mentally ill populations (Liberman et al. 1989), have been turned more recently to problems of head trauma patients (Matson and DiLorenzo 1986). Typically, skills training is conducted in psychoeducational modules with one or two trainers and 5 to 10 participants. Trainers present several learning activities in sequential order to facilitate skill acquisition. Through verbal instructions, the key learning points of the skill are presented to the patient. For example, in an assertiveness module the trainer might say,

> Today we are going to learn how to say "No" using the broken record technique. When someone asks you for a smoke and you

want to keep it, say, "No, I do not want to give you my cigarette." If that person persists, say the same message again, "No, I do not want to give you the cigarette," like a broken record. Keep repeating the same message until the person stops asking.

After being introduced to the learning points, trainees observe a model who demonstrates the skill. This can be done either by using prepackaged videotaped vignettes or by having the trainer model the targeted skills.

Next trainees are encouraged to practice the skill in pre-designed role plays. "Now Jim, I want you to practice saying 'No' when Harry asks you for a dollar." Trainers offer corrective feedback after the role play, focusing especially on successful approximations to the targeted behavior. Liberal rewards are handed out at the end of the session for participating in the module. After trainees have shown some mastery of the skill in the training milieu, they are given homework for practice in the real world:

By next week I want all of you to have practiced the broken record at home where you live. The next time a friend of yours asks you for a dollar and you do not want to give it to him or her, just say no!

These learning activities may be used to improve skill acquisition in several domains of functioning, including self-care, interpersonal, and coping skills (Schade et al. 1990; Spiegler and Agigian 1977). Self-care skills encompass activities for daily living such as grooming, home maintenance skills, shopping, and money management. Interpersonal skill deficits include poor conversation and assertion skills. Deficits in these domains represent a loss in functioning and therefore require a reintroduction to skills. Coping skills are "new" behaviors patients must learn to manage their illness; they include medication management (knowing the therapeutic and side effects of medication and how to talk with the physician when there are problems with these drugs), symptom management (identifying problem behaviors and coping techniques when these behaviors flare up), and stress management (behavioral strategies to handle recurrent tensions).

What accounts for the therapeutic effects of skills training? The operant and social learning components of skills training may yield a direct learning effect. Despite TBI patients' cognitive deficits, they are able to acquire the targeted skills. Alternately, learning points taught in skill-training modules may serve as behavioral prosthetics, much as Gazzaniga (1978) believed. Instead of acquiring skills as they appear in the real world, TBI patients learn manageable behavioral *steps* to help them with the skill domains. For example, D'Zurilla (1986) outlined a seven-step process for resolving interpersonal problems:

1. Adopt a problem-solving attitude.
2. Identify the problem.
3. Brainstorm solutions.
4. Evaluate solutions and pick one out to try.
5. Plan the implementation of this solution.
6. Reevaluate the solution after it has been implemented.
7. Pick another solution if the first was ineffective.

This approach probably does not parallel the way in which people normally solve problems (Bellack et al. 1989). Moreover, it seems to stretch the cognitive limits of most TBI patients. However, by dividing this complex task into manageable steps, the problem-solving method provides a useful tool that helps brain injury patients identify and resolve their interpersonal problems.

Research on the effects of skills training with brain injury patients, although limited mostly to single case designs, has provided some interesting findings. Self-monitoring was added to the traditional package of learning activities to improve the heterosexual conversation skills of four brain damaged men (Gajar et al. 1984; Schloss et al. 1984). In self-monitoring, patients are instructed to keep track of the frequency of specific, jointly defined behaviors. The positive effects of this study were found to generalize to settings outside the training milieu. Similarly, the aggressive behaviors of another patient were significantly reduced as he acquired basic self-care skills (Godfrey and Knight 1988). Results were more limited in a fourth study, however (Brotherton et al.

1988). Training for four patients with severe head injury was more useful on the micro-components of basic social behaviors (e.g., eye contact, posture) than on the macro-skills (e.g., conversation) actually required to interpersonally relate.

Performance

Individuals who have sustained TBI require social and material rewards as incentives to incorporate relearned or newly acquired social, coping, and self-care skills into their everyday behavioral repertoire. The Law of Effect from operant psychology describes the impact of incentives on behaviors; according to this Law, behaviors that are reinforced in specific situations are more likely to occur again in those situations whereas punished behaviors are less likely to be observed in the punished environment (Skinner 1953). Two treatment strategies are based on the Law and have been widely used for treatment of TBI patients: contingency contracts and token economies.

Contingency contracts are defined by if-then rules; if patients perform a targeted response, then they receive desired reinforcers. Targeted responses in research with TBI patients have included verbal abilities, awareness, attention, motivation, social responsiveness, and participation in group activities (Ben-Yishay et al. 1980; Burke and Lewis 1986; Ince 1976; McGlynn 1990; Mueller and Atlas 1972; Prigatano and Altman 1990; Turner et al. 1978; Wehman et al. 1990). Self-care functions such as feeding, bed making, personal hygiene, and clothes maintenance have also been included in these programs (Murphy 1976).

Contingency contracts (for that matter, any reinforcement program) are as effective as the rewards chosen as consequences. Consumables like coffee, candy, other food stuffs, and cigarettes are used as reinforcers.[1] However, what is reinforcing for one

---

[1] Given the health hazards from chronic smoking, what responsibilities should clinicians assume in using cigarettes as reinforcers? For many patients, cigarettes

person may be aversive for another. Several strategies exist for helping clinicians identify reinforcers. Patients can be instructed to identify reinforcing commodities and activities from several self-report surveys (Cautela and Lynch 1983). The reticent patient's reinforcer may be identified by providing a smorgasbord of commodities and opportunities and see what the person selects. Finally, according to principles of operant psychology, any behavior that a person does at a high rate is by definition reinforcing (Premack 1962). For example, washing your hands or sitting in a favorite chair—responses not normally considered to be reinforcers—may be potent rewards for patients' behavior. Therefore, observing rates of various behaviors may provide clues to behavioral reinforcers.

There are also several rules about the manner in which rewards are handed out that affect their reinforcing potential. When a patient is first learning a behavior, rewards should be given immediately after the response has been performed. Staff passing out the rewards should verbally congratulate the patient for meeting the goal by pointing out specifics of the goal that he or she demonstrated:

> Nice job, Harry. You made your bed well by tucking in your sheets and straightening out your blanket. Here's the reward we talked about.

Contingency contracts are sometimes ineffective because the targeted behavior is beyond the patient's response capabilities. For example, TBI patients with a recent history of restlessness would not be able to sit for an hour in skill-training sessions irrespective of the yoked reinforcer. Therefore, clinicians need to shape

---

rank among the most prized commodities and they will work hard to earn them. When not using cigarettes as a reinforcer, a potential control over patient behavior is lost and the opportunity to increase social and coping skills and improve compliance with treatment regimens is diminished. However, if cigarettes are used as a reward, the skill repertoire may improve and perhaps the patients will be better able to learn "quit smoking" strategies (Corrigan 1991).

patients' behaviors toward performance of "macro" targets—in this case, sitting still for an hour—by reinforcing successive approximations to the goals. During the first week of training in the above example, the target would be 5 minutes of sitting. When this is accomplished, the goal would be increased to 10 minutes, and then slowly increased by 10-minute increments until the hour goal is reached.

Token economies are formalized and programmatic forms of contingency contracting that derive their potency from the Law of Effect *and* the Law of Association by Contiguity (Skinner 1953). According to the second Law, previously neutral stimuli (such as tokens) when presented frequently with reinforcing stimuli (such as consumables) will become reinforcing in their own right. Unlike contingency contracts, token economies are typically set up for all members of an inpatient or outpatient program. Three steps are necessary to carry this out. First, unit-wide behaviors that all patients are expected to demonstrate are identified (e.g., daily showering, clean bedroom, talk with peers at meals). Next, token contingencies for accomplishing these behaviors are specified: "If you make your bed by 8:00 A.M., then you will receive 10 tokens." The frequency of inappropriate behaviors can be diminished by specifying response costs for these behaviors (e.g., "If you smoke in your bedroom, then you will lose 10 tokens"). Finally, exchange rules for turning in tokens need to be outlined. When and where do patients swap their tokens for primary reinforcers such as consumables, hygiene products, clothes, and reading material? How many tokens do individual commodities cost?

Token economies have been used extensively in the treatment of TBI patients to increase interpersonal and coping skills or to decrease maladaptive behaviors (Burke and Lewis 1986; Gajar et al. 1984; Horton and Howe 1981; Kushner and Knox 1973; Lira et al. 1983; Mueller and Atlas 1972; Webster and Scott 1983; Wood and Eames 1981). In some token economies, the frequency of inappropriate behaviors has been diminished successfully by penalizing patients for performing these behaviors. Inappropriate responses include interpersonal aggression, treatment noncompliance, and alcohol consumption (Blackerby and Baumgarten 1990;

Franzen and Lovell 1987; Horton and Howe 1981; Kushner and Knox 1973; Lira et al. 1983; McGlynn 1990; Wood and Eames 1981). Despite these successes, several limitations to the technology have been found, including poor generalization from a highly structured treatment setting to the real world (Kazdin and Bootzin 1972). For example, activities of daily living and basic conversation skills in the patient's home setting are not normally maintained by immediate receipt of tokens. Transfer training strategies help to improve the generalization of these effects.

Generalization

Despite great gains in facilitating acquisition and performance of social, coping, and self-care skills, generalization of skills to settings outside the treatment milieu and to behaviors other than those specifically targeted by the behavioral intervention has been lacking (Corrigan et al. 1993a). Generalization of behaviors improved in programs for TBI patients has been especially limited (McGlynn 1990). These negative findings may result from dominance of an older behavioral perspective that views generalization as a naturally occurring phenomenon; that is, some time after key learning events, performance of the skill transfers to similar situations (stimulus generalization) and behaviors (response generalization) in gradient fashion (Skinner 1953). As a result, clinicians have passively sat back waiting for skills to appear in new settings. Others have argued that generalization happens only when it is actively introduced into the rehabilitation program (Kazdin 1982; Stokes and Baer 1977; Stokes and Osnes 1989). Hence, the use of generalization *strategies* significantly enhances transfer effects of token economies and skill-training programs. Examples of some of these strategies are summarized in Table 22–4.

Repeated practice of newly learned skills increases the probability that targeted responses will be performed in situations similar to the practice milieu. Unfortunately, repeating the same task many times is boring and this discourages patients from complying with the task. Multiple training approaches avoid this pitfall by providing different tasks to facilitate skills acquisition. Acquisition of conversational skills can be increased by role plays within a skill-training module, special practice sessions between therapist and patient, and token economy contingencies that reward patients for performing the skill.

Skills transfer more readily from psychoeducational programs when they are practiced in settings other than the training milieu. While the individual is an inpatient, skill-training sessions include in vivo tasks in which patients might be bussed to relevant community settings and assigned a skill-relevant problem (Liberman and Corrigan 1993). For example, TBI patients are instructed at a shopping mall to go to a store, pick out a set of clothes, and determine the cost for the ensemble. Trainers accompany patients and offer prompts and feedback throughout the task. As trainees demonstrate competence, they are given homework assignments to complete independently.

For generalization to occur, patients must be sensitive to the stimulus similarities that define training situations and the rest of the world. TBI patients with cognitive deficits are likely to have diminished sensitivity to social cues and are therefore less likely to readily generalize newly learned skills from treatment programs. Therefore, attention-focusing techniques that improve patients' perception of interpersonal skills should enhance the transfer of

Table 22–4. Strategies that facilitate the transfer of skills to other settings and behaviors

For skill-training programs

Repeatedly practice targeted skill.

Use multiple training approaches to facilitate acquisition.

Practice skill in vivo.

Assign homework to be completed independently.

For token economy programs

Fade from continuous to intermittent schedules.

Target naturally reinforced behaviors.

Teach significant others contingency management.

skills. Similarly, trainers might enhance generalization by pointing out cues present outside the training environment that are similar to cues that signal the skill in the training environment. For example, the trainer may want to point out similarities between the hospital cafeteria and neighborhood diner so that the patient is vigilant to the waitress's statements. As a result, he or she will be ready to give a lunch order, a skill that has been repeatedly practiced at the hospital.

As suggested above, newly learned behaviors maintained by a token economy do not generalize well to settings outside the hospital. Soon after discharge, TBI patients may discover that natural contingencies are not as specific nor as fruitful as econ-omy-defined consequences and the frequency of targeted behaviors may quickly diminish; several strategies avoid this pitfall. As targeted behaviors within the hospital approach "normal" rates, schedules are changed from continuous reinforcement (tokens given immediately after the behavior) to intermittent contingencies, especially variable ratio or variable interval schedules, which are more resistant to extinction (Skinner 1953). For example, Charlene received five tokens for every minute she talked to a peer when she was first admitted to the unit. As behavioral problems remitted and her rate of conversation improved, token schedules were changed such that she received three tokens for talking 15 minutes with someone. As discharge approached, tokens were faded altogether by increasing the ratios and intervals in which they were passed out. In addition, the generalization effects of token economies can be enhanced by extending the program to the community. Family or other caregivers can be trained to continue specific contingencies at home or in vocational training settings (Falloon et al. 1984; Tharp and Wetzel 1969).

Interpersonal and instrumental skills vary in terms of their reinforcement value. Generalization of token economies to situations outside the treatment unit can be facilitated by targeting those skills that are "naturally" reinforced (Ayllon and Azrin 1968; Tharp and Wetzel 1969). For example, patients are more likely to be reinforced in their community for talking politely and showing good hygiene than for demonstrating insight into their injuries or being able to speak about hidden conflicts. Staff must target behaviors in the token economy that are necessary for successful community living.

Case example.

Joe, a 30-year-old, married bus driver, was hospitalized after a major car accident that occurred while he was driving home from work on the expressway. Joe was unconscious for several hours after the accident and sustained injuries to both hemispheres. After a brief hospitalization to manage acute injuries, he underwent intensive treatment at a rehabilitation facility for 6 months. Significant physical sequelae related to the injury had remitted at discharge from this facility.

Despite regaining most physical capabilities, Joe continued to exhibit cognitive and behavioral difficulties at home, which prevented him from returning to work. His wife reported that he seemed less interested in people: for example, he was no longer golfing with his friends or fishing with his family, activities in which he had participated regularly. He tended to sit uncomfortably in a corner during most social functions. "Joe was always such a friendly guy. It's like he doesn't know what to do when he's around others." Family members reported that his grooming had diminished severely and that Joe did little to help keep the house clean. He did not remember to take his medications as prescribed and would frequently skip meals if not prompted. In addition to being frustrated about Joe's loss in social and self-care skills, the family expressed anger at his seeming lack of concern about his change in functioning.

Joe was referred to a behavioral day hospital that specialized in treatment of neuropsychological disorders. Interventions included in the treatment plan that was developed for Joe addressed the processes maintaining the behavioral problems. Joe was enrolled in several psychoeducational classes to help him better understand the course of his disorder, as well as some fundamental skills he might use to cope with day-to-day problems. For example, Joe attended medication management and basic conversation skills modules each day. The medication management module offered exercises emphasizing the benefits of drugs, self-administration, side effects, and medication schedules for adaptation of his medication regimen at the program, at home, and eventually at the workplace. Participation in the basic conversation skills class helped him to relearn verbal and nonverbal communications, as well as active listening skills. Modules incorporated cognitive rehabilitation strategies to help circumvent information processing deficits that might impede learning targeted skills.

The day treatment program used token reinforcement to provide incentive for participants to use newly reacquired skills. Joe was observed to separate himself from peers during social gatherings in the day hospital so his case manager made receipt of 10 tokens contingent on having a friendly talk with a peer in the program for 5 minutes. Because of Joe's highly social premorbid history and his success in the basic conversation skills classes, he quickly met criterion on the 5-minute program, so the case manager raised the goal to 10 minutes. Program participants were also reinforced for completing responsibilities that helped to keep the facilities clean; Joe was assigned to lunch clean up. His case manager instructed him on the specifics of his duties and offered prompts and provided cue cards to guide him through his work. Joe was able to earn his tokens on this job after a short time.

Despite the significant change in prosocial behaviors at the day program, family members reported that he was still asocial and unconcerned at home. The case manager arranged problem-focused family treatment to educate family members regarding Joe's limits. The goal of family treatment, however, was not to get family members to accept Joe's prognosis, but rather to teach them discrete strategies to help Joe improve his behaviors at home. The family learned the basics of problem solving and were encouraged to follow the steps when a management problem occurred. Family members were also taught the basics of contingency contracting so that the rate of particularly recalcitrant behaviors (Joe would not make the bed no matter how they prompted him) could be modified by manipulating key reinforcers (Joe could watch the morning talk show only after he completed the bed).

After several months of participation in the program, Joe's social skills were observed to have increased significantly, both at the day program and at home. Family members still reported times each day when Joe was tired and seemed to withdraw from his wife and children. However, overall his level of interaction was improved and grooming and housekeeping had improved significantly as well. At a recent treatment meeting, Joe, his wife, and the treatment team agreed that Joe was ready to try a work retraining program to prepare for reentry into the work force.

Joe's behavioral problems are typical of those frequently experience by TBI patients. Even though life-threatening aspects of the injury had been resolved and the patient had no significant physical disabilities, Joe and his family had to cope with enduring psychiatric problems that resulted from the accident. Typically, clinicians conducting behavioral programs become involved when physical symptoms have diminished and interpersonal problems are more apparent. Significant impact on these problems was realized by enrolling the patient in a comprehensive, psychoeducational milieu and by involving significant others in carrying out the treatment plan. Resolution of behavioral problems is not usually as dramatic as the resolution following treatments that address physical sequelae of the injury. Behavioral clinicians talk about reductions of inappropriate behaviors or increases of prosocial responses instead of remissions or cures. However, changing the rate of these behaviors can significantly improve the TBI patient's quality of life.

Aggression Management

Aggressive behaviors of TBI patients present a special problem to management and outcome, requiring behavioral interventions that are not subsumed by a process-based rehabilitation program. Aggressive responses are fairly common in psychiatric patients in general (Tardiff and Sweillam 1982) and after brain injury in particular (Silver and Yudofsky 1987). Aggressive behaviors may include verbal outbursts, damage to property, and physical assault. The form of aggression varies across patients and, for the same patient, across situations. Both biological and environmental factors may underlie an individual aggressive episode. Hence, the most effective treatments combine psychopharmacologic and behavioral strategies (Corrigan et al. 1993b; Franzen and Lovell 1987).

Frequently, aggressive behaviors occur because TBI patients, faced with diminished social competence and less tolerance, are more easily frustrated by everyday interpersonal demands. Hence, as they regain some interpersonal and self-care skills, or as they learn various behavioral prosthetics, the frequency of violent behaviors diminishes. However, many aggressive behaviors are of sufficient severity that treatment teams cannot wait for relatively slow, skill-acquisition processes to occur.

Alternative strategies that diminish over-aggressiveness have been divided into "aggression replacement" strategies and "decelerative techniques"; these are reviewed in Table 22–5 (Lennox et al. 1988; Liberman and Wong 1984). Aggressive behaviors may be replaced by other, more specific behaviors such as assertiveness, using the methods and rules of skill-training reviewed above. Content areas include saying "No," making a complaint, and expressing appreciation (Douglas and Mueser 1990).

Table 22–5. Behavioral treatment of aggression

Strategy	Special considerations
Aggression replacement	Must work well in skills training groups.
Assertiveness training: for patients who become angry when they are unable to get their needs met.	Resource requirements may be costly. Can diminish this problem by identifying suitable interfering behaviors.
Differential reinforcement schedules: a nonpunishing strategy to decrease the rate of previolent behavior.	
Decelerative techniques	May not work on schizoid patients.
Social extinction: useful for previolent patients who respond to social reinforcers.	
Contingent observation: provides opportunity for violent responders to model self-control from peers.	Must be sufficiently organized to accurately perceive models.
Self-controlled time-out: advantages of time-out.	May diminish risky attempts to seclude or restrain.
Overcorrection: useful learning experience for relatively docile patients.	Stop if patient struggles with guided practice.
Contingent restraint: this is the last resort for violent patients who do not comply with self-controlled time-out and are resistant to guided practice.	Decreases inadvertent reinforcement of behaviors that covary with seclusion and restraint.

Differential reinforcement strategies comprise another replacement method that helps to decrease aggressive behaviors without using aversive stimuli or response costs. When using Differential Reinforcement of Other Behavior (DRO) for decreasing agitation, staff reinforce *all* behaviors except the aggressive target. In practice, the patient's day is divided into discrete time periods (e.g., 20-minute increments); for each period in which the patient does not show the violent behavior, he or she receives the reward. For example, Hollon (1973) combined reinforcement of positive behavior with ignoring disruptive behavior (e.g., howling, hitting, and scratching) in two women with brain injuries. Within a few weeks the disruptive behaviors decreased significantly and more prosocial behaviors began to appear. Crewe (1980) reported similar results using availability of nurses' attention as the differential reinforcer. Unfortunately, DRO schedules are relatively costly interventions requiring the constant availability of staff to reinforce the relative infinity of a patient's nonaggressive responses. Differential Reinforcement of Incompatible behaviors (DRI) offers a more efficient alternative in which only behaviors that are incompatible with the undesired target are reinforced; for example, a patient might be reinforced each time he or she says "No" rather than yelling angrily at a peer who is begging for a cigarette.

Despite the increase in prosocial, nonhostile behavior that results from aggression replacement strategies, assaultive incidents may still occur and need to be addressed. Decelerative techniques rely on principles of operant psychology to decrease previolent behaviors (i.e., behaviors consistent with being irritable or grumpy that signal impending physical outbursts) and to diminish aggressive episodes when they occur. One such method, social extinction, is effective for patients who actively seek staff approval. Patients are told that acting out aggressively is unacceptable to the milieu and that they will be ignored when they do so again. Effective extinction requires *all* staff to ignore the designated patient during the intervention. The impact of extinction can be augmented by token fines that are levied for antisocial behavior (Horton and Howe 1981).

Whereas social extinction removes some previolent behaviors, the intervention strategy does not include a learning opportunity by which patients can acquire replacement behaviors. Clinicians using contingent observation tell acting-out patients to sit quietly for a predefined time at the edge of the group (Porterfield et al. 1976). While sitting alone, patients are instructed to watch their peers and the staff carefully and to observe alternative responses that they might employ to avoid future angry responses in the situation.

Time-out from reinforcement is an operant technique in which socially inappropriate behaviors can be decreased by short-term removal of patients from overstimulating (and perhaps reinforcing) situations (Wood 1982; Wood and Eames 1981). A time-out chair in a quiet corner of the day room is a place where patients quickly learn to go when prompted by staff. Unlike seclusion, however, self-controlled time-out will probably not evoke as negative a reaction because patients have some control over the process. In this way, time-out offers a less restrictive alternative to seclusion and restraints, engenders less humiliation for the patient, and involves diminished risk of injury to patients, staff, and bystanders (Glynn et al. 1989).

Overcorrection combines time-out and an effort requirement to reduce the rate of offensive behaviors by forcefully replacing these behaviors with more prosocial alternatives (Marholin et al. 1980; Matson and Stephens 1977). The effort requirement compels patients to restore the disturbed situation to a vastly improved condition. For example, after a patient who threw his dinner tray at lunch calmed down in the time-out chair, he was instructed to clean up not only his table but several other tables in the cafeteria as well.

Patients who are unresponsive to all other decelerative techniques may need to be secluded and physically restrained. Contingent restraint is operationally similar to conventional restraining methods; however, it demands immediate and consistent administration of restraint after each severe violent episode. Staff members should not interact verbally with patients during the application of restraints so they do not inadvertently reinforce the maladaptive behavior.

Behavioral Treatment of Emotional Reactions to TBI

The effects of the original injury, the resulting emergency care and hospitalization, the reaction of family members and friends, and the cognitive and behavioral sequelae of the injury are frequently upsetting for the patient. As a result, some TBI patients experience anxiety and panic with their new found inabilities, anger with the frustration that comes with these inabilities, and depression as the road to recovery becomes difficult. Clinical investigators have used various cognitive behavioral strategies to help patients resolve these intense emotional reactions. Lira et al. (1983) used elements of stress inoculation training (Meichenbaum 1975) to improve the frustration tolerance and diminish the anger of a TBI patient. Treatment consisted of the following three phases: 1) education about the phenomena of anger and appropriate ways to express it, 2) training cognitive reappraisal of anger-evoking situations and countering with positive statements, and 3) application training to use skills hierarchically. Results of their study showed that after four weeks of treatment, hostile episodes decreased from 2.75 incidents per week to zero. Moreover, no hostile outbursts were reported at five-month follow-up.

Results from studies on patients with multiple sclerosis (MS) have implications for TBI patients. In one study, stress inoculation training was used to address depression in 20 patients with MS; another group of 20 patients with MS were randomly assigned to "current available care" as a control group (Foley et al. 1987). After six treatment sessions, the patients who received stress inoculation training were significantly less anxious, distressed, and depressed than the control group. Results from a second study were similar; MS subjects in a cognitive-behavior therapy group were significantly less depressed than MS subjects in a waiting-list control group (Larcombe and Wilson 1984). Cognitive-behavior therapy in the second study combined Lewinsohn et al.'s (1976) techniques to increase the number of patients' positive life experiences with Beck et al.'s (1979) strategies to decrease damaging cognitions. In order to improve the number of positive life experiences, patients were taught to identify pleasurable activities, schedule them into their daily lives, and evaluate the efficacy of their schedules. In order to decrease damaging cognitions, patients were taught to identify negative self-statements, to recognize the connection between these self-statements and depression, to examine the evidence against negative statements, and to develop counters to the statements. Most subjects in the cognitive behavior therapy group maintained the therapeutic benefits of treatment at a one-month follow-up. These findings suggest that, in addition to the behavioral rehabilitation goals of increasing lost skills and diminishing antisocial behaviors, clinicians must be sensitive to the emotional reactions to TBI.

Staff Management Issues

Despite the abundance of well-validated behavioral strategies that ameliorate the deficits and excesses that result from TBI, rehabilitation programs for this population are lacking (Bleiberg et al. 1991). Recently, investigators have identified barriers to implementing behavioral interventions in inpatient psychiatric settings in the hope of identifying strategies for increasing the quantity and quality of behaviorally based mental health programs (Corrigan et al. 1992, in press). Although the typical TBI patient is treated at a rehabilitation hospital, many of the insights from these studies are applicable for decisions regarding introduction and implementation of behavioral innovations for brain injury patients. These barriers include lack of necessary supervisory structures to support these programs, insufficient monetary resources to maintain them, and little collegial support to implement them.

One way to overcome barriers to implementation of behavior therapy is to establish training and incentive programs that manage staff behaviors. Training staff members on behavior therapy principles and practices has been shown to markedly improve clinical performance (Carsrud et al. 1980; Milne 1982, 1984; Watson and

Uzell 1980). Training helps inexperienced staff who work with TBI patients to acquire the necessary skills to implement behavior therapy and keeps the skills of experienced workers sharp. For training to be successful, hospital administrators must provide sufficient time for staff to learn behavioral strategies. Moreover, the administration must contract with well-trained behavioral consultants who can provide didactic sessions colored with real-life vignettes (Bernstein 1983; Tharp and Wetzel 1969). The curriculum for the training program should reflect the unique interventions that have been useful to ameliorate the behavioral problems of TBI patients in the specific treatment setting.

Even if trainees learn behavioral strategies well, there is little guarantee that they will use the skills on the unit itself, especially after training has ceased (Bernstein 1979, 1983; Braukman et al. 1975). In the same way that behavioral clinicians provide support, guidance, and incentive for patients to maintain newly acquired behaviors, unit supervisors need to manage the behaviors of the yeoman clinicians charged with daily patient care. Regular clinical supervision assists these professionals and paraprofessionals in maintaining competent levels of behavioral intervention. Clinical supervision includes support and guidance, feedback and ongoing individualized training, and inspiration to continue working with individuals who define a tough patient population.

Unit supervisors can also maintain trainer skills by manipulating the contingencies that affect their staffs' job performance. In a general way, staff salaries, promotions, and vacation days reinforce overall job performance. Unfortunately, receipt of a weekly paycheck is not sufficiently flexible to shape discrete job skills. Research has identified variables other than salary and promotions that are related to job satisfaction, competent work performance, and collegial support (Cullari and Ferguson 1981; Paul and Lentz 1977). These include equal opportunity across staff positions for merit raises and promotion, personal recognition and feedback, small working unit size, good peer group identity, congenial interactions among peers, and high role clarity with much responsibility within these roles. Conversely, several factors lead to staff loss, including unequal workload and little recognition for competent work. In most settings, these variables are not under the direct control of mid-level supervisors. Union rules and hospital-wide job freezes may prevent tampering with merit raises, days off, or staff size. The point of this section, however, is that staff behavior, like patient behavior, is a function of social learning and rewards. Supervisors and administrators must take note of this parallel to develop behavioral programs that are most effective for TBI patients.

Summary

The model of behavioral treatment that we have outlined in this chapter focuses on *rehabilitation;* that is, facilitating the recovery of social and independent living skills so that TBI patients can meet everyday interpersonal and functional needs. As these patients become competent in meeting life demands, frustrations and concomitant behavioral problems diminish in frequency. Clinicians who use a *process* model for setting up behavioral rehabilitation programs have a comprehensive outline for behavioral recovery. Skill-training strategies facilitate acquisition of necessary skills. Contingency management and transfer training methods foster the performance and generalization of newly (re)acquired skills. Cognitive rehabilitation methods help TBI patients overcome learning deficits so they may profit from the program.

The process-based rehabilitation program is proactive in nature. Patients are taught ways not only to cope with current problems but also to avoid future stressors. Behavioral programs must augment these programs with strategies that address patient aggression and extreme emotional responses. We reviewed replacement and decelerative strategies for controlling aggression, and discussed cognitive behavioral interventions to address the emotional reactions to TBI. When combined with the judicious use of medications and physical rehabilitation, behavioral rehabilitation and therapy have significant effects on the TBI patient.

References

Adams JH, Graham DI, Gennarelli TA: Contemporary neuropathological considerations regarding brain damage in head injury, in Central Nervous System Trauma Report. Edited by Becker DP, Povlishock JT. Washington, DC, The National Institute of Neurological and Communicative Disorders and Stroke, National Institutes of Health, 1985, pp 65–67

Ayllon T, Azrin NH: The Token Economy: A Motivational System for Therapy and Rehabilitation. New York, Appleton-Century-Crofts, 1968

Bandura A: Social Learning Theory. Morristown, NJ, General Learning, 1971

Barlow DH, Hersen M: Single Case Experimental Designs: Strategies for Studying Behavior Change, 2nd Edition. New York, Pergamon, 1984

Beck AT, Rush AJ, Shaw BF, et al: Cognitive Therapy of Depression. New York, Guilford, 1979

Bellack AS, Hersen M (eds): Dictionary of Behavior Therapy Techniques. New York, Pergamon, 1985

Bellack AS, Morrison RL, Mueser KT: Social problem solving in schizophrenia. Schizophr Bull 15:101–116, 1989

Ben-Yishay Y, Rattok Y, Ross B, et al: A remedial "module" for the systematic amelioration of basic disturbances in head trauma patients, in Working Approaches to Remediation of Cognitive Deficits in Brain Damaged Persons (Rehabilitation Monograph No. 61). New York, NYU Medical Center, Institute of Rehabilitation Medicine, 1980, pp 71–127

Ben-Yishay Y, Rattok J, Lakin P, et al: Neuropsychologic rehabilitation: Quest for a holistic approach. Semin Neurol 5:252–259, 1985

Bernstein GS: Behavior analysis, professionalization, and deprofessionalization: issues and implications. Behavior Therapist 2:25, 1979

Bernstein GS: Training behavioral change agents: a conceptual overview. Behavior Therapy 13:1–23, 1983

Blackerby WF, Baumgarten A: A model treatment program for the head-injured substance abuser: preliminary findings. Journal of Head Trauma Rehabilitation 5:47–59, 1990

Bleiberg J, Ciulla R, Katz B: Psychological components of rehabilitation programs for brain-injured and spinal-cord-injured patients, in Handbook of Clinical Psychology in Medical Settings. Edited by Sweet JJ, Rozensky RH, Tovian SM. New York, Academic Press, 1991, pp 122–149

Braukman CJ, Fixsen DL, Kirigin KA, et al: Achievement place: the training and certification of teaching parents, in Issues in Evaluating Behavior Modification. Edited by Woods WS. Champaign, IL, Research Press, 1975, pp 157–184

Brotherton FA, Thomas LL, Wisotzek IE, et al: Social skills training in the rehabilitation of patients with traumatic closed head injury. Arch Phys Med Rehabil 69:827–832, 1988

Burke WH, Lewis FD: Management of maladaptive social behavior of a brain injured adult. Int J Rehabil Res 9:335–342, 1986

Carsrud AL, Carsrud KB, Dodd, BG: Randomly monitored staff utilization of behavior modification techniques: long-term effects on clients. J Consult Clin Psychol 48:704–710, 1980

Cautela JR, Lynch E: Reinforcement survey schedules: scoring, administration, and completed research. Psychol Rep 53:447–465, 1983

Cicerone KD, Tupper DE: Cognitive assessment in the neuropsychological rehabilitation of head-injured adults, in Clinical Neuropsychology of Intervention. Edited by Uzzell BP, Gross Y. Boston, MA, Martinus Nijhoff, 1986, pp 155–173

Cone JD, Hawkins RD: Behavioral Assessment: New Directions in Clinical Psychology. Edited by Cone JD, Hawkins RD. New York, Brunner/Mazel, 1977

Corrigan PW: Strategies that overcome barriers to token economies in community programs for severe mentally ill adults. Community Mental Health Journal 27:17–30, 1991

Corrigan PW, Davies-Farmer RM, Lome HB: A curriculum-based, psychoeducational program for the mentally ill. Psychosocial Rehabilitation Journal 12:71–73, 1988

Corrigan PW, Davies-Farmer RM, Lightstone R, et al: An analysis of the behavior components of psychoeducational treatment of persons with chronic, mental illness. Rehabilitation Counseling Bulletin 33:200–211, 1990

Corrigan PW, Kwartarini WY, Pramana W: Barriers to the implementation of behavior therapy. Behav Modif, 16:132–144, 1992

Corrigan PW, Schade ML, Liberman RP: Social skills training, in Rehabilitation of the Psychiatrically Disabled. Edited by Liberman RP. New York, Plenum, 1993a, 95–126

Corrigan PW, Yudofsky SC, Silver JM: Pharmacological and behavioral treatment for aggressive psychiatric patients. Hosp Community Psychiatry 44:125–133, 1993b

Corrigan PW, MacKain SJ, Liberman RP: Skills training modules: a strategy for dissemination and utilization of a rehabilitation innovation, in Intervention Research. Edited by Rothman J, Thomas E. Chicago, IL, Haworth (in press)

Crewe NM: Sexually inappropriate behavior, in Behavioral Problems and the Disabled: Assessment and Management. Baltimore, MD, Williams & Wilkins, 1980, pp 120–141

Cullari S, Ferguson DG: Individual behavior change: problems with programming in institutions for mentally retarded persons. Ment Retard 19:267–270, 1981

Diller L, Gordon WA: Rehabilitation and clinical neuropsychology, in Handbook of Clinical Neuropsychology. Edited by Filskov SB, Boll TJ. New York, Wiley, 1981, pp 702–733

Douglas MS, Mueser KT: Teaching conflict resolution skills to the chronically mentally ill: social skills training groups for briefly hospitalized patients. Behav Modif 14:519–547, 1990

D'Zurilla TJ: Problem-Solving Therapy: A Social Competence Approach. New York, Springer, 1986

Falloon IRH, Boyd JL, McGill C: Family Care of Schizophrenia. New York, Guilford, 1984

Foley FW, Bedell JR, LaRocca NG, et al: Efficacy of stress-inoculation training in coping with multiple sclerosis. J Consult Clin Psychol 55:919–922, 1987

Fordyce DJ, Roueche JR: Changes in perspectives of disability among patients, staff, and relatives during rehabilitation of head injury. Rehabilitation Psychology 31:217–229, 1986

Franzen MD, Lovell MR: Behavioral treatments of aggressive sequelae of brain injury. Psychiatric Annals 17:389–396, 1987

Gajar AH, Schloss PJ, Schloss CN, et al: Effects of feedback and self-monitoring on head trauma youths' conversation skills. J Appl Behav Anal 17:353–358, 1984

Gazzaniga MS: Determinants of cerebral recovery, in Plasticity and Recovery of Function in the Central Nervous System. Edited by Stein DG, Rosen JJ, Butters N. New York, Academic Press, 1974, pp 203–216

Gazzaniga MS: Is seeing believing: notes on clinical recovery, in Recovery from Brain Damage: Research and Theory. Edited by Finger S. New York, Plenum, 1978, pp 409–414

Glasgow RE, Zeiss RA, Barrera M, et al: Case studies on remediating memory deficits in brain damaged individuals. J Clin Psychol 33:1049–1054, 1977

Glynn SM, Bowen LL, Marshall BD, et al: Compliance with less restrictive aggression-control procedures. Hosp Community Psychiatry 40:82–84, 1989

Godfrey HPD, Knight RG: Memory training and behavioral rehabilitation of a severely head-injured adult. Arch Phys Med Rehabil 69:458–460, 1988

Hollon TH: Behavior modification in a community hospital rehabilitation unit. Arch Phys Med Rehabil 54:65–68, 1973

Horton AM, Howe NR: Behavioral treatment of the traumatically brain-injured: a case study. Percept Mot Skills 53:349–350, 1981

Horton AM, Miller WG: Brain damage and rehabilitation, in Current Topics in Rehabilitation Psychology. Edited by Golden CJ. New York, Grune & Stratton, 1984, pp 77–105

Horton AM, Sautter SW: Behavioral neuropsychology: behavioral treatment for the brain-injured, in The Neuropsychology Handbook: Behavioral and Clinical Perspective. Edited by Wedding A, Horton AM, Webster, J. New York, Springer, 1986, pp 259–277

Horton AM, Wedding D: Clinical and Behavioral Neuropsychology. New York, Praeger, 1984

Ince LP: Behavior Modification in Rehabilitation Medicine. Springfield, IL, Charles C Thomas, 1976

Kaufman H: Kaufman Developmental Scale. Chicago, IL, Stoelting, 1975

Kazdin AE: The token economy: a decade later. J Appl Behav Anal 15:431–445, 1982

Kazdin AE, Bootzin RR: The token economy: an evaluation review. J Appl Behav Anal 5:1–30, 1972

Klonoff PS, Snow WG, Costa, LD: Quality of life in patients 2 to 4 years after closed head injury. Neurosurgery 19:735–743, 1986

Kushner H, Knox A: Application of the utilization technique to the behavior of a brain-injured patient. J Commun Disord 6:151–154, 1973

Larcombe NA, Wilson PH: An evaluation of cognitive-behavior therapy for depression in patients with multiple sclerosis. Br J Psychiatry 145:366–371, 1984

Lennox DB, Miltonberger RG, Sprengler P, et al: Decelerative treatment practices with persons who have mental retardation: A review of five years of the literature. Am J Ment Retard 92:492–501, 1988

Levin HS, Benton AL, Grossman RG: Neurobehavioral Consequences of Closed Head Injury. New York, Oxford University Press, 1982

Lewinsohn PM, Biglan BG, Zeiss AM: Behavioral treatment of depression, in Progress in Behavior Modification, Vol 1. Edited by Hersen M, Eisler RM, Miller PM. New York, Pergamon, 1976, pp 184–199

Lewinsohn PM, Danaher BG, Kikel S: Visual imagery as a mnemonic aid for brain injured persons. J Consult Clin Psychol 45:717–723, 1977

Liberman RP, Corrigan PW: Designing new psychosocial treatments for schizophrenia. Psychiatry 56:119–124, 1993

Liberman RP, Wong SE: Behavioral analysis and therapy procedures related to seclusion and restraint, in The Psychiatric Uses of Seclusion and Restraint. Edited by Tardiff K. Washington, DC, American Psychiatric Press, 1984, pp 223–262

Liberman RP, DeRisi WJ, Mueser KT: Social Skills Training for Psychiatric Patients. New York, Pergamon, 1989

Lira FT, Carne W, Masri AM: Treatment of anger and impulsivity in a brain damaged patient: a case study applying stress inoculation. Clinical Neuropsychology 5:159–160, 1983

Marholin DH, Luiselli JK, Townsend NM: Overcorrection: an examination of its rationale and treatment effectiveness, in Progress in Behavior Modification, Vol 10. Edited by Hersen, M, Eisler RM, Miller PM. New York, Academic Press, 1980, pp 56–69

Matson JL, DiLorenzo TM: Social skills training and mental handicap and organic impairment, in Handbook of Social Skills Training: Clinical Applications and New Directions, Vol 2. Edited by Hollin CR, Trower P. New York, Pergamon, 1986, pp 322–343

Matson JL, Stephens RM: Overcorrection of aggressive behavior in a chronic psychiatric patient. Behav Modif 1:559–564, 1977

McGlynn SM: Behavioral approaches to neuropsychological rehabilitation. Psychol Bull 108:420–441, 1990

Meichenbaum D: A self-instructional approach to stress management: a proposal for stress inoculation training, in Stress and Anxiety, Vol 1. Edited by Spielberger C, Sarasen I. New York, Wiley, 1975, pp 237–263

Milne DL: A comparison of two methods of teaching behaviour modification to mental handicap nurses. Behavioural Psychotherapy 10:54–64, 1982

Milne DL: The development and evaluation of structured learning format introduction to behavior therapy for psychiatric nurses. Br J of Clin Psychol 23:175–185, 1984

Mueller DJ, Atlas L: Resocialization of regressed elderly residents: a behavioral management approach. J Gerontol 27:390–392, 1972

Murphy ST: The effects of a token economy program on self-care behaviors of neurologically impaired inpatients. J Behav Ther Exp Psychiatry 7:145–147, 1976

Oddy M, Coughlan T, Tyerman A, et al: Social adjustment after closed head injury: A further follow-up seven years after injury. J Neurol Neurosurg Psychiatry 48:564–568, 1985

Passler MA: A two-phase treatment approach for traumatically brain-injured patients: a case study. Rehabilitation Psychology 32:215–226, 1987

Paul GL, Lentz RJ: Psychosocial Treatment of Chronic Mental Patients. Cambridge, MA, Harvard University Press, 1977

Porterfield JK, Herbert-Jackson E, Risley TR: Contingent observation: an effective and acceptable procedure for reducing disruptive behavior of young children in a group setting. J Appl Behav Anal 9:55–64, 1976

Premack D: Reversibility of the reinforcement relation. Science 136:255–257, 1962

Prigatano GP, Altman IM: Impaired awareness of behavioral limitations after traumatic brain injury. Arch Phys Med Rehabil 71:1058–1064, 1990

Prigatano GP, Fordyce DJ: The neuropsychological rehabilitation program at Presbyterian Hospital, in Neuropsychological Rehabilitation after Brain Injury. Edited by Prigatano GP. Baltimore, MD, Johns Hopkins University Press, 1986, pp 96–118

Sasmor RM: Operant conditioning of a small scale muscle response. J Exp Anal Behav 9:69–85, 1966

Schade ML, Corrigan PW, Liberman RP: Comprehensive psychiatric rehabilitation. New Dir Ment Health Serv 45:3–17, 1990

Schloss PJ, Schloss CN, Gajar AH,: Efficacy of four ratios of questions to text in computer assisted instruction modules. Journal of Computer Based Instruction 11:103–106, 1984

Silver JM, Yudofsky SC: Documentation of aggression in the assessment of the violent patient. Psychiatric Annals 17:375–384, 1987

Skinner BF: Science and Human Behavior. New York, Macmillan, 1953

Spiegler MD, Agigian H: Community Training Center: An Educational-Behavioral-Social Systems Model for Rehabilitating Psychiatric Patients. New York, Brunner/Mazel, 1977

Stokes TF, Baer DM: An implicit technology of generalization. J Appl Behav Anal 10:349–367, 1977

Stokes TF, Osnes PG: An operant pursuit of generalization. Behavior Therapy 20:337–355, 1989

Sunderland A, Harris JE, Baddeley AD: Do laboratory tests predict everyday memory? A neuropsychological study. Journal of Verbal Learning and Verbal Behaviors 22:341–347, 1983

Sunderland A, Harris JE, Gleave J: Memory failures in everyday life following severe head injury. J Clin Neuropsychol 6:127–142, 1984

Tardiff K, Sweillam A: Assaultive behavior among chronic inpatients. Am J Psychiatry 139:212–215, 1982

Tellier A, Adams KM, Walker AE, et al: Long-term effects of severe penetrating head injury on psychosocial adjustment. J Consult Clin Psychol 58:531–537, 1990

Tharp R, Wetzel R: Behavior Modification in the Natural Environment. New York, Academic Press, 1969

Thomsen IV: Late outcome of very severe blunt head trauma: a 10–15 year second follow-up. J Neurol Neurosurg Psychiatry 48:21–28, 1984

Turner SM, Hersen M, Bellack AS: Social skills training to teach prosocial behavior in an organically impaired and retarded patient. J Behav Ther Exp Psychiatry 9:253–258, 1978

Watson LS Jr, Uzell R: A program for teaching behavior modification skills to institutional staff. Applied Research in Mental Retardation 1:41–53, 1980

Webster JS, Scott RR: The effects of self-instructive training on attention deficits following head injury. Clinical Neuropsychology 5:69–74, 1983

Wehman PH, Kreutzer JS, West MD, et al: Return to work for persons with traumatic brain injury: a supported employment approach. Arch Phys Med Rehabil 71:1047–1052, 1990

Weinstein EA, Kahn RL: Denial of Illness: Symbolic and Physiological Aspects. Springfield, IL, Charles C Thomas, 1955

Wood R: Behavioural disturbance and behavioural management, in New Directions in the Neuropsychology of Severe Blunt Head Injury Symposium. Presented at the meeting of the International Neuropsychological Society, Deauville, France, 1982

Wood RL, Eames PG: Application of behavior modification in the rehabilitation of traumatically brain-injured patients, in Applications of Conditioning Theory. Edited by Davey G. New York, Methuen, 1981, pp 81–101

Chapter 23

Neuropharmacological Treatment for Acute Brain Injury

Lawrence S. Honig, M.D., Ph.D.
Gregory W. Albers, M.D.

I t was once commonly assumed that brain damage caused by head trauma occurred instantaneously at the time of injury. However, recent studies have shown that brain tissue destruction evolves over hours to days following the initial insult. Although it is apparent that primary prevention of traumatic brain injury (TBI) is of paramount importance, pharmacological agents may be able to attenuate much of the damage that is produced by secondary processes.

TBI leads to several concurrent pathological processes (see Figure 23–1, and discussion in Chapter 2). Functionally, these may be grouped into neuronal cellular (gray matter) and nerve fiber (white matter) categories (Adams et al. 1985; Langfitt and Zimmerman 1985). Beyond physical destruction of brain tissue directly attributable to mechanical injury, primary neuronal injury may occur from contusion, hemorrhage, or edema. Brain injury may also result from hypoxemia or hypoperfusion, whether systemic

771

from cardiac or pulmonary failure, or local (cerebral) due to tissue pressure effects or disruption and thrombosis of blood vessels. Nerve fiber injury may occur from either the aforementioned factors causing axonal infarction or demyelination, mechanical transection, or disruption of white matter fiber tracts due to shear forces incurred during the trauma (Povlishock 1985). Recovery mechanisms are different for neuronal and axonal injuries, but with the exception of brain matter loss and axonal transection, the above pathologies all seem to trigger a complex set of processes that lead to delayed tissue destruction. This cascade is very similar to that seen following ischemic brain infarction: its elements are diagrammed in Figure 23–1, listed in Table 23–1, and discussed below.

Following injury, acute treatment may be directed toward either primary pathologies (e.g., hematoma removal) or limiting secondary neuronal or demyelinative damage (Table 23–1). Other approaches may be directed toward improving the function or rate of recovery of damaged brain tissue. For example, useful treatments may alter neurotransmitter levels, improve nerve conduction, enhance long-term survival of axotomized or deafferented cells, accelerate axonal regeneration, facilitate nerve remyelination,

---

Table 23–1.   Secondary processes in traumatic brain injury

Ischemia

Acidosis

Excitotoxic neurotransmitter release

Calcium ion influx

Neuronal depolarization

Phospholipase activations

Lipid peroxidation

Free radical generation

Protease activation

Increased membrane permeability

Excitotoxic neurotransmitter leakage

Cytoplasmic swelling (sodium ion influx)

Ion pump failure/Energy failure

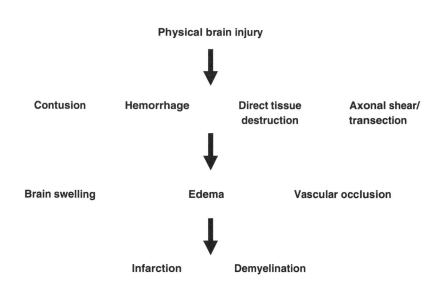

Figure 23–1. Physical brain injury leads to a variety of histopathological processes leading to the common end result of tissue destruction.

or promote plasticity and rewiring of neural connections (Bower 1990). In this chapter, we focus on medical therapies aimed at preventing the early brain damage that results from the secondary processes that follow traumatic injury.

Considerable experimental work has been performed to augment understanding of the pathophysiology of brain injury. A variety of methods have been employed in a diverse array of experimental models. Molecular and cellular processes can be observed in cell culture or brain tissue slices. Other studies, particularly those investigating agents that may be of clinical utility in nervous system injury, have employed models using anesthetized whole small animals. Reproducible ischemia may be induced by experimental vascular occlusion with clips or sutures. Controlled CNS injury can be accomplished by exposing bare brain or spinal cord to fluid percussion damage, defined weight compression or contusion, surgical resection, or cold injury using dry ice or cryogenic probes. Careful biochemical, physiological, and neurological assessment has resulted in the identification of promising agents for clinical use.

The varied histopathological processes of contusion, edema, and hypoxia/ischemia (Figure 23–1) lead to a common set of secondary destructive cellular processes (Figure 23–2). These include excitotoxic neurotransmitter release, intracellular influx of calcium ions, neuronal depolarization, reduction of extracellular calcium ions, tissue acidosis, protease activation, generation of free radicals, lipid peroxidation, autacoid generation, cellular energy depletion, ion pump failure, and alterations in neuronal membrane permeability. Pharmacological treatments have the potential to limit these various processes. Treatments may be grouped into tissue-level therapies (e.g., prevention or reduction of swelling and edema, or improvement of local blood flow) and cellular-level therapies (e.g., preventing excitotoxic damage and lipid peroxidation) (Table 23–2). However, some of the medications discussed below may be effective through mechanisms different from those

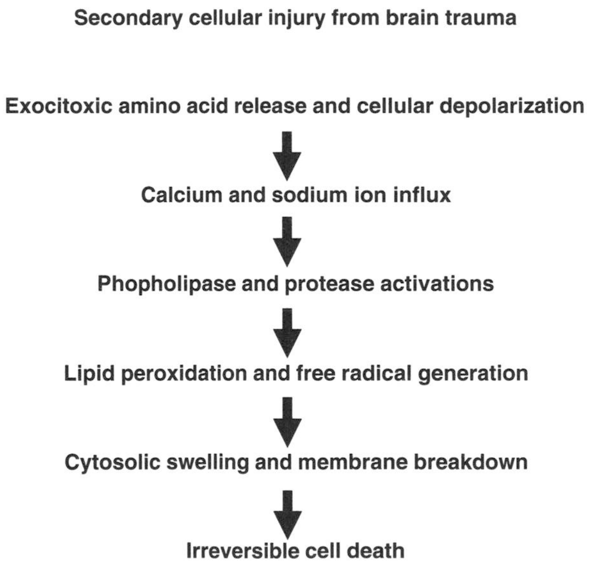

Secondary cellular injury from brain trauma

Exocitoxic amino acid release and cellular depolarization

↓

Calcium and sodium ion influx

↓

Phopholipase and protease activations

↓

Lipid peroxidation and free radical generation

↓

Cytosolic swelling and membrane breakdown

↓

Irreversible cell death

Figure 23–2. Secondary cellular injury from brain trauma results from a cascade of detrimental cellular, biochemical, and electrical processes.

Table 23–2.   Pharmacological therapies

Tissue level
    Antiedema agents
        Osmotic agents (e.g., mannitol and glycerol)
        Glucocorticoids (e.g., methylprednisolone)
    Diuretics (e.g., furosemide)
    Blood flow altering agents
        General anesthetics (e.g., barbiturates and propofol)
        Prostaglandin synthesis inhibitors (e.g., indomethacin)
        Calcium channel antagonists (e.g., nimodipine, verapamil, and flunarizine)
        Thyrotropin-releasing hormone (TRH)/other opiate antagonists
            (e.g., naloxone, nalmefene, and WIN-44441-3)
        Platelet-activating factor (PAF) antagonists (e.g., BIN-52021 and WEB-2086)
Cellular level
    Excitotoxic amino acid antagonists and modulators
        AP5, AP7, CPP, CPPene, CGP-39653, CGP-37849, CGS-19755,
            dizocilpine (MK-801), ketamine, phencyclidine (PCP), dextrorphan,
            glycine inhibitors, magnesium, and polyamine inhibitors
            (e.g., α-difluoro-methylornithine [DFMO])
    Free radical inhibitors
        Superoxide dismutase, α-tocopherol, ebselen (PZ-51),
            allopurinol, oxypurinol, desferoxamine, and 2,3-dihydroxybutyrate
    Lazaroids (21-aminosteroids) (e.g., tirilazad [U74006F])
    Buffering agents (tromethamine [THAM])
    Cholinergic antagonists (e.g., scopalamine); Amphetamines
    Gangliosides (GM1)
    Neurotrophic factors (e.g., NGF, BDNF, NT3, bFGF, EGF, CDF, and CNTF)

---

originally proposed, or have multiple mechanisms of action. For example, steroids reduce vasogenic edema, yet it is likely that much of their efficacy is at a neuronal cellular level through inhibition of lipid peroxidation.

Tissue-Level Therapy

Antiedema Agents

TBI is promptly followed by swelling, with a marked increase in the volume of intracranial soft tissue (Cooper 1985; Tornheim

1985). This swelling consists of several components, including 1) increased intravascular blood volume; 2) increases in intracellular volume due to neuronal and astrocytic cytoplasmic swelling (cytotoxic edema); and 3) increases in extracellular fluid due to blood-brain barrier leakage from increased capillary permeability (vasogenic edema), as well as hydrostatic and osmotic pressure gradients (interstitial edema). Swelling is often evident within 1 hour of injury, and increases over 24–48 hours. Because the volume of the skull is fixed, severe cerebral swelling can result in downward brain herniation through the foramen magnum, or extracranial extrusion in the presence of open fracture or craniectomy. Increased intracranial pressure from swelling causes a significant reduction of blood flow to affected brain areas by reducing cerebral perfusion pressure. Cerebral perfusion pressure (CPP) is the difference between mean arterial pressure (MAP) and intracranial pressure (ICP): CPP = MAP − ICP (Figure 23–3). At low cerebral perfusion pressure, brain vessel autoregulation fails, and blood flow falls below the critical range of 10–20 cc per 100 g brain tissue per minute. The resultant severe ischemia may cause death of otherwise uninjured brain, causing still greater edema. Surgical therapies to reduce intracranial pressure, such as ventricular shunts, may be useful but calvarial decompression is rarely of value, because of increased brain swelling and tissue extrusion (Lyons and Meyer 1990). Medical means of limiting tissue swelling through use of steroids or osmotic agents are potentially beneficial.

Osmotic agents increase serum osmolarity; they include intravenous glycerol and mannitol. An increase in blood osmolarity of even 10 milliosmols/L will cause extraction of water from brain tissue of lower (normal) osmolarity. This decreases intracranial pressure, and may increase cerebral blood flow (providing mean arterial pressure does not decrease from the diuretic effect of the hyperosmolar agent). Unfortunately, osmotic agents such as mannitol do not remain in the vascular compartment but gradually leak into brain tissue. This process is increased following trauma due to blood-brain barrier disruption, thereby limiting any beneficial effects (Cold 1990).

Glucocorticosteroids in some situations are successful in increasing the integrity of the blood-brain barrier and thus decreasing vasogenic tissue edema. Because this effect can be dramatic for brain neoplasms or abscesses, steroids were at one time widely administered following traumatic or ischemic injury. However, studies of patients with stroke and intracerebral hematomas have shown that at standard to high doses, steroids lack efficacy and may even be detrimental (Poungvarin et al. 1987). Adverse effects include hyperglycemia, hypercatabolism, and gastrointestinal hemorrhage. Clinical trials of head injury have also shown no evidence for reduction of intracranial pressure (Gudeman et al. 1979) or improved outcome with steroid treatment (Braakman et al. 1983; Cooper et al. 1979). Their inefficacy may be due to the fact that edema following trauma is of mixed vasogenic, cytotoxic, and interstitial types, as discussed above, and steroids are helpful only for vasogenic edema.

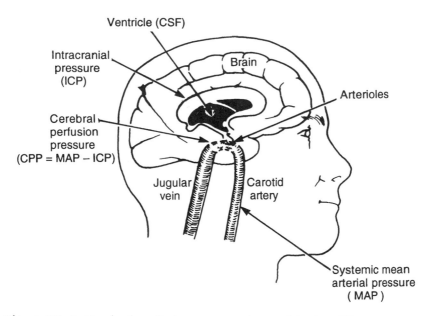

Figure 23–3. Cerebral perfusion pressure is equal to the difference between mean systemic arterial pressure and intracranial pressure.

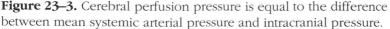

A variety of animal investigations (Hall and Braughler 1987), as well as a recent study of acute human spinal cord injury (Bracken et al. 1990), have shown that truly massive doses of steroids may be beneficial in some situations where conventional doses of steroids are of marginal or no utility. These high doses are much greater than required for stimulation of glucocorticoid receptors and even considerably exceed the "megadoses" previously proposed for reduction of vasogenic edema in other situations. Thus the benefits reported with massive steroid doses may result from non-glucocorticoid-receptor mediated effects such as inhibition of lipid peroxidation (Hall 1989; Hsu and Dimitrijevic 1990). These considerations led to development of the 21-aminosteroid (lazaroid) class of drugs (see below).

Other antiedema agents are under investigation as well. Diuretics such as furosemide and ethacrynic acid may be used to decrease blood volume and brain edema. However, their effects are greater on normal brain than on injured brain with cytotoxic edema; furthermore, systemic hypotension limits their use, particularly because trauma patients often have compromised blood pressure. Nondiuretic derivatives of loop diuretics, including indanyl and fluorenyl ethacrynic relatives, inhibit potassium-stimulated, bicarbonate-dependent glial swelling. Such agents (e.g., MK-474 and L-644711) are under investigation as anti-cytotoxic edema agents in experimental closed head injury (Kimelberg et al. 1990).

Agents That Alter Blood Flow

Decreased blood flow frequently occurs during TBI (Langfitt and Zimmerman 1985; Muizelaar and Obrist 1985). The primary causes of cerebral hypoperfusion following brain trauma include local factors such as arterial dissection or occlusion by foreign body or hematoma, as well as global factors such as systemic hypotension. These conditions should each be treated by specifically directed therapies. However, commonly there are delayed decreases in blood flow that occur during the hours following injury; these occur via a number of secondary mechanisms (Figure 23–4)

(Muizelaar and Obrist 1985; Yamakami and McIntosh 1989; Yuan et al. 1988). As discussed above, global decreases in cerebral perfusion pressure may result from increased intracranial pressure from brain swelling and edema. Local declines in blood flow may occur from the focal mass effects of edema with consequent small vessel occlusion. Vasoconstriction may also be caused by release of vasoactive and inflammatory factors, including leukotrienes and prostaglandins (Ellis et al. 1981, 1989), as well as by changes in vessel autoregulation resulting from injury induced metabolic changes.

Endogenous and exogenous mediators of blood flow

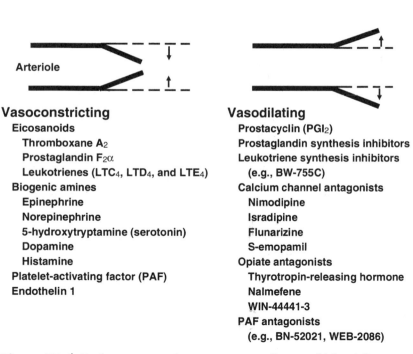

Vasoconstricting
Eicosanoids
　Thromboxane A_2
　Prostaglandin $F_{2\alpha}$
　Leukotrienes (LTC$_4$, LTD$_4$, and LTE$_4$)
Biogenic amines
　Epinephrine
　Norepinephrine
　5-hydroxytryptamine (serotonin)
　Dopamine
　Histamine
Platelet-activating factor (PAF)
Endothelin 1

Vasodilating
Prostacyclin (PGI$_2$)
Prostaglandin synthesis inhibitors
Leukotriene synthesis inhibitors
　(e.g., BW-755C)
Calcium channel antagonists
　Nimodipine
　Isradipine
　Flunarizine
　S-emopamil
Opiate antagonists
　Thyrotropin-releasing hormone
　Nalmefene
　WIN-44441-3
PAF antagonists
　(e.g., BN-52021, WEB-2086)

Figure 23–4. Endogenous and exogenous mediators of blood flow. Mediators of blood flow include endogenous compounds and exogenously administered medications, which can result in either arteriolar vasoconstriction (*left*) or arteriolar vasodilation (*right*).

Pharmacological methods of improving blood flow may be directed toward many of the mechanisms considered above. Brain tissue swelling and edema may be attacked with agents such as steroids and mannitol; the resultant decreased intracranial pressure could lead to increased cerebral blood flow as detailed above (Figure 23–3).

General anesthetics such as barbiturates (Cold 1990) or propofol (Pinaud et al. 1990) may be used to decrease intracranial pressure. Also barbiturates decrease brain electrical activity, thereby reducing cerebral energy demand; these effects are likely due to their strong potentiation of GABA (γ-aminobutyric acid) inhibition at the GABA$_A$ receptor, although barbiturates have been postulated to have a variety of other effects, including inhibition of the AMPA (α-amino-3-hydroxy-5-methyl-4-isoxazoleproprionic acid) or non-NMDA (*N*-methyl-D-aspartate) excitatory amino acid receptor, membrane stabilization, and free radical scavenger action. Because of the hypothesized ability of barbiturates to decrease intracranial pressure, and possibly provide cellular cerebral protection, they have been administered to acute head trauma patients. However, recent clinical trials have documented detrimental side effects, and failed to demonstrate significant improvements in neurological recovery (Cold 1990; Cooper 1985; Moskopp 1991; Ward et al. 1985). The lack of benefits may be related to cardiovascular depression with reduction in mean arterial pressure, thereby precluding increases in cerebral perfusion pressure.

Inhibitors of vasoconstrictive factors have been studied in experimental brain trauma. Lipid peroxidation inhibitors may prevent cytotoxic edema by preventing membrane breakdown (discussed below). Nonsteroidal anti-inflammatory agents inhibit prostaglandin synthetase, and thus could prevent formation of vasoconstrictive prostaglandins and thromboxanes that result from lipid peroxidation. Indeed, indomethacin has been observed to improve cerebral arteriolar vasoreactivity in experimental animals (Becker et al. 1988). Preliminary trials of this medication in fluid-percussion brain-injured rats have shown beneficial effects (Kim et al. 1989).

Calcium channel blockers cause vasodilation through their action on endothelial cells, although they have other physiological effects. In controlled clinical trials, the calcium channel antagonist nimodipine has produced modest but significant improvements in the neurological outcome of patients with subarachnoid hemorrhage (Robinson and Teasdale 1990). However nimodipine has not consistently shown beneficial effects in clinical studies of acute ischemic cerebrovascular disease (American Nimodipine Study Group 1992). In experimental trauma using the rat brain cold-injury model, nimodipine appears to decrease intracranial pressure and edema (Gaab et al. 1990a). However, its mechanism may be through decreasing hydrostatic pressure via reduction in systemic blood pressure. At least one experimental study has suggested that nimodipine may actually worsen tissue edema when the hypotensive effect of the medication is eliminated (Gaab et al. 1990a). A clinical trial of nimodipine in head injury did not demonstrate significant benefit (Bailey et al. 1991).

Thyrotropin-releasing hormone (TRH or protirelin) is a tripeptide hormone that at high concentrations acts as an opiate antagonist and increases blood flow. Some neuroprotective effects have been demonstrated in experimental spinal cord injury (Faden et al. 1989a). The doses used are much higher than those required for its endocrine action; benefits are likely due to improved blood flow. Other opiate antagonists have been tested in trauma and ischemia, including naloxone, nalmefene (Vink et al. 1990), and the compound WIN-44441-3 (McIntosh et al. 1987); the latter two potent drugs are selective for the kappa type opiate receptor. In some experiments these agents have shown neuroprotective effects (Young 1991). However, clinical trials of naloxone, a less selective opiate antagonist, in stroke and human spinal cord injury (Bracken et al. 1990) have not shown beneficial effects.

Platelet-activating factor is an endogenous phospholipid mediator of inflammation with vasoactive, thrombo-occlusive, and edema promoting activities; its production increases after brain ischemia or trauma (Lindsberg et al. 1991). Antagonists such as BN-52021 and WEB-2086 have been reported to improve neurological outcome following experimental ischemia (Lindsberg et al.

1991). However, these compounds have not been shown to be neuroprotective in experimental trauma (Kochanek et al. 1991).

Cellular-Level Therapy

Recent evidence suggests that excitatory amino acids (EAA), especially glutamate, may play a pivotal role in the secondary brain injury that occurs during the hours after trauma (Rothman and Olney 1986). During experimental ischemic injury, substantial elevations of extracellular glutamate occur (Benveniste et al. 1984; Hagberg et al. 1985). This increase is a product of greater synaptic EAA release, cellular EAA leakage, and impaired energy-dependent EAA neurotransmitter reuptake. Increased extracellular glutamate causes excessive activation of glutamate receptors. This "excitotoxic" action causes an increased influx of sodium and calcium ions into neurons. The sodium influx can contribute to neuronal swelling, depolarization, and further build-up of intracellular calcium (Choi 1987).

Calcium ion influx is one of the most critical early steps in secondary neuronal damage (Cheung et al. 1986; Siesjo 1988; Siesjo and Bengtsson 1989; Young 1987). Excessive calcium may enter neurons through agonist-operated cation channels, which are associated with a particular subclass of glutamate receptors—the NMDA receptors (MacDermott et al. 1986), as well as through voltage-dependent channels, which are activated by depolarization (Figure 23–5). Increased intracellular calcium can trigger an array of neurochemical changes, including activation of protein kinases, phosphatases, proteases, and phospholipases; neurons become depolarized and intracellular stores release further calcium. Calcium-stimulated proteases cause conversion of xanthine dehydrogenase to xanthine oxidase (Meldrum 1990) whose action in turn generates free radicals from oxygen. Calcium activation of phospholipase A_2 causes release of arachidonic acid, with production of leukotrienes, prostaglandins, platelet-activating factor, and free radicals (Ikeda and Long 1990; Lindsberg et al. 1991; Meldrum

1990; Siesjo and Bengtsson 1989). Free radicals attack neuronal membranes, releasing lipid peroxides and arachidonic acid. Arachidonic acid metabolites can cause additional neuronal damage, and contribute to local vasoconstriction, breakdown of the blood-brain barrier, and brain edema. This series of events ultimately results in destruction of brain tissue.

Excitatory Amino Acid Antagonists

A considerable body of experimental data has implicated excessive extracellular glutamate as a major contributor to the brain damage that occurs following cerebral ischemia and hypoglycemia (Albers et al. 1989; Choi 1988; Meldrum 1990; Rothman and Olney 1986). Glutamate probably plays a key role in initiating the processes that ultimately lead to secondary neuronal destruction following brain trauma (Faden et al. 1989b; Miller et al. 1990). The neurochemical

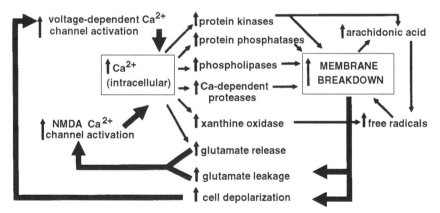

Figure 23–5. Role of intracellular calcium in neuronal injury. Intracellular calcium increases have a central role in secondary brain injury after trauma. Increased (↑) intracellular calcium ion (Ca^{2+}) concentration results in glutamate synaptic release and elevated activity of a number of enzymes, as diagrammed. These processes lead to membrane breakdown processes, and ultimately feedback, causing further increases in calcium. Pharmacological inhibitors at a number of the steps shown may prevent further damage. NMDA = *N*-methyl-D-aspartate.

changes that occur after TBI appear to have much in common with those following brain ischemia and hypoglycemia. Microdialysis studies have documented substantial elevations in extracellular concentration of the excitatory amino acids, glutamate and aspartate, in animal brains after experimental trauma (Faden et al. 1989b). These elevations likely result from direct leakage of excitatory neurotransmitters from traumatized neurons, as well as from synaptic release due to neuronal depolarization, and from failure of glial and presynaptic neuronal reuptake mechanisms (Choi 1988); see Figure 23–6. Trauma may result in excitotoxic damage from both direct excitatory amino acid release and release induced by secondary ischemia.

Glutamate antagonists, agents preventing activation of glutamate receptors, have shown promise in both in vitro and in vivo

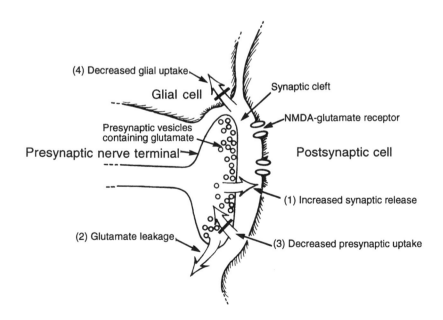

Figure 23–6. Four mechanisms of increased extracellular glutamate during trauma: 1) increased presynaptic vesicular release, 2) increased leakage of neurotransmitter, 3) decreased presynaptic neurotransmitter uptake, and 4) decreased glial uptake. NMDA = *N*-methyl-D-asparate.

models of TBI. Because broad spectrum glutamate antagonists may produce unacceptable suppression of excitatory neurotransmission, most studies have focused on selective NMDA antagonists. It is this subclass of glutamate receptors that is associated with an ion channel with high permeability to calcium. Calcium flux through the NMDA receptor can be reduced by two main categories of specific antagonists—competitive and noncompetitive—and can also be influenced by allosteric agents discussed below (Table 23–3; Figure 23–7). Competitive antagonists interfere with glutamate binding to the endogenous agonist (glutamate) recognition site. Noncompetitive antagonists act at the ion channel, blocking flow through the open NMDA receptor–associated ion channel. Both competitive and noncompetitive antagonists have been shown in studies to attenuate experimental traumatic neuronal injury in vitro using cell culture (Tecoma et al. 1989) and in vivo using animals with experimental brain trauma or spinal

Table 23–3.   NMDA-selective excitatory amino acid (glutamate) receptor antagonists

Competitive
  D-AP5 (APV)
  D-AP7 (APH)
  CPP
  D-CPPene
  CGP-37849
  CGP-39653
  CGS-19755
Noncompetitive
  Dizocilpine (MK-801)
  Phencylidine (PCP)
  Ketamine
  SKF-10047
  Dextrorphan
Other modulating agents
  Magnesium ions (Mg^{2+})
  Zinc ions (Zn^{2+})
  Glycine antagonists (e.g., 7-chlorokynurenate and HA-966)
  Polyamine synthesis inhibitors (e.g., α–difluoro-methylornithine)

Note. NMDA = *N*-methyl-D-aspartate.

cord trauma (Faden et al. 1989b; Hayes et al. 1988).

Competitive NMDA antagonists have the advantage of acting at the binding site for the excitotoxic amino acids. However, because they compete with the endogenous agonist, they may be displaced by high concentrations of endogenous glutamate or aspartate. Furthermore, in general they are polar (water-soluble) molecules that do not penetrate the CNS easily when administered systemically. Synthetic competitive agonists include the aminophosphono-carboxylate analogs of glutamate, and their piperazine and piperidine derivatives. These compounds are best known by their acronymic monikers, including AP5, AP7, CPP, CPPene, CGP-37849, and CGS-19755 (Table 23–3). These agents have shown neuroprotective potential both in vitro and in vivo in ischemia models. In addition, CPP has been shown to attenuate neurological deterioration in an experimental model of brain trauma model (Faden et al. 1989b).

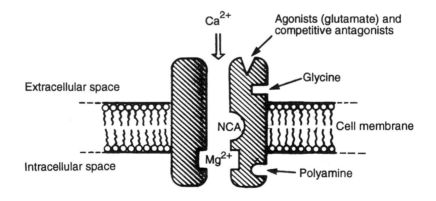

Figure 23–7. The NMDA-type (*N*-methyl-D-aspartate) excitatory amino acid (glutamate) receptor is a transmembrane ion channel protein spanning the lipid bilayer. Glutamate causes increased channel conductivity when bound at its extracellular site. The cotransmitter glycine modulates ion flux through binding at a different extracellular site. Polyamines influence channel conductivity interacting at an intracellular site. Noncompetitive antagonists (NCA) and magnesium ions (Mg^{2+}) apparently act in the channel. Ca^{2+} = calcium ion.

Noncompetitive NMDA antagonists, including dizocilpine (MK-801), dextrorphan, phencyclidine, and ketamine, have been studied extensively. These nonpolar (lipid-soluble) compounds easily penetrate the CNS, and their effects persist or even increase in the presence of excess endogenous agonist. The potent noncompetitive NMDA antagonist dizocilpine reliably prevents damage in experimentally induced focal ischemia (Iversen et al. 1989) and improves postinjury neurological performance when given to rats prior to experimental brain injury induced by fluid percussion (McIntosh et al. 1989a). Even when this agent was administered to rats one hour after a closed head injury, there was improved neurological outcome, and reduction in lesion size (Shapira et al. 1990). The noncompetitive NMDA antagonist, dextrorphan, also limits neurological dysfunction following experimental TBI in rats (Faden et al. 1989b). Dextrorphan, which is undergoing clinical trials in stroke, is the major metabolite of dextromethorphan, a widely used antitussive available on a nonprescription, over-the-counter basis. Another noncompetitive NMDA antagonist is phencyclidine (PCP), used as a veterinary tranquilizer and widely known as a substance of abuse ("angel dust"). Like the previously mentioned antagonists, PCP has been shown to reduce neuronal vulnerability to posttraumatic ischemia (Jenkins et al. 1988).

Many of the above NMDA antagonists appear to have substantial neuroprotective effects when administered in the setting of experimental trauma or ischemia. However, side effects could limit their use in treatment of human brain trauma. Some potential safety concerns have emerged from experimental animal and limited human studies. These include psychotomimetic effects, interference with synaptic plasticity, and the induction of pathological neuronal vacuolization (Albers 1990).

Because glutamate is the major excitatory neurotransmitter in the brain, NMDA antagonists may cause sedation or weakness. These effects probably would be tolerated for short time periods; however, in addition to its function in excitatory neurotransmission, the NMDA receptor plays an important role in neuronal plasticity. For example, its activation seems to be an indispensable part of induction of long-term potentiation, a process of synaptic strengthening that may figure fundamentally in learning and memory (Harris et al. 1984). This has generated concern that NMDA antagonists might interfere with memory function.

Some NMDA antagonists also have psychoactive effects. The noncompetitive NMDA antagonists phencyclidine and ketamine may cause serious dysphoria, agitation, delirium, and hallucinations. It is possible that NMDA antagonists might intrinsically possess adverse psychotomimetic properties. Another effect of NMDA antagonists that is of potential concern is the pathological vacuolization of neuronal cytoplasm produced in the posterior cingulate and retrosplenial neocortex of rats (Olney et al. 1989). These anatomically restricted changes are reversible after treatments with low drug dosages but can be irreversible after high dosages. Although their significance is not clear, it has been shown that concomitant administration of anticholinergic agents or GABAergic drugs such as barbiturates can suppress the pathological changes (Olney et al. 1991). Ongoing clinical investigations of a number of these agents should clarify their safety profile.

Other factors modulating NMDA channels include the amino acid cotransmitter glycine, magnesium ions, zinc ions, and polyamines. Glycine potentiates the activity of NMDA agonists. It acts at an allosteric site on the NMDA receptor—neither at the agonist, nor at the noncompetitive antagonist binding sites. Inhibitors acting at the glycine site, such as 7-chlorokynurenate, may potentially reduce NMDA channel activation; they are under investigation. Magnesium ions block NMDA channel conductance in a voltage dependent manner. Magnesium delivery has been reported to improve long-term neurological outcome when administered to rats after fluid percussion brain injury (McIntosh et al. 1989b). Polyamines—putrescine, spermidine, spermine—also modulate the NMDA channel conductance through action at an allosteric site; they increase the channel flux. Polyamines are cellular molecules that increase in local concentration after ischemia (Ferchmin 1991), most likely due to NMDA receptor stimulation and consequent activation of ornithine decarboxylase (Koenig et al. 1990). This enzyme is responsible for putrescine synthesis, and its inhibitors could potentially ameliorate secondary ischemic injury. One such inhibitor is α-difluoro-methylornithine (DFMO), which is under investigation in experimental trauma.

Free Radical Inhibitors

Generation of free radicals following TBI may contribute to secondary brain injury. Free radicals are atoms or molecules with an unpaired electron in their outer orbit. They are capable of producing substantial damage to biological tissues, both directly by causing peroxidation of neuronal lipids, and indirectly by damaging microvasculature, leading to posttraumatic hypoperfusion and brain edema (Ikeda and Long 1990; McCall et al. 1987a).

Free radicals that appear to be particularly important in TBI include the superoxide radical and the hydroxyl radical. Small quantities of free radicals are produced during normal metabolism but they are neutralized through the actions of the enzymes superoxide dismutase, catalase, and selenium-containing glutathione peroxidase. Following experimental TBI, heightened superoxide radical production has been documented to occur for at least one hour (Ellis et al. 1981; Ikeda and Long 1990; Kontos and Wei 1986).

The central nervous system appears to be uniquely susceptible to damage from free radicals for several reasons. Brain tissue has low levels of catalase, the enzyme responsible for decomposing hydrogen peroxide (H_2O_2) to oxygen and water. The brain is not rich in superoxide dismutase or glutathione peroxidase, two enzymes responsible for intracellular removal of free radicals (Ikeda and Long 1990). In addition, neuronal membranes have a high concentration of lipids that can be attacked by free radicals, yielding reactive lipid peroxides (Hall 1989). Free-radical–induced dissolution of neuronal lysosomes can release hydrolytic enzymes into the cytoplasm, producing autodigestion of neurons. Finally, iron, which can catalyze free radical formation, may accumulate in the brain, particularly following trauma (from decomposition of hemoglobin in red blood cells). The brain has limited mechanisms for removal of iron, and cerebrospinal fluid, unlike serum, does not contain significant iron-binding proteins.

The hydroxyl radical is probably the most important initiator of lipid peroxidation (Ikeda and Long 1990). Increased iron from TBI accelerates the production of hydroxyl radicals through the Haber-Weiss reaction, in which H_2O_2 decomposes to a hydroxyl radical and a hydroxyl ion by receiving an electron from an oxidizable metal ion (Halliwell 1989). A number of pharmacological agents that inhibit the formation or actions of free radicals are available. These include both antioxidants, which actually combine with and eliminate free radicals, and inhibitors of lipid peroxidation.

Superoxide dismutase is an enzyme that specifically scavenges superoxide radicals ($O_2^{\bullet -}$), converting them to hydrogen peroxide and molecular oxygen. Intravenous superoxide dismutase has been administered to animals subjected to experimental brain trauma. Pretreatment with this enzyme produced a substantial reduction in acute mortality in a fluid-percussion model of severe brain injury in rats (Levasseur et al. 1989). Similarly, infusion of lysosome-packaged (to enhance penetration and prolong the half-life) superoxide dismutase prior to dry-ice–freezing injury to rat brain led to reduction in the formation of superoxide radicals, and relative preservation of the blood-brain barrier (Chan et al. 1987). Unfortunately, superoxide dismutase is not an ideal drug due to its short plasma half-life and high molecular weight, which reduce its penetration into the brain.

Other agents that may potentially decrease free radical formation include ebselen, allopurinol, and oxypurinol. Ebselen, also known as PZ-51, is a low-molecular weight, low-toxicity, selenoorganic compound with glutathione peroxidase-like activity (Johshita et al. 1990; Parnham et al. 1991). Allopurinol and oxypurinol both inhibit the action of the enzyme xanthine oxidase, which produces free radicals. Oxypurinol additionally has intrinsic action as a free radical scavenger (Halliwell 1987). Because metals (usually iron derived from blood decomposition) are an important participant in the generation of free radicals, chelating agents such as desferoxamine and 2,3-dihydroxybenzoate may also have therapeutic potential in decreasing radical formation and consequent damage (Halliwell 1987).

Antioxidants include endogenous compounds such as α-tocopherol (vitamin E), which can scavenge free radicals and may play a role in limiting posttraumatic brain damage. Administration of vitamin E to rats within five minutes of a fluid percussion cerebral injury yielded reduced mortality and improved performance on a beam-walking task (Clifton et al. 1989). Using a different experimental trauma model, epidural compression, rats raised on vitamin E-supplemented diets had reductions in brain swelling and improved regional cerebral blood flow compared to vitamin E-deficient rats (Yoshida 1989). Vitamin E therapy in human disease has yielded mixed results (Halliwell 1987), although a recent double-blind study showed some modest benefit in the treatment of tardive dyskinesia (Egan et al. 1992). Despite the fact that vitamin E has high CNS penetration due to its lipophilicity, its entry kinetics are slow, deterring usefulness in acute treatment. Other antioxidants being considered as potential candidates include methyl esters of glutathione and other drugs that could keep cellular glutathione pools in the reduced (protective) state (Halliwell 1987).

Lazaroids (21-Aminosteroids) and Lipid Protective Agents

Lazaroids are a new class of steroids that are potent inhibitors of lipid peroxidation, but devoid of glucocorticoid receptor activity. Their development arose from the considerable controversy regarding the potential mechanisms of effectiveness of glucocorticosteroids in brain trauma. As mentioned above, a number of investigators noted that certain glucocorticosteroids, such as methylprednisolone, could improve recovery following experimental brain or spinal cord injury when repeatedly administered at extremely high doses (Bracken et al. 1990; Hall and Braughler 1987). The fact that the effectiveness of glucocorticoids in this setting appeared to correlate not with their action at glucocorticoid receptors, but rather with some other concentration dependent effects such as inhibition of iron-dependent lipid peroxidation (McCall et al. 1987a), led to the development of the lazaroids. These 21-aminosteroid compounds do not have significant affinity for the cellular glucocorticoid receptor, yet have demonstrated considerable success in reducing experimental traumatic neuronal injury (Anderson et al. 1991; Dimlich et al. 1990; Hall 1987, 1989; Hall and Braughler 1989; Jacobsen et al. 1990).

Lazaroids reduce posttraumatic edema, increase blood flow, and improve neurological recovery in experimental animal models. The mode of action appears to be scavenging of free radicals (lipid peroxides) as well as stabilization of membranes, thereby attenuating arachidonate release after injury. Among dozens of lazaroids synthesized, attention has focused on the compound tirilazad—U74006F (Figure 23–8), an exceptionally potent inhibitor of lipid peroxidation with minimal toxicity in animals (Hall 1987; McCall et al. 1987b).

In a study of experimental compressive injury to the spinal cord (Hall 1989), the tirilazad dose-response curve for improvement of spinal cord blood flow was highly correlated with observed prevention of posttraumatic tissue depletion of endogenous vitamin E. This suggests that the beneficial action may indeed be due to an antioxidant effect (Hall 1989). A major advantage of lazaroids is that they appear to have minimal adverse effects. Specifically, they have no significant glucocorticoid or mineralocorticoid effects and do not suppress the hypothalamic-pituitary-adrenal axis. Clinical trials examining tirilazad for treatment of head injury are already in progress.

CDP-choline, a key intermediate in lipid (phosphatidylcholine) synthesis, reportedly attenuates lipid breakdown. Studies on the cold-injured rabbit brain, and in ischemic rat brain, suggest a beneficial effect on net lipid status. The drug may act through prevention of lipid destruction (Arrigoni et al. 1987) or by improving lipid reconstruction through phospholipid biosynthesis (Kakihana et al. 1988). It is a safe oral medication, and is currently being used for head injury and stroke treatment in Europe and Japan, although objective clinical studies are lacking. Another agent likely acting at the level of improved lipid biosynthesis is S-adenosylmethionine, which acts as a methyl donor during synthesis of phosphatidylcholine. It has been reported to be neuroprotective in a rat model of experimental brain ischemia (Sato et al. 1988).

Inhibitors of Brain Acidosis

Following brain trauma, acidosis ensues due to elevations in lactate (Becker et al. 1988). Low pH is detrimental to neuronal function, and causes channel-dependent cytotoxic glial swelling. However, it should be noted that acidosis may also have neuroprotective effects, shutting off NMDA receptor activation and thus limiting NMDA-mediated damage (Choi et al. 1990). Tromethamine (THAM) is a "nonionic" amine buffering (alkaliniz-

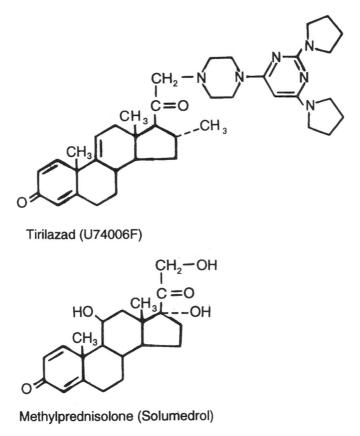

Tirilazad (U74006F)

Methylprednisolone (Solumedrol)

Figure 23–8. Lazaroids are synthetic steroid compounds with antilipid peroxidation activity as described in the text. The structure of tirilazad (also known as *U74006F*) is shown and compared to that of the commonly used synthetic glucocorticoid methylprednisolone (Solumedrol).

ing) agent that can neutralize tissue acidosis and has exhibited protective effects in experimental brain trauma and in preliminary human studies (Gaab et al. 1990b; Muizelaar et al. 1991).

Other Neurotransmitter Agents (Not Glutamate Related)

Various agonists or antagonists acting at neurotransmitter receptors other than glutamate receptors have been reported to be effective in certain models of brain damage or ischemic injury. Some of these may act indirectly by decreasing excitotoxic agonist release, and others, depending on the area of injured brain, may be helpful through increasing preservation of neuronal integrity. The latter action may be due in part to modulation of the functional degeneration and cell death that often follows loss of a neuron's projection target (retrograde degeneration), or loss of its afferent input (anterograde transsynaptic degeneration). For example, following chemically induced lesions of the rat striatum, intraventricular infusion of the GABA agonist muscimol caused sparing of thalamic and substantia nigra cells that otherwise degenerate over two weeks (Schallert 1990).

Anticholinergic drugs have also been studied in experimental TBI (Hayes et al. 1986). Scopolamine treatment prior to or following fluid percussion injury in rats apparently ameliorates initial behavioral deficits and improves motor recovery and survival (Jenkins et al. 1988; Lyeth et al. 1988; Saija et al. 1988). These effects may be mediated by inhibition of the projecting dorsolateral pontine tegmental cholinergic neurons, as well as by muscarinic blockade in the cortex (Saija et al. 1988). Cholinergic-depleting hemicholinium derivatives (A-4 and A-5) also appear to be protective when given as pretreatment (Robinson et al. 1990).

Amphetamine, an indirect catecholamine agonist, has been associated with more rapid and complete functional recovery after experimental stroke (Hurwitz et al. 1988). Limited investigations in humans report similar positive effects after stroke (Crisostomo et al. 1988). Amphetamine may have a stimulatory effect on "masked," alternative neural circuits (Dietrich et al. 1990).

Idazoxan is a selective α_2-adrenergic antagonist, which stimulates locus ceruleus noradrenergic projection neurons, by blocking their autoreceptors; it also blocks cerebral α_2-adrenergic receptors. This drug appears to be relatively free of adverse effects and is neuroprotective in models of rat brain ischemia (Gustafson et al. 1990).

Gangliosides

Gangliosides, sialylated glycosphingolipids, are reported to have beneficial effects on neurons after injury in cell and tissue culture systems, and in some animal experiments (Schengrund 1990). In addition, unconfirmed human clinical trials in stroke and dementia patients have suggested some benefit (Radden et al. 1991). The ganglioside GM_1 appears to have some neuroprotective properties in experimental ischemia (Leon et al. 1990). GM_1 does not affect the NMDA receptor or channel, but may limit "downstream" consequences of excitotoxicity such as cytosolic calcium influx. Treatment with GM_1 after lesions of axonal pathways (mice monoaminergic projections) seems to result in greater nonspecific recovery of the projections over a period of several weeks (Shigemori et al. 1990). This time course suggests an effect on increased sprouting or regeneration. A similar effect may possibly be operative in the case of human spinal cord injury, where a controlled study appeared to demonstrate greater recovery in patients receiving GM_1 treatment (Geisler et al. 1991). There has been much speculation as to possible mechanisms of action, including stimulation of growth factor production, increased lipid synthesis, altered cytoskeletal or cell membrane structure, changed membrane fluidity, or ion fluxes. Further investigation of gangliosides in cell and animal models is needed to clarify their mechanism of action and establish their efficacy.

Nerve Growth Factors and Other Neurotrophic Factors

Neuronal cell death due to transsynaptic degeneration can be prevented in experimental systems by administration of growth factors, and reorganization of neuronal connections can enhance functional recovery (Steward 1989). For example, intracerebral administration of nerve growth factor (NGF) by osmotic pump, or through use of genetically modified cells, can rescue cholinergic septal cells following fimbria fornix transection in rats (Gage et al. 1991). Similarly, ciliary neurotrophic factor (CNTF) can promote survival of axotomized motor neurons (Sendtner et al. 1991). Thus administration of growth factors during the weeks following injury may potentially improve survival of neurons and could stimulate central nervous system axonal regeneration (Thoenen 1991).

Summary

A major portion of the cerebral injury that follows brain trauma derives from a complex cascade of damaging secondary processes. Due to the rapidly increasing understanding of the pathophysiology of excitotoxicity, lipid peroxidation, and other related phenomena, we are at the threshold of having rational therapies that may alleviate some of the devastating consequences of trauma by attenuating secondary damage. As we have outlined in this chapter, many drugs are under development, and a number of agents are already being tested in human trauma protocols. In addition, the future promises continued development of medical therapies designed to prevent degeneration of disconnected neurons, as well as to promote regeneration of axons and reorganization of synaptic connections.

References

Adams JH, Graham DI, Gennarelli TA: Contemporary neuropathological considerations regarding brain damage in head injury, in Central Nervous System Trauma Status Report. Edited by Becker DP, Povlishock JT. Washington, DC, National Institutes of Health, 1985, pp 65–77

Albers GW: Potential therapeutic uses of N-methyl-D-aspartate antagonists in cerebral ischemia. Clin Neuropharm 13:177–197, 1990

Albers GW, Goldberg MP, Choi DW: N-methyl-D-aspartate antagonists: ready for clinical trial in brain ischemia? Ann Neurol 25:398–403, 1989

American Nimodipine Study Group: Clinical trial of nimodipine in acute ischemic stroke. Stroke 23:3–8, 1992

Anderson DK, Hall ED, Braughler JM, et al: Effect of delayed administration of U74006F (tirilazad mesylate) on recovery of locomotor function after experimental spinal cord injury. J Neurotrauma 8:187–192, 1991

Arrigoni E, Averet N, Cohadon F: Effects of CDP-choline on phospholipase A_2 and cholinephosphotransferase activities following a cryogenic brain injury in the rabbit. Biochem Pharm 36:3697–3700, 1987

Bailey I, Bell A, Gray J, et al: A trial of the effect of nimodipine on outcome after head injury. Acta Neurochir (Wien) 110:97–105, 1991

Becker DP, Verity MA, Povlishock J, et al: Brain cellular injury and recovery—horizons for improving medical therapies in stroke and trauma. West J Med 148:670–684, 1988

Benveniste H, Drejer J, Schousboe A, et al: Elevation of the extracellular concentrations of glutamate and aspartate in rat hippocampus during transient cerebral ischemia monitored by intracerebral microdialysis. J Neurochem 43:1369–1374, 1984

Bower AJ: Plasticity in the adult and neonatal central nervous system. Br J Neurosurg 4:253–264, 1990

Braakman R, Schouten HJA, Blaauw-van Dishoeck M, et al: Megadose steroids in severe head injury: results of a prospective double-blind clinical trial. J Neurosurg 58:326–330, 1983

Bracken MB, Shepard MJ, Collins WF, et al: A randomized, controlled trial of methylprednisolone or naloxone in the treatment of acute spinal-cord injury. New Engl J Med 322:1405–1411, 1990

Chan PH, Longar S, Fishman RA: Protective effects of liposome-entrapped superoxide dismutase on posttraumatic brain edema. Ann Neurol 21:540–547, 1987

Cheung JY, Bonventre JV, Malis CD, et al: Calcium and ischemic injury. New Engl J Med 314:1670–1676, 1986

Choi DW: Ionic dependence of glutamate neurotoxicity in cortical cell culture. J Neurosci 7:369–379, 1987

Choi DW: Glutamate neurotoxicity and diseases of the nervous system. Neuron 1:623–634, 1988

Choi DW, Monyer H, Giffard RG, et al: Acute brain injury, NMDA receptors, and hydrogen ions: observations in cortical cell cultures, in Excitatory Amino Acids and Neuronal Plasticity. Edited by Ben-Ari Y. New York, Plenum, 1990, pp 501–504

Clifton GL, Lyeth BG, Jenkins LW, et al: Effect of D-α-tocopheryl succinate and polyethylene glycol on performance tests after fluid percussion brain injury. J Neurotrauma 6:71–81, 1989

Cold GE: Cerebral blood flow in acute head injury. Acta Neurochir (Wien) 49 (Suppl):1–64, 1990

Cooper PR: Delayed brain injury: secondary insults, in Central Nervous System Trauma Status Report. Edited by Becker DP, Povlishock JT. Washington, DC, National Institutes of Health, 1985, pp 217–228

Cooper PR, Moody S, Clark WK, et al: Dexamethasone and severe head injury: a prospective double-blind study. J Neurosurg 51:307–316, 1979

Crisostomo EA, Duncan PW, Propst MA, et al: Evidence that amphetamine with physical therapy promotes recovery of motor function in stroke patients. Ann Neurol 23:94–97, 1988

Dietrich WD, Alonso O, Busto R, et al: Influence of amphetamine treatment on somatosensory function of the normal and infarcted rat brain. Stroke 21 (suppl III):III-147–III-150, 1990

Dimlich RVW, Tornheim PA, Kindel RM, et al: Effects of a 21-aminosteroid (U-74006F) on cerebral metabolites and edema after severe experimental head trauma. Adv Neurol 52:365–375, 1990

Egan MF, Hyde TM, Albers GW, et al: Treatment of tardive dyskinesia with vitamin E. Am J Psychiatry 149:773–777, 1992

Ellis EF, Wright KF, Wei EP: Cyclooxygenase products of arachidonic acid metabolism in cat cerebral cortex after experimental concussive brain injury. J Neurochem 37:892–896, 1981

Ellis EF, Police RJ, Rice LY, et al: Increased plasma PGE2, 6-keto-PGF1a, and 12-HETE levels following experimental concussive brain injury. J Neurotrauma 6:31–37, 1989

Faden AI, Vink R, McIntosh TK: Thyrotropin-releasing hormone and central nervous system trauma. Ann N Y Acad Sci 553:380–384, 1989a

Faden AI, Demediuk P, Panter SS, et al: The role of excitatory amino acids and NMDA receptors in traumatic brain injury. Science 244:799–800, 1989b

Ferchmin PA: Are polyamines modulators of the CNS? Ann N Y Acad Sci 627:354–357, 1991

Gaab MR, Hollerhage HG, Walter GF, et al: Brain edema, autoregulation, and calcium antagonism. Adv Neurol 52:391–400, 1990a

Gaab MR, Seegers K, Smedema RJ, et al: A comparative analysis of THAM (Tris-buffer) in traumatic brain oedema. Acta Neurochir (Wien) 51 (Suppl):320–323, 1990b

Gage FH, Tuszynski MH, Chen KS, et al: Nerve growth factor function in the central nervous system. Curr Top Microbiol Immunol 165:71–93, 1991

Geisler FH, Dorsey FC, Coleman WP: Recovery of motor function after spinal-cord injury—a randomized, placebo-controlled trial with GM-1 ganglioside. New Engl J Med 324:1829–1838, 1991

Gustafson I, Westerberg E, Wieloch T: Protection against ischemia-induced neuronal damage by the α_2-adrenoceptor antagonist idazoxan: influence of time of administration and possible mechanisms of action. J Cereb Blood Flow Metab 10:885–894, 1990

Gudeman SK, Miller JD, Becker DP: Failure of high-dose steroid therapy to influence intracranial pressure in patients with severe head injury. J Neurosurg 51:301–306, 1979

Hagberg H, Lehmann A, Sandberg M, et al: Ischemia-induced shift of inhibitory and excitatory amino acids from intra- to extracellular compartments. J Cereb Blood Flow Metab 5:413–419, 1985

Hall ED: Beneficial effects of the 21-aminosteroid U74006F in acute CNS trauma and hypovolemic shock. Acta Anaesthesiol Belg 38:421–425, 1987

Hall ED: Free radicals and CNS injury. Neurologic Critical Care 5:793–805, 1989

Hall ED, Braughler JM: Non-surgical management of spinal cord injuries: a review of studies with the glucocorticoid steroid methylprednisolone. Acta Anaesthesiol Belg 38:405–409, 1987

Hall ED, Braughler JM: Central nervous system trauma and stroke: physiological and pharmacological evidence for involvement of oxygen radicals and lipid peroxidation. Free Radical Biology and Medicine 6:303–313, 1989

Halliwell B: Oxidants and human disease: some new concepts. FASEB J 1:358–364, 1987

Halliwell B: Oxidants and the central nervous system: some fundamental questions. Acta Neurol Scand 126:23–33, 1989

Harris EW, Ganong AH, Cotman CW: Long-term potentiation in the hippocampus involves activation of N-methyl-D-aspartate receptors. Brain Res 323:132–137, 1984

Hayes RL, Stonnington HH, Lyeth BG, et al: Metabolic and neurophysiologic sequelae of brain injury: a cholinergic hypothesis. Central Nervous System Trauma 3:163–173, 1986

Hayes RL, Jenkins LW, Lyeth BG, et al: Pretreatment with phencyclidine, an N-methyl-D-aspartate antagonist, attenuates long-term behavioral deficits in the rat produced by traumatic brain injury. J Neurotrauma 5:259–274, 1988

Hsu CY, Dimitrijevic MR: Methylprednisolone in spinal cord injury: the possible mechanism of action. J Neurotrauma 7:115–119, 1990

Hurwitz BE, Dietrich WD, McCabe PM, et al: Amphetamine-accelerated recovery from cortical barrel-field infarction: pharmacological treatment of stroke, in Cerebrovascular Disease: Sixteenth Princeton (Research) Conference. Edited by Ginsberg MD, Dietrich WD. New York, Raven, 1988, pp 309–318

Ikeda Y, Long DM: The molecular basis of brain injury and brain edema: the role of oxygen free radicals. Neurosurgery 27:1–11, 1990

Iversen LL, Woodruff GN, Kemp JA, et al: Non-competitive NMDA antagonists as drugs, in The NMDA Receptor. Edited by Watkins JC, Collingridge GL. Oxford, Oxford University Press, 1989, pp 217–226

Jacobsen EJ, McCall JM, Ayer DE, et al: Novel 21-aminosteroids that inhibit iron-dependent lipid peroxidation and protect against central nervous system trauma. J Med Chem 33:1145–1151, 1990

Jenkins LW, Lyeth BG, Lewelt W, et al: Combined ·pretrauma scopolamine and phencyclidine attenuate posttraumatic increased sensitivity to delayed secondary ischemia. J Neurotrauma 5:275–287, 1988

Johshita H, Sasaki T, Matsui T, et al: Effects of ebselen (PZ51) on ischaemic brain oedema after focal ischaemia in cats. Acta Neurochir (Wien) 51 (Suppl):239–241, 1990

Kakihana M, Fukuda N, Suno M, et al: Effects of CDP-choline on neurologic deficits and cerebral glucose metabolism in a rat model of cerebral ischemia. Stroke 19:217–222, 1988

Kim HJ, Levasseur JE, Patterson JL, et al: Effect of indomethacin pretreatment on acute mortality in experimental brain injury. J Neurosurg 71:565–572, 1989

Kimelberg HK, Goderie SK, Higman S, et al: Swelling-induced release of glutamate, aspartate, and taurine from astrocyte cultures. J Neurosci 10:1583–1591, 1990

Kochanek P, Schoettle R, Uhl M, et al: Platelet-activating factor antagonists do not attenuate delayed posttraumatic cerebral edema in rats. J Neurotrauma 8:19–25, 1991

Koenig H, Goldstone AD, Lu CY, et al: Brain polyamines are controlled by N-methyl-D-aspartate receptors during ischemia and recirculation. Stroke 21 (suppl III):III-98–III-102, 1990

Kontos HA, Wei EP: Superoxide production in experimental brain injury. J Neurosurg 64:803–807, 1986

Langfitt TW, Zimmerman RA: Imaging and in vivo biochemistry of the brain in head injury, in Central Nervous System Trauma Status Report. Edited by Becker DP, Povlishock JT. Washington, DC, National Institutes of Health, 1985, pp 53–63

Leon A, Lipartiti M, Seren MS, et al: Hypoxic-ischemic damage and the neuroprotective effects of GM$_1$ ganglioside. Stroke 21 (Suppl III):III-95–III-97, 1990

Levasseur JE, Patterson JL, Ghatak NR, et al: Combined effect of respirator-induced ventilation and superoxide dismutase in experimental brain injury. J Neurosurg 71:573–577, 1989

Lindsberg PJ, Hallenbeck JM, Feuerstein G: Platelet-activating factor in stroke and brain injury. Ann Neurol 30:117–129, 1991

Lyeth BG, Dixon CE, Hamm RJ, et al: Effects of anticholinergic treatment on transient behavioral suppression and physiological responses following concussive brain injury to the rat. Brain Res 448:88–97, 1988

Lyons MK, Meyer FB: Cerebrospinal fluid physiology and the management of increased intracranial pressure. Mayo Clin Proc 65:684–707, 1990

MacDermott AB, Mayer ML, Westbrook GL: NMDA-receptor activation increases cytoplasmic calcium concentration in cultured spinal cord neurones. Nature 321:519–522, 1986

McCall JM, Braughler JM, Hall ED: Lipid peroxidation and the role of oxygen radicals in CNS injury. Acta Anaesthesiol Belg 38:373–379, 1987a

McCall JM, Braughler JM, Hall ED: A new class of compounds for stroke and trauma: effects of 21-aminosteroids on lipid peroxidation. Acta Anaesthesiol Belg 38:417–420, 1987b

McIntosh TK, Hayes RL, DeWitt DS, et al: Endogenous opioids may mediate secondary damage after experimental brain injury. Am J Physiol 253:E565–E574, 1987

McIntosh TK, Vink R, Soares H, et al: Effects of the N-methyl-D-aspartate receptor blocker MK-801 on neurologic function after experimental brain injury. J Neurotrauma 6:247–259, 1989a

McIntosh TK, Vink R, Yamakami I, et al: Magnesium protects against neurological deficit after brain injury. Brain Res 482:252–260, 1989b

Meldrum B: Protection against ischaemic neuronal damage by drugs acting on excitatory neurotransmission. Cerebrovascular and Brain Metabolism Reviews 2:27–57, 1990

Miller LP, Lyeth BG, Jenkins LW, et al: Excitatory amino acid receptor subtype binding following traumatic brain injury. Brain Res 526:103–107, 1990

Moskopp D, Ries F, Wassmann H, et al: Barbiturates in severe head injuries? Neurosurg Rev 14:195–202, 1991

Muizelaar JP, Obrist WD: Cerebral blood flow and brain metabolism with brain injury, in Central Nervous System Trauma Status Report. Edited by Becker DP, Povlishock JT. Washington, DC, National Institutes of Health, 1985, pp 123–137

Muizelaar JP, Marmarou A, Ward JD, et al: Adverse effects of prolonged hyperventilation in patients with severe head injury: a randomized clinical trial. J Neurosurg 75:731–739, 1991

Olney JW, Labruyere J, Price MT: Pathological changes induced in cerebrocortical neurons by phencyclidine and related drugs. Science 244:1360–1362, 1989

Olney JW, Labruyere J, Wang G, et al: NMDA antagonist neurotoxicity: mechanism and prevention. Science 254:1515–1518, 1991

Pinaud M, Lellausque JN, Chetanneau A, et al: Effects of propofol on cerebral hemodynamics and metabolism in patients with brain trauma. Anesthesiology 73:404–409, 1990

Parnham MJ, Leyck S, Graf E, et al: The pharmacology of ebselen. Agents and Actions 32:4–9, 1991

Poungvarin N, Bhoopat W, Viriyavejakul A, et al: Effects of dexamethasone in primary supratentorial intracerebral hemorrhage. New Engl J Med 316:1229–1233, 1987

Povlishock JT: The morphopathologic responses to experimental head injuries of varying severity, in Central Nervous System Trauma Status Report. Edited by Becker DP, Povlishock JT. Washington, DC, National Institutes of Health, 1985, pp 443–452

Robinson MJ, Teasdale GM: Calcium antagonists in the management of subarachnoid haemorrhage. Cerebrovascular and Brain Metabolism Reviews 2:205–226, 1990

Robinson SE, Martin RM, Davis TR, et al: The effect of acetylcholine depletion on behavior following traumatic brain injury. Brain Res 509:41–46, 1990

Radden RA, Wiegandt H, Bauer BL: Gangliosides: the relevance of current research to neurosurgery. J Neurosurg 74:606–619, 1991

Rothman SM, Olney JW: Glutamate and the pathophysiology of hypoxic-ischemic brain damage. Ann Neurol 19:105–111, 1986

Saija A, Robinson SE, Lyeth BG, et al: The effects of scopolamine and traumatic brain injury on central cholinergic neurons. J Neurotrauma 5:161–170, 1988

Sato H, Hariyama H, Moriguchi K: S-adenosyl-L-methionine protects the hippocampal CA1 fields from the ischemic neuronal death in rat. Biochem Biophys Res Commun 150:491–496, 1988

Schallert T, Jones TA, Lindner MD: Multilevel transneuronal degeneration after brain damage: behavioral events and effects of anticonvulsant γ-aminobutyric acid-related drugs. Stroke 21 sSuppl III):III-143–III-146, 1990

Schengrund C-L: The role(s) of gangliosides in neural differentiation and repair: a perspective. Brain Res Bull 24:131–141, 1990

Sendtner M, Kreutzberg GW, Thoenen H: Ciliary neurotrophic factor prevents the degeneration of motor neurons after axotomy. Nature 345:440–441, 1991

Shapira Y, Yadid G, Cotev S, et al: Protective effect of MK-801 in experimental brain injury. J Neurotrauma 7:131–139, 1990

Shigemori M, Okamoto Y, Watanabe T, et al: Effect of monosialoganglioside (GM$_1$) on transected monoaminergic pathways. J Neurotrauma 7:89–97, 1990

Siesjo BK: Historical overview: calcium, ischemia and death of brain cells. Ann N Y Acad Sci 522:638–661, 1988

Siesjo BK, Bengtsson F: Calcium fluxes, calcium antagonists, and calcium-related pathology in brain ischemia, hypoglycemia, and spreading depression: a unifying hypothesis. J Cereb Blood Flow Metab 9:127–140, 1989

Steward O: Reorganization of neuronal connections following CNS trauma: principles and experimental paradigms. J Neurotrauma 6:99–152, 1989

Tecoma E, Monyer H, Goldberg MP, et al: Traumatic neuronal injury in vitro is attenuated by NMDA antagonists. Neuron 2:1541–1545, 1989

Thoenen H: The changing scene of neurotrophic factors. Trends Neurosci 14:165–167, 1991

Tornheim PA: Traumatic edema in head injury, in Central Nervous System Trauma Status Report. Edited by Becker DP, Povlishock JT. Washington, DC, National Institutes of Health, 1985, pp 431–442

Vink R, McIntosh TK, Thomhanyi R, et al: Opiate antagonist nalmefene improves intracellular free Mg^{2+}, bioenergetic state, and neurologic outcome following traumatic brain injury in rats. J Neurosci 10:3524–3530, 1990

Ward JD, Becker DP, Miller JD, et al: Failure of prophylactic barbiturate coma in the treatment of severe head injury. J Neurosurg 62:383–388, 943, 1985

Yamakami I, McIntosh TK: Effects of traumatic brain injury on regional cerebral blood flow in rats as measured with radiolabeled microspheres. J Cereb Blood Flow Metab 9:117–124, 1989

Yoshida S: Brain injury after ischemia and trauma: the role of vitamin E. Ann N Y Acad Sci 570:219–236, 1989

Young W: The post-injury responses in trauma and ischemia: secondary injury or protective mechanisms? Central Nervous System Trauma 4:27–42, 1987

Young W: Pharmacologic therapy of acute spinal cord injury, in Spinal Trauma. Edited by Errico TJ, Bauer RD, Waugh T. Philadelphia, PA, JB Lippincott, 1991, pp 415–433

Yuan X-Q, Prough DS, Smith TL, et al: The effects of traumatic brain injury on regional cerebral blood flow in rats. J Neurotrauma 5:289–301, 1988

Chapter 24

Prevention

Stuart A. Yablon, M.D.
Maritza Cabrera, M.A., C.R.C.
Stuart C. Yudofsky, M.D.
Jonathan M. Silver, M.D.

In this textbook we have focused on the human tragedies and neurobiological complexities that occur subsequent to traumatic brain injury (TBI). Characteristically, therapeutic interventions are agonizingly slow, costly in time and resources, and frequently only partially successful in returning the individual to his or her former functional status. In this chapter, we endeavor to provide information that will be useful for the prevention of TBI. Epidemiological and other data included herein may overlap with those contained in other chapters of the textbook, in order to identify and emphasize key elements that are particularly amenable to intervention. The purpose of this chapter is to elevate the awareness of clinicians and stimulate actions that could prevent TBI in their patients.

Overview

TBI imposes a heavy burden of morbidity and mortality on the citizens of the United States and westernized nations. Every year, there are an estimated 500,000 TBIs in the United States (Kalsbeek et al. 1980; Kraus 1993; Kraus et al. 1975), and this results in approximately 39,000 deaths. Conservative estimates suggest that the annual incidence of TBI in an average community is approximately 200 per 100,000 people (Annegers et al. 1980; Jagger et al. 1984; Kalsbeek et al. 1980; Klauber et al. 1981; Kraus et al. 1984). TBI accounts for 2% of all deaths and 26% of all injury deaths (Sosin et al. 1989). Seventy to ninety thousand TBIs result in individuals' having a permanent disability, including 2,000 people who remain in vegetative states (Committee on Trauma Research 1985).

The relationship between the epidemiology and prevention of TBI is the central theme of this literature review. We discuss technological, educational, and legislative strategies toward TBI prevention. Most of the studies address TBI in adult populations, but we also address pediatric injury prevention issues. Emphasis is directed toward identification of high-risk patients encountered in the clinical setting, so that the physician can initiate interventions with his or her patients, or direct referral to other professionals for appropriate and effective injury prevention actions.

Epidemiology

Complete and accurate data regarding the incidence and prevalence of TBI and its causes are lacking, principally due to the absence of an ongoing data-gathering and -reporting system and ICD-9 (International Classification of Diseases, 9th Revision) codes for brain injuries. Projection-based data are employed to provide estimates of injury prevalence and identification of predisposing factors.

Age

Studies addressing the incidence of TBI in various age groups report generally consistent age distributions (Cooper et al. 1983;

Jagger et al. 1984; Klauber et al. 1981; Kraus et al. 1984; McKenzie et al. 1989). Specifically, a bimodal distribution is observed, with young adults aged 16–24 demonstrating the highest risk of sustaining TBI. Injury risk then declines in people aged 25–59, increasing again in people aged 60 and above. An analysis of death certificates suggests that the incidence of traumatic injuries reported in elderly people may be underestimated (Fife 1987).

▌ **Children.** About 1 in 10,000 children between the ages of 0 and 19 years dies from TBI each year. Annually, this represents 7,000 fatalities, or 30% of all childhood injury fatalities. Another 29,000 people below the age of 20 sustain a permanent disability following TBI (Kraus et al. 1990). Still, the majority of TBI in children tends to be classified as mild. Of the remainder, 14% are classified as moderate to severe, and 5% result in death (Kraus et al. 1990). Motor vehicle crashes are the leading cause of injury fatalities in children in the US. Pedestrian-related injuries are also a significant cause of injury. In fact, for children aged 5–9, pedestrian injuries cause more deaths than any other injury (Rodriguez 1990). In children, injury rates for males increase moderately until age 14, when they increase rapidly through age 19. Rates for females are highest for children under age 4; they then decline and gradually rise again for adolescents 15 to 19 years old (Kraus et al. 1990).

▌ **Adults.** Over half of TBIs occur in people aged 15–44 (Max et al. 1991). Young adults aged 16–24 demonstrate the highest risk of sustaining TBI (Cooper et al. 1983; Kalsbeek et al. 1980; Kraus et al. 1984). This risk then declines past age 25 until late middle age. Motor vehicle crashes and assaults are the leading causes of TBI in young adults (Annegers et al. 1980; Kalsbeek et al. 1980; Klauber et al. 1981). The high rate of TBI caused by motor vehicle crashes in this age group is largely attributed to alcohol use, lack of driving experience, and lack of compliance with seat belt laws (Kraus et al. 1984; Rickert et al. 1990). TBI-associated fatalities due to firearms are observed most frequently in the 24–34 year age group (Goodman et al. 1989; Sosin et al. 1989). As will be noted later, the occurrence of TBI in this age group may thus potentially be influenced by the prevention and early diagnosis and treatment of alcohol abuse, implementation of safety initiatives, and enforcement of more stringent handgun regulations.

∎ **Elderly.** The risk of TBI increases sharply at approximately age 65, and continues to increase rapidly throughout more advanced age (Kraus et al. 1984; Sorensen and Kraus 1991). In elderly people, brain injuries are most frequently due to falls and assaults (Cooper et al. 1983). Males have a higher risk of injury than females. Elderly males also have a higher risk of being involved in motor vehicle crashes (Hogue 1982).

The severity of TBI in elderly people tends to be higher than that observed in other age groups (Sorenson and Kraus 1991). Death rates from unintentional injuries are twice as high for elderly people as for teenagers (Fife et al. 1984). As noted above, the review of death certificates by Fife (1987) suggests that the contribution of traumatic injuries to cause of death in elderly people is often underestimated.

Examples of physician-directed TBI prevention interventions for elderly people include the selection of drugs (e.g., antidepressants) with fewer hypotensive side effects (e.g., serotonin specific reuptake inhibitors), and the education of patients and family members regarding means of preventing falls related to orthostatic hypotension.

Gender

Males are 2–3 times more likely to sustain TBI than females of the same age (Cooper et al. 1983; Galbraith et al. 1976; Kraus and Nourjah 1988; Kraus et al. 1984; Sosin et al. 1989). In addition, males are more likely to sustain injuries of greater severity, and are consequently more likely to die as a result of these injuries (Sosin et al. 1989). Gender differences in risk of sustaining a TBI are most pronounced in children, adolescents, and young adults (Sorenson and Kraus 1991). Lesser differences are observed in mature populations (Kraus and Nourjah 1988).

Socioeconomic Status

Type of employment and overall socioeconomic status appear to be correlated with TBI incidence. In a prospective study of 1,248 patients in central Virginia, the incidence of TBI in "unemployed" patients was almost three times as high as in the general population. Data on educational background revealed that approximately 25% of patients had fewer than 8 years of education, 50% had 8–12 years, and 25% had 12 years or more of education (Rimel et al. 1990).

TBI due to assaults and violence is more prevalent in low socioeconomic, urban areas (Cooper et al. 1983; Kerr et al. 1971). In a study conducted in the Bronx, New York, African Americans and Hispanics had higher rates of TBI than whites. In African American and Hispanic children, the higher incidence of TBI was due to falls from windows. In adults, TBI was largely due to violence. These differences may reflect socioeconomic or sociocultural factors characteristic of the geographic location studied.

Temporal Association

More brain injuries occur during the late spring and summer months, particularly May and June, than during any other season (Cooper et al. 1983; Jagger et al. 1984). The incidence of TBI is lowest during December and January. Seasonal differences vary, however, depending on the region and etiology involved. Weekends, particularly evenings, account for the highest incidence of TBIs (Kraus and Nourjah 1988). Not surprisingly, the rate of motor vehicle crashes is also the highest during these time periods.

Substance Abuse

Investigations consistently find strong associations between alcohol abuse and TBI (National Head Injury Foundation 1988; Rutherford 1977). Fifty percent of all TBIs involve concurrent alcohol abuse (Sparadeo et al. 1990), and a high percentage are associated with drugs other than or in addition to alcohol. TBI occurs about

2–4 times more frequently in people with a history of alcoholism than it does in the general population (Hillbom and Holm 1986).

Alcohol use correlates significantly with acquiring TBI. About half of the patients treated in emergency rooms are intoxicated or have ethanol in their blood, and most reveal a history of alcohol dependence (Galbraith et al. 1976; Parkinson et al. 1985; Rutherford 1977). Serum ethanol levels are associated with cause of injury, with highest levels linked with falls and assaults, and more moderate levels associated with motor vehicle crashes.

The suspicion or presence of alcohol intoxication exerts a confounding influence on the evaluation of TBI severity. Galbraith et al. (1976) noted that an altered mental status or depressed level of consciousness observed following TBI is often attributed to the effects of alcohol intoxication. Consequently, TBI of mild or moderate severity may not be detected, either by the evaluating staff or by the patient. Additionally, an important secondary neurological event, such as an intracranial hematoma, may be overlooked.

TBI severity tends to be higher in alcoholic patients than in nondrinkers (P. F. Waller et al. 1986). In addition, some evidence suggests that alcohol can exacerbate the extent and severity of TBI (Edna 1982) and adversely influence treatment outcome (Sparadeo and Gill 1989).

Etiology

TBI results from a variety of causes. Motor vehicle crashes account for half of all TBI (Kalsbeek et al. 1980; Kraus et al. 1975); the second leading cause is falls (21%). Other causes include assaults (12%), sports and recreation (10%), firearms (6%), and other blunt force (4%). Kraus et al. (1984) noted that 11% of patients with TBI were dead on arrival at the hospital, and 16% were classified as having moderate or severe injuries on admission. Of all patients discharged alive from acute care hospitalization, almost 7% had significant neurological sequelae (Kraus et al. 1984).

■ **Motor vehicles.** Motor vehicle crashes are the leading cause of TBI in the United States. They account for approximately half of all TBI, and 55% of TBI in the 15–19 year age group. Males aged 15–24 have the highest incidence of motor vehicle-related TBI (Klauber et al. 1981; Kraus et al. 1984; Sosin et al. 1989). Young children and infants experience vehicular death rates that are disproportionate to the time spent traveling in motor vehicles (Baker 1979; Decker et al. 1984). They are more vulnerable to injury-related death even when traveling below moderate vehicular speeds (Roberts and Turner 1984). Elderly people drive fewer miles than the average population. However, when the total amount of driving time is considered, drivers aged 65 and older have the second highest motor vehicle crash rates. People 85 and older have the highest crash rates per mile traveled (Hogue 1982; Cerelli 1989).

Motorcyclist injuries represent almost 7% of all motor vehicle deaths. In 1989, there were 3,036 motorcyclist fatalities (Insurance Institute for Highway Safety 1990), mostly due to TBI (Heilman et al. 1982). When considering vehicle miles traveled, the number of deaths in motorcyclists is 17 times greater than the number of deaths in automobile passengers (Insurance Institute for Highway Safety 1992). It has been estimated that for every motorcycle-related death, there are another 37 injuries, and many more that remain unreported to the police (Baker et al. 1984). In the 15–34 year age group, one-tenth of the traffic fatalities involve a motorcycle driver or passenger (United States Department of Transportation 1988).

All-terrain vehicles are associated with a significant risk of injury, particularly TBI (Newman 1987, 1988). These crashes resulted in 1,100 fatalities between 1987 and 1989 (Newman 1988), the overwhelming majority attributable to TBI (Hargarten 1991; Newman 1988). During this same period, another 400,000 injuries were reported, approximately half in children under 16.

❚ **Bicycles.** There are an estimated 570,000 bicycle-related visits to emergency rooms each year, many of them because of TBI (Centers for Disease Control 1987). Every year, 1,300 cyclists are killed in the United States, and at least half of those are school children aged 5–14 (Centers for Disease Control 1987; Sacks et al.

1991). Most fatal injuries result from bicycle crashes with motor vehicles (Kraus et al. 1987). Eighty percent of the fatally injured people suffer TBI. Most pediatric injuries occur in the afternoon hours, between 3:00 and 5:00 P.M. (Insurance Institute for Highway Safety 1989), and usually within one mile of home. Most crashes between young children on bicycles and motor vehicles are caused by the bicyclist. This applies until about age 12, when the trend reverses (Insurance Institute for Highway Safety 1989).

∎ **Falls.** Falls cause one-fifth of all TBI, and are the primary cause of injury for the very young and the very old (Kraus et al. 1984). In infants, over two-thirds of all TBIs result from falls. For children of preschool age, falls account for about half of all TBI (Kraus et al. 1990). In elderly people, falls account for a high rate of TBI (Kraus and Nourjah 1988), and are an underlying cause of about 9,500 deaths each year (Tinetti and Speechley 1989).

The settings from which injurious falls are reported vary with age. Approximately 43% of all fatal falls occur at home. This figure is higher for children, with 67% of their fatal falls occurring at home (Lambert and Sattin 1988). Fall-related injuries in infants usually occur from furniture, such as changing tables, or from walkers, whereas toddlers are usually injured falling from windows or down stairs. Older children are usually injured falling from roofs or playground equipment (National Committee for Injury Prevention and Control 1989). In elderly people over 85, one-fifth of fatal falls occur while in institutional care (Baker et al. 1984). In elderly people, although only a relatively small proportion of falls result in TBI (Tinetti 1987), falls still comprise the single largest cause of TBI in individuals over the age of 70 (Kraus et al. 1984).

∎ **Firearms.** Firearms are involved in 14% of all fatal TBI in the United States, and rank second to motor vehicle crashes as a cause of fatal TBI (Sosin et al. 1989). Handguns are the most common type of firearm involved in gunshot-related deaths in the home, whether accidental or intentional (Kellerman and Reay 1986; Wintemute et al. 1987). Risk factors for firearm-related injury include alcohol abuse, a history of impulsive or emotional behaviors, availability of a loaded gun in the home (Kellerman and Reay 1986), and unsafe storage and locking practices. The availability of guns in the home also appears to increase the risk for suicide within the household (Brent et al. 1991; Kellerman and Reay 1986). Studies in densely populated areas have shown that assaults and assaults with firearms are responsible for the highest incidence of TBI (Kraus 1993).

With increasing prevalence of firearm possession, the incidence of injuries caused by their use is escalating rapidly. Handguns are increasingly available to young people, and the presence of these weapons in high schools is pervasive (Callahan and Rivara 1991). According to the Centers for Disease Control (1991), 1 in 20 students had carried a firearm, usually a handgun, to school in the month prior to the survey. In Louisiana and Texas, the escalating rate of firearm injuries has surpassed the rate of vehicular fatalities, making firearm injuries the leading cause in injury mortality in both states in 1990 (Centers for Disease Control 1992; Zane et al. 1991). Similar trends are appearing throughout the United States.

Clinicians should always include questions regarding the access of their patients to firearms when taking a medical and psychiatric history. Specific safety recommendations should be made to patients who have firearms or have them in their household.

▮ **Assaults and violent crimes.** Assaults account for 12% of TBI (Kraus et al. 1984). Violent acts such as assaults, child and spouse abuse, alcohol and drug abuse, unemployment, and an inability to handle frustration are associated with a high incidence of TBI. Intentional injuries are a leading cause of death in young people, particularly in certain groups (Centerwall 1984; Rosenberg et al. 1987). Suicide is the second leading cause of fatal injury for young white males (Rosenberg et al. 1987). Assaults are the leading cause of death for young black males (Centerwall 1984). Suicide occurs in boys approximately five times more frequently than in girls.

▮ **Sports- and recreation-related injuries.** TBI commonly occurs during contact sports (Kelly et al. 1991). Sports such as boxing, gymnastics, diving, soccer, football, basketball, and hockey are associated with considerable risk of TBI. Each year, an estimated 250,000 concussions (Cantu 1988) and an average of eight deaths (Torg et al. 1987) result from football-related TBI. An estimated 20% of high school football players sustain concussion during a single football season, with some reporting symptoms persisting as long as 6–9 months following the end of the season (Gerberich et al. 1983). Boxing presents a particularly high risk for TBI. One study of adult professional boxers reported that 87% demonstrate clinical, radiological, or electroencephalographic evidence of TBI (Casson et al. 1984).

Overall, population-based studies suggest that 10% of all TBI are the result of sports and recreation injuries. For children 10–14 years, sports and recreational activities account for 43% of TBI. Brain injuries due to sports are more frequent in males than in females, and the peak injury incidence is between 10 and 14 years of age in males, and between 5 and 9 years of age in females (Kraus and Nourjah 1988). For all children under 20, sports and recreational injuries rank third among the causes of TBI.

Prior to concluding discussion of the epidemiology of TBI, one point warrants further elaboration. The leading causes of TBI include events traditionally labeled as "accidents." Studies of the events preceding injury, however, reveal that injuries are frequently associated with specific *modifiable* behaviors and factors, and are *not* merely random occurrences ("accidents") that befall unfortunate individuals. Epidemiologists and other public health professionals now define injuries in terms of host, agent, and environment, employing language commonly used in discussions of disease prevention and public health.

Prevention: Intervention Strategies

Injuries occur as a result of complex interactions between a host (e.g., a young male), an agent (e.g., an automobile), and an environment (e.g., an urban highway). Their prevention is accomplished by interventions focused in three distinct areas: 1) engineering and technology, 2) education and behavior change, and 3) legislation and enforcement (Committee on Trauma Research 1985). Effective injury prevention interventions will usually combine two or more of these approaches, directed to each of the three phases of the "injury-control sequence" (Haddon and Baker 1981). Measures taken to avert injury during the period prior to the potentially injurious event, also known as the "preinjury phase," are categorized as "primary" prevention measures. Wearing bicycle helmets and wearing safety belts are examples of primary prevention measures. "Secondary" prevention measures reduce severity of the injury that has occurred and avoid complications. Rapid response emergency medical services are an example of secondary prevention measures. Finally, "tertiary" prevention measures reduce the impact of injury-related disability through vocational, physical, and social rehabilitation. In this review, we focus on primary prevention strategies.

Environmental or Technological Modification Strategies

Of the primary prevention interventions, "passive" measures generally demonstrate greatest effectiveness, and are preferred (Haddon and Baker 1981; Jagger 1992). Passive measures are those that protect the individual without any action on his or her part, usually through modification of the environment to reduce or eliminate the hazard. Engineering or technological modification strategies are typically employed when designing and implementing passive prevention measures. Airbags, for example, protect drivers and passengers without their active participation, whereas seat belts and child-restraint seats require individual cooperation in order to be effective. A corollary of the principle of passive protection is that neither mechanical failure nor human action should result in injury.

▮ **Motor vehicles.** Automobile crashes are the most common cause of brain trauma in the United States, and account for more than half of all brain injuries reported each year (Annegers et al. 1980; Jagger et al. 1984; Kraus et al. 1984). The head is particularly vulnerable in a crash, and is likely to sustain greater injury than any other body region. A brain injury is also more likely to result in long-term functional deficits than injuries to other body regions. Because TBI and motor vehicle crashes are closely linked, strategies that reduce the likelihood of crash occurrence, or reduce the probability of impact injury to occupants during a crash, will also reduce the occurrence of brain trauma.

Vehicle design significantly influences the injury potential to occupants during a crash. Safety standards have been responsible for the introduction of many structural and interior injury prevention features in passenger vehicles. During a crash, occupants are thrown toward the site of impact. Therefore, the angle of impact determines with which interior structures occupants are likely to collide. Frontal collisions account for about 50% of all crashes in which serious or fatal injuries occur. Side impacts account for about a quarter of such crashes, and rear impacts for about 4% (Jagger 1992). Each vehicular safety feature has a spectrum of effectiveness related to the type of crash in which it provides protection. Rollover crashes are particularly lethal because of the increased likelihood of ejection, when fatality rates are 25 times higher for unrestrained occupants than for those restrained within the vehicle (Jagger 1992).

Safety belts comprise the mainstay of frontal impact and rollover protection in automobile crashes. Front-seat lap-shoulder belts are highly effective in protecting occupants in a crash (Orsay et al. 1988), because they reduce the risk of death by 40%–50% and the risk of moderate to serious injury by 45%–55% (United States Department of Transportation 1984). Frontal collision protection has been significantly upgraded by the installation of automatic occupant restraints, such as airbags (Jagger et al. 1987; Zador and Ciccone 1991) in front seat positions and the mandatory lap-shoulder belts for both front and rear seat positions (Bodiwala et al. 1989). Airbags, which act as a cushion to control deceleration of the brain during an automobile accident, are effective only in frontal collisions, and their efficacy is enhanced when they are used in combination with seat belts (Jagger 1992).

Another effective restraint technology designed for use in automobiles is the child-restraint seat. The National Safety Council (1981) reported that the use of child-restraint seats significantly reduced the number of childhood deaths and injuries. It has been estimated that between 20% and 70% of the serious injuries, and 40%–90% of child fatalities could be avoided with the use of child-restraint seats (Richeldefer 1976; Roberts and Turner 1984). Unfortunately, observational studies suggest that only a small minority of child passengers are safely secured with child-restraint seats (Decker et al. 1984; Margolis et al. 1992).

Many brain injuries occur in side impacts, when the heads of occupants collide with the structural column between the windshield and the side window, known as the "A-pillar." Over 7,000 motor vehicle-related deaths are caused by side impacts, nearly half of which are due to brain trauma (Jagger 1992). Unfortunately, newer side impact regulations do not include criteria for reduction of head and neck injuries, but rather address prevention of chest and pelvic region injuries only (Jagger 1992).

Vehicular design improvements may also contribute to injury prevention by limiting the likelihood of collision, as opposed to limiting injury after collision. The center-mounted brake light has been required as standard equipment in passenger cars since the 1985 model year. It provides a visual cue of an intended stop, and has been credited with a reduction in rear-end collisions (United States Department of Transportation 1989). Antilock braking systems are designed to avoid crashes by preventing a vehicle from going out of control on a slick surface when brakes are suddenly applied. This crash avoidance technology automatically keeps brakes from locking and greatly reduces stopping distances under hazardous circumstances. Increasing numbers of passenger vehicle models are being introduced with this safety feature as standard or optional equipment.

Motorcycles possess characteristics that increase the likelihood of injury to their riders. For example, motorcycles typically have high performance capabilities, including rapid acceleration and high top speeds. Motorcycles, however, are less stable than cars during emergency breaking. The rate of fatal and severe injury is twice as high in drivers of racing design cycles. Motorcycles are also less visible than cars, and are therefore more likely to be involved in crashes. Unlike automobile occupants, riders are totally unprotected.

Motorcycle-related TBIs have been considerably reduced with the use of motorcycle protective wear. The efficacy of helmets in injury prevention is undisputed. Helmets can reduce the risk of on-highway motorcycle fatality by about 25%–28% (Chenier and Evans 1987; Evans and Frick 1988). Death rates from TBI are twice as high in states with weak or nonexistent helmet laws, compared with rates in states with helmet laws that apply to all riders (Sosin et al. 1989). More dramatic differences have been observed when comparing fatality incidence before and after mandatory helmet legislation. When states revoke or relax helmet laws, death rates increase. When mandatory helmet laws were reinstated in Louisiana, death rates decreased from 38 to 29 per 1,000 crashes (United States Department of Transportation 1984).

The safety of all-terrain vehicles has been the subject of substantial controversy. These vehicles are three- and four-wheeled motorized vehicles with motorcycle-type engines intended for off-road use. Because of their poor stability and proneness to tip, the three-wheeled models have been responsible for 87% of the injuries (Newman 1987). Four-wheeled models are more stable but are heavier and more difficult for young people to control.

Reports addressing injuries related to all-terrain vehicles suggest that 30% are alcohol-related (Newman 1987). Other important risk factors include inexperienced riders, lack of seat belt and helmet use, and use on unpaved roads. The risk of fatal or severe TBI is increased by a factor of three for those not wearing helmets (Newman, 1987).

❚ **Bicycles.** Bicycle-related TBI prevention strategies have principally been based on education regarding helmet use. Thompson reported that the risk of sustaining a severe TBI could be reduced 88% with the use of a helmet (Thompson et al. 1989). The combination of injury prevention efficacy and a relatively low cost contributes to prevailing opinion that helmets are the intervention of choice for the prevention of bicycle-related injuries.

In spite of their aforementioned advantages, helmets are used by fewer than 10% of cyclists and less than 2% of children (Weiss 1986). Compliance with the correct and consistent use of helmets has been a problem. Mandatory bicycle helmet legislation has been attempted in several states and counties, but has mostly been directed at children, even though the general population is at risk. For instance, an adolescent's risk of crashing with a motor vehicle while bicycling is 20 times that of a preschool age child and twice that of an elementary school age child (Gallagher et al. 1984). At present, 10 states and several counties have been successful in passing bicycle helmet legislation, and many others have legislation pending.

Bicycle-related TBI prevention methods are not limited to helmet use alone. Other preventive efforts include skills training, segregation of cyclists by the development of bicycle paths, and the use of visibility enhancement devices. Some educational programs have demonstrated effectiveness in raising awareness on the importance of bicycle helmet use, and have contributed to increased helmet use (Bergman et al. 1990). Empirical investigation is needed, particularly regarding educational strategies, to determine which methods are most effective.

Clinicians have the opportunity to contribute to improved cyclist safety by encouraging compliance in the wearing of bicycle helmets. At the very least, physicians should inquire as to whether or not their patients *insist* that their children wear helmets every time they ride bicycles!

❚ **Helmets.** Technical and scientific advances have greatly improved the protective qualities of helmets (Snively and Becker 1991). Improvements in design are still needed to prevent helmets from slipping out of place upon impact. Currently, there are no standards in existence regarding the manufacturing of helmets. Three private organizations have developed standards that individual helmet manufactures can adhere to voluntarily. Helmets meeting those standards often identify such with the Snell Memorial Foundation, American National Standard Institute (ANSI), or American Society for Testing and Materials (ASTM) logos marked on the helmet.

∎ **Roadway design.** Roadway design improvements contribute to reduced risks of crashes and injuries. Crash site identification permits roadway improvement resources to be concentrated at locations where crashes are most likely to occur (Jagger 1992). Roadway design improvements take many forms, and include removal of fixed roadside objects such as trees at high-risk crash sites, and the substitution of breakaway signs and utility poles for rigid ones where vehicles run off the road. Where fixed roadside objects cannot be removed, impact attenuators can be placed in front of unyielding objects such as cement abutments in locations where motorists are likely to collide with them. If a collision occurs, the impact attenuator absorbs the crash forces rather than the vehicle and its occupants (Jagger 1992). Longitudinal barriers redirect errant vehicles away from roadside hazards, and are also used as dividers between opposing lanes of traffic to prevent head-on collisions. Other design improvements include the widening of roadside recovery zones, which provides more unobstructed roadside area for safely regaining control of a vehicle without colliding with fixed objects. Aggressive application of such strategies in the modification and design of new and existing roadways could potentially yield further progress in the prevention of TBI (Jagger 1992).

∎ **Structural adaptations.** Structural adaptations of homes, offices, and public places are often successful, cost-effective strategies in the prevention of TBI. Environmental factors have been estimated to contribute to 18%–50% of falls by elderly people in the home, where nearly half of all fatal falls occur (Lambert and Sattin 1988). A number of environmental adaptations to prevent injuries have been suggested, including the installation of adequate lighting, handrails on stairs and on baths, and nonslip surfaces in bathtubs. Other examples include the installation of window guards, stairway gates, shock absorbing surfaces in playgrounds and nursing homes, and the removal of area rugs and easily overlooked furniture and clutter (National Committee for Injury Prevention and Control 1989).

Impact from falls can also be minimized by shock-absorbing surfaces. Because more than half of all fatal falls involve people 75 and older (Baker et al. 1984), many of whom live in nursing homes, structural adaptations in residential care facilities could prevent many fall-related injuries (National Committee for Injury Prevention and Control 1989).

Psychosocial Strategies

Although often incorrectly considered ineffective (Grossman and Rivara 1992), traditional prevention strategies have relied on education. Educational approaches are based on the premise that a realization of risk and the consequences of identified behaviors can alter the actions and lifestyles of the individual. It further assumes that individuals assume responsibility for the well-being of themselves and others.

Educational injury-prevention strategies are highly complex, and their evaluation requires considerable expertise. Educational approaches, when properly monitored, should comprise an important approach toward injury prevention. Progress toward compliance with proper use of child-restraint seats represents an example on the importance of instructional approaches. All 50 states require the use of child-restraint seats, but the correct use of these devices is contingent upon *successful* education.

Studies on methods to change parental behaviors have yielded promising results. Compliance with the use of child-restraint seats was enhanced when mothers were informed that inappropriate child behavior diminished if child-restraint seats were used properly and consistently (Christofersen and Gyulay 1981). Roberts and Turner (1984) labeled this approach the Behavioral Improvement Emphasis.

Single-session educational programs with high school students have demonstrated success in imparting knowledge, but have not been demonstrated to be effective in changing attitudes or behaviors (Neuwelt et al. 1989).

■ **Substance abuse.** The relationship between substance abuse and TBI is complex, but mounting evidence suggests that substance abuse exerts a negative impact upon the patient with TBI. Substance abuse is a contributing factor to the occurrence of TBI, potentiates the degree of injury sustained (P. F. Waller et al. 1986), and is associated with a worsened outcome following injury (Ruff et al. 1990). Substance abuse presents considerable problems in the diagnosis, treatment, and medication management of the patient with TBI (Sparadeo et al. 1990).

The abuse of alcohol and other drugs plays a major role in the incidence of TBI. Fifty-five percent of all TBI patients in rehabilitation were substance abusers prior to the injury, with alcohol being the most frequently abused substance (Sparadeo et al. 1990). Alcohol is involved in one-third to two-thirds of TBI. In an urban trauma center, 75% of patients tested positive for at least one abused substance (Lindenbaum et al. 1989).

The majority of drivers and pedestrians involved in vehicular fatalities are problem drinkers or alcoholic individuals rather than social drinkers (J. A. Waller and Turkel 1966). Alcoholism is a causative factor in motor vehicle crashes, particularly those involving single-car fatalities (Brenner 1967; Haddon and Brandess 1959).

The influence of TBI on the patient's capacity to tolerate detoxification or drug abuse rehabilitation is unknown. It is recognized that survivors of TBI have lower tolerance for alcohol and drugs (Horton et al. 1992). One may speculate that posttraumatic deficits in impulse control, judgment, memory, and depression may compromise the patient's ability to maintain a substance-abuse–free lifestyle. For example, a social drinker may no longer be able to tolerate alcohol, or recognize the amount consumed or its effect. Conversely, the effect of drug abuse and addiction, and the associated decrease in the person's social and occupational functioning, could have a negative influence on the rehabilitation of the functional losses due to TBI. Further understanding of the interaction of these factors is important for treatment planning and prevention of subsequent drug-related injuries.

▌ **Psychiatric history.** Psychiatric illness has been recognized as a causative factor for TBI as well as for substance abuse. Unlike substance abuse, premorbid personality is difficult to assess. Diagnosis of drug abuse can be facilitated by reports from the patient and the patient's associates, and the assistance of technology, such as breathalizers and blood and urine tests. Without strong documentation of the preinjury events, a careful psychiatric history, a thorough interview with family members, and a combination of psychological and neuropsychological batteries, it is difficult to ascertain the contribution of the psychosocial maladjustment to the injury. Self-reports usually have very limited value in assessing premorbid personality.

A relationship between psychiatric illness and motor vehicle crashes has been established in several studies. Eelkema et al. (1970) found that psychotic patients have a higher-than-average risk of motor vehicle crashes prior to hospitalization, but a better-than-average record after hospitalization. Males diagnosed with personality disorders had the highest crash rate. J. A. Waller (1973) found that nearly half of the crashes that result in serious injury or death involve drivers with medical or psychiatric illness. Patients with diagnoses of neurosis and personality disorders were found to have the highest rates of crashes (Crancer and Quiring 1969; Eelkema et al. 1970). This group also had a significantly higher rate of violations. Early detection by monitoring violations, followed by an evaluation, could identify the high risk populations.

Tsuang et al. (1985) noted that certain personality characteristics, such as low tension tolerance, personality disorders, and paranoid conditions, appear to be risk factors for motor vehicle crashes. Alcoholism strongly correlated with traffic collisions. Evidence suggests that alcoholism exacerbates the existing personality factors and psychiatric disorders. Alcoholic individuals, when intoxicated, are more likely to express underlying illness than nonalcoholic individuals (Selzer et al. 1967; Smart and Schmidt 1969).

The relationship between depression and suicidal intentions as causes for auto crashes has not been well established. Single-car crashes as suicidal attempts have been explored, but results indicate that drivers injured in these crashes tend to abuse alcohol, have more convictions for traffic violations, and have personality traits that predispose them to injuries. These personality traits suggest a high suicide risk, but studies have failed to find suicidal intent in the specific instances of motor vehicle crashes (Schmidt et al. 1977).

▮ Balance dysfunction and other neurological conditions.

Balance impairment in elderly people is a common cause of falls. Balance can be impaired by the degenerative processes associated with aging and by disease involvement (J. A. Waller 1985). Degenerative changes associated with aging that pose the highest risk include worsening of hearing and vision, particularly changes in acuity and in the ability to see in dim light; decrease in muscle mass and strength; and shifting center of gravity.

Medical conditions that can increase the risks of traumatic injury from falls include symptoms of diseases such as diabetes and high blood pressure; disorders of mobility such as Parkinson's disease, multiple sclerosis, arthritis; and disorders involving the parasympathetic nervous system and other neurological functions (Lizardi et al. 1989). The prevalence of disorders of the parasympathetic nervous system increases markedly with old age. Occasional dizziness on rising rapidly, drop attacks, or dizzy spells on reaching upward are common causes of falls. Dementia may contribute to lack of judgment and self-awareness, and is an important risk factor in serious falls (Buchner and Larson 1987).

There is a correlation between the use of medications and falls (Tinetti et al. 1988). The effects of medications, including sedatives and hypnotics, such as benzodiazepines and barbiturates, are frequently associated with falls and motor vehicle crashes. Antidepressants, particularly heterocyclics and monoamine oxidase inhibitors, are frequently associated with orthostatic hypotension and falls in elderly people. Preventive measures include education of the patient and the family on the potential effects of the medication and management planning. Such measures include demonstration on arising from beds, chairs, and bath tubs, in a stable and safe fashion to avoid falls from medication-induced hypotension. Families should be instructed to monitor patient compliance with these safety precautions. Because of increased risk of osteoporosis in elderly people, proper medication management and education to prevent falls is essential.

Legislative and Access Restriction Strategies

Legislation has favorably influenced the prevention of motor-vehicle–related injuries. As early as 1976, Robertson observed that enactment of motorcycle helmet laws was associated with a 30% reduction in motorcyclists' deaths (Robertson 1976).

Legislative approaches to injury prevention, particularly involving restrictive legislation directed at adults, have provoked controversy and strong opposition. The argument of "personal freedom" has been used to oppose the adoption of legislation meant to protect the public good. Legislation has been attacked on the grounds that it infringes on the individual's freedom. In 1972 a federal court in Massachusetts told a cyclist: "The public has an interest in minimizing the resources directly involved. From the moment of injury, society picks the person up off the highways; delivers him to a municipal hospital and municipal doctors; provides him with unemployment compensation if, after recovery, he cannot replace his job lost; and, if the injury causes permanent disability, may assume responsibility for his and his family's subsistence. We do not understand a state of mind that permits plaintiff to think that only he himself is concerned." This decision was affirmed by the U.S. Supreme Court (Simon v. Sargent 1972).

Experiences with motorcycle helmet, seat belt, and firearms statutes exemplify the considerable opposition restrictive legislation can provoke. Measures restricting children have faced less opposition, thus legislators have been much more willing to mandate restrictions for children than for adults.

Drivers 17 years old and younger have the greatest risk of injuries. Raising the minimum age for obtaining a driver's license to 18 could reduce motor vehicle fatalities in drivers of that age group by as much as 85% (Williams et al. 1983). Similarly, because taking driver's education enables minors to drive earlier, its elimination could result in a yearly reduction of over 650 fatalities (Rice et al. 1989). In addition, curfew laws limiting nighttime driving of newly licensed drivers can reduce crashes by 80%.

In the prevention of motor vehicle crashes, legislative efforts directed at access restriction (i.e., driving privileges), combined with passive methods, have proven to be the most effective. Seat belts, child-restraint seats, and airbags are examples of the successful passive approaches. Mandatory license suspension or revocation of individuals convicted of alcohol-related driving violations appears more effective in preventing recurring crashes than fines, jail sentences, or voluntary participation in rehabilitation (Haddon and Baker 1981). For repeated offenders, combining license suspension with treatment has demonstrated success.

Motorcycle restrictions have included the mandatory use of helmets and licensing. However, licensing does not appear to decrease motorcycle injury fatalities. Forty-two percent of all fatally injured motorcyclists either do not have valid licenses, or have had them suspended or revoked (Insurance Institute for Highway Safety 1992). A California study found that only 33% of motorcycle drivers who were killed or severely injured had motorcycle licenses (Kraus et al. 1991). On borrowed motorcycles, 80% of drivers were unlicensed. Improved testing and licensing programs for motorcyclists have been attempted in at least two states, California and New York, but have not demonstrated success in reducing crash or violation rates (Insurance Institute for Highway Safety 1988).

Although not yet thoroughly studied, preventive strategies recommended to control firearm injuries include screening instruments, education, crisis centers, and gun regulation. Of these, the one showing the most promising results is gun regulation. Studies on gun regulation suggest that restrictive regulations can decrease the incidence of suicides and homicides (e.g., Loftin 1991). Firearms restrictions are associated with lower crime rates, including homicides (Deutsch and Alt 1977; O'Carroll et al. 1991; Sloan et al.

1990). Efforts to control firearm injuries in schools have included restrictive measures, searches, and metal detectors.

Banning three-wheel all-terrain vehicles, as recommended by the United States Consumer Product Safety Commission (USCPSC), may be an effective strategy in decreasing traumatic injuries. All-terrain vehicles are unstable, and their use on irregular terrain compounds the risk for serious injury. Also, mandatory registration of these vehicles, restrictions on driver's age, and mandatory licensure of drivers could reduce the risk of injuries. The use of helmets would also significantly reduce the risk of TBI (Rodgers 1990).

Concluding Statements

Physicians bear responsibility in the diagnosis and treatment of disease, as well as responsibility for prevention of disease and injury. Noyes (1985) alerts physicians to be knowledgeable of high-risk groups, and to be skillful in their assessment of people who have sustained injuries in motor vehicle crashes, people with alcohol, personality, and psychiatric disorders, and people receiving medications.

Cushman et al. (1991) suggest that physicians also should have a role in injury prevention, not limited to educating patients but also by becoming involved in the public domains of regulation, legislation, and litigation. Runyan and Runyan (1991) add yet another role: to improve the effectiveness of education and evaluate it as rigorously as other preventive and therapeutic measures, followed by analysis and publication of results.

We agree with the aforementioned sentiments. We encourage clinicians to carefully review the epidemiological risk factor data included in this chapter, and apply this information as an integral component of patient assessment and treatment. Moreover, we urge practitioners to utilize this information during activities related to professional and public education as applied to TBI. Even a cursory review of this textbook will convincingly demonstrate the truth of the aphorism, "an ounce of prevention is worth a pound of cure."

References

Annegers JF, Grabow JD, Kurland LT, et al: The incidence, causes, and secular trends of head trauma in Olmsted County, Minnesota, 1935–1974. Neurology 30:912–919, 1980

Baker SP: Motor vehicle occupant deaths in young children. Pediatrics 64:860–861, 1979

Baker SP, O'Neill B, Karpf RS: The Injury Fact Book. Lexington, MA, DC Heath, 1984

Bergman AB, Rivara FP, Richards DD, et al: The Seattle Children's Bicycle Helmet Campaign. Am J Dis Child 144:727–731, 1990

Bodiwala GG, Thomas PD, Otubushin A: Protective effect of rear-seat restraints during car collisions. Lancet 1:369–371, 1989

Brenner B: Alcoholism and fatal accidents. Quarterly Journal of Studies on Alcohol 28:517–528, 1967

Brent DA, Perper JA, Allman CJ, et al: The presence and accessibility of firearms in the homes of adolescent suicides. JAMA 266:2989–2995, 1991

Buchner DM, Larson EB: Falls and fractures in patients with Alzheimer-type dementia. JAMA 257:1492–1495, 1987

Callahan CM, Rivara FP: Access to handguns among urban adolescents (abstract). Am J Dis Child 145:395, 1991

Cantu RC: When to return to contact sports after a cerebral concussion. Sports Medicine Digest 10:1–2, 1988

Casson IR, Siegel O, Sham R, et al: Brain damage in modern boxers. JAMA 251:2663–2667, 1984

Centers for Disease Control: Bicycle-related injuries: data from the National Electronic Injury Surveillance System. MMWR 36:269–271, 1987

Centers for Disease Control: Weapon-carrying among high school students—United States, 1990. MMWR 40:681–684, 1991

Centers for Disease Control: Firearm-related deaths—Louisiana and Texas, 1970–1990. MMWR 41:213–215, 221, 1992

Centerwall BS: Race, socioeconomic status and domestic violence. Atlanta, 1971–72. Am J Public Health 74:813–815, 1984

Cerelli E: Older drivers, the age factor in traffic safety. United States Department of Transportation, National Highway Traffic Safety Administration DOT HS 807 402, 1989

Chenier TC, Evans L: Motorcyclist fatalities and the repeal of mandatory helmet wearing laws. Accid Anal Prev 19:133–139, 1987

Christofersen ER, Gyulay J: Parental compliance with car seat usage: a positive approach with long-term follow-up. J Pediatr Psychol 6:301–312, 1981

Committee on Trauma Research, National Research Council: Injury in America. Washington, DC, National Academy Press, 1985, p 20

Cooper KD, Tabbador K, Hauser WA, et al: The epidemiology of head injury in the Bronx. Neuroepidemiology 2:70–88, 1983

Crancer A, Quiring DL: The mentally ill as motor vehicle operators. Am J Psychiatry 126:807–813, 1969

Cushman R, James W, Waclawik H: Physicians promoting bicycle helmets for children: a randomized trial. Am J Public Health 81:1044–1046, 1991

Decker MD, Dewey MJ, Hutchenson RH, et al: The use and efficacy of child restraint devices. JAMA 252:2571–2575, 1984

Deutsch SJ, Alt FB: The effect of the Massachusetts gun control law on gun-related crimes in the city of Boston. Evaluation Quarterly 1:543–68, 1977

Edna T: Alcohol influence and head injury. Acta Chir Scand 148:209–212, 1982

Eelkema RC, Brosseau J, Koshnick R, et al: A statistical study on the relationship between mental illness and traffic accidents. Am J Public Health 60:459–469, 1970

Evans L, Frick MC: Helmet effectiveness in preventing motorcycle driver and passenger fatalities. Accid Anal Prev 20:447–458, 1988

Fife D: Injuries and deaths among elderly persons. Am J Public Health 126:936–941, 1987

Fife D, Barancik JI, Chateerjee BF: Northeastern Ohio Trauma Study, II: injury rates by age, sex and cause. Am J Public Health 74:473–478, 1984

Galbraith S, Murray WR, Patel AR, et al: The relationship between alcohol and head injury and its effect on the consciousness level. Br J Surg 63:128–130, 1976

Gallagher SS, Finison K, Guyer B, et al: The incidence of injuries among 87,000 Massachusetts children and adolescents: results of the 1980–81 Childhood Injury Prevention Program Surveillance System. Am J Public Health 74:1340–1347, 1984

Gerberich SG, Priest JD, Boen JR, et al: Concussion incidences and severity in secondary school varsity football players. Am J Public Health 73:1370–1375, 1983

Goodman RA, Herndon MS, Istre GR, et al: Fatal injuries in Oklahoma: descriptive epidemiology using medical examiner data. South Med J 82:1128–1134, 1989

Grossman DC, Rivara FP: Injury control in childhood. Pediatr Clin North Am 39:471–485, 1992

Haddon W, Baker SP: Injury control, in Preventive and Community Medicine, 2nd Edition. Edited by Clark D, MacMahon B. Boston, MA, Little, Brown, 1981, pp 109–140

Haddon W, Brandess VA: Alcohol in single vehicle fatal accidents, experience of Westchester County, New York. JAMA 169:1587–1593, 1959

Hargarten SW: All-terrain vehicle mortality in Wisconsin: a case study in injury control. Am J Emerg Med 9:149–152, 1991

Heilman DR, Weisbuch JB, Blair RW, et al: Motorcycle-related trauma and helmet usage in North Dakota. Ann Emerg Med 11:659–664, 1982

Hillbom ME, Holm L: Contribution of traumatic head injury to neurological deficits in alcoholics. J Neurol Neurosurg Psychiatry 49:1348–1353, 1986

Hogue CH: Injury in late life, I: epidemiology. J Am Geriatr Soc 30:183–190, 1982

Horton AM, Tims FM, Grace WC: Drug abuse and head injury. Journal of Head Injury 3:34–37, 1992

Insurance Institute for Highway Safety: Two Studies Question Value of Motorcycle Licensing Program (Status Report 23). Arlington, VA, 1988, p 8

Insurance Institute for Highway Safety: Fatality Facts 1989. Arlington, VA, 1989

Insurance Institute for Highway Safety: Fatality Facts 1990. Arlington, VA, 1990

Insurance Institute for Highway Safety: Fatality Facts 1992. Arlington, VA, 1992

Jagger J: Prevention of brain trauma by legislation, regulation, and improved technology: a focus on motor vehicles. J Neurotrauma 9 (Suppl 1):S313–S316, 1992

Jagger J, Levine JI, Jane J, et al: Epidemiologic features of head injury in a predominantly rural population. J Trauma 24:40–44, 1984

Jagger J, Verbnerg K, Jane J: Air bags: reducing the toll of brain trauma. Neurosurgery 20:815–817, 1987

Kalsbeek WD, McLaurin RL, Harris BSH, et al: The national head and spinal cord injury survey: major findings. J Neurosurg 53 (Suppl):519–531, 1980

Kellerman AL, Reay DT: Protection or peril? an analysis of firearm related deaths in the home. N Engl J Med 314:1557–1560, 1986

Kelly JP, Nichols JS, Filley CM, et al: Concussions in sports: guidelines for the prevention of catastrophic outcome. JAMA 266:2867–2869, 1991

Kerr TA, Kay WK, Lassman LP: Characteristics of patients, type of accident and mortality in a consecutive series of head injuries admitted to a neurosurgical uni. British Journal of Preventive and Social Medicine 25:179–185, 1971

Klauber MR, Barrett-Connor E, Marshall LF, et al: The epidemiology of head injury: a prospective study of an entire community, San Diego County, California, 1978. Am J Epidemiology 113:500–509, 1981

Kraus JF: Epidemiology of head injury, in Head Injury, 3rd Edition. Edited by Cooper PR. Baltimore, MD, Williams & Wilkins, 1993, pp 1–25

Kraus JF, Nourjah P: The epidemiology of mild, uncomplicated brain injury. J Trauma 28:1637–1643, 1988

Kraus JF, Riggins RS, Franti CE: Some epidemiological features of motorcycle collision injuries: I. Introduction, methods and factors associated with incidence. Am J Epidemiol 102:74–98, 1975

Kraus JF, Black MA, Hessol N, et al: The incidence of acute brain injury and serious impairment in a defined population. Am J Epidemiol 119:186–191, 1984

Kraus JF, Fife D, Conroy C: Incidence, severity, and outcomes of brain injuries involving bicycles. Am J Public Health 77:76–78, 1987

Kraus JF, Rock A, Hemyari P: The causes, impact, and preventability of childhood injuries in the United States: brain injuries among infants, children and adolescents, and young adults in the United States. Am J Dis Child 144:684–691, 1990

Kraus JF, Anderson C, Zaor PL, et al: Motorcycle licensure, ownership, and crash involvement. Am J Public Health 81:172–176, 1991

Lambert DA, Sattin RW: Deaths from falls, 1978–84. MMWR 37 (Suppl 1):21–26, 1988

Lindenbaum GA, Carroll SF, Daskal I, et al: Patterns of alcohol and drug abuse in an urban trauma center: the decreasing role of cocaine abuse. J Trauma 29:1654–1658, 1989

Lizardi JE, Wolfson LI, Whipple RH: Neurological dysfunction in the elderly prone to fall. Journal of Neurologic Rehabilitation 3:113–116, 1989

Loftin C: Effects of restrictive licensing of handguns on homicide and suicide in the District of Columbia. N Eng J Med 325:1615–1620, 1991

Margolis LH, Wagenaar AC, Molnar LJ: Use and misuse of automobile child restraint devices. Am J Dis Child 146361–366, 1992

Max W, MacKenzie EJ, Rice DP: Head injuries: costs and consequences. Journal of Head Trauma Rehabilitation 6(2):76–87, 1991

McKenzie EJ, Edelstein SL, Flynn JP: Hospitalized head-injured patients in Maryland: incidence and severity of injuries. Maryland Medical Journal 38:725–732, 1989

National Committee for Injury Prevention and Control: Injury Prevention: Meeting the Challenge. New York, Oxford University Press, 1989

National Head Injury Foundation Substance Abuse Task Force: White Paper. Southborough, MA, National Head Injury Foundation, 1988

National Safety Council: Policy Update. Washington, DC, 1981

Neuwelt EA, Coe MF, Wilkinson AM, et al: Oregon head and spinal cord injury prevention program and evaluation. Neurosurgery 24:453–458, 1989

Newman R: Hazard analysis: analysis of all terrain vehicles related injuries and deaths. Washington, DC, Division of Hazard Analysis, Directorate for Epidemiology, U.S. Consumer Product Safety Commission, 1987

Newman R: Update of all-terrain vehicle deaths and injuries (technical report). Washington DC, U.S. Consumer Product Safety Commission, 1988

Noyes R Jr: Motor vehicle accidents related to psychiatric impairment. Psychosomatics 26:575–580, 1985

O'Carroll PW, Loftin C, Waller JB, et al: Preventing homicide: an evaluation of the efficacy of a Detroit gun ordinance. Am J Public Health 81:576–581, 1991

Orsay EM, Turnbull TL, Dunne M, et al: Prospective study of the effect of safety belts on morbidity and health care costs in motor-vehicle accidents. JAMA 260:3598–3603, 1988

Parkinson D, Stephensen S, Phillips S: Head injuries: a prospective, computerized study. Can J Surg 28:79–83, 1985

Rice DP, MacKenzie EJ, and Associates: Cost of Injury in the United States: A Report to Congress. Institute for Health and Aging, University of California, San Francisco, California, and the Injury Prevention Center, Johns Hopkins University Press, 1989

Richeldefer TE: Commentaries. Pediatrics 58:307–308, 1976

Rickert VI, Jay S, Gottlieb AA: Adolescent wellness. Med Clin 74:1135–1148, 1990

Rimel RW, Jane JA, Bond MR: Characteristics of the head-injured patient, in Rehabilitation of the Adult and Child with Traumatic Brain Injury, 2nd Edition. Edited by Rosenthal M, Griffith ER, Bond MR, et al. Philadelphia, PA, FA Davis, 1990, pp 8–16

Roberts MC, Turner DS: Preventing death and injury in childhood: a synthesis of child safety seat effects. Health Educ Q 11:181–193, 1984

Robertson LS: An instance of effective legal regulation: motorcyclist helmet and daytime headlamp laws. Law Society Review 10:467–477, 1976

Rodgers GB: The effectiveness of helmets in reducing all-terrain vehicle injuries and deaths. Accid Anal Prev 22:47–58, 1990

Rodriguez JG: Childhood injuries in the United States. Am J Dis Child 144:627–646, 1990

Rosenberg ML, Smith JC, Davidson LE, et al: The emergence of youth suicide: an epidemiologic analysis and public health perspective. Annu Rev Public Health 8:417–440, 1987

Ruff RM, Marshall LF, Klauber MR, et al: Alcohol abuse and neurological outcome of the severely head injured. Journal of Head Trauma Rehabilitation 5(3):21–31, 1990

Runyan CW, Runyan DK: How can physicians get kids to wear bicycle helmets? A prototypic challenge in injury prevention. Am J Public Health 81:972–973, 1991

Rutherford WT: Diagnosis of alcohol ingestion in mild head injuries. Lancet 1:1021–1023, 1977

Sacks JJ, Holmgreen P, Smith SM, et al: Bicycle associated head injuries and deaths in the United States from 1984–1988: how many are preventable? JAMA 266:316–318, 1991

Schmidt CW, Shaffer JN, Zlotowitz H, et al: Suicide by vehicular crash. Am J Psychiatry 134:175–178, 1977

Selzer ML, Payne RE, Westervelt FH, et al: Automobile accidents as an expression of psychopathology in an alcoholic population. Quarter Journal of Studies on Alcohol 28:505–516, 1967

Simon v Sargent: 346 F Supp. 277, 279 (D. Mass. 1972), affirmed 409 U.S. 1020 (1972)

Sloan JH, Rivara FP, Reay DT, et al: Firearm regulations and rates of suicide: a comparison of two metropolitan areas. N Eng J Med 322:369–373, 1990

Smart RG, Schmidt W: Physiological impairment and personality factors in traffic accidents of alcoholics. Quarter Journal of Studies on Alcohol 30:440–445, 1969

Snively SA, Becker EB: Helmet head protection: state of the art and future directions. Journal of Head Trauma Rehabilitation 6(2):11–20, 1991

Sorenson SB, Kraus JF: Occurrence, severity, and outcome of brain injury. Journal of Head Trauma Rehabilitation 6(2):1–10, 1991

Sosin D, Sacks J, Smith S: Head injury-associated deaths in the United States from 1979 to 1986. JAMA 262:2251–2255, 1989

Sparadeo FR, Gill D: Effects of prior alcohol use on head injury recovery. Journal of Head Trauma Rehabilitation 4:75–82, 1989

Sparadeo FR, Strauss D, Barth JT: The incidence, impact and treatment of substance abuse in head trauma rehabilitation. Journal of Head Trauma Rehabilitation 5:1–8, 1990

Speigel CN, Lindaman FC: Children can't fly: a program to prevent childhood morbidity and mortality from window falls. Am J Public Health 67:1143–1147, 1977

Thompson RS, Rivara FP, Thompson DC: A case-control study of the effectiveness of bicycle safety helmets. N Eng J Med 320:1361–1367, 1989

Tinetti ME: Factors associated with serious injury during falls by ambulatory nursing home residents. J Am Geriatr Soc 35:644–648, 1987

Tinetti ME, Speechley M: Prevention of falls among the elderly. N Engl J Med 320:1055–1059, 1989

Tinetti ME, Speechley M, Ginter SF: Risk factors for falls among elderly persons living in the community. N Eng J Med 319:1701–1707, 1988

Torg JS, Vegso JJ, Sennett B, et al: The national football head and neck injury registry: 14-year report on cervical quadriplegia, 1971 through 1984. Clin Sports Med 6(1):61–72, 1987

Tsuang MT, Boor M, Fleming JA: Psychiatric aspects of traffic accidents. Am J Psychiatry 142:538–546, 1985

United States Department of Transportation, National Highway Traffic Safety Administration: Final Regulatory Impact Assessment on Amendments to Federal Motor Vehicle Safety Standard 208, Front Seat Occupant Protection. Publication DOT HS 806 572. Washington, DC, 1984, pp IV–2

United States Department of Transportation, National Highway Traffic Safety Administration: Final rule, FMVSS 208: Occupant crash protection, 49 CPR, part 571. Washington DC, 1988

United States Department of Transportation, National Highway Traffic Safety Administration: An evaluation of center high mounted stop lamps based on 1987 data. NHTSA technical report DOT HS 807 442. Washington, DC, 1989

Waller JA: Medical Impairment to Driving. Springfield, IL, Charles C Thomas, 1973

Waller JA: Injury Control: A Guide to the Causes and Prevention of Trauma. Lexington Books, Lexington, MA, 1985

Waller JA, Turkel HW: Alcoholism and traffic deaths. N Eng J Med 275:523–526, 1966

Waller PF, Stewart JR, Hansen AR, et al: The potentiating effects of alcohol on driver injury. JAMA 256:1461–1466, 1986

Weiss BD: Bicycle helmet use by children. Pediatrics 77:677–679, 1986

Williams AF, Karpf RS, Zador PL: Variations in minimum licensing age and fatal motor vehicle crashes. Am J Public Health 73:1401–1402, 1983

Wintemute GJ, Teret SP, Kraus JF, et al: When children shoot children: 88 unintended deaths in California. JAMA 257:3107–3109, 1987

Zador PL, Ciccone MA: Driver Fatalities in Frontal Impacts: Comparisons Between Cars With Air Bags and Manual Belts. Arlington, VA, Insurance Institute for Highway Safety, 1991

Zane DF, Preece MJ, Patterson PJ, et al: Firearm-related mortality in Texas (1985–1990). Texas Medicine 87:63–65, 1991

Index

*Page numbers printed in **boldface** type refer to tables or figures.*